Cardiovascular Diseases and Depression

Bernhard T. Baune • Phillip J. Tully
Editors

Cardiovascular Diseases and Depression

Treatment and Prevention in Psychocardiology

Springer

Editors
Bernhard T. Baune
Discipline of Psychiatry,
School of Medicine
University of Adelaide
Adelaide
Australia

Phillip J. Tully
The Freemason's Foundation Centre for
Men's Health, Discipline of Medicine,
School of Medicine,
University of Adelaide
Adelaide, SA
Australia

ISBN 978-3-319-32478-4 ISBN 978-3-319-32480-7 (eBook)
DOI 10.1007/978-3-319-32480-7

Library of Congress Control Number: 2016947729

Printed on acid-free paper

This Springer imprint is published by Springer Nature
The registered company is Springer International Publishing AG Switzerland

Contents

Introduction

1

Bernhard T. Baune and Phillip J. Tully

Content

The association between cardiovascular diseases (CVDs) and depression has long been recognized. Reports as early as 1937 suggested that institutionalized psychiatric patients had an eight times higher mortality rate than the general population and "diseases of the heart" accounting for almost 40 % of these deaths (Malzberg 1937).

In the following decades, the comorbidity of depression and CVDs has been rigorously investigated in many cross-sectional and longitudinal studies pointing to an important clinical and societal burden. Current literature suggests that the relationship between CVD and depression is bidirectional. Numerous clinical and epidemiological studies investigating the association between depression and cardiovascular disease have suggested that depression increases the risk of subsequent CVD 1.5-fold on average (Grippo and Johnson 2002; Thombs et al. 2006; Lippi et al. 2009; Nicholson et al. 2006) and that patients with coronary artery disease and depression have a two- to threefold increased risk of future nonfatal and fatal cardiac events compared to those cardiac patients without depression (Goldston and Baillie 2008; Kooy et al. 2007; Rudisch and Charles 2003; Frasure-Smith and

B.T. Baune (✉)
Department of Psychiatry, North Terrace, School of Medicine, University of Adelaide, Adelaide 5005, Australia
e-mail: bernhard.baune@adelaide.edu.au

P.J. Tully
School of Medicine, Discipline of Medicine, The University of Adelaide, Adelaide 5005, Australia

B.T. Baune, P.J. Tully (eds.), *Cardiovascular Diseases and Depression*,
DOI 10.1007/978-3-319-32480-7_1

Lesperance 2010). Moreover, depression has been found to be an independent predictor of a poorer health outcome after an ischemic event (Nicholson et al. 2006; Barth et al. 2004; Meijer et al. 2011).

While the etiology and pathophysiology of the relationship between depression and CVD have been heavily related to various biological mechanisms relating to the hypothalamic-pituitary-adrenal (HPA) axis, pro-inflammatory cytokines, increased sympathetic tone, platelet dysfunction, changes in arterial vessel elasticity, and endothelial function, other reports support important contributions of clinical characteristics of depression (e.g., severity of depression, number of episodes, duration of depression, depression subtype) and sociodemographic factors (marital status, education, and income) to the bidirectional relationship between depression and cardiovascular disease. Whether screening for and treatment of depression are effective in reducing the clinical comorbidity and in improving health outcomes in affected patients, e.g., by using antidepressants, psychotherapy, or anti-inflammatories, became of increasing interest in recent years.

In this most comprehensive book on the topic of cardiovascular disease and depression, expert authors from around the world focus on novel aspects of the clinical and biological etiology and pathophysiology of the comorbidity by extending into new frontiers such as the role of anxiety, neuropsychological and cognitive impairment, emotion processing, and stress and into the underlying neurobiology of the cardiovascular disease and depression comorbidity. To extend the more established knowledge on biological mechanisms of the cardiovascular and depression comorbidity as reviewed here, the book will go beyond in order to review neuroimaging findings, metabolic-inflammation aspects, and the possibility of a genetic overlap between the two conditions. The second main focus of the book is on the topics of treatment and prevention. State-of-the art psychological (e.g., behavioral activation, cognitive training, mobile-app technologies) and pharmacological (e.g., antidepressants, anti-inflammatory agents) as well as complementary alternative and integrative medicine approaches carry promise to improve the short-term and long-term outcomes of this comorbid condition. Finally, the critical topics of screening and prevention will be given extensive consideration.

The broad concept and the comprehensive topics of this book make it a unique reference for the interested student, clinician, and researcher across medical, psychological, public and allied health, and complementary medicine disciplines to better understand the foundations and to clinically improve the conditions of people with cardiovascular and depression comorbidity.

References

Barth J, Schumacher M, Herrmann-Lingen C (2004) Depression as a risk factor for mortality in patients with coronary heart disease: a meta-analysis. Psychosom Med 66(6):802–813

Frasure-Smith N, Lesperance F (2010) Depression and cardiac risk: present status and future directions. Heart 96(3):173–176

Goldston K, Baillie AJ (2008) Depression and coronary heart disease: a review of the epidemiological evidence, explanatory mechanisms and management approaches. Clin Psychol Rev 28(2):288–306

Grippo AJ, Johnson AK (2002) Biological mechanisms in the relationship between depression and heart disease. Neurosci Biobehav Rev 26(8):941–962

Kooy KV et al (2007) Depression and the risk for cardiovascular diseases: a systematic review and meta analysis. Int J Geriatr Psychiatry 22:613–626

Lippi G et al (2009) Mental depression and cardiovascular disease: a multifaceted, bidirectional association. Semin Thromb Hemost 35(3):325–336

Malzberg B (1937) Mortality among patients with evolutionary melancholia. Am J Psychiatry 93(5):1231–1238

Meijer A et al (2011) Prognostic association of depression following myocardial infarction with mortality and cardiovascular events: a meta-analysis of 25 years of research. Gen Hosp Psychiatry 33(3):203–216

Nicholson A, Kuper H, Hemingway H (2006) Depression as an aetiologic and prognostic factor in coronary heart disease: a meta-analysis of 6362 events among 146 538 participants in 54 observational studies. Eur Heart J 27(23):2763–2774

Rudisch B, Charles BN (2003) Epidemiology of comorbid coronary artery disease and depression. Biol Psychiatry 54(3):227–240

Thombs BD et al (2006) Prevalence of depression in survivors of acute myocardial infarction. J Gen Intern Med 21(1):30–38

Epidemiology of Cardiovascular Disease and Depression

2

Tracy Air, Phillip J. Tully, Shaun Sweeney, and John Beltrame

Contents

Abstract

Depression is common in cardiac patients, with 20 % of patients meeting the criteria for major depressive disorder or experiencing depressive symptoms. The relationship between cardiovascular diseases is likely to be bidirectional: people with depression are more likely to develop cardiovascular disease, while patients

T. Air (✉) • S. Sweeney
Discipline of Psychiatry, University of Adelaide, Adelaide, Australia
e-mail: tracy.air@adelaide.edu.au

P.J. Tully • J. Beltrame
Discipline of Medicine, The Queen Elizabeth Hospital, University of Adelaide, Adelaide, Australia

B.T. Baune, P.J. Tully (eds.), *Cardiovascular Diseases and Depression*, DOI 10.1007/978-3-319-32480-7_2

with cardiovascular disease and co-morbid depression have worse cardiac outcomes than those who are not depressed. The influence is not only restricted to cardiovascular outcomes; however, the impact upon psychosocial outcomes such as quality of life and social participation can be just as deleterious. This relationship can also be moderated by socio-demographic and psychosocial risk factors, including gender, age, previous history of depression, social isolation and functional impairment. This chapter will focus on the epidemiology and relationship between depression and cardiovascular disease, the effects on psychiatric and cardiac outcomes and the known risk factors.

2.1 Introduction

Cardiovascular disease (CVD) and depression are significant public health concerns. Both have significant impact with respect to key health system indicators, such as service utilisation and medical costs (Baumeister et al. 2015). More importantly, they also have a profound impact on the quality of life of afflicted individuals.

2.1.1 Cardiovascular Disease

CVD is a collective term for diseases of the heart and blood vessels. The term can refer to a group of disorders, such as coronary heart disease, heart failure, peripheral vascular disease and stroke. CVD is the leading cause of death worldwide, causing more than 17 million deaths per year in 2013, up from 12 million in 1990 (Naghavi et al. 2015). CVD can also result in severe disability. One measure of overall disease burden, disability-adjusted life years (DALYs), combines both mortality and morbidity into a single measurement. Results from the Global Burden of Disease Study report that between 2005 and 2013, DALYs for CVD increased by 6.7 % (Murray et al. 2015). The 2010 Global Burden of Disease Survey estimated that depression accounted for 8.2 % of global years lived with disability (YLD) and 2.5 % of global DALYs (Ferrari et al. 2013). By 2013, ischemic heart disease and cerebrovascular disease were two of the five leading causes of disease burden (Murray et al. 2015).

2.1.2 Depression

Depression (also known as major depressive disorder (MDD), clinical depression or unipolar depression) is a common psychiatric disorder, characterised by a persistent low mood that is accompanied by anhedonia, fatigability and low self-esteem. It has been linked to diminished quality of life, medical morbidity and mortality.

2.2 Depression and Cardiovascular Disease as Co-morbidities: Cause and Effect?

Depression commonly afflicts patients with CVD and contributes to poor cardiovascular and psychosocial outcomes. Two major findings have emerged from the literature: firstly, that depression is associated with an increased risk of development of CVD and other vascular disorders such as vascular dementia. Secondly, depression predicts increased morbidity and mortality in patients with CVD, including those with HF, in individuals following MI or who have undergone coronary artery bypass graft (CABG) surgery. Despite this, depression remains underdiagnosed and undertreated in cardiac populations, even with the availability of safe and effective treatments. The effects of CVD and depression are widespread and harmful, impacting quality of life (Djarv et al. 2012; O'Neil et al. 2013), health service utilisation (Egede 2007), medical costs (Sullivan et al. 2002) and day-to-day functioning (Dickson et al. 2012; Mensah and Brown 2007).

2.2.1 Prevalence of Depression in Cardiovascular Disease Patients

Globally, the lifetime prevalence of depression varies widely, ranging from 1.0% in the Czech Republic to 17% in the United States according to the DSM-IV criteria, while the 12-month prevalence can range between 0.3% (Czech Republic) and 10% (United States) (Kessler and Bromet 2013). Prevalence estimates of depression in the general population also vary by sex with estimates between 5–9% for females and 2–3% among males (American Psychiatric Association 2000). Compare these prevalence estimates to those in cardiovascular populations, and it is clear that the latter chronic disease population are disproportionately affected. Specifically, the prevalence of major depression is most widely documented in coronary heart disease with strikingly similar prevalence rates across CVD subtypes. Thombs et al. showed a 20% prevalence in persons with a recent myocardial infarction (Thombs et al. 2006). Other estimates in acute CVD populations are very similar. Between 15 and 20% major depression prevalence is reported in coronary artery bypass graft (CABG) surgery patients though estimates tend to increase when dysthymia is taken into account (Tully and Baker 2012). Also approximately 20% depression prevalence is evident in heart failure patients (Rutledge et al. 2006). Persons receiving implantable cardioverter defibrillator are an exception, and depression estimates vary considerably 11–26% and may be less reliable since fewer studies have adopted structured clinical interviews to diagnose depression (Magyar-Russell et al. 2011). Putting these collective findings in a clinical context, it can be reliably expected that at least one in five persons with CVD will meet the criteria for major depression.

2.2.2 Prevalence of Cardiovascular Disease in Depressed Patients

People with severe mental illness, including depression, have an increased risk of physical illness, especially CVD. For example, Carter et al. (2014) reported that, in a study of 74,734 psychiatric patients admitted to hospital in the Greater Manchester region between 2001 and 2012, 9.63 % were diagnosed with ischemic heart disease, 6.63 % were diagnosed with atrial fibrillation, 4.6 % had heart failure and 2.31 % reported having an MI. Not surprisingly, similar prevalence rates have been found in samples with major depression. Results from the Medical Outcomes Study (Wells et al. 1989a), in a sample of 11,242 outpatients who either had been diagnosed with depression or reported depressive symptoms, found that 5 % also had current CAD while 4 % currently reported having angina. Other studies have reported a prevalence of 12 % and 5 % of CAD and CHF, respectively, in depressed patients (Lyness et al. 1993), while Diminić-Lisica and colleagues (2010) reported 10.85 % of their depressed sample also had cardiovascular disease. In US adults who reported a diagnosis of depression during their lifetime, the age-standardised prevalence of myocardial infarction, angina and stroke was around 30 %, compared to around 15 % for those who did not (Zhao et al. 2009).

2.2.3 Depression as a CVD Risk Factor

The role of depression in the development of CVD has been examined in numerous studies. In the Baltimore cohort of the Epidemiologic Catchment Area (ECA) Study, patients with a history of dysphoria or depression had 4.5 times the risk of having experienced an acute MI at follow-up when compared to nondepressed patients (Pratt et al. 1996). Rugulies (2002) determined that the risk of developing CVD was approximately 60 % higher in depressed patients, while Wulsin and Singal (2003) reported that MDD was a better predictor for the development of CVD in initially healthy people (Relative risk = 2.69; CI: 1.63–4.43) than depressive symptoms (Relative risk 1.49; CI 1.16–1.92). Furthermore, Rafanelli et al. (2010) reported that patients with dysthymia had a significantly higher risk of developing a cardiac event than patients without dysthymia, while depression has also been found to increase the risk of CVD by 1.5–3 times in otherwise physically healthy individuals (Lett et al. 2004; Xian et al. 2010).

Several population-based studies have also linked MDD in children and young adults to increased risk of premature CVD. A Taiwanese national health insurance study investigated the association of MDD (and other psychiatric disorders) with risk of CVD involving more than one million participants of all age groups including young adults (Huang et al. 2009). The relative risk for CVD among patients less than 20 years old was 2.19 for MDD. Although the prevalence of CVD increased with increasing age, the excessive relative risk for CVD among patients with MDD was greatest among those 20 years old or younger. These results have also been supported by data from meta-analyses. The largest published meta-analysis to date (21 studies N = 124 5,098 participants) indicated that depression was consistently predictive of incident cardiac events in individuals free of CVD (Nicholson et al. 2006), though smoking and exercise were infrequently adjusted for.

Given that depression is associated with major cardiac risk factors, this relationship should be no surprise. For example, numerous cross-sectional and longitudinal studies have found a significant relationship between MDD and smoking (Bakhshaie et al. 2015; Boden et al. 2010; Grant et al. 2004; Hughes et al. 1986; Kinnunen et al. 2006; Lasser et al. 2000). Hypertension is also more prevalent in depressed patients (Adamis and Ball 2000; Kahl et al. 2012; Nakagawara et al. 1987; Wells et al. 1989b, 1991), and MDD has also been associated with reduced physical activity (Aihara et al. 2011; Biddle and Asare 2011; Gallegos-Carrillo et al. 2013; Lampinen et al. 2000; Overdorf et al. 2016).

2.2.4 Risk Factors for Depression in CVD Patients

Determinants of health associated with the development of depression in CVD patients have been identified and aid the recognition of people at high risk of depression. Numerous predictors of depression in physically healthy cohorts can also be a predictor of the development of depression in patients with CVD. These include female gender, age, previous history of depression, social isolation and functional impairment.

2.2.5 Gender

In recent years researchers have made considerable effort to investigate gender differences in CVD. This research recognises the need to improve our understanding of heart disease in women. As in the general population, depression has also been associated with similar increases in cardiovascular risks in both genders with established CVD (Barefoot et al. 1996). Women with CVD are more likely to experience depression when compared to men (Wiklund et al. 1993; Frasure-Smith et al. 1995; Balog et al. 2003; Vaccarino et al. 2003). It has been contended that this partly explains why women face higher mortality rates after MI (Mallik et al. 2006). Smolderen et al. (2015) established a much higher prevalence of prior depression and concurrent depressive symptoms among young women with acute MI than among young men. Even after adjusting for numerous socio-demographic, clinical and disease severity characteristics, young women with an acute MI had 60 % greater odds of having significant depressive symptoms compared with young men.

Numerous studies have found women report more severe and persistent depressive symptoms compared with men (Stern et al. 1977; Drory et al. 2003) with prognosis found to be poorer (Carney et al. 1991; Greenland et al. 1991). Additionally, gender differences in depressive symptoms are greatest among younger female patients (Mallik et al. 2006; Uuskula 1996). In the prospective Community Mental Health Epidemiology Study of Washington County, depression increased cardiovascular risk in women younger than 40 years more than sixfold, while no association was found among men (Wyman et al. 2012).

Even when baseline differences in history of hypertension, congestive heart failure and diabetes are adjusted for, the gender differences in mortality for women persist in some studies (Greenland et al. 1991). This suggests that the reason for these differences may not be entirely due to co-morbidity. Similarly, research by Vaccarino et al. (1999) suggests that depressed women with acute MI may experience an increased risk for adverse outcomes even after adjustment for prognostic variables.

Even though the presence and severity of depressive symptoms following a cardiac event seem to have similar risk factors to depression as in the general population, it should be noted that gender is not always a predictor of depression in these studies. For example, Doyle et al.'s (2015) recent study utilising Cox regression analyses for all-cause mortality demonstrated that the interaction between sex and depression was statistically significant (HR for interaction = 1.12, 95 % CI = 1.05–1.19, $p < 0.001$). This may signify that the association between depression and mortality was stronger for men than for women. The HR associated with depression was 12 % higher in men compared with women (men: HR = 1.38, 95 % CI 1.30–1.47; women: HR = 1.22, 95 % CI 1.14–1.31). Bjerkeset et al. (2005) reported that men and women differed in their long-term outcome after MI. Women showed a higher risk for depression in the first 2 years subsequent to an MI, whereas, in men, the risk for depression increased after 2 years post-MI. This could suggest a difference between the genders in the aetiology for depression in CVD patients.

2.2.6 Age

Studies have found that younger patients are more likely to have depression in the context of CVD. For example, in ACS, age has been identified as a risk factor for the development of depression (Lesperance et al. 1996; Dickens et al. 2004; Schrader et al. 2004; van Melle et al. 2006). In a prospective study of 648 patients at 14 Veterans Affairs (VA) hospitals, Ho and colleagues (2005) established that following cardiac valve surgery, depressed patients were significantly more likely to be younger. In a recent study by Shah et al. (2014), women less than 55 years of age emerged as the group with the highest risks associated with depressive symptoms. Of additional concern (Baumeister et al. 2015), this group also had the highest burden of depression as well, with 27 % exhibiting at least moderate depressive symptoms or higher. Additionally, in the Heart and Soul Study, Whooley and colleagues (2007) found that depressed patients with coronary heart disease were significantly more likely to be younger. Hamo and colleagues (2015) found that in patients with heart failure with preserved ejection fraction and who were also depressed were more likely to be younger than those without depression. Andrikopoulos et al. (2007) reported that the risk ratio in women for in-hospital death was exaggerated among younger patients, aged less than 55 years (RR = 3.84, 95 % CI 1.07–13.74).

However, like gender, not all studies have found age to be a significant risk factor in the development of depression in CVD patients. Doyle and colleagues (2015) determined that age did not have an effect on the prevalence of depression. Given that sex differences between depression and cardiac prognosis may be dependent on postmenopausal status (Vaccarino et al. 2013, 2014), Doyle and colleagues also scrutinised their data to determine if there was a sex-by-age interaction effect in the influence of depression on mortality. The interaction was found to not be significant (HR = 1.00, 95 % CI 0.99–1.01). Supporting this, Krannich et al. (2007) did not find a significant relationship between age and the change in depression pre- and post-CABG surgery.

2.2.7 Prior History

The chronicity of depressive symptoms may be especially relevant considering the onset and progression of CVD during the life course. Smolderen et al. (2015) found that at the time of their acute MI, women with a history of clinical depression were particularly vulnerable to experiencing depressive symptoms when compared with men with a history of depression. Approximately 25 % of women with a history of depression reported current depressive symptoms versus 10 % of men with a history of depression. Lesperance and colleagues' (1996) landmark paper investigated the impact of prior depressive history on 222 acute MI patients. Compared with those without a history of depression, patients with a previous history of depression were more likely to become depressed at some time during the year post discharge. When the data were examined on the basis of whether the depression was a recurrent episode or a first depression, they determined that patients with a recurrent depression were at significantly increased risk of 18-month mortality (40.0 %) when compared with patients who were depressed for the first time in their lives during their index admission.

Leung and colleagues (2012) performed a systematic review and examined the timing of the onset of depression relative to the onset of the CVD. They established that when compared to people who reported never experiencing depression, the risks of poor outcomes (all-cause mortality, cardiac mortality or cardiac morbidity) were increased. This increase was evident in both individuals whose first episode of depression started after the onset of CHD (RR=2.11) and among those whose depression was a recurrence of a previous episode of depression (RR=1.59). Carney and colleagues (1999), in a sample of medically stable patients with coronary artery disease (CAD), found that a higher proportion of depressed subjects experienced a prior history of depression than those who were not depressed.

2.2.8 Functional Impairment

The relationship between depression and functional impairment has been well established in community samples. Depression has been shown to be a strong predictor of difficulties in performing activities of daily living (ADLs) in community-dwelling adults (Mehta et al. 2002; Covinsky et al. 2010). Thus, it is no surprise that similar associations are evident in cardiac populations, specifically HF. For example, in a group of outpatients attending a community heart failure chronic disease management programme, Haworth et al. (2005) established that greater functional impairment as measured by the New York Heart Association (NYHA) classification could predict depression. Sin (2012) reported that high classification on the NYHA at baseline also significantly predicted depression at 6 months. She concluded that people with functional impairment may have slower recovery resulting in less improvement in depression scores at 6 months. Gottlieb and colleagues (2004) also reported a relationship between major depression and functional impairment as measured by NYHA class and also on the physical functioning subscale of a quality of life scale. Several other studies have also employed the NYHA classification as a measure of functional impairment and have found similar results. For example, in a sample of 839 symptomatic HF patients free of depression at baseline, Lossnitzer et al. (2013) found that NYHA class again was a strong predictor of incident depression. Additionally, Freedland et al. (2003) also reported the relationship between MDD and functional impairment.

Similar findings have also been reported in MI populations. Depression following an acute MI has also been shown to correlate with decreased overall functional status (Griego 1993). de Jonge et al. (2006) reported that patients with post-MI depression demonstrated significantly poorer health status on all indicators at 12 months as well as a fourfold increased risk of disability following the MI compared with patients without a post-MI depression.

A possible explanation for these findings could be that increased functional disability may result in reduced activity and social contact. This allows for more time for patients to ruminate about their health conditions and may lead to increased feelings of alienation, helplessness and loneliness (Haworth et al. 2005).

2.2.9 Social Isolation/Participation

An extensive literature has examined the relationship between depression and perceived social support in CVD populations (Krishnan et al. 1998; Bosworth et al. 2000; Horsten et al. 2000; Brummett et al. 2001; Raynor et al. 2002; Bucholz et al. 2014). Prospective studies have provided evidence that low perceived social support can place CVD populations at risk for the development or worsening of MDD (Bucholz et al. 2014; Holahan et al. 1997; Barefoot et al. 2000; Frasure-Smith et al. 2000; Welin et al. 2000). Research has suggested that it is critical to consider the combined effect of depression and social support in predicting CVD prognosis. For example, social support in conjunction with depression has been associated as a predictor. Horsten et al. (2000) reported that CVD patients with high depression scores and who also lacked social support were at the greatest risk for subsequent cardiac events and death. Furthermore, Frasure-Smith and colleagues (2000) found that depressed patients with low perceived social support were at the greatest risk for mortality during the first year following an acute MI. Patients with greater levels of perceived social supports were not at increased risk compared to nondepressed patients given that high perceived social support appeared to buffer the effects of depression on 1-year mortality.

2.2.10 Impact of Depression on CVD Patients

Depression also predicts cardiac morbidity among patients with established CVD. Depression is a particularly significant risk factor for CVD morbidity following acute MI (Tully and Baker 2012; Frasure-Smith et al. 1995; Leung et al. 2012; van Melle et al. 2004; Freedland and Carney 2013). Depressed patients with CVD are at greater risk for readmission or nonfatal cardiac events than nondepressed patients (Barefoot et al. 1996; Carney et al. 1988; Connerney et al. 2001; Tully et al. 2008). Additionally, depression has been shown to predict declines in health status and is associated with worse cardiovascular-specific morbidity. In a study of 460 outpatients with a history of HF and left ventricular ejection fraction, depression was found to be the strongest predictor of decline in health status over a 6-week follow-up period (Rumsfeld et al. 2003). Similarly, Vaccarino and colleagues (2001) also found a graded relationship between the severity of depressive symptoms and a combined end point of functional decline among HF patients.

Numerous studies have demonstrated that the presence of depression predicts all-cause and cardiac mortality following hospitalisation for cardiovascular events (Frasure-Smith et al. 1993; Denollet and Brutsaert 1998; Irvine et al. 1999; Romanelli et al. 2002; Wheeler et al. 2012). For example, Frasure-Smith and colleagues (1993) assessed outcomes following an acute MI in depressed and nondepressed patients. In patients with MDD, the 6-month mortality rate after an MI was 17 %, compared with 3 % among nondepressed patients (HR = 3.44, 95 % CI 2.25–4.63). Similar findings have been reported in larger cohorts of acute coronary syndrome (ACS) patients (Frasure-Smith et al. 1999; Lesperance et al. 2000), as well as in other ischemic heart disease patient cohorts (Barth et al. 2004; Parashar et al. 2006). Depression has also been associated with an increased risk of heart failure readmission and death among HF patients (Jiang et al. 2001; Sherwood et al. 2011). It has also been associated with and increased risk of mortality among patients with prior stoke (Williams et al. 2004; Pan et al. 2011).

Meta-analyses have also found similar results. Barth and colleagues (2004) reported that depressed patients with histories of cardiovascular events were 1.7 times as likely to die within 2 years of initial assessment when compared to nondepressed patients in broad range of CVD conditions (including MI and CABG). In their evaluation of MI patients, van Melle and colleagues (2004) found that post-MI depression was associated with a 2- to 2.5-fold increase in risk of cardiac or all-cause mortality. Finally, in their study of 16,889 MI patients, Meijer and colleagues (2011) reported that post-MI depression was associated with an increased risk of all-cause mortality (OR = 2.25; 95 % CI 1.73–2.93) and cardiac mortality (OR = 2.71; 95 % CI, 1.68–4.36).

Furthermore, a dose-response relationship has been observed between the severity of depression and cardiovascular outcomes. Using data from the Framingham Heart Study, Wulsin and colleagues (2005) also reported a dose-response relationship between severity of depressive symptoms and all-cause mortality. When compared with scores from the lowest tertile of the Center for Epidemiologic Studies Depression Scale (CES-D), the risk of death in the second and third tertiles were 33 % and 88 % higher, respectively. Of course not all findings suggest a positive association (Parashar et al. 2006; Strik et al. 2003; Drago et al. 2007; Thombs et al. 2008). Nicholson et al. showed most studies insufficiently adjusted for confounding variables. For example, left ventricular ejection fraction reduced the purported depression-CVD morbidity link by 65 % (Nicholson et al. 2006).

2.2.11 Impact of CVD on Depressed Patients

The relationship between antecedent depression and subsequent cardiovascular morbidity was investigated in the 1930s, when Malzberg (1937) reported a higher incidence of CVD-related death when compared to control groups. He found the death rates due to cardiac disease were approximately eight times higher in involutional melancholia (depression beginning in midlife or later) than in the general population. In the decades following, numerous studies have observed similar results. For example, Dreyfuss and colleagues (1969) reported the rate of MI was about six times higher among inpatients with depression than among all other inpatients. Prospective studies such as the National Health Examination Follow-Up Study (Anda et al. 1993) found that self-reported depressed mood was associated with a significantly increased risk of fatal ischemic heart disease. In another prospective cohort, Penninx and colleagues (1998) reported that newly depressed older men were approximately twice as likely to have a fatal CVD event than those who were never depressed. Surtees and colleagues (2008) found that participants diagnosed with MDD in the year preceding baseline assessment were 2.7 times more likely to die from IHD in participants free of established heart disease. The severity of depression symptoms has also been found to be an independent risk factor for CVD mortality in prospective cohorts free of CHD at baseline (Ahto et al. 2007; Brown et al. 2011; Whang et al. 2009).

Conclusion

It is important to acknowledge that the association between MDD and CVD is complex and likely bidirectional (Teismann et al. 2014). It should also be considered that the aetiology of depression may differ in certain subgroups within the CVD population (Baune et al. 2012) and that traditional classifications of depression such as melancholia or dysthymia may not be applicable; however, further research is needed to ascertain this.

Given that CVD and depression are among the leading causes of death, disability and disease burden in the developed world, there is the potential for significant harm in ignoring the relationship between the two. The presence of co-morbid CVD and depression not only has the potential to change the prognosis of both clinical and psychosocial outcomes, but it can impact the pathways and responses to treatment.

References

Adamis D, Ball C (2000) Physical morbidity in elderly psychiatric inpatients: prevalence and possible relations between the major mental disorders and physical illness. Int J Geriatr Psychiatry 15(3):248–253

Ahto M, Isoaho R, Puolijoki H, Vahlberg T, Kivela SL (2007) Stronger symptoms of depression predict high coronary heart disease mortality in older men and women. Int J Geriatr Psychiatry 22(8):757–763. doi:10.1002/gps.1735

Aihara Y, Minai J, Aoyama A, Shimanouchi S (2011) Depressive symptoms and past lifestyle among Japanese elderly people. Community Ment Health J 47(2):186–193. doi:10.1007/s10597-010-9317-1

American Psychiatric Association (2000) Diagnostic and statistical manual of mental disorders: DSM-IV-TR. American Psychiatric Association, Washington, DC

Anda R, Williamson D, Jones D, Macera C, Eaker E, Glassman A et al (1993) Depressed affect, hopelessness, and the risk of ischemic heart disease in a cohort of U.S. adults. Epidemiology 4(4):285–294

Andrikopoulos G, Pipilis A, Goudevenos J, Tzeis S, Kartalis A, Oikonomou K et al (2007) Epidemiological characteristics, management and early outcome of acute myocardial infarction in Greece: the HELlenic Infarction Observation Study. Hell J Cardiol 48(6):325–334

Bakhshaie J, Zvolensky MJ, Goodwin RD (2015) Cigarette smoking and the onset and persistence of depression among adults in the United States: 1994-2005. Compr Psychiatry 60:142–148. doi:10.1016/j.comppsych.2014.10.012

Balog P, Janszky I, Leineweber C, Blom M, Wamala SP, Orth-Gomer K (2003) Depressive symptoms in relation to marital and work stress in women with and without coronary heart disease. The Stockholm Female Coronary Risk Study. J Psychosom Res 54(2):113–119. doi:10.1016/S0022-3999(02)00485-3

Barefoot JC, Helms MJ, Mark DB, Blumenthal JA, Califf RM, Haney TL et al (1996) Depression and long-term mortality risk in patients with coronary artery disease. Am J Cardiol 78(6):613–617

Barefoot JC, Brummett BH, Clapp-Channing NE, Siegler IC, Vitaliano PP, Williams RB et al (2000) Moderators of the effect of social support on depressive symptoms in cardiac patients. Am J Cardiol 86(4):438–442

Barth J, Schumacher M, Herrmann-Lingen C (2004) Depression as a risk factor for mortality in patients with coronary heart disease: a meta-analysis. Psychosom Med 66(6):802–813. doi:10.1097/01.psy.0000146332.53619.b2

Baumeister H, Haschke A, Munzinger M, Hutter N, Tully PJ (2015) Inpatient and outpatient costs in patients with coronary artery disease and mental disorders: a systematic review. Biopsychosoc Med 9:11. doi:10.1186/s13030-015-0039-z

Baune BT, Stuart M, Gilmour A, Wersching H, Heindel W, Arolt V et al (2012) The relationship between subtypes of depression and cardiovascular disease: a systematic review of biological models. Transl Psychiat 2:e92. doi:10.1038/tp.2012.18

Biddle SJ, Asare M (2011) Physical activity and mental health in children and adolescents: a review of reviews. Br J Sports Med 45(11):886–895. doi:10.1136/bjsports-2011-090185

Bjerkeset O, Nordahl HM, Mykletun A, Holmen J, Dahl AA (2005) Anxiety and depression following myocardial infarction: gender differences in a 5-year prospective study. J Psychosom Res 58(2):153–161. doi:10.1016/j.jpsychores.2004.07.011

Boden JM, Fergusson DM, Horwood LJ (2010) Cigarette smoking and depression: tests of causal linkages using a longitudinal birth cohort. Br J Psychiatry 196(6):440–446. doi:10.1192/bjp.bp.109.065912

Bosworth HB, Steffens DC, Kuchibhatla MN, Jiang WJ, Arias RM, O'Connor CM et al (2000) The relationship of social support, social networks and negative events with depression in patients with coronary artery disease. Aging Ment Health 4(3):253–258

Brown JM, Stewart JC, Stump TE, Callahan CM (2011) Risk of coronary heart disease events over 15 years among older adults with depressive symptoms. Am J Geriatr Psychiatry 19(8):721–729. doi:10.1097/JGP.0b013e3181faee19

Brummett BH, Barefoot JC, Siegler IC, Clapp-Channing NE, Lytle BL, Bosworth HB et al (2001) Characteristics of socially isolated patients with coronary artery disease who are at elevated risk for mortality. Psychosom Med 63(2):267–272

Bucholz EM, Strait KM, Dreyer RP, Geda M, Spatz ES, Bueno H et al (2014) Effect of Low perceived social support on health outcomes in young patients with acute myocardial infarction: results from the VIRGO (Variation in Recovery: Role of Gender on Outcomes of Young AMI Patients) study. J Am Heart Assoc 3(5):e001252. doi:10.1161/JAHA.114.001252

Carney RM, Rich MW, Freedland KE, Saini J, teVelde A, Simeone C et al (1988) Major depressive disorder predicts cardiac events in patients with coronary artery disease. Psychosom Med 50(6):627–633

Carney RM, Freedland KE, Smith L, Lustman PJ, Jaffe AS (1991) Relation of depression and mortality after myocardial infarction in women. Circulation 84(4):1876–1877

Carney RM, Freedland KE, Veith RC, Cryer PE, Skala JA, Lynch T et al (1999) Major depression, heart rate, and plasma norepinephrine in patients with coronary heart disease. Biol Psychiatry 45(4):458–463

Carter P, Rai G, Aziz A, Mann J, Chandran S, Uppal H et al (2014) Trends of cardiovascular disease amongst psychiatric patients between 2001 and 2012 in Greater Manchester, UK. Int J Cardiol 173(3):573–574. doi:10.1016/j.ijcard.2014.03.116

Connerney I, Shapiro PA, McLaughlin JS, Bagiella E, Sloan RP (2001) Relation between depression after coronary artery bypass surgery and 12-month outcome: a prospective study. Lancet 358(9295):1766–1771

Covinsky KE, Yaffe K, Lindquist K, Cherkasova E, Yelin E, Blazer DG (2010) Depressive symptoms in middle age and the development of later-life functional limitations: the long-term effect of depressive symptoms. J Am Geriatr Soc 58(3):551–556. doi:10.1111/j.1532-5415.2010.02723.x

de Jonge P, Spijkerman TA, van den Brink RH, Ormel J (2006) Depression after myocardial infarction is a risk factor for declining health related quality of life and increased disability and cardiac complaints at 12 months. Heart 92(1):32–39

Denollet J, Brutsaert DL (1998) Personality, disease severity, and the risk of long-term cardiac events in patients with a decreased ejection fraction after myocardial infarction. Circulation 97(2):167–173

Dickens CM, Percival C, McGowan L, Douglas J, Tomenson B, Cotter L et al (2004) The risk factors for depression in first myocardial infarction patients. Psychol Med 34(6):1083–1092. doi:10.1017/S0033291704001965

Dickson VV, Howe A, Deal J, McCarthy MM (2012) The relationship of work, self-care, and quality of life in a sample of older working adults with cardiovascular disease. Heart Lung 41(1):5–14. doi:10.1016/j.hrtlng.2011.09.012

Diminic-Lisica I, Franciskovic T, Janovic S, Popovic B, Klaric M, Nemcic-Moro I (2010) Comorbid chronic diseases in depressed and non-depressed patients in family practice. Psychiatr Danub 22(2):236–240

Djarv T, Wikman A, Lagergren P (2012) Number and burden of cardiovascular diseases in relation to health-related quality of life in a cross-sectional population-based cohort study. BMJ Open 2(5). doi:10.1136/bmjopen-2012-001554

Doyle F, McGee H, Conroy R, Conradi HJ, Meijer A, Steeds R et al (2015) Systematic review and individual patient data meta-analysis of Sex differences in depression and prognosis in persons with myocardial infarction: a MINDMAPS study. Psychosom Med 77(4):419–428. doi:10.1097/PSY.0000000000000174

Drago S, Bergerone S, Anselmino M, Varalda PG, Cascio B, Palumbo L et al (2007) Depression in patients with acute myocardial infarction: influence on autonomic nervous system and prognostic role. Results of a five-year follow-up study. Int J Cardiol 115(1):46–51. doi:10.1016/j.ijcard.2006.04.029

Dreyfuss F, Dasberg H, Assael M (1969) The relationship of myocardial infarction to depressive illness. Psychother Psychosom 17(2):73–81

Drory Y, Kravetz S, Hirschberger G (2003) Israel Study Group on First Acute Myocardial I. Long-term mental health of women after a first acute myocardial infarction. Arch Phys Med Rehabil 84(10):1492–1498

Egede LE (2007) Major depression in individuals with chronic medical disorders: prevalence, correlates and association with health resource utilization, lost productivity and functional disability. Gen Hosp Psychiatry 29(5):409–416. doi:10.1016/j.genhosppsych.2007.06.002

Ferrari AJ, Charlson FJ, Norman RE, Patten SB, Freedman G, Murray CJ et al (2013) Burden of depressive disorders by country, sex, age, and year: findings from the global burden of disease study 2010. PLoS Med 10(11):e1001547

Frasure-Smith N, Lesperance F, Talajic M (1993) Depression following myocardial infarction. Impact on 6-month survival. JAMA 270(15):1819–1825

Frasure-Smith N, Lesperance F, Talajic M (1995) The impact of negative emotions on prognosis following myocardial infarction: is it more than depression? Health Psychol 14(5):388–398

Frasure-Smith N, Lesperance F, Juneau M, Talajic M, Bourassa MG (1999) Gender, depression, and one-year prognosis after myocardial infarction. Psychosom Med 61(1):26–37

Frasure-Smith N, Lesperance F, Gravel G, Masson A, Juneau M, Talajic M et al (2000) Social support, depression, and mortality during the first year after myocardial infarction. Circulation 101(16):1919–1924

Freedland KE, Carney RM (2013) Depression as a risk factor for adverse outcomes in coronary heart disease. BMC Med 11:131. doi:10.1186/1741-7015-11-131

Freedland KE, Rich MW, Skala JA, Carney RM, Davila-Roman VG, Jaffe AS (2003) Prevalence of depression in hospitalized patients with congestive heart failure. Psychosom Med 65(1):119–128

Gallegos-Carrillo K, Flores YN, Denova-Gutierrez E, Mendez-Hernandez P, Dosamantes-Carrasco LD, Henao-Moran S et al (2013) Physical activity and reduced risk of depression: results of a longitudinal study of Mexican adults. Health Psychol 32(6):609–615. doi:10.1037/a0029276

Gottlieb SS, Khatta M, Friedmann E, Einbinder L, Katzen S, Baker B et al (2004) The influence of age, gender, and race on the prevalence of depression in heart failure patients. J Am Coll Cardiol 43(9):1542–1549. doi:10.1016/j.jacc.2003.10.064

Grant BF, Hasin DS, Chou SP, Stinson FS, Dawson DA (2004) Nicotine dependence and psychiatric disorders in the United States: results from the national epidemiologic survey on alcohol and related conditions. Arch Gen Psychiatry 61(11):1107–1115. doi:10.1001/archpsyc.61.11.1107

Greenland P, Reicher-Reiss H, Goldbourt U, Behar S (1991) In-hospital and 1-year mortality in 1,524 women after myocardial infarction. Comparison with 4,315 men. Circulation 83(2):484–491

Griego LC (1993) Physiologic and psychologic factors related to depression in patients after myocardial infarction: a pilot study. Heart Lung 22(5):392–400

Hamo CE, Heitner JF, Pfeffer MA, Kim HY, Kenwood CT, Assmann SF et al (2015) Baseline distribution of participants with depression and impaired quality of life in the Treatment of Preserved Cardiac Function Heart Failure with an Aldosterone Antagonist Trial. Circ Heart Fail 8(2):268–277. doi:10.1161/CIRCHEARTFAILURE.114.001838

Haworth JE, Moniz-Cook E, Clark AL, Wang M, Waddington R, Cleland JG (2005) Prevalence and predictors of anxiety and depression in a sample of chronic heart failure patients with left ventricular systolic dysfunction. Eur J Heart Fail 7(5):803–808. doi:10.1016/j.ejheart.2005.03.001

Ho PM, Masoudi FA, Spertus JA, Peterson PN, Shroyer AL, McCarthy M Jr et al (2005) Depression predicts mortality following cardiac valve surgery. Ann Thorac Surg 79(4):1255–1259. doi:10.1016/j.athoracsur.2004.09.047

Holahan CJ, Moos RH, Holahan CK, Brennan PL (1997) Social context, coping strategies, and depressive symptoms: an expanded model with cardiac patients. J Pers Soc Psychol 72(4):918–928

Horsten M, Mittleman MA, Wamala SP, Schenck-Gustafsson K, Orth-Gomer K (2000) Depressive symptoms and lack of social integration in relation to prognosis of CHD in middle-aged women – The Stockholm Female Coronary Risk Study. Eur Heart J 21(13):1072–1080. doi:10.1053/euhj.1999.2012

Huang KL, Su TP, Chen TJ, Chou YH, Bai YM (2009) Comorbidity of cardiovascular diseases with mood and anxiety disorder: a population based 4-year study. Psychiatry Clin Neurosci 63(3):401–409. doi:10.1111/j.1440-1819.2009.01974.x

Hughes JR, Hatsukami DK, Mitchell JE, Dahlgren LA (1986) Prevalence of smoking among psychiatric outpatients. Am J Psychiatry 143(8):993–997. doi:10.1176/ajp.143.8.993

Irvine J, Basinski A, Baker B, Jandciu S, Paquette M, Cairns J et al (1999) Depression and risk of sudden cardiac death after acute myocardial infarction: testing for the confounding effects of fatigue. Psychosom Med 61(6):729–737

Jiang W, Alexander J, Christopher E, Kuchibhatla M, Gaulden LH, Cuffe MS et al (2001) Relationship of depression to increased risk of mortality and rehospitalization in patients with congestive heart failure. Arch Intern Med 161(15):1849–1856

Kahl KG, Greggersen W, Schweiger U, Cordes J, Balijepalli C, Losch C et al (2012) Prevalence of the metabolic syndrome in unipolar major depression. Eur Arch Psychiatry Clin Neurosci 262(4):313–320. doi:10.1007/s00406-011-0277-4

Kessler RC, Bromet EJ (2013) The epidemiology of depression across cultures. Annu Rev Public Health 34:119

Kinnunen T, Haukkala A, Korhonen T, Quiles ZN, Spiro A 3rd, Garvey AJ (2006) Depression and smoking across 25 years of the Normative Aging Study. Int J Psychiatry Med 36(4):413–426

Krannich JHA, Weyers P, Lueger S, Herzog M, Bohrer T, Elert O (2007) Presence of depression and anxiety before and after coronary artery bypass graft surgery and their relationship to age. BMC Psychiatry 7:47. doi:10.1186/1471-244x-7-47

Krishnan KRR, George LK, Pieper CF, Jiang W, Arias R, Look A et al (1998) Depression and social support in elderly patients with cardiac disease. Am Heart J 136(3):491–495. doi:10.1016/S0002-8703(98)70225-X

Lampinen P, Heikkinen RL, Ruoppila I (2000) Changes in intensity of physical exercise as predictors of depressive symptoms among older adults: an eight-year follow-up. Prev Med 30(5):371–380. doi:10.1006/pmed.2000.0641

Lasser K, Boyd JW, Woolhandler S, Himmelstein DU, McCormick D, Bor DH (2000) Smoking and mental illness: a population-based prevalence study. JAMA 284(20):2606–2610

Lesperance F, Frasure-Smith N, Talajic M (1996) Major depression before and after myocardial infarction: its nature and consequences. Psychosom Med 58(2):99–110

Lesperance F, Frasure-Smith N, Juneau M, Theroux P (2000) Depression and 1-year prognosis in unstable angina. Arch Intern Med 160(9):1354–1360

Lett HS, Blumenthal JA, Babyak MA, Sherwood A, Strauman T, Robins C et al (2004) Depression as a risk factor for coronary artery disease: evidence, mechanisms, and treatment. Psychosom Med 66(3):305–315

Leung YW, Flora DB, Gravely S, Irvine J, Carney RM, Grace SL (2012) The impact of premorbid and postmorbid depression onset on mortality and cardiac morbidity among patients with coronary heart disease: meta-analysis. Psychosom Med 74(8):786–801. doi:10.1097/PSY.0b013e31826ddbed

Lossnitzer N, Herzog W, Stork S, Wild B, Muller-Tasch T, Lehmkuhl E et al (2013) Incidence rates and predictors of major and minor depression in patients with heart failure. Int J Cardiol 167(2):502–507. doi:10.1016/j.ijcard.2012.01.062

Lyness JM, Caine ED, Conwell Y, King DA, Cox C (1993) Depressive symptoms, medical illness, and functional status in depressed psychiatric inpatients. Am J Psychiatry 150(6):910–915. doi:10.1176/ajp.150.6.910

Magyar-Russell G, Thombs BD, Cai JX, Baveja T, Kuhl EA, Singh PP et al (2011) The prevalence of anxiety and depression in adults with implantable cardioverter defibrillators: a systematic review. J Psychosom Res 71(4):223–231. doi:10.1016/j.jpsychores.2011.02.014

Mallik S, Spertus JA, Reid KJ, Krumholz HM, Rumsfeld JS, Weintraub WS et al (2006) Depressive symptoms after acute myocardial infarction: evidence for highest rates in younger women. Arch Intern Med 166(8):876–883. doi:10.1001/archinte.166.8.876

Malzberg B (1937) Mortality among patients with involution melancholia. Am J Psychiatry 93(5):1231–1238

Mehta KM, Yaffe K, Covinsky KE (2002) Cognitive impairment, depressive symptoms, and functional decline in older people. J Am Geriatr Soc 50(6):1045–1050

Meijer A, Conradi HJ, Bos EH, Thombs BD, van Melle JP, de Jonge P (2011) Prognostic association of depression following myocardial infarction with mortality and cardiovascular events: a meta-analysis of 25 years of research. Gen Hosp Psychiatry 33(3):203–216. doi:10.1016/j.genhosppsych.2011.02.007

Mensah GA, Brown DW (2007) An overview of cardiovascular disease burden in the United States. Health Aff (Millwood) 26(1):38–48. doi:10.1377/hlthaff.26.1.38

Murray CJ, Barber RM, Foreman KJ, Ozgoren AA, Abd-Allah F, Abera SF et al (2015) Global, regional, and national disability-adjusted life years (DALYs) for 306 diseases and injuries and healthy life expectancy (HALE) for 188 countries, 1990–2013: quantifying the epidemiological transition. Lancet 386(10009):2145–2191

Naghavi M, Wang H, Lozano R, Davis A, Liang X, Zhou M et al (2015) Global, regional, and national age-sex specific all-cause and cause-specific mortality for 240 causes of death, 1990-2013: a systematic analysis for the Global Burden of Disease Study 2013. Lancet 385(9963):117–171

Nakagawara M, Witzke W, Matussek N (1987) Hypertension in depression. Psychiatry Res 21(1):85–86

Nicholson A, Kuper H, Hemingway H (2006) Depression as an aetiologic and prognostic factor in coronary heart disease: a meta-analysis of 6362 events among 146 538 participants in 54 observational studies. Eur Heart J 27(23):2763–2774. doi:10.1093/eurheartj/ehl338

O'Neil A, Stevenson CE, Williams ED, Mortimer D, Oldenburg B, Sanderson K (2013) The health-related quality of life burden of co-morbid cardiovascular disease and major depressive disorder in Australia: findings from a population-based, cross-sectional study. Qual Life Res 22(1):37–44. doi:10.1007/s11136-012-0128-4

Overdorf V, Kollia B, Makarec K, Szeles CA (2016) The relationship between physical activity and depressive symptoms in healthy older women. Gerontol Geriatr Med 2:2333721415626859

Pan A, Sun Q, Okereke OI, Rexrode KM, Hu FB (2011) Depression and risk of stroke morbidity and mortality: a meta-analysis and systematic review. JAMA 306(11):1241–1249. doi:10.1001/jama.2011.1282

Parashar S, Rumsfeld JS, Spertus JA, Reid KJ, Wenger NK, Krumholz HM et al (2006) Time course of depression and outcome of myocardial infarction. Arch Intern Med 166(18):2035–2043. doi:10.1001/archinte.166.18.2035

Penninx BW, Guralnik JM, Mendes de Leon CF, Pahor M, Visser M, Corti MC et al (1998) Cardiovascular events and mortality in newly and chronically depressed persons > 70 years of age. Am J Cardiol 81(8):988–994

Pratt LA, Ford DE, Crum RM, Armenian HK, Gallo JJ, Eaton WW (1996) Depression, psychotropic medication, and risk of myocardial infarction. Prospective data from the Baltimore ECA follow-up. Circulation 94(12):3123–3129

Rafanelli C, Milaneschi Y, Roncuzzi R, Pancaldi LG (2010) Dysthymia before myocardial infarction as a cardiac risk factor at 2.5-year follow-up. Psychosomatics 51(1):8–13

Raynor DA, Pogue-Geile MF, Kamarck TW, McCaffery JM, Manuck SB (2002) Covariation of psychosocial characteristics associated with cardiovascular disease: genetic and environmental influences. Psychosom Med 64(2):191–203; discussion 4–5

Romanelli J, Fauerbach JA, Bush DE, Ziegelstein RC (2002) The significance of depression in older patients after myocardial infarction. J Am Geriatr Soc 50(5):817–822

Rugulies R (2002) Depression as a predictor for coronary heart disease. A review and meta-analysis. Am J Prev Med 23(1):51–61

Rumsfeld JS, Havranek E, Masoudi FA, Peterson ED, Jones P, Tooley JF et al (2003) Depressive symptoms are the strongest predictors of short-term declines in health status in patients with heart failure. J Am Coll Cardiol 42(10):1811–1817

Rutledge T, Reis VA, Linke SE, Greenberg BH, Mills PJ (2006) Depression in heart failure a meta-analytic review of prevalence, intervention effects, and associations with clinical outcomes. J Am Coll Cardiol 48(8):1527–1537, dx.doi.org/10.1016/j.jacc.2006.06.055

Schrader G, Cheok F, Hordacre AL, Guiver N (2004) Predictors of depression three months after cardiac hospitalization. Psychosom Med 66(4):514–520. doi:10.1097/01.psy.0000128901.58513.db

Shah AJ, Ghasemzadeh N, Zaragoza-Macias E, Patel R, Eapen DJ, Neeland IJ et al (2014) Sex and age differences in the association of depression with obstructive coronary artery disease and adverse cardiovascular events. J Am Heart Assoc 3(3):e000741. doi:10.1161/jaha.113.000741

Sherwood A, Blumenthal JA, Hinderliter AL, Koch GG, Adams KF Jr, Dupree CS et al (2011) Worsening depressive symptoms are associated with adverse clinical outcomes in patients with heart failure. J Am Coll Cardiol 57(4):418–423. doi:10.1016/j.jacc.2010.09.031

Sin MK (2012) Personal characteristics predictive of depressive symptoms in Hispanics with heart failure. Issues Ment Health Nurs 33(8):522–527. doi:10.3109/01612840.2012.687438

Smolderen KG, Strait KM, Dreyer RP, D'Onofrio G, Zhou S, Lichtman JH et al (2015) Depressive symptoms in younger women and men with acute myocardial infarction: insights from the VIRGO study. J Am Heart Assoc 4(4). doi:10.1161/JAHA.114.001424

Stern MJ, Pascale L, Ackerman A (1977) Life adjustment postmyocardial infarction: determining predictive variables. Arch Intern Med 137(12):1680–1685

Strik JJMH, Denollet J, Lousberg R, Honig A (2003) Comparing symptoms of depression and anxiety as predictors of cardiac events and increased health care consumption after myocardial infarction. J Am Coll Cardiol 42(10):1801–1807. doi:10.1016/j.jacc.2003.07.007

Sullivan M, Simon G, Spertus J, Russo J (2002) Depression-related costs in heart failure care. Arch Intern Med 162(16):1860–1866

Surtees PG, Wainwright NW, Luben RN, Wareham NJ, Bingham SA, Khaw KT (2008) Depression and ischemic heart disease mortality: evidence from the EPIC-Norfolk United Kingdom prospective cohort study. Am J Psychiatry 165(4):515–523. doi:10.1176/appi.ajp.2007.07061018

Teismann H, Wersching H, Nagel M, Arolt V, Heindel W, Baune BT et al (2014) Establishing the bidirectional relationship between depression and subclinical arteriosclerosis-rationale, design, and characteristics of the BiDirect study. BMC Psychiatry 14(1):174

Thombs BD, Bass EB, Ford DE, Stewart KJ, Tsilidis KK, Patel U et al (2006) Prevalence of depression in survivors of acute myocardial infarction. J Gen Intern Med 21(1):30–38

Thombs BD, Ziegelstein RC, Parakh K, Stewart DE, Abbey SE, Grace SL (2008) Probit structural equation regression model: general depressive symptoms predicted post-myocardial infarction mortality after controlling for somatic symptoms of depression. J Clin Epidemiol 61(8):832–839. doi:10.1016/j.jclinepi.2007.09.008

Tully PJ, Baker RA (2012) Depression, anxiety, and cardiac morbidity outcomes after coronary artery bypass surgery: a contemporary and practical review. J Geriatr Cardiol 9(2):197–208. doi:10.3724/SP.J.1263.2011.12221

Tully PJ, Baker RA, Turnbull D, Winefield H (2008) The role of depression and anxiety symptoms in hospital readmissions after cardiac surgery. J Behav Med 31(4):281–290. doi:10.1007/s10865-008-9153-8

Uuskula M (1996) Psychological differences between young male and female survivors of myocardial infarction. Psychother Psychosom 65(6):327–330

Vaccarino V, Parsons L, Every NR, Barron HV, Krumholz HM (1999) Sex-based differences in early mortality after myocardial infarction. National Registry of Myocardial Infarction 2 Participants. N Engl J Med 341(4):217–225. doi:10.1056/NEJM199907223410401

Vaccarino V, Kasl SV, Abramson J, Krumholz HM (2001) Depressive symptoms and risk of functional decline and death in patients with heart failure. J Am Coll Cardiol 38(1):199–205

Vaccarino V, Lin ZQ, Kasl SV, Mattera JA, Roumanis SA, Abramson JL et al (2003) Gender differences in recovery after coronary artery bypass surgery. J Am Coll Cardiol 41(2):307–314. doi:10.1016/S0735-1097(02)02698-0

Vaccarino V, Badimon L, Corti R, de Wit C, Dorobantu M, Manfrini O et al (2013) Presentation, management, and outcomes of ischaemic heart disease in women. Nat Rev Cardiol 10(9):508–518. doi:10.1038/nrcardio.2013.93

Vaccarino V, Shah AJ, Rooks C, Ibeanu I, Nye JA, Pimple P et al (2014) Sex differences in mental stress-induced myocardial ischemia in young survivors of an acute myocardial infarction. Psychosom Med 76(3):171–180. doi:10.1097/PSY.0000000000000045

van Melle JP, de Jonge P, Spijkerman TA, Tijssen JG, Ormel J, van Veldhuisen DJ et al (2004) Prognostic association of depression following myocardial infarction with mortality and cardiovascular events: a meta-analysis. Psychosom Med 66(6):814–822. doi:10.1097/01.psy.0000146294.82810.9c

van Melle JP, de Jonge P, Kuyper AM, Honig A, Schene AH, Crijns HJ et al (2006) Prediction of depressive disorder following myocardial infarction data from the Myocardial Infarction and Depression-Intervention Trial (MIND-IT). Int J Cardiol 109(1):88–94. doi:10.1016/j.ijcard.2005.05.053

Welin C, Lappas G, Wilhelmsen L (2000) Independent importance of psychosocial factors for prognosis after myocardial infarction. J Intern Med 247(6):629–639
Wells KB, Stewart A, Hays RD, Burnam MA, Rogers W, Daniels M et al (1989a) The functioning and well-being of depressed patients. Results from the Medical Outcomes Study. JAMA 262(7):914–919
Wells KB, Golding JM, Burnam MA (1989b) Chronic medical conditions in a sample of the general population with anxiety, affective, and substance use disorders. Am J Psychiatry 146(11):1440–1446. doi:10.1176/ajp.146.11.1440
Wells KB, Rogers W, Burnam A, Greenfield S, Ware JE Jr (1991) How the medical comorbidity of depressed patients differs across health care settings: results from the Medical Outcomes Study. Am J Psychiatry 148(12):1688–1696. doi:10.1176/ajp.148.12.1688
Whang W, Kubzansky LD, Kawachi I, Rexrode KM, Kroenke CH, Glynn RJ et al (2009) Depression and risk of sudden cardiac death and coronary heart disease in women: results from the Nurses' Health Study. J Am Coll Cardiol 53(11):950–958. doi:10.1016/j.jacc.2008.10.060
Wheeler A, Beltrame J, Tucker G, Air T, Ling LH, Schrader G (2012) Depression and 5-year mortality in patients with acute myocardial infarction: analysis of the IDACC database. Aust N Z J Psychiatry 46(7):669–675. doi:10.1177/0004867412449875
Whooley MA, Caska CM, Hendrickson BE, Rourke MA, Ho J, Ali S (2007) Depression and inflammation in patients with coronary heart disease: findings from the Heart and Soul Study. Biol Psychiatry 62(4):314–320. doi:10.1016/j.biopsych.2006.10.016
Wiklund I, Herlitz J, Johansson S, Bengtson A, Karlson BW, Persson NG (1993) Subjective symptoms and well-being differ in women and men after myocardial infarction. Eur Heart J 14(10):1315–1319
Williams LS, Ghose SS, Swindle RW (2004) Depression and other mental health diagnoses increased mortality risk after ischemic stroke. Am J Psychiatry 161(6):1090–1095. doi:10.1176/appi.ajp.161.6.1090
Wulsin LR, Singal BM (2003) Do depressive symptoms increase the risk for the onset of coronary disease? A systematic quantitative review. Psychosom Med 65(2):201–210
Wulsin LR, Evans JC, Vasan RS, Murabito JM, Kelly-Hayes M, Benjamin EJ (2005) Depressive symptoms, coronary heart disease, and overall mortality in the Framingham Heart Study. Psychosom Med 67(5):697–702. doi:10.1097/01.psy.0000181274.56785.28
Wyman L, Crum RM, Celentano D (2012) Depressed mood and cause-specific mortality: a 40-year general community assessment. Ann Epidemiol 22(9):638–643. doi:10.1016/j.annepidem.2012.06.102
Xian H, Scherrer JF, Franz CE, McCaffery J, Stein PK, Lyons MJ et al (2010) Genetic vulnerability and phenotypic expression of depression and risk for ischemic heart disease in the Vietnam era twin study of aging. Psychosom Med 72(4):370–375. doi:10.1097/PSY.0b013e3181d28125
Zhao G, Ford ES, Dhingra S, Li C, Strine TW, Mokdad AH (2009) Depression and anxiety among US adults: associations with body mass index. Int J Obes (Lond) 33(2):257–266. doi:10.1038/ijo.2008.268

The Risk Relationship Between Depression and CVD During Ageing

3

Simone Reppermund and Ruby S.M. Tsang

Contents

Late-life depression is one of the most common psychiatric disorders in older adults with a prevalence of 2–10 % in people aged 65 and above. Depression in old age has been associated with functional impairment and many adverse health effects. While there are overlapping symptoms and outcomes of depression throughout the life span, there is evidence for distinct medical, clinical, cognitive, neuroimaging, neuropathological, inflammatory and genetic features for geriatric depression in comparison with depression in young age (see Naismith et al. 2012). Older people with major depression have an increased risk of developing dementia, in particular

S. Reppermund (✉)
Centre for Healthy Brain Ageing, UNSW Medicine, Kensington, NSW, Australia

Department of Developmental Disability Neuropsychiatry, UNSW Medicine, Kensington, NSW, Australia
e-mail: s.reppermund@unsw.edu.au

R.S.M. Tsang
Centre for Healthy Brain Ageing, UNSW Medicine, Kensington, NSW, Australia

B.T. Baune, P.J. Tully (eds.), *Cardiovascular Diseases and Depression*,
DOI 10.1007/978-3-319-32480-7_3

Alzheimer's disease and vascular dementia. There is strong evidence for cardiovascular risk factors being an underlying link between depression and dementia. A recent systematic review and meta-analysis showed that late-life depression is associated with a significant risk of all-cause dementia, Alzheimer's disease and vascular dementia. However, the risk to develop vascular dementia was significantly higher than for Alzheimer's disease (Diniz et al. 2013). Studies suggest that recurrent depression with an onset in midlife may reflect a long-term process of cerebrovascular changes that may be aetiologically related to the development of vascular dementia (Barnes et al. 2012).

The World Health Organization estimates that cardiovascular disease and depression are currently the two most common causes of disability in high-income countries (WHO 2008). The two disorders result in decreased quality of life and in an increase in disability, medical costs and service utilisation. Given the current and projected growth of the elderly population, a better understanding of the link between late-life depression and cardiovascular disease (CVD) is important, especially for possible treatment and prevention strategies.

The following chapter gives an overview of cardiovascular risk factors and their possible relationship with late-life depression.

3.1 Cardiovascular Risk Factors

Cardiovascular risk factors that have been associated with late-life depression include hypertension, diabetes, hypercholesterolemia, heart disease, obesity and smoking (Naismith et al. 2012). Unhealthy lifestyle choices such as smoking, alcohol abuse and inattention to hypertension and other medical conditions may contribute to the development of depression (Vaillant et al. 1996) and represent one possible explanation for the link between depression, CVD and vascular dementia. Depression is further associated with reduced physical activity which in turn is associated with poorer cardiovascular health.

Meta-analyses revealed that depressed patients have a 1.5- to 2-fold increased risk to develop coronary artery disease, even after controlling for other major risk factors for coronary artery disease. A large case-control study with more than 11,000 cases and 13,000 controls from 52 countries showed a 1.5-fold increased risk for myocardial infarction in cases with depression (Rosengren et al. 2004). These findings were consistent in men and women and in different ethnic groups.

3.2 Bidirectional Relationship

Current research findings from epidemiological as well as from clinical studies suggest a bidirectional relationship between CVD and depression, i.e. each condition is associated with an elevated risk of developing the other.

Prior depression has been shown to be related to an increased risk of myocardial infarction and stroke (Barefoot and Schroll 1996; Ferketich et al. 2000;

Liebetrau et al. 2008). In a Danish cohort study, depression was associated with an elevated risk for myocardial infarction and early mortality during a 27-year follow-up even after controlling for traditional risk factors like smoking. Similar results were found in a large US cohort study with more than 7,000 participants by Ferketich et al. (2000). Depression was associated with an increased risk of coronary heart disease and with increased coronary heart disease-related mortality in men. In a population sample of elderly adults in Sweden, depression at baseline was linked to first-ever stroke during a 3-year follow-up (Liebetrau et al. 2008). The authors describe several possible explanations for the relationship between depression and stroke, e.g. increased stress during depression, lower drug compliance and changes in the vascular system that might increase the risk of stroke like myocardial arrhythmia, increased platelet activation and increased insulin resistance.

On the other hand, vascular disease may also promote the development of depression, e.g. white matter lesions can predate and predict the occurrence of late-life depression (Teodorczuk et al. 2007; Reppermund et al. 2014). In a European multicentre study with older adults, the severity of white matter changes predicted the development of depressive symptoms 1 year later (Teodorczuk et al. 2007). In another recent study with community-dwelling elderly participants, reduced white matter integrity was associated with an increase in depressive symptoms 2 years later (Reppermund et al. 2014).

The bidirectional relationship between CVD and late-life depression has important clinical implications. Elderly patients with depressive symptoms should be thoroughly assessed for possible vascular disease and be treated accordingly so that this 'secondary prevention' will improve their long-term outcome and prognosis. A more thorough control of vascular risk factors may help in the prevention of late-life depression.

3.3 Underlying Mechanisms for the Link Between Depression and CVD

Prior depression may be linked to subsequent CVD through unhealthy lifestyle choices like smoking, physical inactivity and non-compliance with treatment but also through biological processes like dysregulation of the hypothalamic-pituitary-adrenal (HPA) axis and resulting elevated cortisol levels and inflammatory cytokines (Byers and Yaffe 2011). High cortisol levels are very common in major depression, and they have been associated with higher levels of circulating cholesterol, hypertension, severity of coronary atherosclerosis (Thomas et al. 2004) and poor verbal memory function (Reppermund et al. 2007). Elevated levels of inflammatory markers (e.g. interleukin 6 and interleukin 8) are associated with late-life depression (Baune et al. 2012a), and interleukin 8 is highly expressed in the brains of patients with Alzheimer's disease (Alsadany et al. 2013), suggesting that it might be specific for long-term changes in neurodegenerative and neuropsychological alterations in the brain (Baune et al. 2012a).

A number of studies have reported associations between arterial stiffness and depression (see Baune et al. 2012b for review). Findings suggest that acute depression may lead to increased arterial stiffness that is related to CVD and mortality.

Another biological mechanism that links depression to CVD is a shared genetic risk factor. In particular, the apolipoprotein E4 allele (APOE 4), which is one of the most robust risk factor genes for Alzheimer's disease, has been associated with coronary disease as well as with late-life depression (Baldwin and O'Brien 2002; McCarron et al. 1999). In a recent 9-year prospective study, the presence of APOE 4 predicted future depression in a population-based sample of older adults, even after excluding individuals who developed dementia later on (Skoog et al. 2015).

In patients with established coronary heart disease, depression is associated with increased cardiac mortality and morbidity. Depressed patients with coronary heart disease have a lower heart rate variability compared to nondepressed patients with coronary heart disease and are, therefore, at a greater risk of ventricular fibrillation (Carney et al. 1995). Potential explanations for these associations are altered autonomic tone, poor adherence and a link with other cardiac risk factors. Some antidepressants (in particular tricyclics and monoamine oxidase inhibitors) may have cardiotoxic side effects, but this accounts only for a very limited number of morbidity and mortality cases in depressed patients as the relationship between depression and cardiovascular disease was observed before antidepressants were developed (Carney et al. 2002).

A recent review on the relationship between depression and CVD highlights the importance to look at different diagnostic subtypes of depression as the association between CVD and depression seems to vary in its strength by subtype (Baune et al. 2012b).

3.4 Vascular Depression

As early as the beginning of the twentieth century, there have already been suggestions that depression with first onset in late life may be secondary to arteriosclerosis (see Post 1962 for a review). Early clinical studies generally reported high comorbidity between vascular risk factors, vascular disease and depression; later silent stroke studies as well as leukoencephalopathy studies highlighted cerebrovascular changes as a possible cause for a subtype of depression commonly observed among the elderly, which Alexopoulos and colleagues (1997) coined *vascular depression*. The vascular depression hypothesis postulates that cerebrovascular disease confers vulnerability to, triggers and maintains a subtype of depression in older adults (Alexopoulos et al. 1997).

While there is still no consensus on the definition of vascular depression to date, it is generally recognised that vascular depression is characterised by a combination of some of the following features (Alexopoulos et al. 1997; Krishnan et al. 1997; Hickie et al. 1995, 1997; Steffens and Krishnan 1998):

- Evidence of vascular disease or vascular risk factors
- Late depression onset or change in the course of depression following development of vascular disease in those with history of early-onset depression

- Neuropsychological impairment including executive dysfunction
- Subcortical neuroimaging abnormalities
- Reduced depressive ideation
- Psychomotor retardation
- Apathy or anhedonia
- Functional disability
- Poorer response to antidepressant treatment
- Absence of family history of mood disorders

Over the years, researchers have tried to further refine the notion of vascular depression by incorporating findings from more recent research. Krishnan et al. (2004) proposed a 'subcortical ischaemic depression' syndrome, which is defined by MRI evidence of confluent deep white matter or subcortical grey matter hyperintensities. In contrast, Alexopoulos et al. (2002) tried to refine the notion based on clinical presentation instead and defined a 'depression-executive dysfunction syndrome' with features of reduced fluency, impaired visual naming, psychomotor retardation, loss of interest in activities and paranoid symptomatology. However, in clinical practice, the same set of criteria used to diagnose major depression is often applied to both younger and older adults, for example, the *Diagnostic and Statistical Manual of Mental Disorders* (DSM-5; American Psychiatric Association 2013), without taking into account effects that biopsychosocial factors in ageing may have on the course and presentation of depression.

McDougall and Brayne (2007) conducted a systematic review of studies that compared symptom profiles of depressed individuals with and without comorbid vascular conditions and found that results have been largely inconsistent. While apathy, lassitude as well as psychomotor change have commonly been reported in these studies, it is unknown whether these behavioural changes are due to depression per se or due to the comorbid vascular conditions.

3.5 White Matter Abnormalities

One of the best replicated findings in neuroimaging studies of late-life depression is the presence of white matter hyperintensities (WMH), also termed leukoaraiosis or leukoencephalopathy in the earlier literature, which are increased signal intensities apparent on T2-weighted fluid-attenuated inversion recovery (FLAIR) magnetic resonance imaging (MRI). These cerebral WM lesions start developing at a relatively young age and both the prevalence and severity are thought to increase with age; community-based cohort studies report around 90 % of older individuals have at least some WM lesions (de Leeuw et al. 2001; Liao et al. 1997; Söderlund et al. 2003). WMH have been found to be associated with a range of poor outcomes, including physical disability and poorer motor function in community-dwelling older adults (Sachdev et al. 2005), as well as a more chronic course of the disorder (Heiden et al. 2005; Hickie et al. 1997; O'Brien et al. 1996) as well as poorer response to treatment (Hickie et al. 1995; Taylor et al. 2003) in those with depression.

WM lesions can be classified by their location in the brain, with periventricular hyperintensities (PVH) located adjacent to the lateral ventricles and deep WMHs (DWMH) located in the subcortical regions, or they can be categorised by severity using visual rating methods such as the Fazekas scale (Fazekas et al. 1987), the Scheltens scale (Scheltens et al. 1993) or Virchow-Robin spaces. DWMH have consistently been reported to be more common and/or more severe in late-life depression (O'Brien et al. 1998; Thomas et al. 2004), but increased and/or more severe PVH was also found in a number of studies (Coffey et al. 1990; de Groot et al. 2000; Herrmann et al. 2008). The exact mechanism linking these WMH with late-life depression is unclear, but the dominant view suggests cerebrovascular disease may contribute to a 'disconnection syndrome' through disruptions in fronto-striato-limbic circuits, which likely underlie both mood and cognitive symptoms observed in late-life depression.

Most studies suggest WMH are non-specific and reflect a heterogeneous assortment of pathologies. Vascular factors were found to differentially influence the development of DWMH and PVH – while the majority of DWMH were associated with small vessel ischaemia, only larger PVH were found to be ischaemic in nature. Other PVH generally reflect ependymal loss, subependymal demyelination, contrasting degrees of myelination in adjacent fibre tracts and astrocytic gliosis (Thomas et al. 2002, 2003; van Swieten et al. 1991). Besides vascular factors, age appears to be the other biggest predictor of total burden of WMH (O'Brien et al. 1996).

Several studies have investigated the specific anatomic localisation and lateralisation of WMH in late-life depression, and lesions disrupting frontal-subcortical projections or the dorsolateral prefrontal circuit have been implicated. Sheline and colleagues (2008) compared WMH burden in individuals with late-life depression to controls matched for vascular risk factors and found increased WMH in the white matter tracts within the dorsolateral prefrontal circuit. Similarly, a neuropathological study by Thomas and colleagues (2002) revealed WMH that are ischaemic in nature were more likely to be found in the dorsolateral prefrontal cortex. More severe WMHs have also been observed in regions including the frontal deep white matter and the putamen in the elderly depressed (Greenwald et al. 1998). While most studies have examined lesion locations only in terms of general brain regions, MacFall et al. (2001) attempted to more precisely study the localisation of these lesions using statistical parametric mapping analyses and identified an increase in lesion density in the medial orbital prefrontal white matter in the elderly depressed individuals.

Few studies have also reported a left lateralisation of WMH in the elderly depressed (Greenwald et al. 1998; Tupler et al. 2002), which is in line with the post-stroke depression literature that found an over-representation of left anterior lesions, particularly those proximal to the frontal pole (e.g. Robinson et al. 1983). However, it is yet unclear what role lesion laterality plays in the vascular depression paradigm. Further research is required to determine whether or how the strategic location of lesions and the total lesion load interact and contribute to the development of depressive symptoms. It is also possible that different lesion locations are associated with different subtypes of depression, for instance, the post-stroke depression study by

Hama and colleagues reported associations between left frontal lesions and *affective* depression and between bilateral basal ganglia lesions and *apathetic* depression (Hama et al. 2007).

Diffusion tensor imaging (DTI) can be used to assess the microstructural integrity of white matter fibre tracts, through the quantification of the magnitude (mean diffusivity, MD) and directionality (fractional anisotropy, FA) of diffusion of water in brain tissues. Reductions in FA have been commonly observed in the frontal and temporal lobes of individuals with late life depression (Bae et al. 2006; Nobuhara et al. 2006; Taylor et al. 2004; Yang et al. 2007), with one study suggesting FA values are inversely related to depression severity (Nobuhara et al. 2006) but another reporting no association (Bae et al. 2006). More recent studies utilising the tract-based spatial statistics technique have demonstrated similar findings (Colloby et al. 2011; Reppermund et al. 2014). Higher FA values in both the bilateral superior frontal gyri and the bilateral anterior cingulate cortices were also found to be associated with failure to remit in a sample of older adults with DSM-IV major depressive disorder without psychosis (Taylor et al. 2008). The pathophysiology underlying these microstructural white matter changes is still largely unknown, as FA values did not appear to be associated with risk factors of late-life depression, such as age, sex, vascular risk factors or hyperintense lesions (Bae et al. 2006; Yang et al. 2007).

3.6 Neuropathology

While neuropathological studies of major depression in younger adults have reported reduced glial cell counts (particularly oligodentrocytes), reduced neuronal size or synaptic proteins (e.g. Cotter et al. 2001; Rajkowska 2000; Uranova et al. 2004), only a handful of neuropathological studies have been conducted in late-life depression, and findings are somewhat inconsistent. The pioneering study by Thomas and colleagues (2001) reported greater frequency of atheromatous disease in individuals with late-life depression, particularly in the cerebral and aortic arteries; however, there was no evidence for increased clinical vascular risk factors or global microvascular disease. Their follow-up studies investigated vascular damage in the dorsolateral prefrontal cortex, anterior cingulate cortex and the occipital cortex. Once again, increased intercellular adhesion molecule-1 (ICAM-1), a marker of ischaemia-induced inflammation, was observed in both grey and white matter of the dorsolateral prefrontal cortex (Thomas et al. 2000, 2002b, 2003), but findings pertaining to vascular cell adhesion molecule-1 expression were inconsistent and there was no evidence of increase microvascular disease in late-life depression (Thomas et al. 2003). More recent studies by Tsopelas et al. (2011) and Xekardaki et al. (2012) reported no association between cerebrovascular pathology (e.g. haemorrhage, large infarcts >10 mm, lacunes or small vessel disease) and late-life depression, even within the subgroup of individuals meeting criteria for vascular depression (Xekardaki et al. 2012). Other types of pathology such as Alzheimer's disease pathology, Lewy bodies and reduced glial and oligodendrocytic density have also been reported in selected studies (e.g. Sweet et al. 2004; Tsopelas et al. 2011), but results were inconsistent. This may be dependent on the characteristics of individuals included in the sample (for instance, some studies included individuals with cognitive impairment and/or dementia) as well as brain regions examined. These findings suggest that not all vascular disease or risk factors may be relevant in the development of late-life depression; for instance, small vessel and microvascular diseases in particular do not appear to be major determinants of late-life depression.

3.7 The Relationship Between Late-Life Depression, CVD and Dementia

Depression and dementia frequently co-occur in older individuals; however, the nature of their relationship is complex and poorly understood. To date, there is no consensus as to whether depression represents a risk factor, a prodrome or a consequence of dementia. The prevalence of depression in Alzheimer's disease reported in the literature varies greatly due to differences in definitions and assessment methods used as well as the populations sampled, but it generally clusters around 20–25 % for major depression and up to 50 % for all depressive syndromes (Lyketsos and Olin 2002; Starkstein et al. 2005). There is also evidence to suggest that depression is more prevalent (Ballard et al. 2000; Newman 1999) as well as more severe (Sultzer et al. 1993) in individuals with vascular dementia. On the other hand, late-life depression is often accompanied by significant cognitive impairment, particularly executive dysfunction. While other neuropsychological deficits may be present as well, some studies suggest these are mediated by deficits in processing speed and working memory (Nebes et al. 2000; Sheline et al. 2006). Two independent meta-analyses reported that a history of depression confers around double the risk for subsequent dementia (Jorm 2001; Ownby et al. 2006). Findings from large cohort studies were also in support of this notion that depression is associated with an increased risk of dementia (Byers et al. 2012; Saczynski et al. 2010).

While much of the attention has focused on examining the relationship between late-life or late-onset depression and dementia, several studies in the past decade have investigated whether early-onset depression is associated with later development of dementia, and the results suggest that early-onset depression is also associated with an increased risk of dementia (see Byers and Yaffe 2011 for a review). In one particular study that studied both mid- and late-life depressive symptoms, Barnes et al. (2012) found that late-life depression alone and late-life depression in combination with midlife depression were associated with an elevated risk of Alzheimer's disease and vascular dementia at the 6-year follow-up. They concluded that recurrent depression over the life course is likely an aetiologic risk factor of vascular dementia, whereas late-onset depression reflects early manifestations of Alzheimer's disease. Moreover, there appears to be a dose-response relationship between cumulative depression burden (as measured in terms of depressive symptom severity, number of prior major depressive episodes or lifetime duration of depression) and later dementia (Kessing and Andersen 2004; Speck et al. 1995).

The two proposed primary pathways linking depression and dementia are grounded in the glucocorticoid cascade hypothesis (Sapolsky et al. 1986) and the vascular depression hypothesis (Alexopoulos et al. 1997). According to the glucocorticoid cascade hypothesis, the HPA axis is activated and glucocorticoid secretion is increased in response to stressors; however, prolonged hypersecretion of glucocorticoids leads to hippocampal damage, which in turn disrupts the hippocampus' negative feedback to the HPA axis and results in further hippocampal damage. Hippocampal atrophy has been shown to be an early marker of Alzheimer's disease, with previous studies reporting such changes predicted subsequent conversion to Alzheimer's disease in individuals with mild cognitive impairment (Apostolova et al. 2006; Jack et al. 1999). Since reduced hippocampal volumes have also been commonly observed in individuals with recurrent depression, the glucocorticoid-hippocampus link may be a common pathway involved in the development of both depression and dementia. On the other hand, ischaemic brain lesions have been consistently reported to be associated with depression in older adults (Herrmann et al. 2008), which if severe enough, can lead to substantial cognitive impairment. It is important to note that the processes involved in these pathways are not necessarily mutually exclusive or sequential, and other factors such as pro-inflammatory cytokines, amyloid plaques, neurofibrillary tangles and neurotrophic factors may contribute to the pathogenesis; in fact, it is most likely the synergistic effect of a range of these processes that results in the development of depression or dementia (Byers and Yaffe 2011). Figure 3.1 provides a

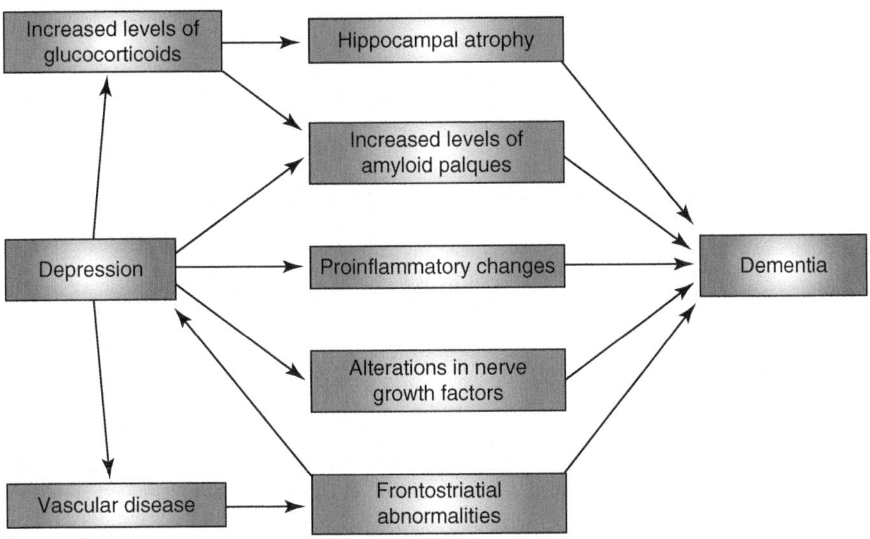

Fig. 3.1 Proposed predominant pathways linking depression to the onset of dementia. The pathways linking depression and dementia are likely to be multifactorial and probably not sequential. Mechanisms that underlie the association between depression and dementia include vascular disease, pro-inflammatory changes and hippocampal atrophy (Reprinted by permission from Macmillan Publishers Ltd: Byers and Yaffe (2011), copyright 2011)

simplified overview of different mechanisms and pathways that may link depression and dementia.

Conclusions

Even though the link between late-life depression and cardiovascular disease is not yet fully understood, accumulating evidence suggests that cardiovascular risk factors and depression have a bidirectional relationship. Proposed mechanisms include unhealthy lifestyle choices, a dysfunction of the HPA axis, pro-inflammatory cytokines, arterial stiffness and genetic risk factors. More research is needed to investigate the mechanisms that link cardiovascular risk factors and depression to develop adequate treatment and prevention strategies. An early control of cardiovascular risk factors may help prevent the development of late-life depression and vice versa; early detection and treatment of depressive symptoms may help prevent CVD later in life. Late-life depression is frequently accompanied by white matter hyperintensities, and further longitudinal studies are required to assess the contribution of white matter hyperintensities to the development of depression. There is growing evidence for depression as a risk factor for dementia and for cardiovascular risk factors being an underlying link between depression and dementia; hence, early treatment of cardiovascular risk factors and depression may be important primary prevention strategies of dementia.

References

Alexopoulos GS, Meyers BS, Young RC, Kakuma T, Silbersweig D, Charlson M (1997) Clinically defined vascular depression. Am J Psychiatr 154(4):562–565

Alexopoulos GS, Kiosses DN, Klimstra S, Kalayam B, Bruce ML (2002) Clinical presentation of the "depression–executive dysfunction syndrome" of late life. Am J Geriatr Psychiatry 10(1):98–106

Alsadany MA, Shehata HH, Mohamad MI, Mahfouz RG (2013) Histone deacetylases enzyme, copper, and IL-8 levels in patients with Alzheimer's disease. Am J Alzheimers Dis Other Dement 28(1):54–61

American Psychiatric Association (2013) Diagnostic and statistical manual of mental disorders, 5th edn. American Psychiatric Association, Washington, DC

Apostolova LG, Dutton RA, Dinov ID et al (2006) Conversion of mild cognitive impairment to Alzheimer disease predicted by hippocampal atrophy maps. Arch Neurol 63(5):693–699

Bae JN, MacFall JR, Krishnan KRR, Payne ME, Steffens DC, Taylor WD (2006) Dorsolateral prefrontal cortex and anterior cingulate cortex white matter alterations in late-life depression. Biol Psychiatry 60(12):1356–1363

Baldwin RC, O'Brien J (2002) Vascular basis of late-onset depressive disorder. Br J Psychiatry 180(2):157–160

Ballard C, Neill D, O'Brien J, McKeith IG, Ince P, Perry R (2000) Anxiety, depression and psychosis in vascular dementia: prevalence and associations. J Affect Disord 59(2):97–106

Barefoot JC, Schroll M (1996) Symptoms of depression, acute myocardial infarction, and total mortality in a community sample. Circulation 93(11):1976–1980

Barnes DE, Yaffe K, Byers AL, McCormick M, Schaefer C, Whitmer RA (2012) Midlife vs late-life depressive symptoms and risk of dementia: differential effects for Alzheimer disease and vascular dementia. Arch Gen Psychiatry 69(5):493–498

Baune BT, Smith E, Reppermund S, Air T, Samaras K, Lux O et al (2012a) Inflammatory biomarkers predict depressive, but not anxiety symptoms during aging: the prospective Sydney Memory and Aging Study. Psychoneuroendocrinology 37(9):1521–1530

Baune BT, Stuart M, Gilmour A, Wersching H, Heindel W, Arolt V et al (2012b) The relationship between subtypes of depression and cardiovascular disease: a systematic review of biological models. Transl Psychiatry 2:e92

Byers AL, Yaffe K (2011) Depression and risk of developing dementia. Nat Rev Neurol 7(6):323–331

Byers AL, Covinsky KE, Barnes DE, Yaffe K (2012) Dysthymia and depression increase risk of dementia and mortality among older veterans. Am J Geriatr Psychiatry: Off J Am Assoc Geriatr Psychiatry 20(8):664–672

Carney RM, Freedland KE, Rich MW, Jaffe AS (1995) Depression as a risk factor for cardiac events in established coronary heart disease: a review of possible mechanisms. Ann Behav Med: Publ Soc Behav Med 17(2):142–149

Carney RM, Freedland KE, Miller GE, Jaffe AS (2002) Depression as a risk factor for cardiac mortality and morbidity: a review of potential mechanisms. J Psychosom Res 53(4):897–902

Coffey CE, Figiel GS, Djang WT, Weiner RD (1990) Subcortical hyperintensity on magnetic resonance imaging: a comparison of normal and depressed elderly subjects. Am J Psychiatr 147(2):187–189

Colloby SJ, Firbank MJ, Thomas AJ, Vasudev A, Parry SW, O'Brien JT (2011) White matter changes in late-life depression: a diffusion tensor imaging study. J Affect Disord 135(1–3):216–220

Cotter DR, Pariante CM, Everall IP (2001) Glial cell abnormalities in major psychiatric disorders: the evidence and implications. Brain Res Bull 55(5):585–595

de Groot J, de Leeuw F, Oudkerk M, Hofman A, Jolles J, Breteler MB (2000) Cerebral white matter lesions and depressive symptoms in elderly adults. Arch Gen Psychiatry 57(11):1071–1076

de Leeuw F-E, de Groot JC, Achten E, Oudkerk M, Ramos LMP, Heijboer R et al (2001) Prevalence of cerebral white matter lesions in elderly people: a population based magnetic resonance imaging study. The Rotterdam Scan Study. J Neurol Neurosurg Psychiatry 70(1):9–14

Diniz BS, Butters MA, Albert SM, Dew MA, Reynolds CF 3rd (2013) Late-life depression and risk of vascular dementia and Alzheimer's disease: systematic review and meta-analysis of community-based cohort studies. Br J Psychiatry: J Ment Sci 202(5):329–335

Fazekas F, Chawluk JB, Alavi A, Hurtig HI, Zimmerman RA (1987) MR signal abnormalities at 1.5 T in Alzheimer's dementia and normal aging. Am J Roentgenol 149(2):351–356

Ferketich AK, Schwartzbaum JA, Frid DJ, Moeschberger ML (2000) Depression as an antecedent to heart disease among women and men in the NHANES I study. National Health and Nutrition Examination Survey. Arch Intern Med 160(9):1261–1268

Greenwald BS, Kramer-Ginsberg E, Krishnan KRR, Ashtari M, Auerbach C, Patel M (1998) Neuroanatomic localization of magnetic resonance imaging signal hyperintensities in geriatric depression. Stroke 29(3):613–617

Hama S, Yamashita H, Shigenobu M, Watanabe A, Kurisu K, Yamawaki S et al (2007) Post-stroke affective or apathetic depression and lesion location: left frontal lobe and bilateral basal ganglia. Eur Arch Psychiatry Clin Neurosci 257(3):149–152

Heiden A, Kettenbach J, Fischer P, Schein B, Ba-Ssalamah A, Frey R et al (2005) White matter hyperintensities and chronicity of depression. J Psychiatr Res 39(3):285–293

Herrmann LL, Le Masurier M, Ebmeier KP (2008) White matter hyperintensities in late life depression: a systematic review. J Neurol Neurosurg Psychiatry 79(6):619–624

Hickie I, Scott E, Mitchell P, Wilhelm K, Austin M-P, Bennett B (1995) Subcortical hyperintensities on magnetic resonance imaging: clinical correlates and prognostic significance in patients with severe depression. Biol Psychiatry 37(3):151–160

Hickie I, Scott E, Wilhelm K, Brodaty H (1997) Subcortical hyperintensities on magnetic resonance imaging in patients with severe depression—a longitudinal evaluation. Biol Psychiatry 42(5):367–374

Jack CR, Petersen RC, Xu YC, O'Brien PC, Smith GE, Ivnik RJ et al (1999) Prediction of AD with MRI-based hippocampal volume in mild cognitive impairment. Neurology 52(7):1397

Jorm AF (2001) History of depression as a risk factor for dementia: an updated review. Aust N Z J Psychiatry 35(6):776–781

Kessing LV, Andersen PK (2004) Does the risk of developing dementia increase with the number of episodes in patients with depressive disorder and in patients with bipolar disorder? J Neurol Neurosurg Psychiatry 75(12):1662–1666

Krishnan KR, Hays JC, Blazer DG (1997) MRI-defined vascular depression. Am J Psychiatry 154(4):497–501

Krishnan KRR, Taylor WD, McQuoid DR, MacFall JR, Payne ME, Provenzale JM et al (2004) Clinical characteristics of magnetic resonance imaging-defined subcortical ischemic depression. Biol Psychiatry 55(4):390–397

Liao D, Cooper L, Cai J, Toole J, Bryan N, Burke G et al (1997) The prevalence and severity of white matter lesions, their relationship with age, ethnicity, gender, and cardiovascular disease risk factors: the ARIC study. Neuroepidemiology 16(3):149–162

Liebetrau M, Steen B, Skoog I (2008) Depression as a risk factor for the incidence of first-ever stroke in 85-year-olds. Stroke 39(7):1960–1965

Lyketsos CG, Olin J (2002) Depression in Alzheimer's disease: overview and treatment. Biol Psychiatry 52(3):243–252

MacFall JR, Payne ME, Provenzale JE, Krishnan KRR (2001) Medial orbital frontal lesions in late-onset depression. Biol Psychiatry 49(9):803–806

McCarron MO, Delong D, Alberts MJ (1999) APOE genotype as a risk factor for ischemic cerebrovascular disease: a meta-analysis. Neurology 53(6):1308–1311

McDougall F, Brayne C (2007) Systematic review of the depressive symptoms associated with vascular conditions. J Affect Disord 104(1–3):25–35

Naismith SL, Norrie LM, Mowszowski L, Hickie IB (2012) The neurobiology of depression in later-life: clinical, neuropsychological, neuroimaging and pathophysiological features. Prog Neurobiol 98(1):99–143

Nebes RD, Butters MA, Mulsant BH, Pollock BG, Zmuda MD, Houck PR et al (2000) Decreased working memory and processing speed mediate cognitive impairment in geriatric depression. Psychol Med 30(3):679–691

Newman SC (1999) The prevalence of depression in Alzheimer's disease and vascular dementia in a population sample. J Affect Disord 52(1–3):169–176

Nobuhara K, Okugawa G, Sugimoto T, Minami T, Tamagaki C, Takase K et al (2006) Frontal white matter anisotropy and symptom severity of late-life depression: a magnetic resonance diffusion tensor imaging study. J Neurol Neurosurg Psychiatry 77(1):120–122

O'Brien J, Desmond P, Ames D, Schweitzer I, Harrigan S, Tress B (1996) A magnetic resonance imaging study of white matter lesions in depression and Alzheimer's disease. Br J Psychiatry: J Ment Sci 168(4):477–485

O'Brien J, Ames D, Chiu E, Schweitzer I, Desmond P, Tress B (1998) Severe deep white matter lesions and outcome in elderly patients with major depressive disorder: follow up study. BMJ 317(7164):982–984

Ownby RL, Crocco E, Acevedo A, John V, Loewenstein D (2006) Depression and risk for Alzheimer disease: systematic review, meta-analysis, and metaregression analysis. Arch Gen Psychiatry 63(5):530–538

Post F (1962) The significance of affective symptoms in old age. Oxford University Press, Oxford

Rajkowska G (2000) Postmortem studies in mood disorders indicate altered numbers of neurons and glial cells. Biol Psychiatry 48(8):766–777

Reppermund S, Zihl J, Lucae S, Horstmann S, Kloiber S, Holsboer F et al (2007) Persistent cognitive impairment in depression: the role of psychopathology and altered hypothalamic-pituitary-adrenocortical (HPA) system regulation. Biol Psychiatry 62(5):400–406

Reppermund S, Zhuang L, Wen W, Slavin MJ, Trollor JN, Brodaty H et al (2014) White matter integrity and late-life depression in community-dwelling individuals: diffusion tensor imaging study using tract-based spatial statistics. Br J Psychiatry: J Ment Sci 205(4):315–320

Robinson RG, Kubos KL, Starr LB, Rao K, Price TR (1983) Mood changes in stroke patients: relationship to lesion location. Compr Psychiatry 24(6):555–566

Rosengren A, Hawken S, Ounpuu S, Sliwa K, Zubaid M, Almahmeed WA et al (2004) Association of psychosocial risk factors with risk of acute myocardial infarction in 11119 cases and 13648 controls from 52 countries (the INTERHEART study): case-control study. Lancet 364(9438):953–962

Sachdev PS, Wen W, Christensen H, Jorm AF (2005) White matter hyperintensities are related to physical disability and poor motor function. J Neurol Neurosurg Psychiatry 76(3):362–367

Saczynski JS, Beiser A, Seshadri S, Auerbach S, Wolf PA, Au R (2010) Depressive symptoms and risk of dementia: the Framingham Heart Study. Neurology 75(1):35–41

Sapolsky RM, Krey LC, McEwen BS (1986) The neuroendocrinology of stress and aging: the glucocorticoid cascade hypothesis. Endocr Rev 7(3):284–301

Scheltens P, Barkhof F, Leys D, Pruvo JP, Nauta JJP, Vermersch P et al (1993) A semiquantative rating scale for the assessment of signal hyperintensities on magnetic resonance imaging. J Neurol Sci 114(1):7–12

Sheline YI, Barch DM, Garcia K, Gersing K, Pieper C, Welsh-Bohmer K et al (2006) Cognitive function in late life depression: relationships to depression severity, cerebrovascular risk factors and processing speed. Biol Psychiatry 60(1):58–65

Sheline YI, Price JL, Vaishnavi SN, Mintun MA, Barch DM, Epstein AA et al (2008) Regional white matter hyperintensity burden in automated segmentation distinguishes late-life depressed subjects from comparison subjects matched for vascular risk factors. Am J Psychiatr 165(4):524–532

Skoog I, Waern M, Duberstein P, Blennow K, Zetterberg H, Borjesson-Hanson A et al (2015) A 9-year prospective population-based study on the association between the APOE*E4 Allele and late-life depression in Sweden. Biol Psychiatry 78:730–736

Söderlund H, Nyberg L, Adolfsson R, Nilsson L-G, Launer LJ (2003) High prevalence of white matter hyperintensities in normal aging: relation to blood pressure and cognition. Cortex 39(4–5):1093–1105

Speck CE, Kukull WA, Brenner DE, Bowen JD, McCormick WC, Teri L et al (1995) History of depression as a risk factor for Alzheimer's disease. Epidemiology 6(4):366–369

Starkstein SE, Jorge R, Mizrahi R, Robinson RG (2005) The construct of minor and major depression in Alzheimer's disease. Am J Psychiatr 162(11):2086–2093

Steffens DC, Krishnan KRR (1998) Structural neuroimaging and mood disorders: recent findings, implications for classification, and future directions. Biol Psychiatry 43(10):705–712

Sultzer DL, Levin HS, Mahler ME, High WM, Cummings JL (1993) A comparison of psychiatric symptoms in vascular dementia and Alzheimer's disease. Am J Psychiatry 150(12):1806–1812

Sweet RA, Hamilton RL, Butters MA, Mulsant BH, Pollock BG, Lewis DA et al (2004) Neuropathologic correlates of late-onset major depression. Neuropsychopharmacol: Off Publ Am Coll Neuropsychopharmacol 29(12):2242–2250

Taylor WD, Steffens DC, MacFall JR, McQuoid DR, Payne ME, Provenzale JM et al (2003) White matter hyperintensity progression and late-life depression outcomes. Arch Gen Psychiatry 60(11):1090–1096

Taylor WD, MacFall JR, Payne ME, McQuoid DR, Provenzale JM, Steffens DC et al (2004) Late-life depression and microstructural abnormalities in dorsolateral prefrontal cortex white matter. Am J Psychiatry 161(7):1293–1296

Taylor WD, Kuchibhatla M, Payne ME, MacFall JR, Sheline YI, Krishnan KR et al (2008) Frontal white matter anisotropy and antidepressant remission in late-life depression. PLoS ONE 3(9):e3267

Teodorczuk A, O'Brien JT, Firbank MJ, Pantoni L, Poggesi A, Erkinjuntti T et al (2007) White matter changes and late-life depressive symptoms: longitudinal study. Br J Psychiatry: J Ment Sci 191:212–217

Thomas AJ, Ferrier IN, Kalaria RN, Woodward SA, Ballard C, Oakley A et al (2000) Elevation in late-life depression of intercellular adhesion molecule-1 expression in the dorsolateral prefrontal cortex. Am J Psychiatr 157(10):1682–1684

Thomas AJ, Ferrier IN, Kalaria RN, Perry RH, Brown A, O'Brien JT (2001) A neuropathological study of vascular factors in late-life depression. J Neurol Neurosurg Psychiatry 70(1):83–87
Thomas AJ, Ferrier IN, Kalaria RN, Davis S, O'Brien JT (2002a) Cell adhesion molecule expression in the dorsolateral prefrontal cortex and anterior cingulate cortex in major depression in the elderly. Br J Psychiatry 181(2):129–134
Thomas AJ, O'Brien JT, Davis S et al (2002b) Ischemic basis for deep white matter hyperintensities in major depression: a neuropathological study. Arch Gen Psychiatry 59(9):785–792
Thomas AJ, O'Brien JT, Barber R, McMeekin W, Perry R (2003) A neuropathological study of periventricular white matter hyperintensities in major depression. J Affect Disord 76(1–3):49–54
Thomas AJ, Kalaria RN, O'Brien JT (2004) Depression and vascular disease: what is the relationship? J Affect Disord 79(1–3):81–95
Tsopelas C, Stewart R, Savva GM, Brayne C, Ince P, Thomas A et al (2011) Neuropathological correlates of late-life depression in older people. Br J Psychiatry 198(2):109–114
Tupler LA, Krishnan KRR, McDonald WM, Dombeck CB, D'Souza S, Steffens DC (2002) Anatomic location and laterality of MRI signal hyperintensities in late-life depression. J Psychosom Res 53(2):665–676
Uranova NA, Vostrikov VM, Orlovskaya DD, Rachmanova VI (2004) Oligodendroglial density in the prefrontal cortex in schizophrenia and mood disorders: a study from the Stanley Neuropathology Consortium. Schizophr Res 67(2–3):269–275
Vaillant GE, Orav J, Meyer SE, McCullough Vaillant L, Roston D (1996) 1995 IPA/Bayer Research Awards in Psychogeriatrics. Late-life consequences of affective spectrum disorder. Int Psychogeriatr IPA 8(1):13–32
van Swieten JC, van den Hout JHW, van Ketel BA, Hijdra A, Wokke JHJ, van Gijn J (1991) Periventricular lesions in the white matter on magnetic resonance imaging in the elderly: a morphometric correlation with arteriolosclerosis and dilated perivascular spaces. Brain 114(2):761–774
World Health Organization (2008) The global burden of disease: 2004 update. WHO Press, Geneva
Xekardaki A, Santos M, Hof P, Kovari E, Bouras C, Giannakopoulos P (2012) Neuropathological substrates and structural changes in late-life depression: the impact of vascular burden. Acta Neuropathol 124(4):453–464
Yang Q, Huang X, Hong N, Yu X (2007) White matter microstructural abnormalities in late-life depression. Int Psychogeriatr 19(04):757–766

Mechanisms Linking Depression to Cardiovascular Disease: What Do Epidemiological Studies Tell Us?

4

Brenda W.J.H. Penninx

Contents

Abstract

The burden of disease for depression goes beyond functioning and quality of life and extends to somatic health. Depression has shown to subsequently increase the risk of cardiovascular morbidity and mortality. These somatic consequences can be partly explained by mediating mechanisms such as unhealthy lifestyle (smoking, excessive alcohol use, physical inactivity, unhealthy diet) or unfavorable pathophysiological disturbances (metabolic, immuno-inflammatory, autonomic, and HPA-axis dysregulations). This chapter presents epidemiological evidence for the existence of these plausible underlying mechanisms that link

B.W.J.H. Penninx, PhD
Department of Psychiatry, EMGO+ Institute for Health and Care Research and Neuroscience Campus Amsterdam, VU University Medical Center,
AJ Ernststraat 1187, Amsterdam 1081 HL, The Netherlands
e-mail: b.penninx@vumc.nl

B.T. Baune, P.J. Tully (eds.), *Cardiovascular Diseases and Depression*,
DOI 10.1007/978-3-319-32480-7_4

depression to cardiovascular disease. However, alternative explanations for an increased cardiovascular risk in depressed persons are also discussed, namely, the confounding hypothesis, iatrogenic effects, or noncausal "third factors."

4.1 Somatic Consequences of Depression

The impact of depression on health extends beyond mental health. Over the last 20 years, many studies illustrated the adverse impact of depression on somatic health as well. As described previously, the evidence is convincing that depression increases the subsequent risk of cardiovascular disease development. Cardiovascular disease refers to those conditions that affect the heart and blood vessels, including among others coronary heart disease, cerebrovascular disease, and peripheral artery disease. Meta-analyses integrating longitudinal evidence concluded that depression results in an at least 80 % increased risk of cardiovascular disease onset (Nicholson et al. 2006; van der Kooy et al. 2007). In line with a dose-response association, the cardiovascular morbidity risk is higher among persons with major depressive disorder than among those with subthreshold depressive symptoms, but the risk is also significantly increased in the latter group. This epidemiological evidence also extends to subclinical cardiovascular processes. Depressed persons are also at increased risk for peripheral atherosclerosis as indicated through, e.g., coronary or aortic calcification, impaired endothelial function, and increased arterial stiffness (Seldenrijk et al. 2010, 2011; Hamer et al. 2010).

This chapter will mainly focus on evidence that considers depression to be an etiological risk factor for cardiovascular disease. However, it is good to note that this is only a small part of the complex interaction between depression and cardiovascular disease. First, beyond increasing the risk of cardiovascular disease onset, depression also increases the risk of cardiovascular mortality when cardiovascular disease has already emerged (Doyle et al. 2015). So, there is extensive evidence that depression contributes not only to the onset but also to the progression of cardiovascular disease. Several of the underlying mechanisms discussed in this chapter are not specific for explaining why depression is an etiological risk factor but may also explain why depression is a prognostic risk factor among patients with clinically overt cardiovascular disease. Second, although I focus mainly on the mechanisms through which depression can increase subsequent cardiovascular risk, it is clear that a bidirectional link exists. Cardiovascular disease itself can – either through direct physical consequences or through indirect biological, bodily, or psychosocial changes – also increase the risk of developing depressive symptoms and disorders.

Furthermore, it is good to realize that the impact of depression on somatic health is not restricted to cardiovascular disease alone. There are various meta-analyses that have shown similar evidences when integrating results from longitudinal studies among initially somatic disease-free subjects. Depression also increases the onset risk of overall mortality (relative risk (RR) = 1.81), diabetes (RR = 1.60), hypertension (RR = 1.42), stroke (RR = 1.34), obesity (RR = 1.58), Alzheimer's disease (RR = 1.66), and to a lesser extent even cancer (RR = 1.29) (Penninx et al. 2013). To even provide a larger picture, the increased cardiovascular risk associated with depression is not specific for depression either. For various other psychiatric conditions, similar observations have been described. In a large-scale population-based study incorporating data from over 50,000 subjects across the world, also panic disorder, specific phobia, post-traumatic stress disorder, and alcohol use disorders were found to predict subsequent heart disease onset (Scott et al. 2013). For nonspecific anxiety disorder, a recent meta-analysis summarizing a total of 37 papers including 1,565,699 persons also indicated a 50 % increased risk of cardiovascular disease onset (Batelaan et al. 2016).

The fact that depression is not only associated with the onset of cardiovascular disease but also that of various other somatic conditions combined with the fact that this association extends to other psychiatric conditions as well already illustrates that it is not likely that underlying mechanisms are very disease specific. In the paragraphs below, I will describe which underlying mechanisms may likely contribute to the increased cardiovascular risk in depressed individuals. For this purpose I will mainly focus on results provided by large-scale epidemiological studies.

4.2 The "Confounding Hypothesis" as Mechanism Linking Depression to Cardiovascular Health

Subjects with depression are usually older, more often female, and have a lower socioeconomic status, and their general health is worse than that of their non-depressed peers. This leads to the hypothesis that age, sex, sociodemographics, and baseline health conditions rather than depression per se might be responsible for the differential subsequent cardiovascular health patterns between depressed and non-depressed subjects. This "confounding hypothesis" (see Table 4.1) is likely to contribute to finding worse cardiovascular outcomes among the depressed. Generally, most longitudinal population studies that examined the risk of cardiovascular events in depressed persons have found that the risk associated with depression declined with 20–30 % after considering these sociodemographic and baseline health conditions (Nicholson et al. 2006; van der Kooy et al. 2007). However, after adjustment for these potential confounding variables in statistical analyses, the cardiovascular risk in depressed persons remained significantly increased compared to that of non-depressed persons illustrating that the link does not seem to be completely due to simply confounding. Of course, it can be that in some cases depression may be a prodrome of not yet discovered and diagnosed (and therefore not measurable) subclinical or medical conditions that affect subsequent cardiovascular disease onset. However, it is unlikely that this completely explains the increased cardiovascular risk as results are rather consistent across studies, not restricted to older samples only (in which other health conditions may be present), and have also been found for major depressive disorders with an early age of onset.

Table 4.1 Summary of proposed mechanisms linking depression to increased cardiovascular risk

Causal mediating mechanisms	
Unhealthy lifestyle	Smoking
	Excessive alcohol use
	Physical inactivity
	Unhealthy diet
Worse medical care	Inadequate medical attention
	Lower (e.g., somatic) treatment compliance
Pathophysiology	Metabolic dysregulations
	Immuno-inflammatory dysregulations
	Autonomic dysregulations
	HPA-axis dysregulations
Noncausal mechanisms	
Confounding	Depression picks up or is a prodrome of not yet discovered or measured (sub)clinical conditions
Iatrogenic effects	Pharmacological effect of, e.g., antidepressants increase cardiovascular risk
"Third underlying factors[a]"	Childhood stressors
	Personality
	Genetic pleiotropy

However, alternative explanations for an increased cardiovascular risk in depressed persons are also discussed, namely, the confounding hypothesis, iatrogenic effects, or noncausal "third factors"

[a]Factors that influence both cardiovascular risk and depression risk but rather independently from each other

4.3 Unhealthy Lifestyle as Mechanism Linking Depression to Cardiovascular Health

Increased behavioral risk profiles in depressed persons may explain their higher risk for adverse health consequences. Behavioral risk factors appear to cluster in the same individuals. Increased smoking and alcohol consumption are well documented in depression. Depressed persons not only smoke more often, they are found to be less likely to quit smoking and might inhale more deeply and smoke more of the cigarette than non-depressed smokers (Anda et al. 1990). In addition, the food intake of depressed persons has shown to be less adequate, healthy, and nutritious than that of non-depressed persons. It has been shown that depressed persons have a higher 24-h caloric intake than non-depressed persons (Sanhueza et al. 2013). On the other hand, certain vitamin deficiencies, such as vitamin D, B12, and folate deficiencies, are more prevalent in depressed older persons (Penninx et al. 2000; Milaneschi et al. 2014), which illustrates that certain depressed persons may not get adequate nutrition. Depressed persons also engage less in physical activities such as walking, gardening, and vigorous exercise activities such as sports. So, physical inactivity is common among depressed persons

(Stephens 1988), partly because their attitudes toward exercise and exercise self-efficacy may be more negative. These unhealthy lifestyles can contribute to the fact that depressed individuals are more at risk for adverse health outcomes, since these constitute the most important risk factors for the onset of cardiovascular disease. This is especially an important observation, since, e.g., the level of physical activity is potentially modifiable through an exercise regimen. There are several clinical trials that – although not consistent across all trials – illustrate that when depressed persons are randomized to an exercise intervention, their depressed mood significantly improves (Rosenbaum et al. 2014). Other lifestyle changing programs, such as nutritional interventions or smoking cessation, may also be relevant in depressed persons and may positively impact not just on mental health but also on cardiovascular health (Ward et al. 2015).

Finally, depressed mood has shown to impede recovery processes by discouraging persons from obtaining adequate medical attention and rehabilitation and following treatment regimens. It has been described that depressed persons are generally at least twice less compliant in taking medications or following up on certain lifestyle regimens provided by health-care professionals (DiMatteo et al. 2000). This lower compliance and poorer self-care with general health regimens could in part be due to lack of a supportive social network which has more often been observed in depressed than in non-depressed persons (Penninx et al. 1998). One study indeed confirmed that depressed cardiac patients received lower quality of care than their non-depressed peers and that this contributed to their higher mortality risk (Druss et al. 2001).

Meta-analyses on cardiovascular consequences of depression have reported pooled effect sizes for adjusted associations which considered potential mediating variables such as lifestyle indicators. This is possible as many – but not all – of the conducted longitudinal studies associating depression to incident cardiovascular morbidity have adjusted for lifestyle differences. These lifestyle-adjusted pooled effect sizes are only slightly lower than unadjusted ones, suggesting that the increased morbidity risks are not simply due to lifestyle differences (Nicholson et al. 2006; van der Kooy et al. 2007). However, considering the fact that, e.g., nutritional and physical activity patterns are not easy to assess in detail in large-scale observational studies, residual impact of these behavioral factors may still exist.

4.4 Biological Dysregulation Linking Depression to Cardiovascular Health

In addition to the above provided explanations, depression-related biological dysregulations that also constitute risk factors for somatic illnesses could further contribute to the observed depression and cardiovascular disease link. The next section describes evidence for biological dysregulations examined in this context. I focused on the most commonly examined biological dysregulations in this respect, namely, metabolic, immuno-inflammatory, autonomic, and HPA-axis dysregulations.

4.4.1 Metabolic Dysregulation

Often clinical metabolic dysregulations are assessed in the context of the metabolic syndrome: a clustering of general metabolic risk factors including abdominal obesity, increased blood glucose (hyperglycemia), elevated blood pressure, increased triglycerides, and decreased high-density lipoprotein (HDL) cholesterol. Metabolic dysregulations are well-established risk factors for the development of various somatic conditions, especially cardiovascular disease and diabetes (Mottillo et al. 2010). Pan et al. (2012) systematically reviewed 29 cross-sectional studies and found depression and the metabolic syndrome to be modestly associated (unadjusted odds = 1.42; adjusted odds = 1.34). Some reviewed prospective studies confirmed a bidirectional association with depression predicting the onset of metabolic syndrome, which in turn predicted depression onset over time. However, the metabolic syndrome is a heterogeneous concept: pathophysiological mechanisms of elevated blood pressure, dyslipidemia, and hyperglycemia are not necessarily similar. Consequently, various studies have tested consistency of associations with depression across different metabolic syndrome components. The most consistent evidence seems to exist between depression and obesity-related components (abdominal obesity, low HDL cholesterol, hypertriglyceridemia), whereas associations between depression with hyperglycemia and hypertension are less often confirmed (Pan et al. 2012). Also when evidence from longitudinal studies was pooled, consistent associations were only confirmed for the obesity-related components. The association between depression and metabolic dysregulations seems to follow a dose-response association as larger dysregulations were found with increasing level of depression severity (Van Reedt Dortland et al. 2010). Two longitudinal studies among depressed patients found that a combination of multiple metabolic dysregulations contributed to sustained chronicity of depression (Vogelzangs et al. 2011, 2014). Taken together, literature suggests that abdominal obesity and lipid disturbances are the driving force behind the relationship between depression and metabolic syndrome. Once both are present, abdominal obesity might give rise to multiple metabolic dysregulations, which in turn might be responsible for remaining in a depressed state.

Indeed, depression is a heterogeneous condition with multiple, diverging symptoms defining the concept. Metabolic dysregulations have found to be more specifically present in "atypical depression," a subtype present in 20–30 % of all depressed cases and marked by hypersomnia and fatigue, increased appetite and weight gain, mood reactivity, and interpersonal rejection sensitivity (Penninx et al. 2013). Two studies directly comparing atypical versus melancholic depressed persons both confirmed that metabolic syndrome were more present in atypical than in melancholic depression (Seppälä et al. 2012; Lamers et al. 2010). Also when examining longitudinal associations with abdominal obesity-related outcomes in a large-scale population sample, it was mainly atypical depression that was found to be predictive (Lasserre et al. 2014).

How could metabolic dysregulations in depression arise? White adipose tissue, especially in the abdominal area, is an active endocrine organ producing inflammatory cytokines and hormones (e.g., leptin) and, therefore, a major contributor to pathogenic immune-metabolic responses both in the central nervous system and brain and in the rest of the body. For instance, leptin has shown to affect hippocampal and cortical structure through its actions on neurogenesis, axon growth, synaptogenesis, and dendritic morphology regulation (Paz-Filho et al. 2010). Another possible mechanism linking metabolic dysregulation and depression may be represented by cerebrovascular damage associated with metabolic syndrome, which according to the so-called "vascular depression" hypothesis predispose to depression especially in late life (Alexopoulos 2006). Finally, other depression-related biological dysregulations discussed below may constitute shared underlying pathways to metabolic alterations.

4.4.2 Immuno-Inflammatory Dysregulation

A consistent body of evidence indicates that depression is associated with dysregulated inflammation, an immune response that derives from activation of the innate immune system. The inflammatory mediator network is represented by a bewildering array of molecules, the most prominent of which are pro-inflammatory cytokines (e.g., interleukin (IL)-6 and TNF-α) produced within innate immune cells in response to immunologic challenge. Other cytokines, known as anti-inflammatory, oppose this response by attenuating the production of pro-inflammatory cytokine (e.g., IL-10) or by antagonizing their action at the receptor level (e.g., IL-1RA). The actions of pro-inflammatory cytokines on peripheral cellular targets such as hepatocytes lead to the synthesis of acute phase proteins (e.g., C-reactive protein (CRP)) responsible for the systemic inflammatory response. Chronic, low-grade systemic elevations of these molecules are considered abnormal and have shown to increase the onset of cardiovascular morbidity and mortality (Cesari et al. 2003; Kaptoge et al. 2010). There is a strong interconnection between metabolic abnormalities and inflammation illustrated by the facts that abdominal fat tissue produces cytokines, and these subsequently increase metabolic syndrome development (Visser et al. 1999).

Three recent meta-analyses reported significantly higher levels of the inflammatory markers TNF-α, sIL-2R, IL-6, and IL-1RA in drug-naïve depressed subjects compared to controls (Dowlati et al. 2010; Liu et al. 2012; Howren et al. 2009). Overall, effect sizes were modest (ranging from a Cohen's d of 0.15–0.35) with slightly stronger effect sizes for studies using clinical diagnoses of depression instead of symptom reports (Penninx et al. 2013). Although systemic inflammation has been found for both melancholic and atypical depressed subjects, it appears to be more strongly present in atypical depression (Lamers et al. 2013; Penninx et al. 2013). An essential role was found for body mass index (BMI) as a covariate: studies adjusting for BMI found much lower effect sizes, likely due to the fact that adipose tissue is an important source of cytokines. However, even after adjustment for BMI, elevated inflammation levels in the depressed were observed, indicating that immune and metabolic dysregulations are partly complementary.

Most meta-analyzed studies were cross-sectional which makes it hard to draw any causal inferences. However, several lines of research indicate that the link between inflammation and depression is likely bidirectional. It has been demonstrated that immunotherapy with IFN-α can precipitate depression (Bonaccorso et al. 2002). In turn, cytokines produced peripherally can access the brain – either directly crossing the blood-brain barrier through saturable active transport systems or indirectly via microglia activation – which can result in decreased neurogenesis also in emotion-regulating brain structures (Shelton and Miller 2010). Cytokines also catalyze the synthesis of kynurenine from tryptophan, which may result in reduced synthesis of serotonin and increased synthesis of tryptophan catabolites, which could all perturb neurotransmission and result in hippocampal neuron damage (Sublette and Postolache 2012). Finally, depression may facilitate weight gain – partly as a result of sedentary behavior and unhealthy dietary choice – which in turn promotes inflammation that ultimately may reinforce depression, creating a deleterious vicious cycle for physical and mental health.

4.4.3 Autonomic Dysregulation

Acute stress results into immediate activation of sympathetic nerves and reduction of parasympathetic nerves in order to prepare the body for a fight and flight response. A direct measurement method for autonomic tone is assessing noradrenaline spillover to plasma. Unfortunately, such invasive spillover studies are not implementable in large psychiatric cohorts, restricting our insights into generalizability of results and the role of potential confounding factors. That is why researchers have used noninvasive, but more indirect, indicators of autonomic tone obtained from electrical and impedance cardiography assessments. A noninvasive method for autonomic dysregulation assessment is heart rate variability (HRV), particularly in the respiratory frequency range, as an indicator of cardiac vagal control. HRV reflects an individual's capacity for parasympathetic inhibition of autonomic arousal and is an important predictor for cardiovascular disease and mortality (Dekker et al. 2000; Tsuji et al. 1996). Autonomic dysregulation is involved in cardiovascular somatic symptoms such as tachycardia, blood pressure liability, and tendencies toward hypertension and predicts the onset of metabolic dysregulations over time (Licht et al. 2013).

Depression is hypothesized to involve an autonomic nervous system that is in a relative state of more sympathetic and less parasympathetic activation. According to the polyvagal theory, this is partly due to the fact that impairments of low vagal tone are associated with reduced social engagement and a less flexible behavioral response to environmental changes (Porges 2001). Rottenberg (2007) summarized 13 studies including 312 depressed patients and 374 controls and found indeed a significantly reduced HRV in depression (Cohen's $d=0.33$). Four years later, Kemp et al. (2010) repeated a meta-analysis in which only power-domain analyses were allowed to measure HRV, and all included subjects were free of cardiovascular disease. Meta-analyzing results of 14 studies (302 patients, 424 controls) yielded again a modest but significant pooled effect size indicating a lower HRV among the depressed. Contrary to these results were studies by Licht et al. (2008) and Kemp et al. (2014) with a sample size that was by far larger than the total number of participants in the meta-analyses and could adjust for lifestyle. In these studies, more than 1,000 major depressive disorder patients without antidepressants did not consistently show differences in HRV as compared to control subjects, and in a 2-year follow-up, depression state (changes) was not associated with HRV (Licht et al. 2010). On the contrary, in both large-scale studies (Licht et al. 2008; Kemp et al. 2014), significantly lower HRV was found among antidepressant users, especially those using tricyclic antidepressants and serotonergic-noradrenergic reuptake inhibitors. This led to the authors' conclusion that it is not depressed state but use of antidepressants that changes autonomic tone. The TCA effect on HRV – likely through direct anticholinergic effects – was confirmed in a meta-analysis (Kemp et al. 2010). So, it remains rather unclear whether depression itself is associated with a reduced vagal tone. Of note is that studies included in these meta-analyses measured autonomic tone during resting condition. Depression could be more strongly associated with reduced parasympathetic tone when persons are exposed to stress conditions.

4.4.4 Hypothalamic-Pituitary-Adrenal (HPA) Axis Dysregulation

Hyperactivity of the HPA-axis in depression has been considered one of the most reliable findings in biological psychiatry. Chronic stress is perceived by the cortex of the brain and transmitted to the hypothalamus, where corticotropin-releasing hormone is released onto pituitary receptors, ultimately resulting in release of cortisol into the blood. To assess HPA-axis activity, salivary measures are increasingly used to reflect the active unbound form of cortisol. The cortisol awakening response assesses the natural response of the HPA-axis to awakening; evening cortisol levels reflect basal activity. In a meta-analysis by Knorr et al. (2010) summarizing 20 case-control studies including 1,354 depressed patients and 1,052 controls, salivary cortisol levels were on average 2.58 nmol/l increased in the morning and 0.27 nmol/l in the evening for depressed patients. In an even larger meta-analysis by Stetler and Miller (2011), evidence for higher cortisol levels across various bodily fluids (plasma, urine, saliva) was summarized. Again, this evidence illustrated that depressed individuals displayed increased cortisol levels ($d = 0.60$), although the effect size was considerably less – and rather modest – when only high methodological quality studies were included ($d = 0.33$). Vreeburg and colleagues (2009) showed that these findings were consistent among 701 current as well as among 579 remitted depressed cases, suggesting that HPA-axis hyperactivity represents a vulnerability rather than a state indicator. In line with this, HPA-axis hyperactivity has also been observed among non-affected offspring of depressed patients, suggesting that it may partly reflect a genetic vulnerability marker or endophenotype of depression (Vreeburg et al. 2010).

HPA-axis dysregulation appears to be more prevalent especially in persons with melancholic depression, characterized by a disturbance in affect marked by anhedonia and nonreactive mood, by psychomotor disturbance, and by vegetative and cognitive symptoms of insomnia, loss of appetite and weight, diurnal mood variation, and impaired concentration. When summarizing several studies directly that compared cortisol levels across melancholic and atypical depression, we showed that in fact, cortisol levels among individuals with atypical depression may not be reliably higher than cortisol levels among healthy non-depressed persons (Lamers et al. 2013; Penninx et al. 2013). In line with this, a sub-analysis in Stetler and Miller's meta-analysis (2011) described that the effect size of the cortisol-depression association is higher when more melancholic depressed cases were included in studies and lower when more atypical depressed cases were included. Melancholic features were associated with 54 % larger effect sizes compared with depression without melancholic features.

Some studies have used a dexamethasone test to evaluate the sensitivity of the hypothalamus to feedback signals for the shutdown of CRH release, but results are more inconsistent. Nelson and Davis (1997) summarized that dexamethasone suppression studies found that the normal cortisol-suppression response is absent in about half of the patients with very severe symptoms (e.g., those hospitalized or those with psychotic symptoms). However, the non-suppression rate in outpatients with major depression was found to be much lower and not differential between 1,280 depressed outpatients and 308 controls (Vreeburg et al. 2009). So, the indicated larger non-suppression of the HPA-axis in depression is likely restricted to only the most severe (psychotic) cases.

Several mechanisms may underlie the relationship between HPA-axis dysregulation and depression. Depression research has focused mainly on the role of mineral corticoid and glucocorticoid receptors, acting as transcriptional regulators of cortisol effects on the initiation and termination of the stress response. Alterations of this regulating network, defined glucocorticoid resistance, may determine a chronic activation of the stress response resulting in atrophy of hippocampal cells, reduced neurogenesis, and synaptic plasticity and altered monoaminergic signaling, all of which may lead to a depressive state (De Kloet et al. 2005). Other factors such as early-life epigenetic programming of glucocorticoid genes and inflammatory processes may also be involved in the dysregulation of HPA-axis responsiveness in depressed subjects (Silverman and Sternberg 2012).

HPA-axis dysregulation has also been implicated in the onset and progression of cardiovascular disease, although evidence for this is not extensive. In two longitudinal observational studies, higher morning cortisol levels and a flatter slop in cortisol levels across the day were found to increase the risk of subsequent cardiovascular mortality in nonclinical populations (Vogelzangs et al. 2010; Kumari et al. 2011).

4.5 Iatrogenic Effects Linking Depression to Cardiovascular Risk

To what extent can antidepressant utilization contribute to an increased cardiovascular risk among depressed individuals? A few observational large-scale studies have reported increased cardiovascular risks among persons using antidepressants (Whang et al. 2009; Hamer et al. 2011). It is an easy step to then point at the antidepressants as driving the increased cardiovascular risk. However, this type of finding cannot simply be interpreted as evidence for cardiovascular-induced risks through pathophysiological effects of antidepressants themselves mainly because such findings are heavily biased through "confounding by indication." In observational studies, subjects using antidepressants are likely to be different in many ways from subjects not using antidepressants: they are likely the most severe and chronic depression cases, or they may have other (mental or physical) reasons to be treated with antidepressants. Even if observational analyses adjust for presence and severity of depression, confounding by indication may still be present, and therefore one should be cautious with research interpretations of observational studies regarding effects of medications.

As described above, there is more and more consistent evidence that antidepressant medications, especially the tricyclic antidepressants and the serotonergic-noradrenergic reuptake inhibitors, may increase cardiac vagal tone (Licht et al. 2008, 2010; Kemp et al. 2014). However, whether this in the end may truly contribute to an increased subsequent cardiovascular disease risk remains unknown. Autonomic tone differences were generally completely diminished when antidepressant medication use was stopped (Licht et al. 2010), and it could simply be that detrimental effects of depressed mood status itself may be larger than that of antidepressants. In addition, experimental intervention results, however, do indicate that several antidepressants may in fact contribute to reduction of other specific pathophysiological disturbances such as inflammation and cortisol levels (Hannestad et al. 2011; Hinkelmann et al. 2012). In all, it is difficult to use epidemiological observational data to draw definitive conclusions of the presence of iatrogenic effects of antidepressants, and whether these truly contribute to cardiovascular disease risks. In order to formally test this, one would require a very large, long-term experimental trial, which is difficult, if not impossible, to conduct.

4.6 Other Noncausal Factors Linking Depression to Cardiovascular Risk

Alternative explanations for the link between depression and increased cardiovascular morbidity development could be "third underlying factors" that increase the risk of depression as well as the risk of cardiovascular disease but rather independently from each other (see Table 4.1). Several examples for such noncausal mechanisms exist. First, childhood maltreatment including emotional, physical, or sexual abuse has shown to be a very strong risk factor for the later onset of depression (Teicher and Samson 2013). However, childhood maltreatment has also found to be associated with both subclinical cardiovascular processes and an increased cardiovascular event risk, partly independent from depression (Bomhof-Roordink et al. 2015; Sumner et al. 2015). Consequently, if the same at-risk persons share increased risks for two conditions, associations would become apparent, but this does not have to reflect a causal, temporal association between the two conditions. Second, personality traits such as neuroticism, introversion, and type D personality have shown to be linked to both the development of depression and cardiovascular events and could therefore constitute such a "third factor" that indirectly links both outcomes (Grande et al. 2012; Jokela et al. 2014).

Finally, an often ignored "third factor" is genetic vulnerability. If two conditions share similar genetic risk variants, persons with those high-risk genes could develop both conditions. The phenomenon of shared genetic effects is called genetic pleiotropy (de Geus 2006). This is an area that has not received a lot of research attention yet. However, it is not hard to imagine that the phenomenon of genetic pleiotropy may occur. Utilizing twin data, de Moor et al. (2008) and Bartels et al. (2012) illustrated that the link between reduced exercise behavior and mood symptoms is for a large extent due to shared genetic risks. Also for several of the biological mechanisms described above, for instance, inflammation or metabolic dysregulations, strong genetic influences have been described. These genetic influences may make persons vulnerable for biological dysregulations, which could then result in both depression as well as cardiovascular disease and in (longitudinal) relationships between both outcomes.

Conclusions

This review summarized longitudinal evidence indicating that depression increased the onset risk of cardiovascular disease onset. As summarized in Table 4.1, epidemiological evidence indicates that underlying mechanisms likely involve unhealthy lifestyles as well as a multitude of biological dysregulations that are more prevalent among depressed persons as compared to their non-depressed peers. To what extent each of these mediating mechanisms contribute to the observed increased cardiovascular risk among the depressed remains to be determined as hardly any studies have examined and quantified the mediating mechanisms in the link between depression and cardiovascular disease in a comprehensive manner. In addition, using an epidemiological observational study design for this has its limitations since the confounding hypothesis and the influence of noncausal "third factors" are hard to exclude. Nevertheless, considering the consistency of findings over multiple studies, there is convincing evidence that unhealthy lifestyles and various biological dysregulations interplay in reinforcing the vicious cycle through which depression and cardiovascular disease reinforce each other.

Acknowledgements Penninx was supported through a VICI grant (NWO grant 91811602).

Competing Interests The author has no conflict of interest to report.

References

Alexopoulos GS (2006) The vascular depression hypothesis: 10 years later. Biol Psychiatry 60:1304–1305

Anda RF, Williamson DF, Escobedo LG, Mast EE, Giovino GA, Remington PL (1990) Depression and the dynamics of smoking. A national perspective. JAMA 264:1541–1545

Bartels M, de Moor MH, van der Aa N, Boomsma DI, de Geus EJ (2012) Regular exercise, subjective wellbeing, and internalizing problems in adolescence: causality or genetic pleiotropy? Front Genet 3:4

Batelaan N, Seldenrijk A, Bot M, van Balkom A, Penninx BW (2016) Anxiety and new-onset of cardiovascular disease: a critical review and meta-analysis. Br J Psychiatry 208(3):223–231

Bomhof-Roordink H, Seldenrijk A, van Hout HP, van Marwijk HW, Diamant M, Penninx BW (2015) Associations between life stress and subclinical cardiovascular disease are partly mediated by depressive and anxiety symptoms. J Psychosom Res 78:332–339

Bonaccorso S, Marino V, Puzella A, Pasquini M, Biondi M, Artini M et al (2002) Increased depressive ratings in patients with hepatitis C receiving interferon-alpha-based immunotherapy are related to interferon-alpha-induced changes in the serotonergic system. J Clin Psychopharmacol 22:86–90

Cesari M, Penninx BWJH, Newman AB, Kritchevsky SB, Nicklas BJ, Sutton-Tyrrell K et al (2003) Inflammatory markers and onset of cardiovascular events: results from the Health ABC study. Circulation 108:2317–2322

de Geus EL (2006) Genetic pleiotropy in depression and coronary artery disease. Psychosom Med 8:185–186

de Kloet ER, Joels M, Holsboer F (2005) Stress and the brain: from adaptation to disease. Nat Rev Neurosci 6:463–475

De Moor MH, Boomsma DI, Stubbe JH, Willemsen G, de Geus EJ (2008) Testing causality in the association between regular exercise and symptoms of anxiety and depression. Arch Gen Psychiatry 65:897–905

Dekker JM, Crow RS, Folsom AR, Hannan PJ, Liao D, Swenne CA et al (2000) Low heart rate variability in a 2-minute rhythm strip predicts risk of coronary heart disease and mortality from several causes: the ARIC Study. Atherosclerosis Risk In Communities. Circulation 102:1239–1244

DiMatteo MR, Lepper HS, Croghan TW (2000) Depression is a risk factor for noncompliance with medical treatment: meta-analysis of the effects of anxiety and depression on patient adherence. Arch Intern Med 160:2101–2107

Dowlati Y, Herrmann N, Swardfager W, Liu H, Sham L, Reim EK et al (2010) A meta-analysis of cytokines in major depression. Biol Psychiatry 67:446–457

Doyle F, McGee H, Conroy R, Conradi HJ, Meijer A, Steeds R, Sato H, Stewart DE, Parakh K, Carney R, Freedland K, Anselmino M, Pelletier R, Bos EH, de Jonge P (2015) Systematic review and individual patient data meta-analysis of sex differences in depression and prognosis in persons with myocardial infarction: a MINDMAPS study. Psychosom Med 77:419–428

Druss BG, Bradford WD, Rosenheck RA, Radford MJ, Krumholz HM (2001) Quality of medical care and excess mortality in older patients with mental disorders. Arch Gen Psychiatry 58:565–572

Grande G, Romppel M, Barth J (2012) Association between type D personality and prognosis in patients with cardiovascular diseases: a systematic review and meta-analysis. Ann Behav Med 43:299–310

Hamer M, Kivimaki M, Lahiri A, Marmot MG, Steptoe A (2010) Persistent cognitive depressive symptoms are associated with coronary artery calcification. Atherosclerosis 210:209–213

Hamer M, Batty GD, Seldenrijk A, Kivimaki M (2011) Antidepressant medication use and future risk of cardiovascular disease: the Scottish Health Survey. Eur Heart J 32:437–442

Hannestad J, DellaGioia N, Bloch M (2011) The effect of antidepressant medication treatment on serum levels of inflammatory cytokines: a meta-analysis. Neuropsychopharmacology 36:2452–2459

Hinkelmann K, Mortiz S, Botzenhardt J, Muhtz C, Wiedemann K, Kellner M, Otte C (2012) Changes in cortisol secretion during antidepressive treatment and cognitive improvement in patients with major depression: a longitudinal study. Psychoneuroendocrinology 37:685–692

Howren MB, Lamkin DM, Suls J (2009) Associations of depression with C-reactive protein, IL-1, and IL-6: a meta-analysis. Psychosom Med 71:171–186

Jokela M, Pulkki-Raback L, Elovainio M, Kivimaki M (2014) Personality traits as risk factors for stroke and coronary heart disease mortality: pooled analysis of three cohort studies. J Behav Med 37:881–889

Kaptoge S, Di Angelantonio E, Lowe G, Pepys MB, Thompson SG, Collins R et al (2010) C-reactive protein concentration and risk of coronary heart disease, stroke, and mortality: an individual participant meta-analysis. Lancet 375:132–140
Kemp AH, Quintana DS, Gray MA, Felmingham KL, Brown K, Gatt JM (2010) Impact of depression and antidepressant treatment on heart rate variability: a review and meta-analysis. Biol Psychiatry 67:1067–1074
Kemp AH, Brunoni AR, Santos IS, Nunes MA, Dantas EM, Carvalho de Figueiredo R, Pereira AC, Ribeiro AL, Mill JG, Andreão RV, Thayer JF, Benseñor IM, Lotufo PA (2014) Effects of depression, anxiety, comorbidity, and antidepressants on resting-state heart rate and its variability: an ELSA-Brasil cohort baseline study. Am J Psychiatry 171:1328–1334
Knorr U, Vinberg M, Kessing LV, Wetterslev J (2010) Salivary cortisol in depressed patients versus control persons: a systematic review and meta-analysis. Psychoneuroendocrinology 35:1275–1286
Kumari M, Shipley M, Stafford M, Kivimaki M (2011) Association of diurnal patterns in salivary cortisol with all-cause and cardiovascular mortality: findings from the Whitehall II study. J Clin Endocrinol Metab 96:1478–1485
Lamers F, De Jonge P, Nolen WA, Smit JH, Zitman FG, Beekman ATF et al (2010) Identifying depressive subtypes in a large cohort study: results from the Netherlands Study of Depression and Anxiety (NESDA). J Clin Psychiatry 71:1582–1589
Lamers F, Vogelzangs N, Merikangas K, de Jonge P, Beekman A, Penninx B (2013) Evidence for a differential role of HPA-axis function, inflammation and metabolic syndrome in melancholic versus atypical depression. Mol Psychiatry 18:692–699
Lasserre AM, Glaus J, Vandeleur CL, Marques-Vidal P, Vaucher J, Bastardot F, Waeber G, Vollenweider P, Preisig M (2014) Depression with atypical features and increase in obesity, body mass index, waist circumference, and fat mass: a prospective, population-based study. JAMA Psychiatry 71:880–888
Licht CMM, de Geus EJC, Zitman FG, Hoogendijk WJG, van Dyck R, Penninx BWJH (2008) Association between major depressive disorder and heart rate variability in the Netherlands Study of Depression and Anxiety (NESDA). Arch Gen Psychiatry 65:1358–1367
Licht CMM, de Geus EJC, van Dyck R, Penninx BWJH (2010) Longitudinal evidence for unfavorable effects of antidepressants on heart rate variability. Biol Psychiatry 68:861–868
Licht CMM, de Geus EJC, Penninx BW (2013) Dysregulation of the autonomic nervous system predicts the development of the metabolic syndrome. J Clin Endocr Metab 98:2484–2493
Liu Y, Ho RC-M, Mak A (2012) Interleukin (IL)-6, tumour necrosis factor alpha (TNF-alpha) and soluble interleukin-2 receptors (sIL-2R) are elevated in patients with major depressive disorder: a meta-analysis and meta-regression. J Affect Disord 139:230–239
Milaneschi Y, Hoogendijk W, Lips P, Heijboer AC, Schoevers R, van Hemert AM, Beekman ATF, Smit JH, Penninx BW (2014) The association between low vitamin D and depressive disorders. Mol Psychiatry 19:444–451
Mottillo S, Filion KB, Genest J, Joseph L, Pilote L, Poirier P et al (2010) The metabolic syndrome and cardiovascular risk a systematic review and meta-analysis. J Am Coll Cardiol 56:1113–1132
Nelson JC, Davis JM (1997) DST studies in psychotic depression: a meta-analysis. Am J Psychiatry 154:1497–1503
Nicholson A, Kuper, Hemingway H (2006) Depression as an aetiologic and prognostic factor in coronary heart disease: a meta-analysis of 6362 events among 146538 participants in 54 observational studies. Eur Heart J 27:2763–2774
Pan A, Keum N, Okereke OI, Sun Q, Kivimaki M, Rubin RR et al (2012) Bidirectional association between depression and metabolic syndrome: a systematic review and meta-analysis of epidemiological studies. Diabetes Care 35:1171–1180
Paz-Filho G, Wong ML, Licinio J (2010) The procognitive effects of leptin in the brain and their clinical implications. Int J Clin Pract 64:1808–1812
Penninx BW, van Tilburg T, Boeke AJ, Deeg DJ, Kriegsman DM, van Eijk JT (1998) Effects of social support and personal coping resources on depressive symptoms: different for various chronic diseases? Health Psychol 17:551–558

Penninx BW, Guralnik JM, Ferrucci L, Fried LP, Allen RH, Stabler SP (2000) Vitamin B(12) deficiency and depression in physically disabled older women: epidemiologic evidence from the Women's Health and Aging Study. Am J Psychiatry 157:715–721

Penninx BW, Milaneschi Y, Lamers F, Vogelzangs N (2013) Understanding the somatic consequences of depression: biological mechanisms and the role of depression symptom profile. BMC Med 11:129

Porges SW (2001) The polyvagal theory: phylogenetic substrates of a social nervous system. Int J Psychophysiol 42:123–146

Rosenbaum S, Tiedemann A, Sherrington C, Curtis J, Ward PB (2014) Physical activity interventions for people with mental illness: a systematic review and meta-analysis. J Clin Psychiatry 75:964–974

Rottenberg J (2007) Cardiac vagal control in depression: a critical analysis. Biol Psychol 74:200–211

Sanhueza C, Ryan L, Foxcroft DR (2013) Diet and the risk of unipolar depression in adults: systematic review of cohort studies. J Hum Nutr Diet 26:56–70

Scott KM, de Jonge P, Alonso J, Viana MC, Liu Z, O'Neill S, Aguilar-Gaxiola S, Bruffaerts R, Caldas-de-Almeida JM, Stein DJ, de Girolamo G, Florescu SE, Hu C, Taib NI, Lépine JP, Levinson D, Matschinger H, Medina-Mora ME, Piazza M, Posada-Villa JA, Uda H, Wojtyniak BJ, Lim CC, Kessler RC (2013) Associations between DSM-IV mental disorders and subsequent heart disease onset: beyond depression. Int J Cardiol 168:5293–5299

Seldenrijk A, Vogelzangs N, van Hout HP, van Marwijk HW, Diamant M, Penninx BW (2010) Depressive and anxiety disorders and risk of subclinical atherosclerosis: findings from the Netherlands Study of Depression and Anxiety (NESDA). J Psychosom Res 69:203–210

Seldenrijk A, van Hout HP, van Marwijk HW, de Groot E, Gort J, Rustemeijer C, Diamant M, Penninx BW (2011) Depression, anxiety, and arterial stiffness. Biol Psychiatry 69:795–803

Seppälä J, Vanhala M, Kautiainen H, Eriksson J, Kampman O, Mantyselka P et al (2012) Prevalence of metabolic syndrome in subjects with melancholic and non-melancholic depressive symptoms. A Finnish population-based study. J Affect Disord 136:543–549

Shelton RC, Miller AH (2010) Eating ourselves to death (and despair): the contribution of adiposity and inflammation to depression. Prog Neurobiol 91:275–299

Silverman MN, Sternberg EM (2012) Glucocorticoid regulation of inflammation and its functional correlates: from HPA axis to glucocorticoid receptor dysfunction. Ann N Y Acad Sci 1261:55–63

Stephens T (1988) Physical activity and mental health in the United States and Canada: evidence from four population surveys. Prev Med 17:35–47

Stetler C, Miller GE (2011) Depression and hypothalamic-pituitary-adrenal activation: a quantitative summary of four decades of research. Psychosom Med 73:114–126

Sublette ME, Postolache TT (2012) Neuroinflammation and depression: the role of indoleamine 2,3-dioxygenase (IDO) as a molecular pathway. Psychosom Med 74:668–672

Sumner JA, Kubzansky LD, Elkind MS, Roberts AL, Agnew-Blais J, Chen Q, Cerdá M, Rexrode KM, Rich-Edwards JW, Spiegelman D, Suglia SF, Rimm EB, Koenen KC (2015) Trauma exposure and posttraumatic stress disorder symptoms predict onset of cardiovascular events in women. Circulation 132:251–259

Teicher MH, Samson JA (2013) Childhood maltreatment and psychopathology: a case for ecophenotypic variants as clinically and neurobiologically distinct subtypes. Am J Psychiatry 170:1114–1133

Tsuji H, Larson MG, Venditti FJJ, Manders ES, Evans JC, Feldman CL et al (1996) Impact of reduced heart rate variability on risk for cardiac events. The Framingham Heart Study. Circulation 94:2850–2855

Van der Kooy K, van Hout H, Marwijk H, Marten H, Stehouwer C, Beekman A (2007) Depression and the risk for cardiovascular diseases: systematic review and meta-analysis. Int J Geriatr Psychiatry 22:613–626

van Reedt Dortland AK, Giltay EJ, Zitman FG, van VT, Penninx BW (2010) Metabolic syndrome abnormalities are associated with severity of anxiety and depression and with tricyclic antidepressant use. Acta Psychiatr Scand 122:30–39

Visser M, Bouter LM, McQuillan GM, Wener MH, Harris TB (1999) Elevated C-reactive protein levels in overweight and obese adults. JAMA 282:2131–2135

Vogelzangs N, Beekman AT, Milaneschi Y, Bandinelli S, Ferrucci L, Penninx BW (2010) Urinary cortisol and six-year risk of all-cause and cardiovascular mortality. J Clin Endocr Metab 95:4959–4964

Vogelzangs N, Beekman AT, Boelhouwer IG, Bandinelli S, Milaneschi Y, Ferrucci L et al (2011) Metabolic depression: a chronic depressive subtype? Findings from the InCHIANTI study of older persons. J Clin Psychiatry 72:598–604

Vogelzangs N, Beekman ATF, van Reedt-Dortland AKB, Schoevers R, Giltay E, de Jonge P, Penninx BW (2014) Inflammatory and metabolic dysregulation and the 2-year course of depressive disorders. Neuropsychopharmacology 39:1624–1634

Vreeburg SA, Hoogendijk WJG, van Pelt J, Derijk RH, Verhagen JCM, van Dyck R et al (2009) Major depressive disorder and hypothalamic-pituitary-adrenal axis activity: results from a large cohort study. Arch Gen Psychiatry 66:617–626

Vreeburg SA, Hartman CA, Hoogendijk WJG, van Dyck R, Zitman FG, Ormel J et al (2010) Parental history of depression or anxiety and the cortisol awakening response. Br J Psychiatry 197:180–185

Ward MC, White DT, Druss BG (2015) A meta-review of lifestyle interventions for cardiovascular risk factors in the general medical population: lessons for individuals with serious mental illness. J Clin Psychiatry 76:e477–e486

Whang W, Kubzansky LD, Kawachi I, Rexrode KM, Kroenke CH, Glynn RJ, Garan H, Albert CM (2009) Depression and risk of sudden cardiac death and coronary heart disease in women: results from the Nurses' Health Study. J Am Coll Cardiol 53:950–958

5 Anxiety and the Effects on Cardiovascular Disease

Phillip J. Tully and Bernhard T. Baune

Contents

Abstract

Anxiety disorders have been implicated with the development and progression of cardiovascular diseases (CVD) for more than 100 years; however, empirical research and intervention efforts have largely been overshadowed by a focus on depression in recent times. This chapter focuses on anxiety disorders' prevalence in CVDs. The associations between anxiety disorder subtypes with major clinical outcomes pertinent to cardiovascular function are also described. An emerging literature indicates that anxiety disorders increase the risk for development of CVD and major cardiovascular complications in persons already with CVD.

P.J. Tully (✉)
The Freemason's Foundation Centre for Men's Health, Discipline of Medicine, The School of Medicine, The University of Adelaide, Adelaide, SA, Australia
e-mail: phillip.tully@adelaide.edu.au

B.T. Baune
Discipline of Psychiatry, School of Medicine, University of Adelaide, Adelaide, SA, Australia

B.T. Baune, P.J. Tully (eds.), *Cardiovascular Diseases and Depression*,
DOI 10.1007/978-3-319-32480-7_5

The risk for cardiovascular events is independent from depression. Anxiety disorders therefore hold relevance for uncovering discrete mechanisms of cardiopathogenesis, novel therapeutic strategies, and initiating clinical interventions in the population at risk of developing heart disease or those already diagnosed with cardiovascular diseases.

5.1 Introduction

Anxiety disorders are a heterogeneous category in the prevailing *Diagnostic and Statistical Manual of Mental Disorders* (Craske et al. 2009). In the broadest sense, anxiety disorders described herein focus on panic disorder, generalized anxiety disorder (GAD), social phobia, and specific phobia, but might also refer to agoraphobia, obsessive-compulsive disorder (OCD), and anxiety due to a general medical condition. Such distinction between subtypes is imperative in order to identify potentially unique cardiovascular pathogenic pathways that might be leveled out on a group level (Baune et al. 2012). For example, each disorder is characterized by varying physiological symptoms (palpitations, dyspnea, restlessness, and tension), behavioral patterns (avoidance, safety behaviors, compulsions), and cognitive profiles (worry, thought suppression, catastrophizing, obsessions). Clearly given such breadth in anxiety phenotypes, there is also a widespread scope in potential correlates of cardiovascular functioning (Thayer et al. 1996; Kawachi et al. 1995). Along these lines, both the American (Lichtman et al. 2014) and German Heart Association (Ladwig et al. 2014) recommended that further research must strive to identify the independent contribution of anxiety disorders to CVD prognosis. Extending further, the recognition and treatment of anxiety disorder subtypes is therefore integral to expanding efforts to improve psychosocial function in heart disease populations.

Anxiety symptoms have been implicated in arterial hypertension, coronary heart disease (CHD), and open heart surgery outcomes for more than 100 years (Miles and Cobb 1951; Fish 1964; Weiss et al. 1957). Despite the inextricable relevance of anxiety to cardiovascular function and CVDs, surprisingly, the etiological and prognostic links between anxiety disorders and CHD is only beginning to emerge. Recent empirical advances point to the strong likelihood that anxiety disorders are a risk factor for the development of CVDs (Garfield et al. 2014; Seldenrijk et al. 2015; Scott et al. 2013; Nabi et al. 2010; Janszky et al. 2010; Tully et al. 2015c). Likewise, anxiety disorders confer a prognostic risk for subsequent major adverse coronary events (MACE, e.g., myocardial infarction [MI], left ventricular failure, coronary revascularization procedure, stroke) in persons with established CVDs (Tully et al. 2014a). In this chapter the epidemiological evidence relating to different anxiety disorders and CVDs is described while closely examining anxiety disorders' association with clinical outcomes pertinent to cardiovascular function.

5.2 Epidemiological Studies Reporting Anxiety Disorders in Cardiovascular Disease Populations

The prevalence of anxiety disorders and clinically relevant anxiety symptoms ranges from 15 to 40 % in patients with CHD (Sardinha et al. 2013; Liang et al. 2013; Bunevicius et al. 2013; Bankier et al. 2008; Tully and Cosh 2013), 10–60 % in coronary revascularization patients undergoing coronary artery bypass graft (CABG) or percutaneous coronary intervention (Rymaszewska et al. 2003; Tully and Baker 2012; Tully et al. 2010; Williams et al. 2013; Dao et al. 2012; McKenzie et al. 2010; Damen et al. 2011), up to 30 % in heart failure (Sherbourne et al. 1996; Haworth et al. 2005; Cully et al. 2009; Pudlo et al. 2009; Tully et al. 2014b), 8–63 % in implantable cardioverter defibrillator therapy (Magyar-Russell et al. 2011), and 12–17 % in arterial hypertension (Wiltink et al. 2011; Carroll et al. 2010). Overall, these studies indicate that the prevalence of anxiety in patients with CVD is higher than that typically found in general population epidemiological surveys (Wittchen et al. 2011; Baxter et al. 2014). In fact several large epidemiological surveys have corroborated high comorbidity between anxiety disorders and CVDs in Taiwan (Chen and Lin 2011), the United States of America (Goodwin et al. 2009), Australia (Teesson et al. 2011), the Netherlands (Vogelzangs et al. 2010), Germany (Tully and Baune 2014), and most recently the World Mental Health Survey (Scott et al. 2013). However, in these epidemiological surveys, CVD is typically ascertained by patient self-report only and unfortunately not confirmed by an independent medical examiner. This methodology, though pragmatic for large epidemiological surveys, is problematic given that anxiety disorder patients display a tendency to misreport medical illnesses (Burch 1991; Schwarz et al. 2015).

To overcome these limitations, our recent meta-analysis pooled together studies utilizing structured psychiatric interview in persons with CHD verified by a health professional (e.g., 50 % stenosis in one or more coronary arteries, coronary revascularization, documented MI by serum assays) (Tully et al. 2014a). In the meta-analysis of 40 studies, the point prevalence of any anxiety disorder was 15.5 %. Thus, anxiety disorders appear to be at least as common as unipolar depression disorder in the population with acute coronary syndrome (ACS) (Thombs et al. 2013; Di Benedetto et al. 2006; Carney and Freedland 2009; Marchesi et al. 2014) and CABG surgery (Tully and Baker 2012; Rafanelli et al. 2006; Dao et al. 2011; Mitchell et al. 2005). In fact, anxiety disorders were comorbid with depression disorders in 49 % of cases suggesting strong intraindividual comorbidity in CHD patients, parallel to what is known in psychiatric and community samples (Dilsaver et al. 2006; Simon et al. 2003; Watson 2009). Identifying depression-anxiety comorbidity is perhaps especially important in CVDs. Recent evidence indicates that ACS patients with an anxiety disorder are more likely to have insufficiently treated depression and, in turn, be at higher risk for subsequent MI (Scherrer et al. 2012).

It is essential to also describe anxiety disorder subtypes in CVDs. It appears that GAD is the most common anxiety disorder in CHD (8 %) parallel to reports from heart failure populations (Tully and Cosh 2013; Haworth et al. 2005; Cully et al. 2009).

The prevalence of anxiety disorder subtypes in descending prevalence from our systematic review were panic disorder (7 %), social phobia (5 %), simple phobia (4 %), agoraphobia (4 %), and obsessive-compulsive disorder (2 %) (see Table 5.1 for further data regarding the pooled prevalence estimates) (Tully et al. 2014a).

It should be pointed out that anxiety disorder prevalence fluctuates based on the inpatient and outpatient setting, the sample age, gender, and whether the examiner was blinded to CHD status (Tully et al. 2014a). Thus, it appears that making an anxiety disorder diagnosis in CVDs is not straightforward, corresponding to case-diagnostic findings evaluating the confounds of somatic depression symptoms (Angermann et al. 2011). Of course, the pitfalls of somatic symptoms confounding a psychiatric diagnosis in chronic diseases are well known (Katon et al. 2007). Indeed, the clinical presentation of CVDs and anxiety frequently overlaps in the acute setting, especially atypical chest pain, dyspnea, palpitations, and arrhythmias (Tully et al. 2011a, 2014a; Barsky et al. 1994, 1996; Fleet et al. 1997, 1998). This substantial symptom overlap is illustrated quite clearly in the case of panic disorder which is described in Table 5.2 (Tully et al. 2015a). In light of this significant somatic overlap, it is hardly surprising that the nexus between panic disorder and CHD remains the most tenuous among all of the anxiety disorders (Fleet et al. 2000; Katerndahl 2008; Katon et al. 1988). Yet it is important to point out that depression also shares significant somatic overlap with the symptoms commonly experienced in CHD and heart failure (Smolderen et al. 2009) and that cognitive depression symptoms appear to have lower prognostic predictive value (de Jonge et al. 2006) (see Table 5.1).

Table 5.1 The prevalence of anxiety disorder subtypes in the population with verified coronary heart disease

Type of anxiety disorder	Studies *N*	Pooled prevalence in CHD	95 % CI	Sources of heterogeneity
Comorbid anxiety and depression disorders	12	49.06	34.28–64.01	–
Any anxiety disorder	13	15.52	10.34–22.64	Outpatients, rater qualification
Generalized anxiety disorder		7.97	5.42–11.57	Pre DSM-IV, sex
Panic disorder	29	6.81	4.09–11.14	Pre DSM-IV, rater blinding, rater qualification, sex
Agoraphobia	17	3.62	1.78–7.21	Pre DSM-IV, sex
Social phobia	10	4.62	2.31–9.02	Rater qualification, sex
Specific phobia	11	4.21	2.23–8.15	Rater qualification, sex
Obsessive-compulsive disorder	6	1.80	1.23–2.65	–

Sources of heterogeneity between prevalence estimates were identified by meta-regression
CHD coronary heart disease, *CI* confidence interval, *DSM-IV Diagnostic and Statistical Manual of Mental Disorders-IV*

Table 5.2 Characteristic symptoms of a panic attack and cardiovascular disease

Number	Panic disorder symptom	Relevance to cardiovascular disease
1	Palpitations, pounding heart, or accelerated heart rate	Common in ACS, arrhythmia
2	Sweating	Common in ACS, arrhythmia, HF
3	Trembling or shaking	
4	Sensations of shortness of breath or smothering	Common in ACS, arrhythmia, HF
5	Feelings of choking	Uncommon
6	Chest pain or discomfort	Common in ACS, arrhythmia, HF
7	Nausea or abdominal distress	Common in ACS
8	Feeling dizzy, unsteady, light-headed, or faint	Common in ACS, arrhythmia, HF
9	Chills or heat sensations	Uncommon
10	Paresthesias (numbness or tingling sensations)	Common in ACS, arrhythmia, HF
11	Derealization (feelings of unreality) or depersonalization (being detached from oneself)	Uncommon
12	Fear of losing control or "going crazy"	Uncommon
13	Fear of dying	Common in ACS

Panic disorder/panic attack symptoms adapted from the *Diagnostic and Statistical Manual of Mental Disorders Fifth Edition*

Additional qualifiers:

A. A panic attack is an abrupt surge of intense fear or intense discomfort that reaches a peak within minutes and during which time four (or more) of the above symptoms occur

B. At least one of the attacks has been followed by 1 month (or more) of one or both of the following:

1. Persistent concern or worry about additional panic attacks or their consequences (e.g., losing control, having a heart attack, "going crazy")

2. A significant maladaptive change in behavior related to the attacks (e.g., behaviors designed to avoid having panic attacks, such as avoidance of exercise or unfamiliar situations)

A. The disturbance is not attributable to the physiological effects of a substance (e.g., a drug of abuse, a medication) or another medical condition (e.g., hyperthyroidism, cardiopulmonary disorders)

B. The disturbance is not better explained by another mental disorder (e.g., the panic attacks do not occur only in response to feared social situations, as in social anxiety disorder; in response to circumscribed phobic objects or situations, as in specific phobia; in response to obsessions, as in obsessive-compulsive disorder; in response to reminders of traumatic events, as in post-traumatic stress disorder; or in response to separation from attachment figures, as in separation anxiety disorder)

ACS acute coronary syndromes including unstable angina and myocardial infarction, *HF* heart failure and cardiomyopathy

5.3 Panic Disorder and the Development of Cardiovascular Diseases

The etiological and prognostic effects of panic disorder are controversial and debated among scholars (Fleet et al. 2000; Katerndahl 2008). Recent evidence however reveals a plethora of biobehavioral mechanisms of cardiopathogenesis.

Behavioral factors that may lead to CVD include a preponderance to smoking (Isensee et al. 2003), alcohol use (Hoertel et al. 2013), and avoidance of exercise attributed to fear of bodily symptoms (Muotri and Bernik 2014). Likewise, clinical factors evident in cardiovascular monitoring studies include myocardial ischemia during panic attack (Fleet et al. 2005, 2014), diminished heart rate variability (HRV) (Yeragani et al. 1993), change in the QT-interval (Sullivan et al. 2004; Yeragani et al. 2002; Pohl and Yeragani 2001), coronary slow-flow (Vural et al. 2009), microvascular angina (Roy-Byrne et al. 1989), and arterial stiffness (Cicek et al. 2012). Thus, there appears to be strong biological plausibility for panic disorder potentiating cardiopathogenesis and aggravating existing coronary disease. Supporting this assertion, Goodwin et al. (2009) showed that CVDs were more strongly associated with panic disorder ($_{adj}$ odds ratio [OR] 1.29) by comparison to unipolar depression ($_{adj}$OR 1.22) or dysthymia (nonsignificant) in cross-sectional analysis. Reports of others corroborate close links between panic disorder and CVD (Chen and Lin 2011; Chen et al. 2009; Walters et al. 2008; Muller-Tasch et al. 2008; Gomez-Caminero et al. 2005; Tully 2015). Strong evidence was recently provided in a meta-analysis of 1,131,612 persons and 58,111 cardiac events showing that panic disorder significantly increased the risk for subsequent CHD (Tully et al. 2015c). Panic disorder increased the risk for subsequent CHD by 47 %, increased risk for MACE by 40 %, and MI by 36 %. Surprisingly, stronger risk estimates were evident after excluding depression (64 % CHD risk) than after depression adjustment (38 % CHD risk). However, unfortunately, reverse causality cannot be ruled out, and it was possible that panic represented an as yet undiagnosed cardiac condition (Fig. 5.1).

Covariate	Events(*n*)	Analysis(*n*)	$_{ADJ}$HR (95 % CI)	I^2
Depression excluded	57,331	446,540	1.64 (1.45–1.85)	73
Depression adjusted	40,346	507,362	1.38 (1.03–1.87)	98
Comorbid depression	6,205	100,253	1.79 (0.85–3.76)	99
Out-patients	44,758	699,752	1.50 (1.22–1.85)	95
In-patients	13,353	431,860	1.39 (1.17–1.65)	68
Panic only	55,015	1,003,773	1.42 (1.16–1.74)	95
Anxiety Neurosis	3,096	127,839	1.58 (1.39–1.79)	0
Panic disorders	54,910	951,805	1.46 (1.21–1.77)	95
Panic symptoms	1,307	130,486	1.45 (1.02–2.07)	49
Prospective	3,212	179,974	1.54 (1.12–2.11)	48
Retrospective	54,899	951,638	1.44 (1.18–1.76)	96

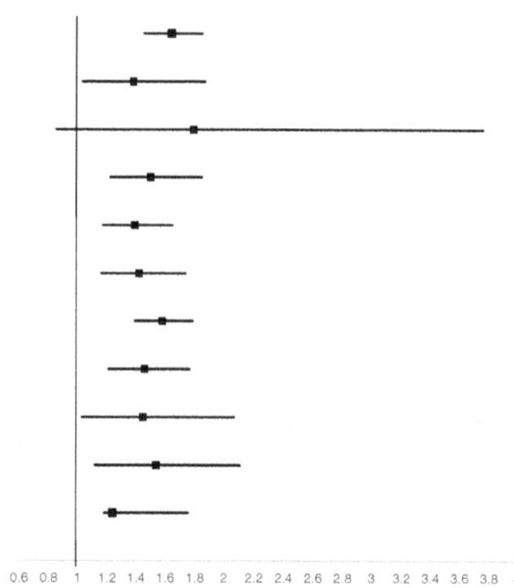

Fig. 5.1 Forest plot of adjusted hazard ratios (aHR) for incident coronary heart disease (CHD) by psychiatric-level panic disorder (PD) study characteristics. aHR with 95 % confidence intervals (CI) that exceed 1 (*vertical line*) indicate an increased CHD risk for persons with PD (Republished with permission from Cambridge Press. Original citation Tully et al. (2015c))

5.4 Anxiety Disorders and Adverse Clinical Outcomes

The prognostic association between anxiety disorder subtypes and CVD is only beginning to emerge. There is an accumulating body of evidence to suggest that anxiety disorders exacerbate existing CVDs; however, these findings are most commonly reported for GAD and panic disorder. In the following paragraphs, we describe recent findings indicating that anxiety disorders predict MACE in these patients (summary provided in Table 5.3).

The largest body of prognostic evidence relates to GAD. Frasure-Smith and Lespérance (2008) first reported the incident MACE risk attributable to GAD in a prospective cohort of 804 ACS outpatients. Participants underwent a baseline interview with the SCID to determine affective disorder diagnoses, and interviewers were blinded to self-reported depression and anxiety symptoms. A total of 115 MACEs occurred over 2 years. The authors found that GAD increased the risk of MACE twofold. These initial findings were later confirmed in the Heart and Soul longitudinal cohort study of 1,015 stable CHD outpatients by Martens et al. (2010). The authors evaluated the association between GAD and incident MACE with mean 5.6-year follow-up. GAD was associated with a 74 % risk of MACE. Together, these (Frasure-Smith and Lespérance 2008; Martens et al. 2010) and more recent confirmations (Goodwin et al. 2009; Tully et al. 2011b; 2013; Roest et al. 2012) indicate GAD is a risk factor for adverse CVD prognosis. Plausible mechanisms of cardiopathogenesis identified in GAD patients include disturbance in heart rate variability, hypertension, lower ω–3 fatty acid levels, tobacco smoking, sedentary activity levels, and lower adherence to medications (Bankier et al. 2008; Martens et al. 2010; Tully et al. 2013; Barger and Sydeman 2005; Parker et al. 2011).

Other studies reporting anxiety disorders on a group level confirm that anxiety disorders are associated with adverse prognosis (Goodwin et al. 2009; Dao et al. 2012; Abrams et al. 2009). Thus, it appears that by comparison to depression, relatively limited attention has been focused on anxiety disorder subtypes which might uncover discrete patterns of association. Rather, studies tend to favor the more heterogeneous any anxiety disorder category. It is likely however that a mixture of these analytical methods would be most informative. As an example, Selendrijk et al. (2015) evaluated incident CVDs (MI, CABG, percutaneous coronary intervention) at 6-year follow-up in the Netherlands Study of Anxiety and Depression. A total of 2,451 community-dwelling individuals underwent structured Composite International Diagnostic Interview (Wittchen 1994) and were free from CVD at baseline. The authors showed that the collective group of any anxiety disorders was not associated with incident CVD, nor were the subtypes of agoraphobia, GAD, and social phobia. Yet in contrast, panic disorder significantly increased incident CVD risk ($_{adj}$hazard ratio [HR] 2.12; 95 % confidence interval [CI] 1.27–3.55) (Seldenrijk et al. 2015). These findings serve to underscore the importance of delineating anxiety subtypes in relation to CVD that might be missed on a group level and bolster evidence implicating panic disorder in cardiopathogenesis.

Table 5.3 The association between anxiety disorders and adverse clinical outcome in patients with cardiovascular disease

Study	Sample and design	Anxiety disorder assessment	CVD	Association between AD and CVDs (95 % CI)
Abrams et al. (2009)	Retrospective case registry of 21,745 AMI patients	ICD-9 CM codes (300.00–300.02, 293.84, 309.28, 309.21–309.23); in- and outpatients	30-day F/U for mortality	(+) inpatient AD: OR 1.44
				(+) outpatient AD: OR 1.36
Chen and Lin (2011)	Cross-sectional database registry of 22,032 patients in NHIRD	Three consecutive panic disorder diagnoses ICD-9 CM (300.01)	MI, CHD	(+) PD for AMI: $_{adj}$OR 6.55 (2.86–14.97)
				(+) PD for CHD: $_{adj}$OR 7.69 (6.78–8.71)
Frasure-Smith and Lespérance (2008)	Prospective cohort of 804 ACS outpatients	SCID DSM-IV	2 year F/U for cardiac death, survived MI, survived cardiac arrest, or nonelective revascularization	(+) GAD: $_{adj}$OR 2.09 (1.08–4.05)
Goodwin et al. (2009)	Cross-sectional survey of 43,093 community-dwelling individuals	AUDADIS-IV	Self-reported CVD including MI in past 12 months	(+) Any AD: $_{adj}$OR 1.43 (1.20–1.71)
				(+) GAD: $_{adj}$OR 1.48 (1.09–2.01)
				(+) Panic disorder: $_{adj}$OR 1.46 (1.12–1.91)
				(−) Social phobia: $_{adj}$OR 0.90 (0.66–1.23)
				(+) Specific phobia: $_{adj}$OR 1.29 (1.04–1.59)
Martens et al. (2010)	Prospective cohort study of 1,015 ACS patients	DIS DSM-IV	5.6 year F/U for MI, stroke, heart failure, mortality	(+) GAD: $_{adj}$HR 1.74 (1.13–2.67)

Parker et al. (2011)	Prospective cohort study of 489 ACS patients	CIDI DSM-IV	Five-year F/U for death or CVD readmission	(−) Agoraphobia: OR 1.72 (0.55–5.42)
				(−) Panic: OR 1.42 (0.43–4.74)
				(−) Social phobia: OR 1.27 (0.68–2.37)
				(−) GAD: OR 0.63 (0.36–1.10)
				(−) OCD: OR 3.05 (0.88–10.58)
Seldenrijk et al. (2015)	Prospective cohort study of 2,510 patients free from CVD at baseline	CIDI DSM-IV	Self-reported CHD (CHD; angina pectoris, MI, PCI, CABG)	(+) any AD $_{adj}$HR1.48 (0.74–2.96)
				Comorbid AD-depression $_{adj}$HR 2.86 (1.49–5.49)
				Panic disorder $_{adj}$HR 2.12 (1.27–3.55)
				Agoraphobia $_{adj}$HR 0.71 (0.25–2.03) 0.81
				Social phobia $_{adj}$HR (0.45–1.45)
				GAD 1.28 (0.71–2.30)
Tully and Baune (2014)	Cross-sectional epidemiological survey	CIDI DSM-IV	CVD, hypertension, PVD, cerebrovascular disease	(+) Panic disorder: OR 3.50 (1.87–6.56)
				(+) Phobia: OR 1.43 (1.08–1.88)
				(+) Phobia and depression: OR 1.89 (1.27–2.82)

+ denotes increased risk of CVD; – denotes null findings or reduced risk of CVD

ACS acute coronary syndrome, *AD* anxiety disorder, *AUDADIS-IV Alcohol Use Disorder and Associated Disabilities Interview Schedule-DSM-IV*, *CABG* coronary artery bypass graft surgery, *CHD* coronary heart disease, *CI* confidence interval, *CIDI* Composite International Diagnostic Interview, *CVD* cardiovascular disease, *DSM-IV Diagnostic and Statistical Manual of Mental Disorders Fourth Edition*, *F/U* follow-up, *HR* hazard ratio, *ICD* international classification of disease, *MI* myocardial infarction, *NHIRD* Taiwan National Health Insurance Research Database, *OR* odds ratio, *PCI* percutaneous coronary intervention, *PVD* peripheral vascular disease

5.5 Does Anxiety and Depression Disorder Comorbidity Affect Cardiovascular Prognosis?

Explicating the independent and conjoint effects of anxiety and depression disorders upon CVD outcomes is an important empirical pursuit to better understand putative risk factors and inform psychosocial interventions. Concurrent and lifetime comorbidity between anxiety and depression is common (Fava et al. 2014), and some studies have reported that comorbid anxiety and depression disorder is associated with a higher CHD risk than either disorder in isolation (Gomez-Caminero et al. 2005).

In a retrospective cohort design, Scherrer and colleagues (2010) evaluated 355,999 individuals free from CHD at baseline in the Veteran Administration database. For over 7 years of follow-up, 12,304 incident MIs occurred. They stratified analysis by anxiety disorder subtype and depression comorbidity. It was found that panic disorder and anxiety disorder unspecified, each conferred a higher risk for incident MI irrespective of depression comorbidity ($_{adj}$HRs range 1.11–1.43). Curiously, in the absence of depression, OCD was associated with a lower risk for MI ($_{adj}$HR 0.32; 95 % CI 0.12–0.84). Taking further the issue of anxiety comorbidity in a nationally representative German cohort, we recently evaluated whether comorbid depression and anxiety disorders mediated the more commonly accepted association between depression and CVD (Tully and Baune 2014). We found that comorbid phobia and depression was significantly associated with cerebrovascular disease ($_{adj}$OR 1.61; 95 % CI 1.04–2.50). Surprisingly, unique associations between depression alone and CVDs were not evident. By contrast, isolated panic disorder was associated with cerebrovascular disease, peripheral vascular disease, and the combined CVD end point (OR range 2.28–2.97).

A remaining pivotal task to moving this area forward is firmly establishing the independent and additive cardiopathogenic effects of anxiety and depression disorders. Although many studies have assessed the prognostic impact of comorbid depression and anxiety symptoms, largely disparate findings have been reported (Meyer et al. 2014; Linke et al. 2009; Frasure-Smith et al. 2002; Wang et al. 2013; van Dijk et al. in press; Kornerup et al. 2011; Huffman et al. 2008; Pedersen et al. 2006; Kubzansky et al. 2006; Watkins et al. 2006) suggesting this question remains to be answered.

5.6 Clinical Treatment of the Anxiety Disorders in CVDs

In relation to CHD, anxiety disorder subtypes have been rendered somewhat in obscurity when compared to depression which remains at the forefront of recent intervention efforts (Tully et al. 2014a; Huffman et al. 2014). In this context, however, it is important to emphasize that antidepressant and psychotherapy interventions have not led to a significant reduction in MACE as might be anticipated (Baumeister et al. 2011; Sheps et al. 2003). These findings point to the necessity to revise and expand our intervention efforts to incorporate anxiety. In doing so, interventions may align more closely to cardiovascular patients' clinical needs and open up opportunities for novel therapeutics.

The frontline treatments for anxiety disorders in CVDs include CVD risk factor management (Pogosova et al. 2015), exercise (Asmundson et al. 2013), cognitive-behavioral therapy (Roy-Byrne et al. 2008; Merswolken et al. 2011), serotonergic reuptake inhibitors (Lesperance et al. 2007; Glassman et al. 2002), and benzodiazepines (Mendels et al. 1986; Freeman et al. 1986), though recent data with respect to the latter is lacking. The use of internet-based interventions is still emerging (Norlund et al. 2015) but initial findings with chronic diseases show promise (Charova et al. 2015). Several studies encourage the use of combined intervention strategies (Tully et al. 2015b) delivered by multiple cooperating health professionals given the heterogeneity in physical and mental health needs that would be evident across different anxiety disorder subtypes and CVDs. Collaborative care, for example, has emerged as a particularly promising package of interventions involving coordinated care by multiple health professionals (Katon et al. 2010). Two recent RCTs conducted in primary care populations encouragingly point to the feasibility of collaborative care in populations with substantial cardiovascular comorbidity (Huffman et al. 2014; Roy-Byrne et al. 2010).

Recently several authors have noted that treatment of anxiety disorders co-occurring with depression, and anxiety disorder treatment in its own right, is a possible step toward improving existing mental health care among CHD populations (Lichtman et al. 2014; Tully et al. 2014a; Rollman and Huffman 2013). Remaining challenges to initiating anxiety disorder interventions in CHD populations include the lower priority by comparison to depression interventions (Frasure-Smith and Lespérance 2008) and the relative paucity of prognostic evidence.

Conclusion

A contemporary body of work indicates that anxiety disorders are highly prevalent and associated with adverse prognosis, including an increased risk of MACE across CVD patient groups. Discrete mechanisms of cardiopathogenesis for GAD and panic disorder serve to make these the primary candidates to direct future clinical interventions. However, limited empirical attention has been paid to other anxiety subtypes. Unfortunately, shifting diagnostic boundaries over time (e.g., neurasthenia revised into multiple psychosomatic disorders (Taylor 2001); anxiety neurosis delineated into panic disorder and GAD (Noyes et al. 1978); the exclusion of OCD and post-traumatic stress disorder from anxiety disorders (American Psychiatric Association 2013)), combined with very limited etiological and prognostic data, precludes a definitive assessment of all anxiety disorder subtypes. Yet, perhaps, a more general conclusion can be reached as it appears that emotional disorders in general increase CVD risk. Along these lines, emotional disorders including anxiety should be elevated to the level of clinical priority afforded to depression.

References

Abrams TE, Vaughan-Sarrazin M, Rosenthal GE (2009) Psychiatric comorbidity and mortality after acute myocardial infarction. Circ Cardiovasc Qual Outcomes 2(3):213–220. doi:10.1161/circoutcomes.108.829143

American Psychiatric Association (2013) The diagnostic and statistical manual of mental disorders DSM-V. American Psychiatric Association, Washington, DC

Angermann CE, Gelbrich G, Störk S, Schowalter M, Deckert J, Ertl G et al (2011) Somatic correlates of comorbid major depression in patients with systolic heart failure. Int J Cardiol 147(1):66–73, doi:http://dx.doi.org/10.1016/j.ijcard.2009.07.044

Asmundson GJ, Fetzner MG, Deboer LB, Powers MB, Otto MW, Smits JA (2013) Let's get physical: a contemporary review of the anxiolytic effects of exercise for anxiety and its disorders. Depress Anxiety 30(4):362–373. doi:10.1002/da.22043

Bankier B, Barajas J, Martinez-Rumayor A, Januzzi JL (2008) Association between C-reactive protein and generalized anxiety disorder in stable coronary heart disease patients. Eur Heart J 29(18):2212–2217. doi:10.1093/eurheartj/ehn326

Barger SD, Sydeman SJ (2005) Does generalized anxiety disorder predict coronary heart disease risk factors independently of major depressive disorder? J Affect Disord 88(1):87–91

Barsky AJ, Cleary PD, Sarnie MK, Ruskin JN (1994) Panic disorder, palpitations, and the awareness of cardiac activity. J Nerv Ment Dis 182(2):63–71

Barsky AJ, Delamater BA, Clancy SA, Antman EM, Ahern DK (1996) Somatized psychiatric disorder presenting as palpitations. Arch Intern Med 156(10):1102–1108

Baumeister H, Hutter N, Bengel J (2011) Psychological and pharmacological interventions for depression in patients with coronary artery disease. Cochrane Database Syst Rev (9):CD008012. doi:10.1002/14651858.CD008012.pub3

Baune BT, Stuart M, Gilmour A, Wersching H, Heindel W, Arolt V et al (2012) The relationship between subtypes of depression and cardiovascular disease: a systematic review of biological models. Transl Psychiatry 2:e92. doi:10.1038/tp.2012.18

Baxter AJ, Vos T, Scott KM, Norman RE, Flaxman AD, Blore J et al (2014) The regional distribution of anxiety disorders: implications for the Global Burden of Disease Study, 2010. Int J Methods Psychiatr Res 23(4):422–438

Bunevicius A, Staniute M, Brozaitiene J, Pop VJ, Neverauskas J, Bunevicius R (2013) Screening for anxiety disorders in patients with coronary artery disease. Health Qual Life Outcomes 11(1):37. doi:10.1186/1477-7525-11-37

Burch EA Jr (1991) Increased risk of stroke in patients with panic attacks: real or perceived? Am J Psychiatry 148(10):1420–1421

Carney RM, Freedland KE (2009) Treatment-resistant depression and mortality after acute coronary syndrome. Am J Psychiatr 166(4):410–417

Carroll D, Phillips AC, Gale CR, Batty GD (2010) Generalized anxiety and major depressive disorders, their comorbidity and hypertension in middle-aged men. Psychosom Med 72(1): 16–19

Charova E, Dorstyn D, Tully PJ, Mittag O (2015) Web-based interventions for comorbid depression and chronic illness: a systematic review. J Telemed Telecare 21:189–201

Chen YH, Lin HC (2011) Patterns of psychiatric and physical comorbidities associated with panic disorder in a nationwide population-based study in Taiwan. Acta Psychiatr Scand 123(1): 55–61

Chen YH, Tsai SY, Lee HC, Lin HC (2009) Increased risk of acute myocardial infarction for patients with panic disorder: a nationwide population-based study. Psychosom Med 71(7):798–804. doi:10.1097/PSY.0b013e3181ad55e3

Cicek Y, Durakoglugil ME, Kocaman SA, Guveli H, Cetin M, Erdogan T et al (2012) Increased pulse wave velocity in patients with panic disorder: independent vascular influence of panic disorder on arterial stiffness. J Psychosom Res 73(2):145–148

Craske MG, Rauch SL, Ursano R, Prenoveau J, Pine DS, Zinbarg RE (2009) What is an anxiety disorder? Depress Anxiety 26(12):1066–1085

Cully JA, Johnson M, Moffett ML, Khan M, Deswal A (2009) Depression and anxiety in ambulatory patients with heart failure. Psychosomatics 50(6):592–598. doi:10.1176/appi.psy.50.6.592

Damen NL, Pelle AJ, van Geuns RJ, van Domburg RT, Boersma E, Pedersen SS (2011) Intraindividual changes in anxiety and depression during 12-month follow-up in percutaneous coronary intervention patients. J Affect Disord 134(1–3):464–467. doi:10.1016/j.jad.2011.05.026

Dao TK, Youssef NA, Armsworth M, Wear E, Papathopoulos KN, Gopaldas R (2011) Randomized controlled trial of brief cognitive behavioral intervention for depression and anxiety symptoms preoperatively in patients undergoing coronary artery bypass graft surgery. J Thorac Cardiovasc Surg 142(3):e109–e115

Dao TK, Voelkel E, Presley S, Doss B, Huddleston C, Gopaldas R (2012) Gender as a moderator between having an anxiety disorder diagnosis and coronary artery bypass grafting surgery (CABG) outcomes in rural patients. J Rural Health 28(3):260–267. doi:10.1111/j.1748-0361.2011.00395.x

de Jonge P, Ormel J, van den Brink RH, van Melle JP, Spijkerman TA, Kuijper A et al (2006) Symptom dimensions of depression following myocardial infarction and their relationship with somatic health status and cardiovascular prognosis. Am J Psychiatr 163:138–144

Di Benedetto M, Lindner H, Hare DL, Kent S (2006) Depression following acute coronary syndromes: a comparison between the cardiac depression scale and the beck depression inventory II. J Psychosom Res 60(1):13–20. doi:10.1016/j.jpsychores.2005.06.003

Dilsaver SC, Akiskal HS, Akiskal KK, Benazzi F (2006) Dose-response relationship between number of comorbid anxiety disorders in adolescent bipolar/unipolar disorders, and psychosis, suicidality, substance abuse and familiality. J Affect Disord 96(3):249–258

Fava GA, Tossani E, Bech P, Berrocal C, Chouinard G, Csillag C et al (2014) Emerging clinical trends and perspectives on comorbid patterns of mental disorders in research. Int J Method Psychiatr Res 23(Suppl 1):92–101. doi:10.1002/mpr.1412

Fish F (1964) The psychiatric aspects of paroxysmal tachycardia. Br J Psychiatry 110(1):205–210

Fleet RP, Dupuis G, Marchand A, Burelle D, Beitman BD (1997) Detecting panic disorder in emergency department chest pain patients: a validated model to improve recognition. Ann Behav Med 19(2):124–131

Fleet RP, Dupuis G, Marchand A, Kaczorowski J, Burelle D, Arsenault A et al (1998) Panic disorder in coronary artery disease patients with noncardiac chest pain. J Psychosom Res 44(1):81–90

Fleet R, Lavoie K, Beitman BD (2000) Is panic disorder associated with coronary artery disease? A critical review of the literature. J Psychosom Res 48(4–5):347–356

Fleet R, Lesperance F, Arsenault A, Gregoire J, Lavoie K, Laurin C et al (2005) Myocardial perfusion study of panic attacks in patients with coronary artery disease. Am J Cardiol 96(8):1064–1068. doi:10.1016/j.amjcard.2005.06.035

Fleet R, Foldes-Busque G, Grégoire J, Harel F, Laurin C, Burelle D et al (2014) A study of myocardial perfusion in patients with panic disorder and low risk coronary artery disease after 35% CO2 challenge. J Psychosom Res 76(1):41–45

Frasure-Smith N, Lespérance F (2008) Depression and anxiety as predictors of 2-year cardiac events in patients with stable coronary artery disease. Arch Gen Psychiatry 65(1):62–71. doi:10.1001/archgenpsychiatry.2007.4

Frasure-Smith N, Lesperance F, Gravel G, Masson A, Juneau M, Bourassa MG (2002) Long-term survival differences among low-anxious, high-anxious and repressive copers enrolled in the Montreal heart attack readjustment trial. Psychosom Med 64(4):571–579

Freeman AM 3rd, Fleece L, Folks DG, Sokol RS, Hall KR, Pacifico AD et al (1986) Alprazolam treatment of postcoronary bypass anxiety and depression. J Clin Psychopharmacol 6(1):39–41

Garfield LD, Scherrer JF, Hauptman PJ, Freedland KE, Chrusciel T, Balasubramanian S et al (2014) Association of anxiety disorders and depression with incident heart failure. Psychosom Med 128–36(2):128–136

Glassman AH, O'Connor CM, Califf RM, Swedberg K, Schwartz P, Bigger JT Jr et al (2002) Sertraline treatment of major depression in patients with acute MI or unstable angina. JAMA 288(6):701–709

Gomez-Caminero A, Blumentals WA, Russo LJ, Brown RR, Castilla-Puentes R (2005) Does panic disorder increase the risk of coronary heart disease? A cohort study of a national managed care database. Psychosom Med 67(5):688–691. doi:10.1097/01.psy.0000174169.14227.1f, 67/5/688 [pii]

Goodwin RD, Davidson KW, Keyes K (2009) Mental disorders and cardiovascular disease among adults in the United States. J Psychosom Res 43(3):239–246

Haworth JE, Moniz-Cook E, Clark AL, Wang M, Waddington R, Cleland JGF (2005) Prevalence and predictors of anxiety and depression in a sample of chronic heart failure patients with left ventricular systolic dysfunction. Eur J Heart Fail 7(5):803–808

Hoertel N, Le Strat Y, De Maricourt P, Limosin F, Dubertret C (2013) Are subjects in treatment trials of panic disorder representative of patients in routine clinical practice? Results from a national sample. J Affect Dis 146(3):383–389. doi:10.1016/j.jad.2012.09.023

Huffman JC, Smith FA, Blais MA, Januzzi JL, Fricchione GL (2008) Anxiety, independent of depressive symptoms, is associated with in-hospital cardiac complications after acute myocardial infarction. J Psychosom Res 65(6):557–563. doi:10.1016/j.jpsychores.2008.08.001

Huffman JC, Mastromauro CA, Beach SR, Celano CM, Dubois CM, Healy BC et al (2014) Collaborative care for depression and anxiety disorders in patients with recent cardiac events: The Management of Sadness and Anxiety in Cardiology (MOSAIC) randomized clinical trial. JAMA Intern Med 174(6):927–936. doi:10.1001/jamainternmed.2014.739

Isensee B, Wittchen HU, Stein MB, Hofler M, Lieb R (2003) Smoking increases the risk of panic: findings from a prospective community study. Arch Gen Psychiatry 60(7):692–700

Janszky I, Ahnve S, Lundberg I, Hemmingsson T (2010) Early-onset depression, anxiety, and risk of subsequent coronary heart disease: 37-year follow-up of 49,321 young Swedish men. J Am Coll Cardiol 56(1):31–37. doi:10.1016/j.jacc.2010.03.033

Katerndahl DA (2008) The association between panic disorder and coronary artery disease among primary care patients presenting with chest pain: an updated literature review. J Clin Psychiatry 10(4):276–285

Katon W, Hall ML, Russo J, Cormier L, Hollifield M, Vitaliano PP et al (1988) Chest pain: relationship of psychiatric illness to coronary arteriographic results. Am J Med 84(1):1–9

Katon W, Lin EH, Kroenke K (2007) The association of depression and anxiety with medical symptom burden in patients with chronic medical illness. Gen Hosp Psychiatry 29(2):147–155

Katon WJ, Lin EH, Von Korff M, Ciechanowski P, Ludman EJ, Young B et al (2010) Collaborative care for patients with depression and chronic illnesses. N Engl J Med 363(27):2611–2620. doi:10.1056/NEJMoa1003955

Kawachi I, Sparrow D, Vokonas PS, Weiss ST (1995) Decreased heart rate variability in men with phobic anxiety (data from the Normative Aging Study). Am J Cardiol 75(14):882–885

Kornerup H, Zwisler AD, Prescott E (2011) No association between anxiety and depression and adverse clinical outcome among patients with cardiovascular disease: findings from the DANREHAB trial. J Psychosom Res 71(4):207–214. doi:10.1016/j.jpsychores.2011.04.006

Kubzansky LD, Cole SR, Kawachi I, Vokonas P, Sparrow D (2006) Shared and unique contributions of anger, anxiety, and depression to coronary heart disease: a prospective study in the normative aging study. Ann Behav Med 31(1):21–29

Ladwig KH, Lederbogen F, Albus C, Angermann C, Borggrefe M, Fischer D et al (2014) Position paper on the importance of psychosocial factors in cardiology: update 2013. Ger Med Sci 12:Doc09. doi:10.3205/000194

Lesperance F, Frasure-Smith N, Koszycki D, Laliberte MA, van Zyl LT, Baker B et al (2007) Effects of citalopram and interpersonal psychotherapy on depression in patients with coronary artery disease: the Canadian Cardiac Randomized Evaluation of Antidepressant and Psychotherapy Efficacy (CREATE) trial. JAMA 297(4):367–379. doi:10.1001/jama.297.4.367

Liang JJ, Tweet MS, Hayes SE, Gulati R, Hayes SN (2013) Prevalence and predictors of depression and anxiety among survivors of myocardial infarction due to spontaneous coronary artery dissection. J Cardiopulm Rehabil Prev 34(2):138–142. doi:10.1097/hcr.0000000000000030

Lichtman JH, Froelicher ES, Blumenthal JA, Carney RM, Doering LV, Frasure-Smith N et al (2014) Depression as a risk factor for poor prognosis among patients with acute coronary syndrome: systematic review and recommendations: a scientific statement from the American Heart Association. Circulation 129(12):1350–1369. doi:10.1161/cir.0000000000000019

Linke SE, Rutledge T, Johnson BD, Vaccarino V, Bittner V, Cornell CE et al (2009) Depressive symptom dimensions and cardiovascular prognosis among women with suspected myocardial ischemia: a report from the National Heart, Lung, and Blood Institute-sponsored Women's

Ischemia Syndrome Evaluation. Arch Gen Psychiatry 66(5):499–507. doi:10.1001/archgen-psychiatry.2009.27, 66/5/499 [pii]
Magyar-Russell G, Thombs BD, Cai JX, Baveja T, Kuhl EA, Singh PP et al (2011) The prevalence of anxiety and depression in adults with implantable cardioverter defibrillators: a systematic review. J Psychosom Res 71(4):223–231. doi:10.1016/j.jpsychores.2011.02.014
Marchesi C, Ossola P, Scagnelli F, Paglia F, Aprile S, Monici A et al (2014) Type D personality in never-depressed patients and the development of major and minor depression after acute coronary syndrome. J Affect Disord 155:194–199. doi:10.1016/j.jad.2013.10.052
Martens EJ, de Jonge P, Na B, Cohen BE, Lett H, Whooley MA (2010) Scared to death? Generalized anxiety disorder and cardiovascular events in patients with stable coronary heart disease: the heart and soul study. Arch Gen Psychiatry 67(7):750–758. doi:10.1001/archgenpsychiatry.2010.74
McKenzie LH, Simpson J, Stewart M (2010) A systematic review of pre-operative predictors of post-operative depression and anxiety in individuals who have undergone coronary artery bypass graft surgery. Psychol Health Med 15(1):74–93
Mendels J, Chernoff RW, Blatt M (1986) Alprazolam as an adjunct to propranolol in anxious outpatients with stable angina pectoris. J Clin Psychiatry 47(1):8–11
Merswolken M, Siebenhuener S, Orth-Gomer K, Zimmermann-Viehoff F, Deter HC (2011) Treating anxiety in patients with coronary heart disease: a randomized controlled trial. Psychother Psychosom 80(6):365–370. doi:10.1159/000329177
Meyer T, Hussein S, Lange HW, Herrmann-Lingen C (2014) Anxiety is associated with a reduction in both mortality and major adverse cardiovascular events five years after coronary stenting. Eur J Prev Cardiol. doi:10.1177/2047487313505244
Miles HHW, Cobb S (1951) Neurocirculatory asthenia, anxiety and neurosis. NEJM 245(19):711–719. doi:10.1056/NEJM195111082451901
Mitchell RH, Robertson E, Harvey PJ, Nolan R, Rodin G, Romans S et al (2005) Sex differences in depression after coronary artery bypass graft surgery. Am Heart J 150(5):1017–1025
Muller-Tasch T, Frankenstein L, Holzapfel N, Schellberg D, Lowe B, Nelles M et al (2008) Panic disorder in patients with chronic heart failure. J Psychosom Res 64(3):299–303. doi:10.1016/j.jpsychores.2007.09.002
Muotri RW, Bernik MA (2014) Panic disorder and exercise avoidance. Rev Bras Psiquiatr 36:68–75
Nabi H, Hall M, Koskenvuo M, Singh-Manoux A, Oksanen T, Suominen S et al (2010) Psychological and somatic symptoms of anxiety and risk of coronary heart disease: the health and social support prospective cohort study. Biol Psychiatry 67(4):378–385. doi:10.1016/j.biopsych.2009.07.040, S0006-3223(09)01031-2 [pii]
Norlund F, Olsson EM, Burell G, Wallin E, Held C (2015) Treatment of depression and anxiety with internet-based cognitive behavior therapy in patients with a recent myocardial infarction (U-CARE Heart): study protocol for a randomized controlled trial. Trials 16(1):154. doi:10.1186/s13063-015-0689-y
Noyes R, Clancy J, Hoenk PR, Slymen DJ (1978) Anxiety neurosis and physical illness. Compr Psychiatry 19(5):407–413
Parker G, Hyett M, Hadzi-Pavlovic D, Brotchie H, Walsh W (2011) GAD is good? Generalized anxiety disorder predicts a superior five-year outcome following an acute coronary syndrome. Psychiatry Res 188(3):383–389. doi:10.1016/j.psychres.2011.05.018
Pedersen SS, Denollet J, Spindler H, Ong AT, Serruys PW, Erdman RA et al (2006) Anxiety enhances the detrimental effect of depressive symptoms on health status following percutaneous coronary intervention. J Psychosom Res 61(6):783–789
Pogosova N, Saner H, Pedersen SS, Cupples ME, McGee H, Höfer S et al (2015) Psychosocial aspects in cardiac rehabilitation: From theory to practice. A position paper from the Cardiac Rehabilitation Section of the European Association of Cardiovascular Prevention and Rehabilitation of the European Society of Cardiology. Eur J Prev Cardiol 22:1290–1306. doi:10.1177/2047487314543075
Pohl R, Yeragani VK (2001) QT interval variability in panic disorder patients after isoproterenol infusions. Int J Neuropsychopharmacol 4(1):17–20

Pudlo R, Piegza M, Zakliczynski M, Zembala M (2009) The occurrence of mood and anxiety disorders in heart transplant recipients. Transplant Proc 41(8):3214–3218. doi:10.1016/j.transproceed.2009.09.031

Rafanelli C, Roncuzzi R, Milaneschi Y (2006) Minor depression as a cardiac risk factor after coronary artery bypass surgery. Psychosomatics 47(4):289–295, doi:http://dx.doi.org/10.1176/appi.psy.47.4.289

Roest AM, Zuidersma M, de Jonge P (2012) Myocardial infarction and generalised anxiety disorder: 10-year follow-up. Br J Psychiatry 200(4):324–329. doi:10.1192/bjp.bp.111.103549

Rollman BL, Huffman JC (2013) Treating anxiety in the presence of medical comorbidity: calmly moving forward. Psychosom Med 75(8):710–712. doi:10.1097/psy.0000000000000011

Roy-Byrne PP, Schmidt P, Cannon RO, Diem H, Rubinow DR (1989) Microvascular angina and panic disorder. Int J Psychiatry Med 19(4):315–325

Roy-Byrne PP, Davidson KW, Kessler RC, Asmundson GJ, Goodwin RD, Kubzansky L et al (2008) Anxiety disorders and comorbid medical illness. Gen Hosp Psychiatry 30(3):208–225

Roy-Byrne P, Craske MG, Sullivan G, Rose RD, Edlund MJ, Lang AJ et al (2010) Delivery of evidence-based treatment for multiple anxiety disorders in primary care: a randomized controlled trial. JAMA 303(19):1921–1928. doi:10.1001/jama.2010.608

Rymaszewska J, Kiejna A, Hadrys T (2003) Depression and anxiety in coronary artery bypass grafting patients. Eur Psychiatry 18(4):155–160

Sardinha A, Nardi AE, Araujo CG, Ferreira MC, Eifert GH (2013) Brazilian portuguese validated version of the cardiac anxiety questionnaire. Arq Bras Cardiol. doi:10.5935/abc.20130207

Scherrer JF, Chrusciel T, Zeringue A, Garfield LD, Hauptman PJ, Lustman PJ et al (2010) Anxiety disorders increase risk for incident myocardial infarction in depressed and nondepressed veterans administration patients. Am Heart J 159(5):772–779

Scherrer JF, Chrusciel T, Garfield LD, Freedland KE, Carney RM, Hauptman PJ et al (2012) Treatment-resistant and insufficiently treated depression and all-cause mortality following myocardial infarction. Br J Psychiatry 200(2):137–142. doi:10.1192/bjp.bp.111.096479

Schwarz J, Prashad A, Winchester DE (2015) Prevalence and implications of severe anxiety in a prospective cohort of acute chest pain patients. Crit Pathw Cardiol 14(1):44–47. doi:10.1097/hpc.0000000000000038

Scott KM, de Jonge P, Alonso J, Viana MC, Liu Z, O'Neill S et al (2013) Associations between DSM-IV mental disorders and subsequent heart disease onset: beyond depression. Int J Cardiol 168(6):5293–5299. doi:10.1016/j.ijcard.2013.08.012

Seldenrijk A, Vogelzangs N, Batelaan NM, Wieman I, van Schaik DJ, Penninx BJ (2015) Depression, anxiety and 6-year risk of cardiovascular disease. J Psychosom Res 78(2):123–129. doi:10.1016/j.jpsychores.2014.10.007

Sheps DS, Freedland KE, Golden RN, McMahon RP (2003) ENRICHD and SADHART: implications for future biobehavioral intervention efforts. Psychosom Med 65(1):1–2

Sherbourne CD, Jackson CA, Meredith LS, Camp P, Wells KB (1996) Prevalence of comorbid anxiety disorders in primary care outpatients. Arch Fam Med 5(1):27–35

Simon NM, Smoller JW, Fava M, Sachs G, Racette SR, Perlis R et al (2003) Comparing anxiety disorders and anxiety-related traits in bipolar disorder and unipolar depression. J Psychiatr Res 37(3):187–192

Smolderen KG, Spertus JA, Reid KJ, Buchanan DM, Krumholz HM, Denollet J et al (2009) The association of cognitive and somatic depressive symptoms with depression recognition and outcomes after myocardial infarction. Circ Cardiovasc Qual Outcomes 2(4):328–337

Sullivan GM, Kent JM, Kleber M, Martinez JM, Yeragani VK, Gorman JM (2004) Effects of hyperventilation on heart rate and QT variability in panic disorder pre- and post-treatment. Psychiatry Res 125(1):29–39

Taylor RE (2001) Death of neurasthenia and its psychological reincarnation: a study of neurasthenia at the National Hospital for the Relief and Cure of the Paralysed and Epileptic, Queen Square, London, 1870-1932. Br J Psychiatry: J Mental Sci 179:550–557

Teesson M, Mitchell PB, Deady M, Memedovic S, Slade T, Baillie A (2011) Affective and anxiety disorders and their relationship with chronic physical conditions in Australia: findings of the

2007 National Survey of Mental Health and Wellbeing. Aust N Z J Psychiatry 45(11):939–946. doi:10.3109/00048674.2011.614590
Thayer JF, Friedman BH, Borkovec TD (1996) Autonomic characteristics of generalized anxiety disorder and worry. Biol Psychiatry 39(4):255–266. doi:10.1016/0006-3223(95)00136-0, 0006-3223(95)00136-0 [pii]
Thombs BD, Roseman M, Coyne JC, de Jonge P, Delisle VC, Arthurs E et al (2013) Does evidence support the American Heart Association's recommendation to screen patients for depression in cardiovascular care? An updated systematic review. PLoS One 8(1):e52654. doi:10.1371/journal.pone.0052654
Tully PJ (2015) A good time to panic? Premorbid and postmorbid panic disorder in heart failure affects cardiac and psychiatric cause admissions. Australas Psychiatry 23(2):124–127
Tully PJ, Baker RA (2012) Depression, anxiety, and cardiac morbidity outcomes after coronary artery bypass surgery: a contemporary and practical review. J Geriatr Cardiol 9(2):197–208. doi:10.3724/SP.J.1263.2011.12221
Tully PJ, Baune BT (2014) Comorbid anxiety disorders alter the association between cardiovascular diseases and depression: the German National Health Interview and Examination Survey. Soc Psych Psychiatr Epidemiol 49(5):683–691
Tully PJ, Cosh SM (2013) Generalized anxiety disorder prevalence and comorbidity with depression in coronary heart disease: a meta analysis. J Health Psychol 18(12):1601–1616. doi:10.1177/1359105312467390
Tully PJ, Baker RA, Winefield HR, Turnbull DA (2010) Depression, anxiety disorders and type D personality as risk factors for delirium after cardiac surgery. Aust N Z J Psychiatry 44(11):1005–1011
Tully PJ, Bennetts JS, Baker RA, McGavigan AD, Turnbull DA, Winefield HR (2011a) Anxiety, depression, and stress as risk factors for atrial fibrillation after cardiac surgery. Heart Lung 40(1):4–11
Tully PJ, Pedersen SS, Winefield HR, Baker RA, Turnbull DA, Denollet J (2011b) Cardiac morbidity risk and depression and anxiety: a disorder, symptom and trait analysis among cardiac surgery patients. Psychol Health Med 16(3):333–345. doi:10.1080/13548506.2011.553960
Tully PJ, Cosh SM, Baune BT (2013) A review of the affects of worry and generalized anxiety disorder upon cardiovascular health and coronary heart disease. Psychol Health Med 18(6):627–644. doi:10.1080/13548506.2012.749355
Tully PJ, Cosh SM, Baumeister H (2014a) The anxious heart in whose mind? A systematic review and meta-regression of factors associated with anxiety disorder diagnosis, treatment and morbidity risk in coronary heart disease. J Psychosom Res 77(6):439–448
Tully PJ, Wittert GA, Selkow T, Baumeister H (2014b) The real world mental health needs of heart failure patients are not reflected by the depression randomized controlled trial evidence. PLoS One 9(1):e85928. doi:10.1371/journal.pone.0085928
Tully PJ, Wittert GA, Turnbull DA, Beltrame JF, Horowitz JD, Cosh S et al (2015a) Panic disorder and incident coronary heart disease: a systematic review and meta-analysis protocol. Syst Rev 4:33
Tully PJ, Selkow T, Bengel J, Rafanelli C (2015b) A dynamic view of comorbid depression and generalized anxiety disorder symptom change in chronic heart failure: discrete effects of cognitive behavioral therapy, exercise rehabilitation, and psychotropic medication. Disabil Rehabil 37(7):585–592
Tully PJ, Turnbull DA, Beltrame JF, Horowitz JD, Cosh S, Baumeister H et al (2015c) Panic disorder and incident coronary heart disease: a systematic review and meta-regression in 1,131,612 persons and 58,111 cardiac events. Psychol Med 45:2909–2920
van Dijk MR, Utens EMWJ, Dulfer K, Al-Qezweny MNA, van Geuns RJ, Daemen J et al (2016) Depression and anxiety symptoms as predictors of mortality in PCI patients at 10 years of follow-up. Eur J Prev Cardiol 23(5):552–558
Vogelzangs N, Seldenrijk A, Beekman ATF, Van Hout HPJ, De Jonge P, Penninx BWJH (2010) Cardiovascular disease in persons with depressive and anxiety disorders. J Affect Disord 125(1–3):241–248
Vural M, Satiroglu O, Akbas B, Goksel I, Karabay O (2009) Coronary artery disease in association with depression or anxiety among patients undergoing angiography to investigate chest pain. Tex Heart Inst J 36(1):17–23

Walters K, Rait G, Petersen I, Williams R, Nazareth I (2008) Panic disorder and risk of new onset coronary heart disease, acute myocardial infarction, and cardiac mortality: cohort study using the general practice research database. Eur Heart J 29(24):2981–2988. doi:10.1093/eurheartj/ehn477

Wang G, Cui J, Wang Y, Deng B, Liang X, Bai J et al (2013) Anxiety and adverse coronary artery disease outcomes in Chinese patients. Psychosom Med 75(6):530–536. doi:10.1097/PSY.0b013e3182984317

Watkins LL, Blumenthal JA, Davidson JR, Babyak MA, McCants CB Jr, Sketch MH Jr (2006) Phobic anxiety, depression, and risk of ventricular arrhythmias in patients with coronary heart disease. Psychosom Med 68(5):651–656. doi:10.1097/01.psy.0000228342.53606.b3

Watson D (2009) Differentiating the mood and anxiety disorders: a quadripartite model. Annu Rev Clin Psychol 5:221–247

Weiss E, Dolin B, Rollin HR, Fischer HK, Bepler CR (1957) Emotional factors in coronary occlusion. I. Introduction and general summary. Arch Int Med 99(4):628–641

Williams JB, Alexander KP, Morin J-F, Langlois Y, Noiseux N, Perrault LP et al (2013) Preoperative anxiety as a predictor of mortality and major morbidity in patients aged >70 years undergoing cardiac surgery. Am J Cardiol 111(1):137–142, doi:http://dx.doi.org/10.1016/j.amjcard.2012.08.060

Wiltink J, Beutel ME, Till Y, Ojeda FM, Wild PS, Munzel T et al (2011) Prevalence of distress, comorbid conditions and well being in the general population. J Affect Disord 130(3):429–437. doi:10.1016/j.jad.2010.10.041, S0165-0327(10)00670-1 [pii]

Wittchen HU (1994) Reliability and validity studies of the WHO - composite international diagnostic interview (CIDI): a critical review. J Psychiatr Res 28(1):57–84

Wittchen HU, Jacobi F, Rehm J, Gustavsson A, Svensson M, Jonsson B et al (2011) The size and burden of mental disorders and other disorders of the brain in Europe 2010. Eur Neuropsychopharmacol 21(9):655–679. doi:10.1016/j.euroneuro.2011.07.018

Yeragani VK, Pohl R, Berger R, Balon R, Ramesh C, Glitz D et al (1993) Decreased heart rate variability in panic disorder patients: a study of power-spectral analysis of heart rate. Psychiatry Res 46(1):89–103

Yeragani VK, Pohl R, Balon R, Jampala VC, Jayaraman A (2002) Twenty-four-hour QT interval variability: increased QT variability during sleep in patients with panic disorder. Neuropsychobiology 46(1):1–6

A Clinical Cardiology Perspective of Psychocardiology

6

John F. Beltrame and Rosanna Tavella

Contents

6.1 Contemporary Medical Practice

The human body is organised into a number of bodily systems that each serve a key function. Since diseases tend to predominantly afflict one of these physiological-based systems, the practice of medicine has evolved into the management of diseased-based systems. Consequently, cardiac disease is primarily under the care of cardiologists and psychological disorders under psychiatrists. This specialty-based

J.F. Beltrame (✉) • R. Tavella
Discipline of Medicine, The University of Adelaide, Adelaide, SA, Australia

The Queen Elizabeth Hospital, Central Adelaide Local Health Network, SA Health, Adelaide, SA, Australia
e-mail: John.Beltrame@adelaide.edu.au

B.T. Baune, P.J. Tully (eds.), *Cardiovascular Diseases and Depression*,
DOI 10.1007/978-3-319-32480-7_6

approach has given clinicians the opportunity to focus their skills on one system and therefore more thoroughly address and treat the disease process.

However, this approach is limited since the body systems are highly integrated so that the disease process and/or its treatment may impact on other systems. Accordingly, there is a risk that the patient may not receive optimal medical care because of the specialty clinician's inattention to other systems. The purpose of this chapter is to address these cross-specialty issues particularly focussing upon when the psychiatrist should consider cardiological issues in their patients and vice versa.

The interaction between psychiatry and cardiology involves consideration of three areas. Firstly, the patient who has a past history of concurrent disease may influence the problem at hand. Secondly, the pathophysiology for the clinical presentation may interact with the other system. Finally, the treatment of one condition may impact on the alternate system. These will be systematically discussed in the following text.

6.2 Cardiological Issues in the Psychiatry Patient

6.2.1 Premorbid Cardiac Conditions

The prevalence of cardiovascular disease within both developed and developing countries is high, particularly with advancing age. As outlined previously, depression is also prevalent within the community so that it is common for the two to occur in unison. Thus, it is important to consider this possibility when the psychiatrist is managing the depressed patient.

The impact of premorbid cardiac disease on the depressed patient warrants close consideration. Firstly, the cardiac disease may be a precipitant or aggravating factor for an episode of depression, especially when the patient has experienced a life-threatening cardiac event. Secondly, the underlying pathophysiology may have a common link between the cardiac and psychological disorder. For example, inflammation plays an important role in the pathogenesis of acute coronary syndromes as it does in depression; therefore, it is not surprising that the two frequently coexist. Thirdly, the physical disability resulting from the cardiac disease may limit the efficacy of some therapies required for the psychiatric disease. For example, end-stage cardiac failure with its associated dyspnoea at rest may make it difficult for patients to focus on psychotherapy for the treatment of their depression.

6.2.2 Cardiac Considerations in Psychological Disorders

In some patients it may be difficult to delineate if the presenting symptoms are attributable to psychological or cardiological dysfunction. Panic attacks are a good example where the recurrent presentations with chest pain may be a manifestation of psychological stress with no cardiac abnormalities or alternatively an occult cardiac disorder that has been misdiagnosed as being of psychological origin in a patient with an anxious predisposition.

The general approach in psychiatry is to exclude organic causes for the presenting symptoms and evaluate the underlying psychopathology. If a patient with 'suspected panic attacks' is referred to a cardiologist for exclusion of a cardiac cause for the recurrent episodes of chest pain, an exercise stress test and possibly even a coronary angiogram may be undertaken. If these were normal, it is possible that the cardiologist may conclude that the patient does not have significant coronary artery disease and discharge the patient form their care. However, it is possible that these symptoms may arise from coronary vasomotor disorders such as vasospastic angina or microvascular dysfunction (Di Fiore and Beltrame 2013).

Vasospastic angina is a cardiac condition attributable to coronary artery spasm with the hallmark manifestation of recurrent episodes of chest pain at rest, promptly responsive to sublingual nitrates (Beltrame et al. 2015). Associated features include episodes of nocturnal chest pain and episodes precipitated by hyperventilation (Beltrame et al. 2015). If an ECG is performed during a spontaneous episode of chest pain, the diagnosis may be readily confirmed with the documentation of ischaemic ECG changes such as transient ST elevation (Beltrame et al. 2015). However, frequently an ECG is not obtained during the episode of chest pain so that cardiac investigations including exercise testing and angiography are performed. In patients with vasospastic angina, these are frequently normal and do not preclude the diagnosis. Definitive testing requires provocative spasm testing, which is undertaken in specialised centres and involves the administration of spasm-inducing stimuli during invasive coronary angiography. The importance of diagnosing vasospastic angina is evident from its associated risk of cardiac events (including sudden death) and the fact that effective therapies are readily available to prevent these events.

Case reports have detailed patients thought to have panic disorder but subsequently shown to have a coronary disorder (Mansour et al. 1998). Whilst vasospastic angina is an important treatable cause for recurrent chest pain with a normal angiogram, other possible causes include coronary microvascular disorders (Mansour et al. 1998) and takotsubo cardiomyopathy (Neil et al. 2012). Thus, the psychiatrist must entertain the possibility that the patient's symptoms may arise from an organic cause. This should be particularly considered if the clinical presentation is not consistent with a panic disorder.

The clinical similarities between panic disorder and coronary syndromes may account for the increased events reported in patients with panic disorder (Tully et al. 2015). In a meta-analysis of 12 studies involving over a million patients with panic disorder, the hazard ratio of these patients experiencing a major adverse cardiac event (cardiac death or non-fatal myocardial infarction) was 1.40 (95% confidence intervals 1.16–1.69). Although cause cannot be attributed in this association, especially considering the data heterogeneity, the possibility remains that some patients may have had an organic cardiac cause for their chest pain symptoms rather than the ascribed panic disorder diagnosis.

For the above reasons, the psychiatrist must be constantly vigilant for organic causes of chest pain in patients who have been diagnosed with mental disorders and not merely attribute them to a psychiatric disorder such as panic disorder, hypochondriasis or a conversion reaction. In particular, they should be aware that exclusion of *structural coronary artery disease* by coronary angiography does not exclude *functional coronary disorders* such as coronary artery spasm and microvascular dysfunction, which require specific evaluation by provocative spasm testing and coronary blood flow assessment. Thus, if the psychiatrist is concerned that the clinical presentation is not consistent with a psychiatric disorder, these differential diagnoses should be considered and referred for further cardiac assessment.

6.2.3 Cardiac Effects of Antidepressant Therapies

Many treatments initiated by psychiatrists have potential cardiac effects that need to be considered, especially in patients with premorbid cardiac conditions. Antidepressant medications may produce a prolong QT syndrome, orthostatic hypotension or unusual class-specific cardiovascular adverse effects (Table 6.1) (Teply et al. 2015; Ramamurthy et al. 2013). The tricyclic antidepressants have been available for many years, and their use for the treatment of depression should generally be avoided in patients with significant cardiac disease considering their potential adverse effects and the availability of newer agents.

Prolongation of the QT interval predisposes patients to the life-threatening malignant arrhythmia and torsades de pointes (a specific form of ventricular tachycardia) and may account for the increased sudden death in patients prescribed with antidepressant medications (Honkola et al. 2012; Leonard et al. 2011). An antidepressant may precipitate this arrhythmia especially if there are other predisposing conditions such as (1) co-administration of other QT prolongation medications (e.g. sotalol, amiodarone, fluconazole,

Table 6.1 Adverse cardiac effects of antidepressant medications

Antidepressant class	Cardiac effects
Tricyclic antidepressants (TCAD) Amitriptyline, desipramine, doxepin, imipramine, nortriptyline, clomipramine, maprotiline, trimipramine, protriptyline	Orthostatic hypotension QT prolongation
Atypical antidepressants Bupropion, mirtazapine, trazodone	QT prolongation
Monoamine oxidase inhibitor Phenelzine, selegiline, tranylcypromine, moclobemide	Hypertensive crisis Peripheral oedema (moclobemide) Orthostatic hypotension
Selective serotonin reuptake inhibitors (SSRIs) Fluoxetine, fluvoxamine, escitalopram, paroxetine, citalopram, sertraline	QT prolongation (citalopram) Serotonin syndrome Orthostatic hypotension
Serotonin-norepinephrine reuptake inhibitors (SNRIs) Desvenlafaxine, duloxetine, venlafaxine, milnacipran, levomilnacipran	QT prolongation (venlafaxine)
'Natural' antidepressants St John's wort, 5-hydroxytryptophan, fish oil	Serotonin syndrome (St John's wort, 5-hydroxytryptophan) Drug interactions (St John's wort) Bleeding (fish oils)

azithromycin, roxithromycin, trimethoprim-sulphamethoxazole, domperidone), (2) predisposing metabolic conditions (e.g. hypokalaemia, hypomagnesaemia, hypocalcaemia) or (3) associated cardiac disorders (congenital long QT syndrome, recent myocardial infarction, cardiomyopathy). The tricyclic antidepressants are well recognised for their QT prolongation effects, but clinicians should also be aware of this effect with some of the newer agents especially high-dose citalopram (Castro et al. 2013), escitalopram, fluoxetine, venlafaxine, bupropion, trazodone and mirtazapine.

Orthostatic hypotension is a less often recognised problem with many of the antidepressants but nonetheless a significant issue particularly in elderly patients and those with cardiac disease. Thus, the introduction of antidepressants associated with this effect (Table 6.1) may result in falls or syncope, producing significant morbidity and even mortality. Elderly patients with cardiac disease are of particular concern since many cardiac medications also lower blood pressure.

Several studies have implicated tricyclic antidepressants in the development of ischaemic heart disease (Cohen et al. 2000; Hamer et al. 2011; Hippisley-Cox et al. 2001). This may further account for the increased mortality reported in patients prescribed these medications. However, further prospectively randomised trials are required to confirm this relationship.

Several classes of antidepressants have unique adverse effects that have cardiovascular manifestations, which may inadvertently be ascribed to cardiac disease. Hence, a hypertensive crisis precipitated by tyramine consumption in a patient prescribed with monoamine oxidase inhibitors may induce an acute coronary syndrome or acute pulmonary oedema in a patient with underlying cardiac disease. The serotonin syndrome associated with the selective serotonin reuptake inhibitors (potentially aggravated with concomitant use of St John's wort or 5-hydroxytryptophan) may also be confused with a cardiac problem with its associated tachycardia and hypertension. Moclobemide use is associated with peripheral oedema, which may be misinterpreted as heart failure.

Given the above concerns with antidepressant medications, the questions arises as to which can be safely used in cardiac patients. From an evidence base perspective, the most extensively studied antidepressant in cardiac patients is sertraline (O'Connor et al. 2010; Xiong et al. 2012), which had an excellent safety profile in the SADHART study (Glassman et al. 2002).

6.3 Psychiatric Issues in the Cardiology Patient

Traditionally, psychiatry has embodied a holistic approach in assessing and managing patients, not only considering the psychological disorder but also medical conditions, psychosocial issues and patient global functioning. In contrast, cardiology has traditionally adopted a 'disease-specific' philosophy in the management of cardiac patients, with a focus merely on structural aspects of the disease. Fortunately the later approach is changing with the influence of cardiac outcomes research, where the focus is shifting from merely 'disease outcomes' to also incorporating 'patient-reported outcomes' and the concept of health status.

As illustrated in Fig. 6.1, the treatment of coronary artery disease could be focussed exclusively on the disease process by undertaking coronary angiography

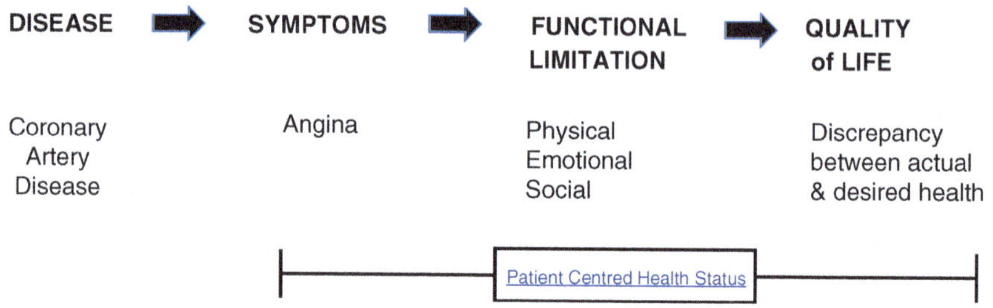

Fig. 6.1 Health Status in Cardiovascular Disease

and tests evaluating myocardial ischaemia. However, health status should also be evaluated where the angina symptoms the patient experiences with the resulting impact on physical capacity, associated emotional concerns and social impairment should also be considered (Rumsfeld 2002). Moreover, quality of life, with the patient's health expectations being relative to their actual impairment, should also be considered especially since depression is a major determinant of this factor (Xiong et al. 2012). This approach is more consistent with the psychiatric approach and will result in closer links between psychiatrists and cardiologists, thus resulting in better patient care.

6.3.1 Premorbid Psychological Conditions

Considering the high prevalence of depression within the community and its association with cardiovascular disease, it is not surprising that many patients will be afflicted by both disorders (Hare et al. 2014). Furthermore, since depression is associated with an increased risk of rehospitalisation and mortality in patients with cardiovascular disease (Jiang et al. 2001), the cardiologist should actively promote the treatment of this risk factor, much the same as they would treat blood pressure, lipids and glycaemic levels in affected patients. Indeed psychological factors such as depression double the risk of experiencing a myocardial infarction (Yusuf et al. 2004).

The importance of premorbid health status is exemplified by a recent study evaluating potential factors contributing to the two- to threefold higher in-hospital mortality in young women (<55 years) who experience a myocardial infarct, compared with their male counterparts (Dreyer et al. 2015). This study demonstrated that compared to men, these young women had poorer premorbid physical and mental quality of life parameters, as well as experiencing more angina and physical limitation from their disease (Dreyer et al. 2015). Whether treatment of these mental and psychosocial factors results in an improved prognosis requires further evaluation.

In addition to depression, patients with premorbid psychoses require close attention considering their increased risk of cardiovascular disease. Moreover, many of the antipsychotic medications have adverse cardiovascular effects including clozapine-associated myocarditis/cardiomyopathy (Alawami et al. 2014), orthostatic hypotension and QT prolongation, as well as producing unfavourable effects on cardiovascular risk factors such as cholesterol, glucose and weight.

6.3.2 Psychological Considerations in Cardiac Disorders

Several cardiac disorders may be precipitated or adversely affected by psychological stress. Examples include stress cardiomyopathy and coronary microvascular disorders.

Stress cardiomyopathy (also referred to as takotsubo cardiomyopathy or apical ballooning syndrome) has attracted particular interest in the cardiology literature (Akashi et al. 2015) and exemplifies the nexus between heart and mind. This condition typically occurs in postmenopausal women who experience an acute emotional stress (e.g. watching their house on fire) precipitating an episode of chest pain that mimics an acute myocardial infarct (including ECG changes and small rise in troponin). However, subsequent angiography reveals no occluded blood vessels and left ventriculography classically reveals akinesis and ballooning of cardiac apex but maintained a vigorous contraction of the cardiac base. This intriguing syndrome is attributed to excessive adrenergic discharge although the precise mechanism involved remains elusive (Neil et al. 2012). Further investigation of this syndrome should provide further insights on how mental stress can impact on cardiac function.

Coronary microvascular disorders, such as syndrome X, microvascular angina, microvascular spasm and the coronary slow flow phenomenon, are clinically characterised as patients with recurrent chest pain mimicking angina but in the absence of obstructive coronary artery disease on angiography (Di Fiore and Beltrame 2013). These conditions are difficult to assess so that symptoms are attributed to psychosomatic manifestations rather than cardiac dysfunction. Moreover, the delay and ambiguity in making the diagnosis frequently promotes anxiety in the patient as to the nature of their illness so that the encounter with the medical process may produce depression per se. Yet another layer of complexity in these conditions is the demonstration of altered pain perception in some affected patients and whether the syndromes represent a defective pain pathway (Cannon et al. 1994). Accordingly, considerable research is still required to understand these elusive disorders and multidisciplinary assessment will be of benefit to the patient.

6.3.3 Psychological Effects of Cardiac Therapies

The nature of cardiac disorders may produce far-reaching psychological effects, which can be exacerbated by suboptimal cardiac management, especially if a holistic approach is not adopted. This can be further complicated by some of cardiac therapies instituted including drugs and devices.

Several cardiac medications have been implicated as depression-inducing medications; however, the evidence base for these assertions is not substantiated in the literature. Beta-blockers can cause fatigue and erectile dysfunction but have not been shown to precipitate depression. In a prospectively conducted study, van Melle et al. (2006) demonstrated a similar prevalence of depression in post-infarct patients independent whether or not they were prescribed beta-blockers. Similarly, statins have also been implicated in depression but two systematic analyses of the literature have refuted this assertion (Macedo et al. 2014; Parsaik et al. 2014).

The evolution of cardiac devices has improved cardiac outcomes but also created novel scenarios that impact on patient psyche. For example, the implantable cardiac defibrillator (ICD) can terminate life-threatening arrhythmias and save lives in high-risk patients. These patients are often those with heart failure, and although the 'electrical issues' can be managed with the ICD, the 'pump failure' continues to progress with depression ensuing given the inevitable outcome. Thus not surprisingly, there is a high prevalence of anxiety and depression in patients with ICDs (Bilge et al. 2006). Other issues that these devices may cause are inappropriate shocks and recurrent multiple shocks for 'electrical storms' (i.e. incessant malignant arrhythmias resulting in multiple shocks). Both of these may lead to post-traumatic stress disorder, anxiety and depressed mood in affected individuals and warrant consultation with psychological therapy.

6.4 The Future of Psychocardiology

The above discussion outlines the important interface between cardiac and psychological issues in patient management, particularly in relation to depression. In the future, it will be important to integrate management strategies between these clinical disciplines with the use of multidisciplinary clinics in patient assessment. The evolution of this field may even entice young clinicians to train in both psychiatry and cardiology and thus develop the discipline of psychocardiology.

References

Akashi YJ, Nef HM, Lyon AR (2015) Epidemiology and pathophysiology of Takotsubo syndrome. Nat Rev Cardiol 12:387–397

Alawami M, Wasywich C, Cicovic A, Kenedi C (2014) A systematic review of clozapine induced cardiomyopathy. Int J Cardiol 176:315–320

Beltrame JF, Crea F, Kaski JC, Ogawa H, Ong P, Sechtem U et al (2015) International standardization of diagnostic criteria for vasospastic angina. Eur Heart J pii: ehv351. [Epub ahead of print]

Bilge AK, Ozben B, Demircan S, Cinar M, Yilmaz E, Adalet K (2006) Depression and anxiety status of patients with implantable cardioverter defibrillator and precipitating factors. Pacing Clin Electrophysiol 29:619–626

Cannon RO 3rd, Quyyumi AA, Mincemoyer R, Stine AM, Gracely RH, Smith WB et al (1994) Imipramine in patients with chest pain despite normal coronary angiograms. N Engl J Med 330:1411–1417

Castro VM, Clements CC, Murphy SN, Gainer VS, Fava M, Weilburg JB et al (2013) QT interval and antidepressant use: a cross sectional study of electronic health records. BMJ 346:f288

Cohen HW, Gibson G, Alderman MH (2000) Excess risk of myocardial infarction in patients treated with antidepressant medications: association with use of tricyclic agents. Am J Med 108:2–8

Di Fiore DP, Beltrame JF (2013) Chest pain in patients with 'normal angiography': could it be cardiac? Int J Evid Based Healthc 11:56–68
Dreyer RP, Smolderen KG, Strait KM, Beltrame JF, Lichtman JH, Lorenze NP et al (2015) Gender differences in pre-event health status of young patients with acute myocardial infarction: a VIRGO study analysis. Eur Heart J Acute Cardiovasc Care 5(1):43–54
Glassman AH, O'Connor CM, Califf RM, Swedberg K, Schwartz P, Bigger JT Jr et al (2002) Sertraline treatment of major depression in patients with acute MI or unstable angina. JAMA 288:701–709
Hamer M, Batty GD, Seldenrijk A, Kivimaki M (2011) Antidepressant medication use and future risk of cardiovascular disease: the Scottish Health Survey. Eur Heart J 32:437–442
Hare DL, Toukhsati SR, Johansson P, Jaarsma T (2014) Depression and cardiovascular disease: a clinical review. Eur Heart J 35:1365–1372
Hippisley-Cox J, Pringle M, Hammersley V, Crown N, Wynn A, Meal A et al (2001) Antidepressants as risk factor for ischaemic heart disease: case-control study in primary care. BMJ 323:666–669
Honkola J, Hookana E, Malinen S, Kaikkonen KS, Junttila MJ, Isohanni M et al (2012) Psychotropic medications and the risk of sudden cardiac death during an acute coronary event. Eur Heart J 33:745–751
Jiang W, Alexander J, Christopher E, Kuchibhatla M, Gaulden LH, Cuffe MS et al (2001) Relationship of depression to increased risk of mortality and rehospitalization in patients with congestive heart failure. Arch Intern Med 161:1849–1856
Leonard CE, Bilker WB, Newcomb C, Kimmel SE, Hennessy S (2011) Antidepressants and the risk of sudden cardiac death and ventricular arrhythmia. Pharmacoepidemiol Drug Saf 20:903–913
Macedo AF, Taylor FC, Casas JP, Adler A, Prieto-Merino D, Ebrahim S (2014) Unintended effects of statins from observational studies in the general population: systematic review and meta-analysis. BMC Med 12:51
Mansour VM, Wilkinson DJ, Jennings GL, Schwarz RG, Thompson JM, Esler MD (1998) Panic disorder: coronary spasm as a basis for cardiac risk? Med J Aust 168:390–392
Neil CJ, Nguyen TH, Sverdlov AL, Chirkov YY, Chong CR, Stansborough J et al (2012) Can we make sense of takotsubo cardiomyopathy? An update on pathogenesis, diagnosis and natural history. Expert Rev Cardiovasc Ther 10:215–221
O'Connor CM, Jiang W, Kuchibhatla M, Silva SG, Cuffe MS, Callwood DD et al (2010) Safety and efficacy of sertraline for depression in patients with heart failure: results of the SADHART-CHF (Sertraline Against Depression and Heart Disease in Chronic Heart Failure) trial. J Am Coll Cardiol 56:692–699
Parsaik AK, Singh B, Murad MH, Singh K, Mascarenhas SS, Williams MD et al (2014) Statins use and risk of depression: a systematic review and meta-analysis. J Affect Disord 160:62–67
Ramamurthy G, Trejo E, Faraone SV (2013) Depression treatment in patients with coronary artery disease: a systematic review. Prim Care Companion CNS Disord 15(5)
Rumsfeld JS (2002) Health status and clinical practice: when will they meet? Circulation 106:5–7
Teply RM, Packard KA, White ND, Hilleman DE, DiNicolantonio JJ (2015) Treatment of depression in patients with concomitant cardiac disease. Prog Cardiovasc Dis 58(5):514–528
Tully PJ, Turnbull DA, Beltrame J, Horowitz J, Cosh S, Baumeister H et al (2015) Panic disorder and incident coronary heart disease: a systematic review and meta-regression in 1 131 612 persons and 58 111 cardiac events. Psychol Med 45:1–12
van Melle JP, Verbeek DE, van den Berg MP, Ormel J, van der Linde MR, de Jonge P (2006) Beta-blockers and depression after myocardial infarction: a multicenter prospective study. J Am Coll Cardiol 48:2209–2214
Xiong GL, Fiuzat M, Kuchibhatla M, Krishnan R, O'Connor CM, Jiang W (2012) Health status and depression remission in patients with chronic heart failure: patient-reported outcomes from the SADHART-CHF trial. Circ Heart Fail 5:688–692
Yusuf S, Hawken S, Ounpuu S, Dans T, Avezum A, Lanas F et al (2004) Effect of potentially modifiable risk factors associated with myocardial infarction in 52 countries (the INTERHEART study): case-control study. Lancet 364:937–952

The Validity of Vascular Depression as a Diagnostic Construct

7

Lauren Taylor, Adith Mohan, and Perminder S. Sachdev

Contents

L. Taylor
School of Psychiatry, University of New South Wales Medicine,
Barker St, Randwick, NSW 2031, Australia

Neuropsychiatric Institute (NPI), Euroa Centre Prince of Wales Hospital, Sydney, Australia

A. Mohan • P.S. Sachdev, MD, PhD, FRANZCP (✉)
Centre for Healthy Brain Ageing (CHeBA), Barker St, Randwick, NSW 2031, Australia

School of Psychiatry, University of New South Wales Medicine,
Barker St, Randwick, NSW 2031, Australia

Neuropsychiatric Institute (NPI), Euroa Centre Prince of Wales Hospital, Sydney, Australia
e-mail: p.sachdev@unsw.edu.au; http://www.cheba.unsw.edu.au

B.T. Baune, P.J. Tully (eds.), *Cardiovascular Diseases and Depression*,
DOI 10.1007/978-3-319-32480-7_7

Abstract

The 'vascular depression' (VaD) construct initially proposed a relationship between late-life depression (LLD) and vascular disease and stimulated significant investigation into this nature of this relationship. The construct became synonymous with an aetiological proposition that vascular disease or risk factors are central in the pathogenesis of LLD. Validity of the VaD construct warrants consideration. This chapter reviews strategies that have been used to demonstrate an aetiological relationship between vascular disease and depression and considers the evidence for this association from various perspectives including (i) clinical features and the specificity of a VaD clinical phenotype, (ii) neuroimaging findings, (iii) proposed mechanisms for the aetiological role of vascular disease in depression, (iv) prognostic implications with a focus on treatment response and (v) shared pathomechanisms underlying both depression and vascular pathology. Our review suggests that the evidence in support of a causal relationship between depression and vascular disease, and thus the validity of the VaD construct, is not consistent. Whilst strong associations exist, the agnostic ascription of vascular disease as *causative* in LLD is potentially misleading, particularly in light of emerging evidence for diverse and interrelated pathomechanisms.

7.1 Introduction

The 'vascular depression' (VaD) construct was proposed nearly two decades ago (Alexopoulos et al. 1997a; Krishnan and McDonald 1995), broadly defined as a depressive disorder with late-life onset or an alteration in the nature of an earlier onset depressive disorder, in the presence of vascular disease or vascular risk factors. Significant interest in the relationship between vascular disease and depression has ensued. As such, the validity of the VaD construct warrants closer examination. In this chapter, strategies that have been used to demonstrate an aetiological relationship between vascular disease and depression will be reviewed and evidence for this association considered from various perspectives, including (i) clinical features and the specificity of a VaD clinical phenotype, (ii) neuroimaging findings, (iii) proposed mechanisms for the aetiological role of vascular disease in depression, (iv) prognostic implications with a focus on treatment response and (v) shared pathomechanisms underlying both depression and vascular pathology.

Evaluation of the VaD construct necessitates differentiation between risk factors for vascular disease and the presence of vascular disease itself, as the putative 'vascular' risk factors could arguably influence depression through mechanisms other than vascular disease. The spectrum of severity, anatomical location of cerebrovascular disease and the techniques used to evaluate it merit attention. The field has evolved such that hypotheses regarding the nature of the relationship and potential causative mechanisms have been refined. This chapter aims to synthesise the literature and draw conclusions as to the validity of the VaD construct.

7.2 The VaD Hypothesis: Concept and Evolution

The VaD construct (Alexopoulos et al. 1997a) hypothesised that cerebrovascular disease may predispose, precipitate or perpetuate some depressive syndromes and was suggested by the contemporaneous findings of several authors (Krishnan and McDonald 1995; Krishnan 1993). Epidemiologic, neuroimaging and clinical data underpinned the hypothesis. High prevalence rates of coronary disease (Carney et al. 1987), stroke (Robinson et al. 1984a; Lipsey et al. 1986) and risk factors for vascular disease (Rabkin et al. 1983) in late-life depression (LLD) have been observed, as have the frequent occurrence of white matter hyperintensities in LLD (Coffey et al. 1990; Krishnan et al. 1988; Figiel et al. 1991) and infrequent family history of mood disorder in post-stroke depression (Fujikawa et al. 1994). Vascular disease-mediated disruption of frontal-subcortical pathways central in mood regulation was the proposed mechanism (Alexopoulos et al. 2002a; Lyness et al. 1998; Krishnan et al. 1997). Alexopoulos et al. (1997b) outlined a 'threshold' concept, with the accumulation of vascular lesions to a level sufficient to either disrupt neuronal circuits critical for mood regulation *or* confer sufficient vulnerability to the development of depression in conjunction with non-biological factors. A clinical phenotype distinguishable from 'non-vascular depression' was proposed (Alexopoulos et al. 1997a). Despite the breadth of the VaD hypothesis, it became synonymous with an *aetiological* proposition, a hybrid of nominalist (Krishnan 2005) and essentialist approaches to taxonomy. The proposed cardinal features were (1) depression onset after the age of 65 years, or a change in the course of depression (increased frequency or duration), and (2) clinical and/or laboratory evidence of vascular disease or vascular risk factors (Alexopoulos et al. 1997a). 'Secondary features', deemed suggestive of a VaD phenotype, were (i) dysexecutive syndrome, (ii) psychomotor retardation, (iii) limited depressive ideation, (iv) limited insight, (v) disability (disproportionate to the depression severity) and (vi) absent family history of mood disorder (Alexopoulos et al. 1997a) (see Table 7.1). Krishnan and colleagues (2004) proposed that VaD be defined by the presence of characteristic MRI white matter hyperintensities (WMHs). Efforts to characterise the specific pattern of cognitive dysfunction in LLD gave rise to the related and poorly defined offspring of the original VaD construct, subcortical ischaemic depression (SID) (Krishnan et al. 2004) and depression-executive dysfunction syndrome (DED) (Kelly and Alexopoulos 2009).

The concept of VaD thus evolved to be a 'diagnostic subtype' defined primarily by executive dysfunction and demonstrable MRI white matter lesions. The VaD construct has been limited by poor clinical sensitivity and specificity. Small vessel disease (SVD) is associated with a range of neuropsychiatric presentations including cognitive impairment (Sachdev et al. 2004), psychosis (Breitner et al. 1990) and bipolar disorder (McDonald et al. 1999). Additionally, the VaD construct agnostically ascribed cerebrovascular disease as causative in all individuals with co-occurring cerebrovascular disease and depression. Concurrently, methodological limitations in detecting cerebrovascular disease, specifically SVD, created the challenge of the construct not being sufficiently inclusive (Kelly and Alexopoulos

Table 7.1 Proposed vascular depression criteria

Proposed cardinal features	1. Depression onset after age 65 years *or* change in nature of depression of earlier onset, with more frequent or persistent episodes
	2. Clinical and/or laboratory evidence of vascular disease *or* risk factors
	For example, history of CVA, TIA, myocardial infarction, IHD, history of hypertension, hyperlipidaemia, neurologic signs or carotid bruit, radiological evidence of white matter hyperintensities in perforating artery territory, cerebral infarct or carotid stenosis
Proposed secondary vascular depression features, i.e. distinctive clinical phenotype	(i) Cognitive impairment characterised by but not limited to executive dysfunction
	(ii) Psychomotor retardation
	(iii) Minimal or absent depressive ideation (e.g. guilt)
	(iv) Poor insight
	(v) Disability
	(vi) Negative family history of mood disorders

Modified from Kelly and Alexopoulos (2009)

2009). For the purposes of this review, the presence of cerebrovascular disease is predominantly identified by neuroimaging, specifically MRI, rather than by neuropathology. This is appropriate given the methodological limitations that arise with attempts to correlate post-mortem neuropathology (e.g. lacunar infarcts, microbleeds and non-infarct white matter ischaemic changes) with pre-mortem psychiatric disorder (Sachdev and Reutens 2014). Substantive methodological flaws also arise when a clinical history of vascular risk factors is used as a proxy for cerebral small vessel disease as the two cannot be neatly equated (Sheline et al. 2008), and this is therefore cautioned against when considering the literature.

As outlined by Sachdev and Reutens (2014), technical evolution in neuroimaging modalities has added complexity to operational research definitions of VaD and to the interpretation of MRI abnormalities as they relate to the VaD construct. Much of the focus has been on white matter lesions (WMLs), identified as *leukoaraiosis* or hypodensity on CT or T1-weighted images or white matter hyperintensities (WMHs) on T2-weighted MRI, in particular using fluid-attenuated inversion recovery (FLAIR) sequences. Ascribing significance to WMHs, however, has been complicated by reportedly high prevalence and lack of aetiological specificity. WMHs have been described in almost one-half of healthy 40-year-olds (Wen et al. 2009) and the majority of 60- to 64-year-old individuals (Wen and Sachdev 2004). Data from the Rotterdam Study of a large representative community sample aged between 60 and 90 years demonstrated periventricular or subcortical WMHs in 95% (Almeida 2008). In addition to ischaemia, WMHs may reflect such diverse aetiologies as inflammation, demyelination, oedema, developmental abnormality or degeneration (Ovbiagele and Salver 2006). Impaired cerebral vasomotor reactivity and autoregulatory dysfunction (Taylor et al. 2013a) have also been cited as potential contributory factors in WMH development. There is consensus, however, that incidental WMHs (especially *deep* white matter hyperintensities and large periventricular hyperintensities (Thomas 2013)) in older individuals most likely reflect ischaemic change (Pantoni and Garcia 1997), thereby supporting their use as an (imperfect) proxy for cerebral SVD. FLAIR enables differentiation of WMHs from dilated perivascular (Virchow-Robin) spaces and detailed characterisation of lacunar infarcts. T2*-weighted MRI utilising gradient-echo sequencing allows the application of susceptibility-weighted imaging (SWI) which is highly sensitive for identifying cerebral microbleeds (Chavhan et al. 2009). Diffusion tensor imaging (DTI) has recently enabled more sensitive interrogation of white matter integrity than is possible on T2-weighted imaging (Nucifora et al. 2007) and furthered evaluation of the frontal-subcortical disconnection hypothesis. Blood oxygen level-dependent (BOLD) functional MRI, magnetic resonance spectroscopy (MRS) and perfusion MRI (pMRI) have been less prominent in the VaD literature.

7.3 Strategies to Evaluate Validity of the VaD Construct

Broad strategies that have been applied to investigate the nature of the relationship between cerebrovascular disease and depression and therefore have utility in evaluating validity of the VaD construct will be considered below.

7.3.1 Prevalence Estimates and Epidemiological Data

High rates of co-occurrence of cerebral SVD and depression have been established bidirectionally (Thomas et al. 2004), and there is strong evidence that the relationship is a reciprocal one (Valkanova and Ebmeier 2013). Cerebral SVD is frequent in older depressed individuals and depression frequent in those with cerebral SVD. This has been particularly evident in the stroke (Salaycik et al. 2007; Jonas and Mussolino 2000) and myocardial infarct (Ford et al. 1998; Pratt et al. 1996) literature, with two- to threefold incidence (of cerebral SVD) reported in individuals with a history of depression. Depression is common in the heritable disorder cerebral autosomal dominant arteriopathy with subcortical infarcts and leukoencephalopathy (CADASIL) (Valenti et al. 2008), which is characterised by extensive cerebral SVD. A compelling epidemiological argument is that older individuals with depression are more likely to have subcortical lesions compared with nondepressed control subjects (Taylor et al. 2003a). Additionally, those with later onset depression, when compared with earlier onset depression, have greater frequency of subcortical WMHs (up to fivefold), including when age is considered as a covariate in analysis (Krishnan et al. 1997; Lavretsky et al. 1998). Community-based studies have also demonstrated an association between depressive symptoms and subcortical WMHs (Jorm et al. 2005; Steffens et al. 2002). Epidemiological data, however, has shown that an exponential increase in cardiovascular disease prevalence with age is *not* paralleled by a similar increase in depression prevalence (Almeida 2008).

A potential confounding factor accounting for both increased WMHs and depression is the influence of chronic illness. An early study found the relationship between WMHs and depression was no longer significant after adjustment for poor physical health (Stewart and Hirani 2010). Subsequent authors similarly concluded that the strength of association between vascular disease and depression was significantly attenuated by controlling for chronic disease (Jorm et al. 2005; Lyness et al. 2000; Sanders et al. 2006; Stewart and Hirani 2010). A prospective cohort study by Kivimaki et al. (2012) further supported the chronic illness hypothesis, finding equivalent risk of depressive symptoms in vascular and non-vascular conditions. Baune and colleagues (2012) evaluated the effect of clinical characteristics of depression, including depression severity, and sociodemographic factors on the association between depression and cardiovascular disease. Reviewing longitudinal evidence, they concluded that further studies were required but that these variables required integration into future models of the relationship.

Risk factors for vascular disease, including hypertension, diabetes and elevated homocysteine (Khan et al. 2007) have been independently associated with depression in some studies.

Developing unifying hypotheses of the depression/vascular disease relationship incorporating these risk factors however remains challenging given the complexity of these associations. To illustrate this, the association between depressive symptoms and type 2 diabetes (T2D) and consideration of shared pathophysiological processes were recently considered by Doyle and colleagues (2014). Epidemiological data was found to support a bidirectional relationship between T2D and depressive symptoms, the strength of association between depressed mood and risk of incident diabetes being reported as particularly robust. The authors (Doyle et al. 2014) highlighted emerging evidence of reduced neuroplasticity as a common biological feature of both depression and T2D. Both depression and T2D appear significantly correlated with reduced neuroplasticity, with proposed mechanisms including inflammation, poor glycaemic control, HPA dysregulation and endothelial dysfunction (Doyle et al. 2014). Hippocampal and prefrontal cortex volume reduction and neurocognitive deficits in patients with T2D align with those reported in the depression literature (Doyle et al. 2014). Alijore et al.'s (2010) finding of greater volumetric deficits in samples with T2D *and* MDD compared with *nondepressed* T2D suggests a synergistic effect, although the direction of any association with reduced neuroplasticity remains unclear. On analysing the association between depression and traditional cardiovascular risk factors, a recent meta-analysis (Valkanova and Ebmeier 2013) found no significant correlation between depression and hypertension, dyslipidaemia or Framingham stroke risk score and a weak association with smoking. Robust association was evident however between depression and the disease states diabetes, stroke and cardiovascular disease and between depression and Risk Factor Composite Scores (RFCS). It is unclear as to why an association with the composite risk score was evident; however, the authors highlight that the use of *peripheral* vascular disease and vascular *risk factors* as evidence of *cerebro*vascular disease complicates interpretation of the epidemiological data and recommends the inclusion of neuroimaging data in future epidemiologic studies to address this (Valkanova and Ebmeier 2013).

Whilst useful, high prevalence rates of vascular disease in depression and vice versa are insufficient to establish a *causal* association. Critique of the association supported by epidemiological data requires consideration of (1) a potential confounding factor common to both SVD and depression, (2) a common pathophysiological process underlying both the SVD and depression and (3) complex relationships between covariates, of which there are a multitude given the complexity and heterogeneity of both depression and small vessel disease. Epidemiological evidence that certain individual risk factors, including hypertension, do not share an independent association with depression is helpful in consideration of pathophysiologic models.

7.3.2 Temporal Association

The likelihood of an aetiological relationship between a factor of known association (vascular disease) and outcome (depression) is increased if occurrence of the latter is clearly *temporally* related to the former. Temporality has been clearly established in relation to depression and acute, focal vascular events, as in post-stroke depression (Robinson and Spalletta 2010; Wade et al. 1987; Whyte and Mulsant 2003). Embedded within the Rotterdam Study was the first large (over 5,000 participants) longitudinal prospective study to consider incident depression following a TIA (Luijendijk et al. 2011). Confirming the findings of an earlier cross-sectional study, Luijendijk and colleagues concluded that TIA was independently associated with a near threefold increased risk of incident DSM-IV major depressive disorder (Luijendijk et al. 2011). The risk of developing depression was positively correlated with the *number* of TIAs, suggestive of a dose-response effect; however, the mean time to onset of depression was a considerable 3.8 years, suggesting the influence of other significant variables affects temporal onset of depression in addition to TIA occurrence. The relationship between stroke, TIA and depression is complicated by the likelihood of cerebral SVD preceding the symptomatic neurological event. Thus, controlling for baseline cerebral SVD would be ideal in future studies to distil TIA association effect and SVD association effect.

Examination of the temporal relationship between cerebral SVD and depression is limited by methodological problems. Typically, WMHs cannot be dated with the same accuracy as stroke lesions (Robinson 2005), except in symptomatic lacunar infarction. A recent meta-analysis (Egeto et al. 2014) considered the association between lacunar infarcts and depression. No statistically significant association was found between volume or location of lacunes and depression. The authors commented that the small number of studies, heterogeneity in comparison groups within and between studies, posed significant problems, recommending the separation of deep WMH and lacunar stroke patients, larger sample sizes and healthy controls in future studies. Given the paucity of robust data regarding the temporal relationship between symptomatic lacunar infarct and depression, it is not possible to reliably extrapolate any temporal correlation between the two. Thus, whilst tight temporal fit is a useful and robust indicator of aetiological association, methodological and data limitations prevent determination of temporality between WMHs and incident depression in the current literature.

7.3.3 Is There a Distinct 'VaD' Clinical Phenotype?

Late-life depression (LLD) is a broad term encompassing heterogenous syndromes of unipolar depression that occur in older adults (typically defined as 65 years and older (Vu and Aizenstein 2013)). The LLD group is often differentiated by those with 'late-onset' LLD, confusingly, often identified in the literature as onset over the age of 50 (Vu and Aizenstein 2013) as distinct from 'earlier onset' LLD, which is characterised by recurring depressive episodes in later life. The concept of VaD is as a proposed *subtype* of LLD. Conceptual and methodological problems with 'late-onset' LLD as a criterion for VaD have been reported by several authors (Alexopoulos 2005; Krishnan et al. 2004; Sneed 2011) and mirror the problems encountered in attempting to delineate differing profiles of 'early-onset' and 'late-onset' LLD more broadly. In reviewing this literature, the most consistent distinction is that of 'early-onset' LLD with presence of a positive family history (Brodaty et al. 2001; Devanand et al. 2004; Baldwin and Tomenson 1995), but this is not reported by other studies, (Hickie et al. 2001; Greenwald and Kramer-Ginsberg 1988; Janssen et al. 2006). No consistent phenomenological or clinical characteristics reliably distinguish late-onset from early-onset LLD. Clinical phenomena observed with greater frequency in late-onset LLD have included increased loss of interest and fewer guilty cognitions (Krishnan et al. 1995), frequent hypochondriasis and greater severity of guilty cognitions (Brodaty et al. 2005), increased anhedonia (Rapp et al. 2005) and more lassitude (Corruble et al. 2008; McDougall and Brayne 2007). Lower rates of family history of mood or other psychiatric disorder have been reported in those with SVD and depression (Taylor et al. 2003b; Simpson et al. 1997).

'Subcortical ischaemic depression' (SID) and the 'depression-executive dysfunction syndrome' (DED) are constructs related closely to VaD. The DED syndrome (Alexopoulos 2001) was proposed as a syndromal characterisation of the frontal-executive dysfunction that has been frequently noted in LLD (Sexton et al. 2011), clinically manifesting as planning, sequencing, organising and abstraction deficits. In characterising the neuropsychological profile in LLD subjects, one group (Sexton et al. 2011) reported core neuropsychological deficits to be in information processing speed and executive dysfunction, which mediate performance in multiple other cognitive domains including memory retrieval. The neural circuitry of these cognitive functions localise to a series of parallel prefrontal pathways that project from the frontal lobe to ventral striatum, then globus pallidus and substantia nigra, through the thalamus and back to the frontal lobe. Aberrant dorsolateral circuit function is implicated in executive dysfunction, the anterior cingulate circuit in apathy and the orbitofrontal circuit in mood lability and disinhibition (Taylor et al. 2006). The DED and SID proposals hypothesised that vascular lesions were pathogenic in frontal-subcortical circuit dysfunction. Thus it would follow that the clinical phenotype would have some correlation with lesion location (insofar as determining which circuit is impacted) and severity. Kohler and colleagues (2010) investigated the association between WMHs and cognition. They found severity of WMHs to be correlated with executive dysfunction and episodic memory in depressed, but not nondepressed, patients. This pattern of deficits, however, is by no means specific to LLD and occurs in a wide range of neurocognitive disorders including bipolar disorder (McDonald et al. 1999) and psychosis (Breitner et al. 1990; Tonkonogy and Geller 1999). The specificity of symptoms conveyed by the DED and SID constructs is poor, and the validity of specific VaD, SID and DED clinical phenotypes remains controversial (Baldwin 2005).

7.3.4 Longitudinal Course, Prognostic Implications and Treatment Response

Longitudinal studies are more likely to establish an aetiological relationship if cerebral small vessel disease and depression can be demonstrated to covary over time. As summarised by Thomas (2013), prospective studies have investigated the role of WMH burden and reported predictive validity of incident depressive symptoms (at 1 and 3 years (Krishnan et al. 2006; Teodorczuk et al. 2010)), deterioration in depressive symptoms (at 4 years (Steffens et al. 2002)) and emergent major depressive episodes at 3 and 4 years (Kohler et al. 2010). Meta-analytic analysis found that effect sizes for increases in WMH burden ranged from 0.39 to 0.9 (Herrmann et al. 2008). However, data regarding incident depression is conflicting. Ikram and colleagues (2010) found no association between neuroimaging data and incident depression, proposing that WMH burden may be associated with persistence rather than incidence of depression. If the difference in response to treatment and/or long-term outcome is demonstrated in individuals with cerebral SVD in comparison to those without, it is likely that the SVD plays at least a partial aetiological role in the pathogenesis of depression. The findings of WMH burden effect on acute antidepressant treatment response have been discrepant and are difficult to reconcile (Thomas 2013).

Whilst there have been frequent findings of greater overall WMH burden being associated with poorer response to maintenance antidepressant therapy (Hickie et al. 1995; Taylor et al. 2003a; Simpson et al. 1997), typically studies have considered static cross-sectional WMH burden rather than rate of change or *progression*, and few have combined total *severity* of WMH with *location* in investigating treatment response.

Taylor and colleagues (2003b) reported a positive association between WMH volume and clinical outcome, concluding that subjects with DSM-IV major depressive disorder who sustained remission over a 2-year follow-up had lower total WMH volume than those who did not sustain remission, including when baseline depression severity was controlled for. They calculated a 7 % increased risk of poor outcome with every 1 % increase of WMH volume (Taylor et al. 2003b).

Godin and colleagues (2008) replicated this finding in a 4-year longitudinal study, reporting positive correlation reported between lifetime major depression and WMH volume and between WMH progression and lifetime major depression. Notably, however, the PROSPER study (Verslius et al. 2006) found no association between progression of cerebral WMLs and incident depression, with the authors concluding that clearly delineated treatment and control groups are necessary in future longitudinal studies in order to address this question.

Longitudinal studies investigating treatment and prognostic effects of WMHs have found an association between WMHs and increased treatment resistance (Simpson et al. 1998), lower remission rates at 2 years (Taylor et al. 2003b) and less favourable chronic course (Taylor et al. 2013a). A meta-analytic review found executive dysfunction to correlate with poorer acute antidepressant response, lower remission and higher relapse rates (McLennan and Mathias 2010). Executive dysfunction in LLD was reported by one group to have predictive validity for antidepressant response (Taylor et al. 2013a). In addition to poorer response to antidepressants (Taylor et al. 2003a) and poorer response to ECT, an increased likelihood of developing delirium has been reported in those with subcortical WMLs (Steffens et al. 2001; Coffey et al. 1988; Figiel et al. 1990). There is literature, however, that supports the antidepressant efficacy of ECT in patients with evidence of SVD (Figiel et al. 1990). The VaD construct has utility in informing intervention research, with interventions targeting vascular disease variables being shown to have antidepressant utility. Detailed review of this evidence is beyond the scope of this chapter; however, to illustrate, nimodipine has been shown to positively augment antidepressant treatment response in subjects with 'VaD' (Taragano et al. 2001).

Whilst the association between WMHs and greater cognitive dysfunction is consistent (Carvalho et al. 2014), the relationship is unlikely to be one of linear causation. Depressive states are associated with hypothalamic-pituitary-adrenal (HPA) hyperactivity resulting in chronic glucocorticoid exposure, which is demonstrably neurotoxic, associated with hippocampal atrophy (Bae et al. 2006; Zou et al. 2008) and increased dementia risk (Vu and Aizenstein 2013). Kohler and colleagues (2010) assessed executive dysfunction and episodic memory whilst controlling for cortisol levels and brain atrophy and found these to be positively correlated in depressed individuals. Diniz et al. (2013) examined the incident risk of all-cause, Alzheimer's and vascular dementia in LLD with the inclusion of only community-based prospective cohort studies in a recent meta-analysis. In subgroup analysis with risk measures adjusted for confounders, including sociodemographic, cognitive and biological indicators, a significant pooled risk of 2.02 was found for vascular dementia, 1.55 for Alzheimer's dementia and 1.59 for all-cause dementia. Whilst only five studies were included in the vascular dementia analysis, the findings remained significant with differentially elevated vascular, compared with Alzheimer's dementia risk.

7.3.5 Anatomical Specificity

The presence of fit between anatomical site of pathology and clinical presentation is another consideration in the evaluation of an aetiological relationship between vascular disease and depression. Indeed, the VaD hypothesis has been credited with promoting the investigation of mechanisms by which vascular disease influences brain circuitry (Taylor et al. 2013a). The approach, however, of correlating anatomical site of pathology and clinical phenotype remains problematic with regard to psychiatric disorder given that dysfunction of neuronal circuits rather than discrete neuronal regions is understood to give rise to psychiatric symptomatology. Knowledge regarding constituents of these circuits as they relate to depressive symptoms currently remains an area of active study with emerging methods allowing the study of brain function in vivo as never before. Prominent examples include functional neuroimaging data regarding constituent circuitry that have emerged from deep brain stimulation (DBS) studies (Seminowicz et al. 2004). The application of novel technologies including CLARITY (Deisseroth and Schnitzer 2013) and optogenetics (Steinberg et al. 2015) is ongoing in animal models.

Given that the location of stroke was long viewed as the determinant of post-stroke depression (PSD), we briefly review this literature in considering anatomical lesion location. Initially the postulated PSD mechanism was interruption of ascending brainstem and midbrain projections by acute ischaemia with resultant reduction in bioavailability of the biogenic amine serotonin, noradrenalin and dopamine (Loubinoux et al. 2012). Early MRI studies reported an increased risk of PSD in left-sided frontal lesions, compared with left hemisphere posterior lesions or right hemisphere lesions (Robinson et al. 1984b) and numerous MRI studies ensued. The positive correlation between left prefrontal-subcortical lesion location, volume size and PSD was supported in several reviews, including by Vataja and colleagues (2004), but was subsequently challenged. Bhogal and collaborators (2004) cited methodological flaws including small sample sizes and inconsistent ischaemic lesion characterisation and PSD definitions, as undermining the left-sided association. In addition, sample source was identified as a determinant of lesion association; hospital-based and population-based studies found significant association between PSD and left hemisphere lesions whilst community-based samples found association with right hemisphere lesions. Thus, following a period of controversial association, lesion lateralisation was not consistently borne out as being predictive of PSD. Brodaty and colleagues (2007) postulated *cumulative burden* of micro- and macrovascular lesions as being more predictive of PSD than lesion location or lateralisation, an assertion supported by some studies that found the burden of deep WMHs and cerebral microbleeds as predictive of PSD in a 'dose-dependent' manner (Tang et al. 2011a, b; Xiong et al. 2011).

In cerebral SVD, the diffuse nature of WMHs poses significant challenges to meaningful correlation between site of pathology and clinical presentation. SVD-mediated damage to frontal-subcortical circuits implicated in mood regulation and cognition (Dieguez et al. 2004) has been a prevailing model given the prevalence of subcortical lesions in LLD. Contrasting with the aforementioned evidence, several studies have reported a correlation between strategic location of WMHs, particularly frontal lobe lesions, and the development of depression (Greenwald et al. 1998; MacFall et al. 2006, 2001). Compared with control subjects, elderly depressed subjects were found by Taylor et al. to have prefrontal bilateral frontal WMHs (Taylor et al. 2003a), in addition to parietotemporal regions, noted in both depressed and controls. Poorer prognosis was reported where WMLs were located in the frontal lobes, basal ganglia and pons (Franklin et al. 2012). The neuroimaging literature has evolved to plausibly localise WMLs to neuronal tracts putatively involved in depression and cognitive function (Vu and Aizenstein 2013), albeit in the context of incomplete models of the relevant neuronal circuitry. WMLs were reported to converge on the uncinate fasciculus, inferior longitudinal fasciculus, superior longitudinal fasciculus and cingulum such that location correlated with depression severity (Taylor et al. 2013b). The superior longitudinal fasciculus and uncinate fasciculus have demonstrated particular significance as sites of WMLs in LLD subjects with more severe executive deficits on neuropsychological assessment (Mettenburg et al. 2012).

DTI studies have demonstrated correlation between fractional anisotropy as a marker of white matter damage and depressive symptoms in SVD (Brookes et al. 2014). In applying DTI in a whole-brain study, Sexton and colleagues (2012) found fractional anisotropy reductions (indicative of impaired white matter integrity) in frontal-subcortical and limbic tracts, with particular signal in the uncinate fasciculus in depressed subjects. In reviewing this data, Vu and Aizenstein (2013) concluded that *location* and *severity* of WMLs were of equal salience in relation to cognitive impairment in LLD. DTI studies have also demonstrated correlation between impaired white matter integrity in the presence of WMLs with depression severity, treatment response and prognosis and found poorer treatment response in association with frontal white matter tract disruption (Alexopoulos et al. 2002b).

Increasing evidence, particularly from DTI studies, supports anatomical specificity of WMLs as correlating with depressive features. Overall, this data remains limited, given incomplete modalities of clinically interrogating the structure and function of cerebral white matter tracts in vivo in humans.

7.3.6 Neuropathological Studies

Post-mortem biopsies in patients with a history of depressive symptoms have demonstrated cellular alterations including hippocampal atrophy and changes in neuronal and glial cell size, shape and density (Stockmeier et al. 2004). Whilst review of all neuropathological studies is beyond the aims of the authors, a large neuropathology autopsy series reported by Tsopelas and colleagues (2011) (including 153 community participants, 36 with a history of LLD) supported initial work by Thomas and colleagues (2001, 2002, 2003) and found hippocampal volume loss in non-demented depressed post-mortem subjects. No association was found between neuropathological correlates of dementia (neuritic plaques, neurofibrillary tangles, Lewy bodies) and depression in the presence of hippocampal volume loss. This finding supported hippocampal grey matter changes as being independent of a pathogenic dementia process. A notable limitation of this study was the exclusion of autopsy subjects with prior history of dementia. These findings could be interpreted as being supportive of depression as a neurotoxic state, explored below in the context of the glucocorticoid hypothesis. Cellular morphometric studies of depression have reported discrepant findings in younger/middle-aged and late-life cohorts (Khundakar and Thomas 2014). In the former, reduction in glial populations in cortical regions has been consistently reported, whereas in the latter, layer-specific pyramidal neuron pathology in cortical regions has been reported, suggesting different pathophysiological mechanisms, with the possibility that vascular factors may be more relevant to late-life depression (Thomas et al. 2003).

7.4 Potential Common Processes Underpinning Depression and Vascular Pathology

There has been substantive interest in potential common processes that underpin both depression and vascular pathology. Such processes include immune dysfunction and inflammation, oxidative stress, HPA axis dysfunction and genetic variation. Ageing-related changes in the immune, endocrine and neurological systems have all been implicated in LLD (Taylor et al. 2013a). Increasing evidence is emerging of complex and intertwined pathophysiological processes occurring across the inflammatory, immune and neuroendocrine systems as potentially underpinning both depression and vascular pathology. The roles of oxidative stress and genetic polymorphisms have also seen increasing investigation as potentially underlying both depression and SVD (Wright et al. 2014). Brief consideration of this evidence is relevant in evaluating validity of the VaD construct, as significant developments have occurred since the original model was proposed.

7.4.1 Inflammation

Aberrant inflammatory processes, and specifically the role of pro-inflammatory cytokines (Alexopoulos and Morimoto 2011), are emerging as an area of interest in LLD. This interest parallels the more developed adult depression literature, which has outlined complex and as yet unresolved relationships between cytokines (Raison et al. 2005), monoamine neurotransmitter regulation (Harrison et al. 2009), glucocorticoid receptors (Pace et al. 2007) and neurotrophic function (Koo and Duman 2008). The ‘inflammatory hypothesis’ proposes that pro-inflammatory cytokines are central to the association between depression and cerebrovascular disease-mediated ischaemic injury, with both precipitating and maintaining roles (Wright et al. 2014). Li and colleagues (2014) considered the inflammatory hypothesis in the context of post-stroke depression, and arguably these principles can be applied to the vascular depression construct. There is substantive evidence that ischaemic neuronal injury triggers a pro-inflammatory cytokine cascade with downstream effects on neurotransmitter metabolism, neuroendocrine function (particularly HPA regulation) and neuroplasticity. These effects are highly biologically relevant with regard to models of depression. Administration of the pro-inflammatory cytokine interferon-α (IFN-α) has been reported to induce depressive symptoms including depressed mood and cognitive dysfunction (Dantzer et al. 2011). IL-1 and TNF-α have been demonstrated to increase serotonin, norepinephrine and dopamine metabolism in hypothalamic nuclei and limbic sites (Anisman and Hayley 2012). In addition, serotonergic tone is altered by pro-inflammatory cytokines via enhanced expression of the gene encoding for a tryptophan-degrading enzyme (indoleamine 2,3-dioxygenase, IDO). Downstream effects of the increase in IDO-mediated conversion of tryptophan to kynurenine include reduced serotonin concentrations in paralimbic regions and increased production of neurotoxic tryptophan catabolites (TRYCATs) (quinolinic acid, 3-hyrdroxykynurenine, kynurenic acid). Several groups have implicated reduced tryptophan and TRYCATs in the pathogenesis of depression (Maes et al. 2011; Dantzer et al. 2011). Pro-inflammatory cytokines have a reciprocal role in models of depression and vascular disease. They are both *triggered by* ischaemic cell damage and *contribute to* vascular disease. To illustrate this, IL-18, a marker of cardiovascular disease, has been implicated in atherosclerotic plaque development.

Glucocorticoids (GCs) significantly influence CNS neuronal function and are recognised as being active in neurodegenerative processes, including hippocampal neuronal degeneration. Increasing evidence suggests that GCs exact a greater effect in the context of excitotoxic or metabolic neuronal insult, including ischaemic injury. This is highly relevant to hypotheses of the interrelationship between depression, vascular disease, ischaemia and neuronal degeneration. Whilst the mechanisms of GC actions are yet to be fully elucidated, their role in glutamatergic tone, NMDA-receptor signalling and neuronal plasticity has been described (Franklin et al. 2012). Furthermore, experimental and clinical evidence has demonstrated that GC elevation may result in an increase in pro-inflammatory cytokines (Dantzer et al. 2011), thus establishing a critical link between the inflammatory and glucocorticoid pathways. The reciprocal relationship has also been described, with IL-1, IL-6 and TNF-a reported to directly stimulate HPA activity (Turnbull and Rivier 1999).

The glucocorticoid hypothesis as relevant to the VaD construct proposes that the state of LLD itself may be inherently neurotoxic and increase dementia risk via HPA chronic activity and chronic glucocorticoid exposure (Vu and Aizenstein 2013). Specifically, reduced hippocampal neuroplasticity has been proposed (Pittenger and Duman 2008) and supported by meta-analysis of MRI studies in LLD, which found the hippocampus to be one of the areas most associated with grey matter volume loss (Vu and Aizenstein 2013). In a comparison of hippocampal volume loss, greater volume loss was found in late-onset LLD compared with early-onset LLD (Hickie et al. 2005), potentially differentially supporting the GC hypothesis in the late-onset LLD group from the early-onset LLD group. Together with the aforementioned post-mortem neuropathological study by Tsopelas and colleagues (2011), which found hippocampal grey matter changes in LLD independent of neuropathological correlates of dementia, this evidence provides indirect support for the GC hypothesis.

7.4.2 Oxidative Stress

Oxidative stress and neuroinflammation have been pathophysiologically linked, via neurovascular dysfunction and altered blood-brain barrier hyperpermeability, with neurological disorders including Alzheimer's disease, epilepsy, multiple sclerosis, traumatic brain injury and stroke. Given the high rates of depression in these neurological disorders and the fact that depression is an independent risk factor for morbidity and mortality in disorders characterised by vascular endothelial dysfunction (Serlin et al. 2011) (including cerebrovascular disease), the role of oxidative stress in depression has been actively pursued. Meta-analytic data support a robust and bidirectional relationship between medical disorders characterised by endothelial dysfunction and major depressive disorder (MDD) (Valkanova and Ebmeier 2013). An evidence base has emerged that implicates oxidative stress in the neurobiology of depression. Specifically, experimental and clinical evidence increasingly supports the role of oxidative stress, endothelial nitric oxide synthase (eNOS) uncoupling and lowered levels of endothelial nitric oxide (NO) in the pathogenesis of peripheral vascular endothelial dysfunction that has been associated with depression (Najjar et al. 2013). Najjar and colleagues (2013) proposed putative mechanisms of oxidative stress and neuroinflammation in major depression mediated via neurovascular unit dysfunction with blood-brain barrier hyperpermeability. These mechanisms have already stimulated investigation of novel treatment targets (Scapagnini et al. 2012) for the effects of oxidative stress in vascular endothelial dysfunction as relevant to depression and other 'core' neurological disorders.

7.4.3 Genetics

Genetic polymorphisms that increase vascular risk with LLD (Taylor et al. 2013a) represent another exponentially expanding area of interest. The most widely cited are genetic variations associated with the renin-angiotensin system (RAS) (Kondo et al. 2007). RAS polymorphisms may have effects on hypothalamic-pituitary-adrenal (HPA) axis function (Annerbrink et al. 2010), monoamine neurotransmitter modulation (Baghai et al. 2002) and frontotemporal brain structure (Taylor et al. 2012), in addition to vascular effects mediated via blood pressure regulation and fluid homeostasis. Associations have been reported between RAS AGTR1 variants and severity of WMH progression and antidepressant response. The possibility of earlier life depression resulting in epigenetic modifications of genes implicated in vascular homeostasis (Zill et al. 2012) and pro-inflammatory activity (Miller et al. 2009; Surtees et al. 2008) has also been raised. Further studies are required to clarify the potential role of genetic polymorphisms and epigenetics in the VaD territory.

Conclusion

The concept of vascular depression as it was proposed initially implied an aetiological relationship between cerebrovascular disease and major depression and later became synonymous with an aetiological proposition. Our review suggests that the evidence in support of the VaD construct is not consistent. The supportive and nonsupportive evidence is summarised in Table 7.2. Epidemiological data demonstrating a bidirectional association between vascular disease and depression is robust, but this alone is insufficient to establish a causal relationship. A close temporal fit between diffuse cerebral SVD and incident depression is difficult to establish given methodological limitations, and there is limited evidence for a discrete VaD clinical phenotype. Evidence for heterogenous and interconnected pathomechanisms involving genetic, neurotransmitter, immune, oxidative and inflammatory systems (Najjar et al. 2013) support new explanatory models of the association between depression and vascular disease whilst also opening the doors for the future development of novel therapeutic targets and interventions. In light of the evidence that has emerged since its initial proposal,

Table 7.2 Summary table evaluating supportive and equivocal/nonsupportive evidence for validity of the 'vascular depression' hypothesis

Supportive evidence	Equivocal and nonsupportive evidence
Subcortical ischaemic depression affects clinical presentation, long-term outcomes and response to antidepressant therapy, arguing that it is a valid diagnostic entity worth further study (Taylor et al. 2006)	The exponential increase age-related CVD prevalence is not paralleled by an exponential increase in depression prevalence in epidemiological studies
There is an increased frequency of subcortical WMHs in older people with depression compared with nondepression age-matched control subjects (Taylor et al. 2003a)	Delineation of a specific clinical phenotype of vascular depression has not been possible. Whilst vascular depression is reported as more frequently associated with psychomotor retardation, executive dysfunction, anhedonia, reduced motivation and fatigue, these findings have not been consistently replicated
Subcortical WMHs are more frequent in late-onset LLD when compared to early-onset LLD even following adjustment for age (Krishnan et al. 1997; Lavretsky et al. 1998)	The mechanism by which SVD directly results in depression has not been clarified; current mechanistic hypotheses propose that immune and other non-vascular systems are of equal import to vascular disease. These systems are complex and integrated and do not function in isolation
Prospective studies have reported WMH burden to have predictive validity in relation to deterioration in depressive symptoms/long-term course (Steffens et al. 2002) and emergent depressive episodes (Godin et al. 2008)	A threshold model whereby vulnerability to depression is conferred by WMLs and precipitated by other biological and non-biological triggers is plausible
A meta-analytic review found depressive-executive dysfunction to correlate with poor antidepressant response, lower remission and higher relapse rates (McLennan and Mathias 2010)	No correlation has been demonstrated between manipulation of WMH lesion progression and depression outcomes (Taylor et al. 2006); thus, strictly WMHs cannot be defined as causal in relation to depression
Strategic location of WMHs has been reported to influence severity of depression	There is an absence of evidence (from secondary analysis of RCTs) that modification or treatment of vascular risk factors, including hypertension, hyperlipidaemia and hyperhomocystinaemia, reduces the incidence of depression or reduces the severity of existing depressive symptoms (Almeida 2008)

Table 7.2 (continued)

Supportive evidence	Equivocal and nonsupportive evidence
WMHs located in the frontal lobes, basal ganglia and pons (Steffens et al. 2002; Taylor et al. 2003a; MacFall et al. 2006; Alexopoulos et al. 2002b) have been correlated with poorer depression prognosis	The chronic illness hypothesis: the prevalence of depression in other chronic illnesses is elevated to similar levels as seen in post-stroke and myocardial infarct, including in neurological (Rickards 2005) and rheumatological (Dickens et al. 2002) disorders and in chronic obstructive pulmonary disease (Krishnan 2002). When physical health has been included as a covariate, the relationship between depression and WMHs has been found non-significant in some studies (Jorm et al. 2005)
WMHs located in specific white matter tracts have also demonstrated an association with severity of depression, including the superior longitudinal fasciculus, cingulum and uncinate fasciculus (Sheline et al. 2008; Taylor et al. 2013b; Dalby et al. 2010). These same tracts have been implicated in adult studies of depression	
Lower rates of positive familial mood or psychiatric disorder have been reported in those with SVD and depression (Taylor et al. 2003a)	

as a diagnostic construct, 'vascular depression' is arguably now somewhat misleading in its agnostic ascription of vascular disease as *causative* of depression. Utility is however purpose dependent, and the construct has contributed significantly to lines of research that have enabled the complexity of the association to begin to be disentangled. It is hoped that further development of such lines of research will deliver future novel therapeutic targets.

References

Ajilore O, Narr K, Rosenthal J, Pham D, Hamilton L, Watari K et al (2010) Regional cortical grey matter thickness differences associated with type 2 diabetes and major depression. Psychiatry Res 184(2):63–70

Alexopoulos GS (2001) 'The Depression-Executive Dysfunction Syndrome of Late Life': a specific target for D3 agonists? Am J Geriatr Psychiatry 9(1):22–29

Alexopoulos GS (2005) Depression in the elderly. Lancet 365(9475):1961–1970

Alexopoulos GS, Morimoto SS (2011) The inflammation hypothesis in geriatric depression. Int J Geriatr Psychiatry 26(11):1109–1118

Alexopoulos GS, Meyers BS, Young RC, Kakuma T, Silbersweig D, Charlson M (1997a) Clinically defined vascular depression. Am J Psychiatry 154(4):562–565

Alexopoulos GS, Meyers BS, Young RC, Campbell S, Silbersweig D, Charlson M (1997b) 'Vascular depression' hypothesis. Arch Gen Psychiatry 54(10):915–922

Alexopoulos GS, Kiosses DN, Klimstra S, Kalayam B, Bruce ML (2002a) Clinical presentation of the "depression-executive dysfunction syndrome" of late life. Am J Geriatr Psychiatry 10(1):98–106

Alexopoulos GS, Klosses DN, Choi SJ, Murphy CF, Lim KO (2002b) Frontal white matter microstructure and treatment response of late-life depression: a preliminary study. Am J Psychiatry 159(11):1929–1932

Almeida OP (2008) Vascular depression: myth or reality? Int Psychogeriatr 20(4):645–652

Anisman H, Hayley S (2012) Inflammatory factors contribute to depression and its comorbid conditions. Sci Signal 5(244):pe45
Annerbrink K, Jonsson EG, Olsson M, Nilsson S, Sedvall GC, Anckarster H et al (2010) Associations between the angiotensin-converting enzyme insertion/deletion polymorphism and monoamine metabolite concentrations in cerebrospinal fluid. Psychiatry Res 179(2):231–234
Bae JN, MacFall, Krishnan KR, Payne ME, Steffens DC, Taylor WD (2006) Dorsolateral prefrontal cortex and anterior cingulate cortex white matter alterations in late-life depression. Biol Psychiatry 60(12):1356–1363
Baghai TC, Schule C, Zwanzger P, Minov C, Zill P, Ella R et al (2002) Hypothalamic-pituitary-adrenocortical axis dysregulation in patients with major depression is influenced by the insertion/deletion polymorphism in the angiotensin 1-converting enzyme gene. Neurosci Lett 328(3):299–303
Baldwin RC (2005) Is vascular depression a distinct sub-type of depressive disorder? A review of causal evidence. Int J Geriatr Psychiatry 20(1):1–11
Baldwin RC, Tomenson B (1995) Depression in later life. A comparison of symptoms and risk factors in early and late onset cases. Br J Psychiatry 167(5):649–652
Baune B, Stuart M, Gilmour A, Wersching H, Arolt V, Berger K (2012) Moderators of the relationship between depression and cardiovascular disorders: a systematic review. Gen Hosp Psychiatry 34(5):478–492
Bhogal SK, Teasell R, Foley N, Speechley M (2004) Lesion location and poststroke depression: systematic review of the methodological limitations of the literature. Stroke 35(3):794–802
Breitner C, Husain MM, Figiel GS, Krishnan KR, Koyko OB (1990) Cerebral white matter disease in late-onset paranoid psychosis. Biol Psychiatry 28(3):266–274
Brodaty H, Luscombe G, Parker G, Wilhelm K, Hickie I, Austin MP, Mitchell P (2001) Early and late onset depression in old age: different aetiologies, same phenomenology. J Affect Disord 66(2–3):225–236
Brodaty H, Cullen B, Thompson C, Mitchell P, Parker G, Wilhelm K, Austin MP, Mahli G (2005) Age and gender in the phenomenology of depression. Am J Geriatr Psychiatry 13(7):589–596
Brodaty H, Withall A, Altendorf A, Sachdev PS (2007) Rates of depression at 3 and 15 months poststroke and their relationship with cognitive decline: the Sydney Stroke Study. Am J Geriatr Psychiatry 15(6):477–486
Brookes RL, Herbert VH, Lawrence AJ, Morris RG, Markus HS (2014) Depression in small-vessel disease relates to white matter ultrastructural damage, not disability. Neurology 83(16):1417–1423
Carney RM, Rich WM, Tevelde A, Saini J, Clark K, Jaffe AS (1987) Major depressive disorder in coronary artery disease. Am J Cardiol 140(16):1072–1074
Carvalho AF, Miskowiak KK, Hyphantis TN et al (2014) Cognitive dysfunction in depression – pathophysiology and novel targets. CNS Neurol Disord Drug Targets 13(10):1819–1835
Chavhan GB, Babyn PS, Thomas B, Shroff MM, Haacke EM (2009) Principles, techniques, and applications of T2-based MR imaging and its special applications. Radiographics 29(5):1433–1449
Coffey CE, Figiel GS, Djang WT, Sullivan DC, Herfkens RJ, Weiner RD (1988) Effects of ECT on brain structure: a pilot prospective magnetic resonance imaging study. Am J Psychiatry 17(8): 701–706
Coffey CE, Figiel GS, Djang WT, Weiner RD (1990) Subcortical hyperintensity on magnetic resonance imaging: a comparison of normal and depressed elderly subjects. Am J Pyschiatry 147(2):187–189
Corruble E, Gorwood P, Falissard B (2008) Association between age of onset and symptom profiles in late-life depression. Act Psychiatr Scand 118(5):389–394
Dalby RB, Chakravarty MM, Ahdidan J et al (2010) Localisation of white-matter lesions and effect of vascular risk factors in late-onset major depression. Psychol Med 40(8):1389–1399
Dantzer R, O'Connor JC, Lawson MA, Kelley KW (2011) Inflammation-associated depression: from serotonin to kynurenine. Psychoneuroendocrinology 36(3):426–436

Deisseroth K, Schnitzer MJ (2013) Engineering approaches to illuminating brain structure and dynamics. Neuron 80(3):568–577

Devanand DP, Adorno E, Cheng J, Burt T, Pelton GH, Roose SP, Sackheim HA (2004) Late onset dysthymic disorder and major depression differ from early onset dysthymic disorder and major depression in elderly outpatients. J Affect Disord 78(3):259–267

Dickens C, McGowan L, Clark-Carter D, Creed F (2002) Depression in rheumatoid arthritis: a systematic review of the literature with meta-analysis. Psychosom Med 64(1):52–60

Dieguez S, Staub F, Brugginmann L, Bogousslavsky J (2004) Is poststroke depression a vascular depression? J Neurol Sci 226(1–2):53–58

Diniz BS, Butters MA, Albert SM, Dew MA, Reynolds CF (2013) Late-life depression and risk of vascular dementia and Alzheimer's disease: systematic review and meta-analysis of community-based cohort studies. Br J Psychiatry 202(5):329–335

Doyle T, Halaris A, Rao M (2014) Shared neurobiological pathways between type 2 diabetes and depressive symptoms: a review of morphological and neurocognitive findings. Curr Diabet Rep 14(12):560. doi:10.1007/s11892-014-0560-7

Egeto P, Fischer CE, Ismail Z, Smith EE, Schweizer TA (2014) Lacunar stroke, deep white matter disease and depression: a meta-analysis. Int Psychogeriatr 26(7):1101–1109

Figiel GS, Krishnan KR, Doraiswamy PM (1990) Subcortical structural changes in ECT-induced delirium. J Geriatr Psychiatry Neurol 3(3):172–176

Figiel GS, Krishnan KRR, Doraiswamy PM, Rao VP, Nemeroff CB, Boyko OB (1991) Subcortical hyperintensities on brain magnetic resonance imaging: a comparison between late age onset and early onset elderly depressed subjects. Neurobiol Aging 12(3):245–247

Ford DE, Mead LA, Chang PP, Cooper-Patrick L, Wang NY, Klag MJ (1998) Depression is a risk factor for coronary artery disease in men: the precursors study. Arch Intern Med 158(13):1422–1426

Franklin TB, Saab BJ, Mansuy IM (2012) Neural mechanisms of stress resilience and vulnerability. Neuron 75(5):747–761

Fujikawa T, Yamawaki S, Touhouda Y (1994) Background factors and clinical symptoms of major depression with silent cerebral infarction. Stroke 25(4):798–801

Godin O, Dufouil C, Maillard P, Delcroix N, Mazoyer B, Crivello F, Alpérovitch A, Tzourio C (2008) White matter lesions as a predictor of depression in the elderly: the 3C-Dijon study. Biol Psychiatry 63(7):663–669

Greenwald BS, Kramer-Ginsberg E (1988) Age at onset in geriatric depression: relationship to clinical variables. J Affect Disord 15(1):61–68

Greenwald BS, Kramer-Ginsberg E, Krishnan KR, Ashtari M, Auerback C, Patel M (1998) Neuroanatomic localisation of magnetic resonance imaging signal hyperintensities in geriatric depression. Stroke 29(3):613–617

Harrison NA, Brydon L, Walker C, Gray MA, Steptoe A, Crtichley HD (2009) Inflammation causes mood changes through alterations in subgenual cingulate activity and mesolimbic connectivity. Biol Psychiatry 66(5):407–414

Herrmann IL, Le Masurier M, Ebmeier KP (2008) White matter hyperintensities in late life depression: a systematic review. J Neurol Neurosurg Psychiatry 79(6):619–624

Hickie I, Scott E, Mitchell P et al (1995) Subcortical hyperintensities on magnetic resonance imaging: clinical correlates and prognostic significance in patients with severe depression. Biol Psychiatry 37(3):151–160

Hickie I, Scott E, Naismith S, Ward PB, Turner K, Parker G, Mitchell P, Wilhelm K (2001) Late-onset depression: genetic, vascular and clinical contributions. Psychol Med 31(8):1403–1412

Hickie I, Naismith S, Ward PB et al (2005) Reduced hippocampal volumes and memory loss in patients with early- and late-onset depression. Br J Psychiatry 186:197–202

Ikram MA, Luijendijk HJ, Vernooij MW, Hofman A, Niessen WJ, van der Lujt A, Tiemeier H, Breteler MM (2010) Vascular brain disease and depression in the elderly. Epidemiology 21(1):78–81

Janssen J, Beekman AT, Comijs HC, Deeg DJ, Heeren TJ (2006) Late-life depression: the differences between early- and late-onset illness in a community-based sample. Int J Geriatr Psychiatry 21(1):86–93

Jonas BS, Mussolino ME (2000) Symptoms of depression as a prospective risk factor for stroke. Psychosom Med 62(4):463–471

Jorm AF, Anstey KJ, Christensen H, de Plater G, Kumar R, Wen W, Sachdev P (2005) MRI hyperintensities and depressive symptoms in a community sample of individuals 60–64 years old. Am J Psychiatry 162(4):699–705

Kelly RE, Alexopoulos GS (2009) The vascular depression concept and its implications. In: Ellison JM, Kyomen HH, Verma S (eds). Mood disorders in later life. 2nd ed. Informa Healthcare, New York, pp 161–178

Khan U, Porteous L, Hassan A, Markus HS (2007) Risk factor profile of cerebral small vessel disease and its subtypes. J Neurol Neurosurg Psychiatry 78(7):702–706

Khundakar AA, Thomas AJ (2014) Am J Geriatr Psychiatry 22(2):122–132

Kivimaki M, Shipley MJ, Allan CL, Sexton CE, Jokela M, Virtanen M et al (2012) Vascular risk status as a predictor of later-life depressive symptoms: a cohort study. Biol Psychiatry 72(4):324–330

Kohler S, Thomas AJ, Lloyd A et al (2010) White matter hyperintensities, cortisol levels, brain atrophy and continuing cognitive deficits in late-life depression. Br J Psychiatry 196(2):143–149

Kondo DG, Speer MC, Krishnan KR, McQuoid DR, Slifer SH, Pieper CF, Billups AV, Steffens DC et al (2007) Association of AGTR1 with 18-month treatment outcome in late-life depression. Am J Geriatr Psychiatry 15(7):564–572

Koo JW, Duman RS (2008) IL-1 beta is an essential mediator of the antineurogenic and anhedonic effects of stress. Proc Natl Acad Sci U S A 105(2):751–756

Krishnan KRR (1993) Neuroanatomic substrates of depression in the elderly. J Geriatr Psychiatry Neurol 6(1):39–58

Krishnan KR (2002) Comorbidity of depression with other medical diseases in the elderly. Biol Psychiatry 15(6):559–588

Krishnan KR (2005) Psychiatric disease in the genomic era: rational approach. Mol Psychiatry 10(11):978–974

Krishnan KRR, McDonald WM (1995) Arteriosclerotic depression. Med Hypotheses 44(2):111–115

Krishnan KRR, Goli V, Ellinwood EH, France RD, Blazer DG, Nemeroff CB (1988) Leukoencephalopathy in patients diagnosed as major depressive. Biol Psychiatry 23(5):519–522

Krishnan KR, Hays JC, Tupler LA, George LK, Blazer DG (1995) Clinical and phenomenological comparisons of late-onset and early-onset depression. Am J Psychiatry 152(5):785–788

Krishnan KR, Hays JC, Blazer DG (1997) MRI-defined vascular depression. Am J Psychiatry 154(4):497–501

Krishnan KR, Taylor WD, Dr McQuoid et al (2004) Clinical characteristics of magnetic resonance imaging-defined subcortical ischaemic depression. Biol Psychiatry 55(4):390–397

Krishnan MS, O'Brien JT, Firbank MJ, Pantoni L, Carlucci G, Erkinjutti T et al (2006) Relationship between periventricular and deep white matter lesions and depressive symptoms in older people: the LADIS Study. Int J Geriatr Psychiatry 21(10):983–989

Lavretsky H, Lesser IM, Wohl M, Miller BL (1998) Relationship of age, age at onset, and sex to depression in older adults. Am J Geriatr Psychiatry 6(3):248–256

Li W, Ling S, Yang Y, Hu Z, Davies H, Fang M (2014) Systematic hypothesis for post-stroke depression caused inflammation and neurotransmission and resultant on possible treatments. Neuroendocrinol Lett 35(2):104–109

Lipsey JR, Spencer WC, Rabins PV, Robinson RG (1986) Phenomenological comparison of post-stroke depression and functional depression. Am J Psychiatry 143(4):527–529

Loubinoux I, Kronenberg G, Endres M, Schumann-Bard P, Freret T, Filipkowski RK, Kaczmarek L, Popa-Wagner A (2012) Poststroke depression: mechanisms, translation and therapy. J Cell Mol Med 16(9):1961–1969

Lujjendijk HJ, Stricker BH, Wieberdink RG, Koudstaal PJ, Hofman A, Breteler MM, Tiemeier H (2011) Transient ischaemic attack and incident depression. Stroke 42(7):1857–1861

Lyness JM, Caine ED, Cox C, King DA, Conwell Y, Olivares T (1998) Cerebrovascular risk factors and later-life major depression. Testing a small-vessel brain disease model. Am J Geriatr Psychiatry 6(1):5–13

Lyness JM, King DA, Conwell Y, Cox C, Caine ED (2000) Cerebrovascular risk factors and 1-year depression outcome in older primary care patients. Am J Psychiatry 157(9):1499–1501

MacFall JR, Payne ME, Provenzale JM, Krishnan KR (2001) Medial orbital frontal lesions in late-onset depression. Biol Psychiatry 49(9):803–806

MacFall JR, Taylor WD, Rex DE, Pieper S, Payne ME, McQuoid D et al (2006) Lobar distribution of lesion volumes in late-life depression: the Biomedical Information Research Network (BIRN). Neuropsychopharmacology 31(7):1500–1507

Maes M, Leonard B, Myint A, Kubera M, Verkerk R (2011) The new '5-HT' hypothesis of depression: cell-mediated immune activation induces indoleamine 2, 3-dioxygenase, which leads to lower plasma tryptophan and an increased synthesis of detrimental tryptophan catabolites (TRYCATs), both of which contribute to the onset of depression. Prog Neuro-Psychopharmacol Biol Psychiatry 35(3):702–721

McDonald WM, Tupler LA, Marsteller FA, Figiel GS, DiSouza S, Nemeroff CB et al (1999) Hyperintense lesions on magnetic resonance images in bipolar disorder. Biol Psychiatry 45(8):965–971

McDougall F, Brayne C (2007) Systematic review of the depressive symptoms associated with vascular conditions. J Affect Disord 104(1–3):25–35

McLennan SN, Mathias JL (2010) The depression-executive dysfunction (DED) syndrome and response to antidepressants: a meta-analytic review. Int J Geriatr Psychiatry 25(10):933–944

Mettenburg JM, Benzinger TL, Shimony JS et al (2012) Diminished performance on neuropsychological testing in late life depression is correlated with microstructural white matter abnormalities. Neuroimage 60(4):2182–2190

Miller AH, Maletic V, Raison CL (2009) Inflammation and its discontents: the role of cytokines in the pathophysiology of major depression. Biol Psychiatry 65(9):732–741

Najjar S, Pearlman DM, Devinsky O, Najjar A, Zagzag D (2013) Neurovascular unit dysfunction with blood-brain barrier hyperpermeability contributes to major depressive disorder: a review of clinical and experimental evidence. J Neuroinflammation 10:142

Nucifora PG, Verma R, Lee SK, Melhem ER (2007) Diffusion-tensor MR imaging and tractography: exploring brain microstructure and connectivity. Radiology 245(2):367–384

Ovbiagele B, Salver JL (2006) Cerebral white matter hyperintensities on MRI: current concepts and therapeutic implications. Cerebrovasc Dis 22(2–3):83–90

Pace TW, Hu F, Miller AH (2007) Cytokine effects on glucocorticoid receptor function: relevance to glucocorticoid resistance and the pathophysiology and treatment of major depression. Brain Behav Immun 21(1):9–19

Pantoni L, Garcia JH (1997) Pathogenesis of leukoaraiosis: a review. Stroke 28(3):652–659

Pittenger C, Duman RS (2008) Stress, depression, and neuroplasticity: a convergence of mechanisms. Neuropsychopharmacology 33(1):88–109

Pratt LA, Ford DE, Crum RM, Armenian HK, Gallo JJ, Eaton WW (1996) Depression, psychotropic medication, and risk of myocardial infarction. Prospective data from the Baltimore ECA follow-up. Circulation 94(12):3123–3129

Rabkin JG, Charles E, Kass F (1983) Hypertension and DSM-III depression in psychiatric outpatients. Am J Psychiatry 140(8):1072–1074

Raison CL, Demetrashvili M, Caproun L, Miller AH (2005) Neuropsychiatric adverse effects of interferon-alpha: recognition and management. CNS Drugs 19(2):105–123

Rapp MA, Dahlman K, Sano M, Grossman HT, Haroutunian V, Gorman JM (2005) Neuropsychological differences between late-onset and recurrent geriatric major depression. Am J Psychiatry 162(4):691–698

Rickards H (2005) Depression in neurological disorders: Parkinson's disease, multiple sclerosis, and stroke. J Neurol Neurosurg Psychiatry 76(Suppl.1):i48–i52

Robinson RG (2005) Vascular depression and poststroke depression where do we go from here? Am J Geriatr Psychiatry 13(2):85–87

Robinson RG, Spalletta G (2010) Poststroke depression: a review. Can J Psychiatry 55(6):341–349
Robinson RG, Kubo KL, Starr LB, Rao K, Price TR (1984a) Mood disorders in stroke patients: importance of location of lesion. Brain 107(Pt 1):81–93
Robinson RG, Starr LB, Lipsey JR, Rao K, Price TR (1984b) A two-year longitudinal study of post-stroke mood disorders: dynamic changes in associated variables over the first six months of follow-up. Stroke 15(3):510–517
Sachdev PS, Reutens S (2014) Psychiatric consequences of small vessel disease. In: Pantoni L, Gorlick PB (eds) Clinical aspects of cerebral small vessel disease. Cambridge Univ Press, Cambridge, pp 261–272
Sachdev PS, Brodaty H, Valenzuela MJ, Lorentz L, Looi JC, Wen W, Zagami AS (2004) The neuropsychological profile of vascular cognitive impairment in stroke and TIA patients. Neurology 62(6):912–919
Salaycik KJ, Kelly-Hayes M, Beiser A, Nguyen A-H, Brady SM, Kase CS (2007) etal. Depressive symptoms and risk of stroke: the Framingham Study. Stroke 79(6):619–624
Sanders ML, Lyness JM, Eberly S, King DA, Caine ED (2006) Cerebrovascular risk factors, executive dysfunction, and depression in older primary care patients. Am J Geriatr Psychiatry 14(2):145–152
Scapagnini G, Davinelli S, Drago F, De Lorenzo A, Oriani G (2012) Antioxidants as antidepressants: fact or fiction? CNS Drugs 26(6):477–490
Seminowicz DA, Mayberg HS, McIntosh AR et al (2004) Limbic-frontal circuitry in major depression: a path modeling meta-analysis. NeuroImage 22(1):409–418
Serlin Y, Levy J, Shalev H (2011) Vascular pathology and blood-brain barrier disruption in cognitive and psychiatric complications of type 2 diabetes mellitus. Cardiovasc Psychiatry Neurol 2011:609202
Sexton CE, McDermott L, Kalu UG, Hermann LL, Bradley KM, Allan CL et al (2011) Exploring the pattern and neural correlates of neuropsychological impairment in late-life depression. Psychol Med 42(6):1195–1202
Sexton CE, Allan CL, Le Masurier M et al (2012) Magnetic resonance imaging in late-life depression: multimodal examination of network. Arch Gen Psychiatry 69(7):680–689
Sheline YI, Price JL, Vaishnavi SN, Mintun MA, Barch DM, Epstein AA et al (2008) Regional white matter hyperintensity burden in automated segmentation distinguishes late-life depressed subjects from comparison subjects matched for vascular risk factors. Am J Psychiatry 165(4):524–532
Simpson SW, Jackson A, Baldwin RC, Burns A (1997) Subcortical hyperintensities in late-life depression: acute response to treatment and neuropsychological impairment. Int Psychogeriatr 9(3):257–275
Simpson S, Baldwin RC, Jackson A, Burns AS (1998) Is subcortical disease associated with a poor response to antidepressants? Neurological, neuropsychological and neuroradiological findings in late life depression. Psychol Med 28(5):1015–1026
Sneed JR, Culang-Reinlieb (2011) The vascular depression hypothesis: an update. Am J Geriatr Psychiatry 19(2):99–103
Steffens DC, Conway CR, Dombeck CB, Wagner HR, Tupler LA, Weiner RD (2001) Severity of subcortical gray matter hyperintensity predicts ECT response in geriatric depression. J ECT 17(1):45–49
Steffens DC, Krishnan KRR, Crump C, Burke GL (2002) Cerebrovascular disease and evolution of depressive symptoms in the cardiovascular health study. Stroke 33(6):1636–1644
Steinberg EE, Christoffel DJ, Deisseroth K, Malenka RC (2015) Illuminating circuitry relevant to psychiatric disorders with optogenetics. Curr Opin Neurobiol 30:9–16
Stewart R, Hirani V (2010) General health status and vascular disorders as correlates of late-life depressive symptoms in a national survey sample. Int J Geriatr Psychiatry 25(5):483–488
Stockmeier CA, Mahajan GJ, Konick LC, Overholser JC, Jurjus GJ, Meltzer HY et al (2004) Cellular changes in the post-mortem hippocampus in major depression. Biol Psychiatry 56(9):640–650

Surtees PG, Wainwright NM, Boekholdt SM, Luben RN, Wareham NJ, Khaw KT (2008) Major depression, C-reactive protein, and incident ischaemic heart disease in healthy men and women. Psychosom Med 70(8):850–855
Tang WK, Chen YK, Lu JY, Chu WC, Mok VC, Ungvari GS, Wong KS (2011a) Cerebral microbleeds and symptom severity of post-stroke depression: a magnetic resonance imaging study. J Affect Disord 129(1–3):354–358
Tang WK, Lu JY, Chen JK, Chu WC, Mok V, Ungvari GS, Wong KS (2011b) Association of frontal subcortical circuit infarcts in poststroke depression: a magnetic resonance imaging study of 591 Chinese patients with ischaemic stroke. J Geriatr Psychiatry Neurol 24(1):44–49
Taragano FE, Allegri R, Vicario A, Bagnatti P, Lyketsos CG (2001) A double blind, randomised clinical trial assessing the efficacy and safety of augmenting standardised antidepressant therapy with nimodipine in the treatment of "vascular depression". Int J Geriatr Psychiatry 16(3):254–260
Taylor WD, MacFall JR, Steffens DC, Payne ME, Provenzale JM, Krishnan KR (2003a) Localisation of age-associated white matter hyperintensities in late-life depression. Prog Neurospcyhopharmacol Biol Psychiatry 27(3):539–544
Taylor WD, Steffens DC, MacFall JR, McQuoid DR, Payne ME, Provenzale JM, Krishnan KRR (2003b) White matter hyperintensity progression and late life depression outcomes. Arch Gen Psychiatry 60(11):1090–1096
Taylor WD, Steffens DC, Krishnan KR (2006) Psychiatric disease in the twenty-first century: the case for subcortical ischaemic depression. Biol Psychiatry 60(12):1299–1303
Taylor WD, Benjamin S, McQuoid DR, Payne ME, Krishnan RR, MacFall JR et al (2012) AGTR1 gene variation: association with depression and frontotemporal morphology. Psychiatry Res 202(2):104–109
Taylor WD, Aizenstein HJ, Alexopoulos GS (2013a) The vascular depression hypothesis: mechanisms linking vascular disease with depression. Mol Psychiatry 18(9):963–974
Taylor WD, Zhao Z, Ashley-Koch A et al (2013b) Fiber tract specific white matter lesion severity. Findings in late life depression and by AGTR1 A1166C genotype. Hum Brain Mapp 34(2):295–303
Teodorczuk A, Firbank MJ, Pantoni L, Pggessi A, Erkinjuntti T, Wallin A et al (2010) Relationship between baseline white-matter changes and development of late-life depressive symptoms:3-year results from the LADIS study. Psychol Med 40(4):603–610
Thomas AJ (2013) Vascular depression. In: Ferro FM (ed) Neuropsychiatric symptoms of cerebrovascular diseases. Springer, London, pp 299–305
Thomas AJ, Ferrier IN, Kalaria RN, Perry RH, Brown A, O'Brien JT (2001) A neuropathological study of vascular factors in late-life depression. J Neurol Neurosurg Psychiatry 70(1):83–87
Thomas AJ, O'Brien JT, Davis S, Ballard C, Barber R, Kalaria RN, Perry RH (2002) Ischaemic basis for deep white matter hyperintensities in major depression: a neuropathological study. Arch Gen Psychiatry 59(9):785–792
Thomas AJ, Perry R, Kalaria RN, Oakley A, McMeekin W, O'Brien JT (2003a) Neuropathological evidence for ischaemia in the white matter of the dorsolateral prefrontal cortex in late-life depression. Int J Geriatr Psychiatry 18(1):7–13
Thomas AJ, Kalaria RN, O'Brien JT (2004) Depression and vascular disease: what is the relationship? J Affect Disord 79(1–3):81–95
Tonkonogy JM, Geller JL (1999) Late-onset paranoid psychosis as a distinct clinicopathologic entity: magnetic resonance imaging data in elderly patients with paranoid psychosis of late onset and schizophrenia of early onset. Neuropsychiatry Neuropsychol Behav Neurol 12(4):230–235
Tsopelas C, Stewart R, Sawa GM et al (2011) Neuropathological correlates of late-life depression in older people. Br J Psychiatry 198(2):109–114
Turnbull AV, Rivier CL (1999) Regulation of the hypothalamic-pituitary-adrenal axis by cytokines: actions and mechanisms of action. Physiol Rev 79(1):1–71
Valenti R, Poggesi A, Pescini F, Inzitari D, Pantoni L (2008) Psychiatric disturbances in CADASIL: a brief review. Acta Neurol Scand 118(5):291–295
Valkanova V, Ebmeier K (2013) Vascular risk factors and depression in later life: a systematic review and meta-analysis. Biol Psychiatry 73(5):406–413

Vataja R, Leppavuori A, Pohjasvaara T, Mantyla R, Aronen HJ, Salonen O, Kaste M, Erkinjuntti T (2004) Poststroke depression and lesion location revisited. J Neuropsychiatry Clin Neurosci 16(2):156–162

Verslius CE, van der Mast RC, van Buchem MA, Bollen MA, Bollen EL, Blauw GJ, Eekhof JA et al (2006) Progression of cerebral white matter lesions is not associated with development of depressive symptoms in elderly subjects at risk of cardiovascular disease: the PROSPER study. In J Geriatr Psychiatry 21(4):375–381

Vu NQ, Aizenstein HJ (2013) Depression in the elderly: brain correlates, neuropsychological findings, and role of vascular lesion load. Curr Opin Neurol 26(6):656–661

Wade DT, Legh-Smith J, Hewer RA (1987) Depressed mood after stroke. A community study of its frequency. Br J Psychiatry 151:200–205

Wen W, Sachdev PS (2004) The topography of white matter hyperintensities on brain MRI in healthy 60- to 64-year-old individuals. Neuroimage 22(1):144–154

Wen W, Sachdev PS, Li JJ, Chen X, Anstey KJ (2009) White matter hyperintensities in the forties: their prevalence and topography in an epidemiological sample aged 44–48. Hum Brain Mapp 30(4):1155–1167

Whyte EM, Mulsant BH (2003) Poststroke depression: prevalence, diagnosis, treatment, and disease progression. Biol Psychiatry 54(3):376–387

Wright L, Simpson W, Van Lieshout RJ (2014) Steiner. Depression and cardiovascular disease in women: is there a common immunological basis? A theoretical synthesis. Ther Adv Cardiovasc Dis 8(2):56–69

Xiong YY, Wong A, Mok VC, Tang WK, Lam WW, Kwok TC, Chu WC, Chan AY, Wong LK (2011) Frequency and predictors of proxy-confirmed post-stroke cognitive complaints in lacunar stroke patients without major depression. Int J Geriatr Psychiatry 26:1144–1151

Zill P, Baghai TC, Schule C, Born C, Frustuck C, Buttner A et al (2012) DNA methylation analysis of the angiotensin converting enzyme (ACE) in major depression. PLoS ONE 7(7):e40479

Zou K, Huang X, Li T, Gong Q, Li Z, Ou-yang L et al (2008) Alterations of white matter integrity on adults with major depressive disorder: a magnetic resonance imaging study. Psychiatry Neurosci 33(6):525–530

Mental Stress-Induced Myocardial Ischemia

8

Viola Vaccarino

Contents

Abstract

Acute psychological stress induced in the laboratory can provoke myocardial ischemia in a substantial proportion of cardiac patients. This phenomenon, known as mental stress-induced myocardial ischemia (MSIMI), represents a "proof-of-concept" of the adverse effects of acute psychological stress on the heart in susceptible individuals. MSIMI clearly demonstrates that ischemic responses can be induced by relatively mild behavioral challenges similar to

This work was supported in part by grants from the National Institutes of Health (K24 HL077506, R21 HL093665, R01 HL109413 and P01 HL101398).

V. Vaccarino, MD, PhD
Department of Epidemiology, Rollins School of Public Health, Emory University, 1518 Clifton Rd NE, Room 3011, Atlanta, GA 30322, USA
e-mail: viola.vaccarino@emory.edu

B.T. Baune, P.J. Tully (eds.), *Cardiovascular Diseases and Depression*,
DOI 10.1007/978-3-319-32480-7_8

those that might be encountered in everyday life and not merely by extreme emotional stress. MSIMI has considerable prognostic significance, since it is linked to about twofold increased risk of cardiac events and mortality. Despite this, MSIMI remains relatively understudied and underappreciated. Some subgroups of patients, such as women and individuals with depression, appear to be especially vulnerable to MSIMI for reasons that are not yet clear; whether MSIMI plays a role in the adverse outcomes associated with depression needs further study. MSIMI is clearly distinct from ischemia induced by conventional stress testing, such as exercise or pharmacological stress testing. It is typically without pain, generally not related to severity of coronary artery disease, and occurs at lower levels of oxygen demand. Stress-induced vascular changes, particularly increases in systemic vascular resistance, coronary artery vasomotion, and microvascular function, may all contribute to this pattern of ischemia. While evidence of effective interventions for MSIMI is still limited, emerging data suggest that selective serotonin reuptake inhibitors and perhaps angiotensin-converting enzyme inhibitors might be beneficial in patients with MSIMI, as well as behavioral interventions for stress reduction.

8.1 Psychological Stress and Coronary Heart Disease

There is growing evidence that psychological stress can increase the risk of coronary heart disease (CHD) or accelerate its natural course. Psychological stress can affect CHD risk factors such as hypertension and hyperinsulinemia, can promote progression of atherosclerosis, and can impair prognosis, recovery, and quality of life of patients who have survived an acute coronary syndrome such as a myocardial infarction (Steptoe and Kivimaki 2013). In a large international case-control study, stress was associated with a greater than twofold increase in the risk for myocardial infarction (Rosengren et al. 2004).

Acute stress, in particular, has been implicated in heart disease for more than a century and has been investigated using a number of approaches, from epidemiological research to mechanistic studies, animal models, psychophysiological experiments, and clinical investigations. From human studies there is evidence that bouts of anger, acute bereavement, intense fear, and extreme excitement can trigger an acute myocardial infarction or sudden cardiac death in susceptible individuals (Bhattacharyya and Steptoe 2007; Mostofsky et al. 2012, 2013; Steptoe and Kivimaki 2013). In addition, animal models, particularly nonhuman primates, have provided direct experimental evidence of the adverse cardiovascular effects of psychological stress (Kaplan et al. 2009; Shively et al. 2009).

The autonomic nervous system is thought to be the mediator of such effects through its complex actions on cardiovascular hemodynamics, cardiac conduction, endothelial function, metabolism, immunity, coagulation, and inflammation. In terms of acute stress, a sudden increase in sympathetic nervous system activation and/or acute vagal withdrawal may cause a rise in cardiac oxygen demands or acute coronary vasoconstriction predisposing to myocardial ischemia and left ventricular dysfunction in susceptible individuals. Severe stress, accompanied by exaggerated sympathetic nervous system stimulation, can also induce myocardial stunning with severe, reversible left ventricular dysfunction (Wittstein et al. 2005). Furthermore, stress-induced autonomic changes can affect myocardial electrical stability increasing the risk for cardiac arrhythmias (Lampert et al. 2002; Lane et al. 2005).

Acute physiological responses to a laboratory stressor predict cardiovascular risk status in longitudinal studies, suggesting that repeated exposure to acute stressors in everyday life can affect cardiovascular health and the risk for acute coronary syndromes in a cumulative fashion (Chida and Steptoe 2010; Treiber et al. 2003). Thus, several pathophysiological processes underlie the link between stress and an acute coronary event. Indeed, the current paradigm for the etiology of acute coronary syndromes is that of a "perfect storm," i.e., the joint presence of many co-occurring pathophysiologic processes, in conjunction with environmental exposures, such as stressful situations, that confer vulnerability to a clinical event (Arbab-Zadeh et al. 2012).

8.2 Mental Stress Testing and Cardiovascular Reactivity

Despite the available evidence from animal models and human observational studies, the demonstration of a causal link between stress and CHD in humans has been difficult to prove conclusively, due to variations in the definitions of stress, difficulties in accurately measuring stressful exposures, and the complexities of determining cause and effect when dealing with naturally occurring stressful events. A useful method of assessing the influence of stress and emotion on cardiac function is to measure transient cardiovascular responses to a standardized psychological stress challenge in the laboratory, also known as "mental stress test," by using techniques such as mental arithmetic, public speeches, or anger recall. This methodology has the advantage of experimental manipulation allowing the control of possible confounding factors and thus direct investigation of causal factors and mechanisms. Despite these advantages, this technique could have limited translational significance since it is based on eliciting short-term responses to an acute stressor artificially administered in the laboratory. However, results of longitudinal studies have provided face validity to a possible link between mental stress-induced cardiovascular responses and future cardiovascular events. A recent systematic review concluded that greater cardiovascular reactivity to mental stress (mostly defined as acute changes in blood pressure and heart rate with stress) and poor recovery from stress (defined as sustained cardiovascular activation above baseline levels during the post-task period) are associated longitudinally with poor cardiovascular risk status, with the most consistent associations being with incident hypertension and increases in systolic and diastolic blood pressure (Chida and Steptoe 2010). Neuroendocrine responses to mental stress, including changes in cortisol (Hamer et al. 2012; Hamer and Steptoe 2012) and catecholamines (Flaa et al. 2008), have also been related to future hypertension and other cardiovascular end points.

Mental stress may affect the electrical properties of the heart; a mental stress task in CHD patients with defibrillators was associated with an increase in T-wave alternans (a marker of myocardial electrical instability) and other measures of abnormal cardiac repolarization that have been related to arrhythmogenesis and sudden cardiac death (Kop et al. 2004; Lampert et al. 2009). Mental stress is also associated with a decrease in heart rate variability (Hamer and Steptoe 2007), a measure of the beat-to-beat changes in heart rate in response to various stimuli, which is an accepted noninvasive measure of overall cardiac autonomic function. Reduced heart rate variability predicts coronary heart disease in population studies, as well as mortality, particularly sudden death, following an acute myocardial infarction (Thayer and Lane 2007).

8.3 Mental Stress-Induced Myocardial Ischemia

Within the mental stress-testing paradigm, one aspect that has drawn particular attention is myocardial ischemia induced by mental stress, defined as an imbalance between myocardial oxygen demand and supply. In clinical medicine, this imbalance is traditionally thought to occur when there is an increase in demand due to physical exertion which cannot be met by an increase in myocardial blood flow because of an obstructive coronary stenosis. Yet this imbalance may also occur during psychological stress and can be captured through a mental stress test, a phenomenon called mental stress-induced myocardial ischemia (MSIMI). The approach of using mental stress to test for inducible myocardial ischemia mirrors conventional exercise or pharmacological stress testing in clinical cardiovascular medicine, except that the stimulus employed is psychological rather than physical (Holmes et al. 2006; Strike and Steptoe 2003).

MSIMI has been assessed with a variety of techniques, including stress-induced regional or global parameters of left ventricular dysfunction (drops in ejection fraction or new wall motion abnormalities) using radionuclide ventriculography or echocardiography, electrocardiographic changes, or, more recently, stress-induced perfusion abnormalities or reductions in blood flow using myocardial perfusion imaging (Strike and Steptoe 2003). The latter is considered the gold standard for ischemia detection, although echocardiographic assessments remain popular due to low cost and lack of radiation exposure. In general, however, there is limited correspondence between indicators of regional/global left ventricular dysfunction and myocardial perfusion, and these may be measuring different processes (Arrighi et al. 2003; Krantz and Burg 2014).

A range of different stressful stimuli have also been used for mental stress testing, mostly including public speaking, anger recall, mental arithmetic, or a combination of these. Overall, this literature indicates that MSIMI can be induced in 20 % to over 60 % of CHD patients, depending on study enrollment criteria and assessment methods (Strike and Steptoe 2003; Wei et al. 2014). MSIMI is typically painless and occurs at lower levels of oxygen demand than ischemia due to physical exertion (Burg et al. 1993; Deanfield et al. 1984; Gottdiener et al. 1994; Modena et al. 1989; Rozanski et al. 1988). In addition, MSIMI is generally not related to the severity of coronary artery disease (Blumenthal et al. 1995; Gottdiener et al. 1994; Jain et al. 1998; Krantz et al. 1991; Ramadan et al. 2013), suggesting that it is not simply a reflection of coronary disease severity, but an indicator of susceptibility to psychological factors (Strike and Steptoe 2003). Patients may develop ischemia with mental stress but not with exercise or pharmacological stress (Jain et al. 1998; Ramachandruni et al. 2006; Ramadan et al. 2013; Stone et al. 1999), and only about 10–20 % of patients will be positive to both (Jiang et al. 2013; Ramadan et al. 2013).

Mental stress-induced (but not exercise-induced) myocardial ischemia correlates with ischemia measured in daily life ambulatory monitoring (Blumenthal et al. 1995; Stone et al. 1999). In addition, despite being usually silent when induced in the laboratory, MSIMI is associated with self-reported angina symptoms in everyday life (Pimple et al. 2015). A recent study also found that propensity toward MSIMI in patients with CHD was related to an integrated measure of resting myocardial velocities measured with Doppler echocardiography, as an indicator of subclinical left ventricular dysfunction (Ersboll et al. 2014). This finding suggests that a more chronic form of asymptomatic ischemia could be present in these patients, extending the data mentioned above linking MSIMI to "silent" ambulatory ischemia and angina symptoms in daily life. As a whole, these data suggest that mental stress testing could provide a means for the identification of patients vulnerable to myocardial ischemia or chest pain syndromes due to emotional stress in everyday life.

8.4 Prognostic Implications

All the results published to date have indicated that MSIMI is a predictor of poor prognosis. Several patient series followed from 1 to 5 years have found substantial increases, between 70 % and threefold, in cardiovascular events, revascularization procedures, and death comparing CHD patients with MSIMI with those without, independent of coronary disease severity and CHD risk factors (Burg et al. 1993; Jain et al. 1995; Jiang et al. 1996; Krantz et al. 1999; Sheps et al. 2002). For example, in the Psychophysiological Investigations of Myocardial Ischemia (PIMI) study of 196 patients with CHD, the all-cause mortality rates were 16.2 % in mental stress-positive and 6.6 % in mental stress-negative patients, a difference that remained significant after adjusting for age, history of myocardial infarction and diabetes, baseline ejection fraction, hypertension, and duration of exercise tolerance tests. Similarly, in the study by Jiang et al. ($n=126$), patients with MSIMI had a 2.8-fold increased risk for a cardiac event during a 5-year follow-up, while there was no significant increase in risk with exercise-induced ischemia (Jiang et al. 1996). Although the numbers of patients followed longitudinally are small, a recent meta-analysis pooled these data (Wei et al. 2014). The pooled five prospective studies included a total of 555 patients with CHD (85 % male) and 117 events with a range of follow-up from 35 days to 8.8 years. In the pooled analysis, MSIMI was associated with a twofold increased risk of a combined end point of cardiac events or total mortality (relative risk 2.2, 95 % confidence interval 1.6–3.1). No heterogeneity was detected, since the effect estimate was similar across the studies (Fig. 8.1).

Study or Subgroup	MSIMI Events	MSIMI Total	No MSIMI Events	No MSIMI Total	Weight	Risk Ratio IV, Fixed, 95% CI	Year
Jain 1995	10	15	4	15	14.2%	2.50 [1.00, 6.23]	1995
Jiang 1996	23	84	5	42	14.8%	2.30 [0.94, 5.62]	1996
Krantz 1999	20	45	8	34	24.9%	1.89 [0.95, 3.76]	1999
Sheps 2002	6	37	9	145	12.6%	2.61 [0.99, 6.88]	2002
Babyak 2010	11	26	21	112	33.6%	2.26 [1.25, 4.08]	2010
Total (95% CI)		207		348	100.0%	2.24 [1.59, 3.15]	
Total events	70		47				

Heterogeneity: $Chi^2 = 0.39$, df = 4 (P = 0.98); $I^2 = 0\%$
Test for overall effect Z = 4.60 (P < 0.00001)

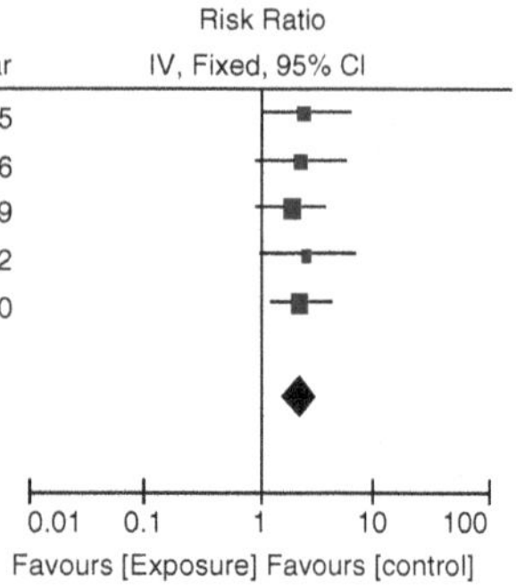

Fig. 8.1 Forest plot of five cohort studies included in a meta-analysis of mental stress-induced myocardial ischemia and subsequent cardiac events in patients with coronary artery disease. *Squares* indicate risk ratio estimates for individual studies; *square* size is proportional to the weight of the corresponding study in the meta-analysis. *Horizontal* lines represent 95 % confidence intervals. The *diamond* represents the pooled relative risk and 95 % confidence interval (Wei et al. 2014) (Reproduced with publisher's permission)

Thus, although larger prospective studies, including more diverse patient populations, are clearly needed, current evidence suggests that myocardial ischemic responses to standardized mental stress are clinically significant, may be an index of ambulatory ischemia occurring in everyday life, and carry a prognostic significance similar to exercise-induced ischemia.

8.5 Potential Mechanisms

The mechanisms behind MSIMI are not entirely clear. As mentioned above, MSIMI is not related to severity of obstructive coronary artery disease (Blumenthal et al. 1995; Gottdiener et al. 1994; Jain et al. 1998; Krantz et al. 1991; Ramadan et al. 2013), which is an important difference as compared with myocardial ischemia induced by conventional methods such as exercise stress testing.

8.5.1 Hemodynamic Workload

MSIMI may be the result of heightened hemodynamic workload during psychological stress in susceptible individuals, such as a rapid increase in blood pressure and heart rate. It is clear, however, that myocardial ischemia in response to mental stress occurs at a lower rate-pressure product than exercise-induced ischemia in the same patients, although stress-induced increases in blood pressure and heart rate tended to be larger in patients who developed MSIMI than those who did not in some studies (Goldberg et al. 1996; L'Abbate et al. 1991; Miller et al. 1993; Rozanski et al. 1988; Schiffer et al. 1980). Thus, other factors besides increased hemodynamic load with stress must be implicated in MSIMI.

8.5.2 Increased Peripheral Vascular Resistance

The PIMI study clearly demonstrated that CHD patients who develop MSIMI have increase in systemic vascular resistance, and the drop in left ventricular ejection fraction (an indicator of myocardial ischemia) during mental stress was inversely correlated with the changes in systemic vascular resistance (Goldberg et al. 1996). These findings, which have been replicated in other studies (Jain et al. 1998; Ramadan et al. 2013), suggest that MSIMI is secondary to an increase in afterload caused by peripheral vasoconstriction. By contrast, systemic vascular resistance is decreased by exercise (Goldberg et al. 1996; Jain et al. 1998). Even among healthy volunteers, left ventricular ejection fraction reductions with mental stress were negatively correlated with systemic vascular resistance (Becker et al. 1996). Thus, both in people with and without CHD, MSIMI is associated with increases in systemic vascular resistance and afterload. These effects may be secondary to centrally mediated neurogenic peripheral vasoconstriction. Indeed, plasma catecholamines increase rapidly with mental stress (Becker et al. 1996; Goldberg et al. 1996) and correlate with hemodynamic changes (Goldberg et al. 1996). Others have found that the rise in plasma catecholamines correlate with decreases in ejection fraction during mental stress (Kuroda et al. 2000). However, elevation in catecholamines tends to be lower with mental stress than with exercise stress, and their relationship with MSIMI is not entirely consistent across studies (Goldberg et al. 1996).

Recent investigations have directly measured peripheral arterial tone in relation with MSIMI using a peripheral arterial tonometry (PAT) device (Burg et al. 2009; Hassan et al. 2009; Ramadan et al. 2013). This device measures changes in digital microvascular tone with stress as the ratio of pulse wave amplitude during mental stress compared with baseline (pre-stress). In these studies, the peripheral arterial tonometry ratio during mental stress was consistently lower in patients who developed MSIMI compared with those who did not develop MSIMI, therefore confirming that MSIMI is associated with peripheral vasoconstriction.

8.5.3 Abnormal Coronary Artery Function

In addition to increasing myocardial ischemia risk by affecting afterload, peripheral vasoconstriction may be a correlate of abnormal vasomotion in the coronary territory, which may induce ischemia through coronary vasoconstriction or a slow-flow phenomenon. Indeed, mental stress has been associated with paradoxical vasoconstriction or reduced blood flow in coronary vessels (Kop et al. 2001). However, reported responses are highly variable, varying from constriction to dilation (Dakak et al. 1995; Kop et al. 2001; L'Abbate et al. 1991; Lacy et al. 1995; Yeung et al. 1991). Coronary artery responses to mental stress correlate with the response to an infusion of acetylcholine, suggesting that coronary endothelial dysfunction plays a role (Yeung et al. 1991). That endothelial function is implicated is also shown by the finding that, peripherally, even a brief period of mental stress induces prolonged endothelial dysfunction in the brachial artery (Ghiadoni et al. 2000).

Although vasoconstriction in the epicardial coronary arteries as a result of mental stress may reduce myocardial blood flow and thus result in myocardial ischemia, the degree of constriction of epicardial coronary arteries may not be sufficient to explain the decrease in coronary flow during mental stress. It has been proposed that vasomotor abnormalities in the coronary microvasculature also play a role, secondary to stress-induced sympathetic nervous system activation via adrenergic receptors in the vascular system (Arrighi et al. 2000; Dakak et al. 1995; Kop et al. 2001). Abnormalities in coronary microvascular flow can be reversed by α-adrenergic blockade via intracoronary administration of phentolamine, suggesting that the sympathetic nervous system plays a role (Dakak et al. 1995).

8.5.4 Confluence of Mechanisms

The current mechanistic model for MSIMI suggests a complex etiology resulting from a confluence of factors, including coronary vasomotor abnormalities (inadequate dilation and/or constriction) and microvascular dysfunction in the setting of augmented oxygen demands. The latter may include stress-induced increase in blood pressure and heart rate and stress-induced increase in afterload due to peripheral vasoconstriction. CHD risk factors might contribute through oxidative stress and inflammation, although most studies have not found an association between MSIMI and unfavorable CHD risk factor profile (Jiang et al. 2013; Ramadan et al. 2013). Although few data are available, it is possible that dysregulation of the autonomic nervous system and of the hypothalamic-pituitary-adrenal axis may predispose to MSIMI, especially in subjects with early life traumas or with chronic or repeated daily stressors, depression, and other psychosocial risk factors. While the exact biochemical pathways are not known, a recent metabolomic analysis from the REMIT (Responses of Mental Stress-Induced Myocardial Ischemia to Escitalopram Treatment) trial has implicated several compounds, including kynurenine, uric acid, tyrosine, and methionine (Boyle et al. 2015). Increased hypercoagulability may also play a role, as heightened mental stress-induced platelet aggregation responses to collagen, epinephrine, and serotonin have been described during mental stress in patients who developed MSIMI compared with those who did not develop MSIMI (Jiang et al. 2015).

8.6 Sex Differences

Unfortunately, most studies of MSIMI were carried out predominantly in men, and if women were included, the sample was often too small to allow comparisons by sex (Strike and Steptoe 2003; Wei et al. 2014). In addition, the study populations mostly included patients with broad coronary disease diagnoses and few patients with a previous myocardial infarction, a subgroup where women face higher risks. Recent studies where more women were included, however, suggest that MSIMI is more common in women than in men. In a sample of patients with stable coronary artery disease, Jiang et al. reported that there was a higher prevalence of MSIMI, assessed by echocardiography, in women than in men (Jiang et al. 2013; Samad et al. 2014). In a study of young patients with a recent myocardial infarction designed to specifically address sex differences in MSIMI, women up to age 50 years had twice the rate of MSIMI compared with age-matched men, a difference that was not observed among older patients (Vaccarino et al. 2014). Myocardial ischemia was assessed with myocardial perfusion imaging, and results were not explained by traditional cardiovascular risk factors, severity of coronary artery disease, or even behavioral and psychosocial factors.

It is unclear why MSIMI is more common in women, especially young women. This finding is not due to greater hemodynamic responses to stress in female patients, since hemodynamic changes with mental stress are similar in women and men (Becker et al. 1996; Steptoe et al. 1996; Vaccarino et al. 2014). A possible mechanism is the higher burden of psychosocial risk factors in women, especially young women, including depression, early life adversities, and low socioeconomic resources (Mallik et al. 2006; Samad et al. 2014; Vaccarino et al. 1999, 2014). Furthermore, vasomotor tone could play a role, since women are thought to be more susceptible to abnormal vasomotor reactivity and microvascular dysfunction in the coronary bed than men, mechanisms that are thought to play a role in MSIMI (Pepine et al. 2010; von Mering et al. 2004; Wong et al. 2002).

8.7 Depression and Other Psychological Correlates

There is increasing evidence that MSIMI is associated with certain psychological traits. Emotional reactivity in everyday life (exhibiting substantial variations of self-reported tension levels) (Carels et al. 1999), as well as anxiety and depression, has been correlated with myocardial ischemia during mental stress but, in general, not with exercise (Boyle et al. 2013; Burg et al. 2014; Carels et al. 1999; Wei et al. 2014). Aggressive responding, hostile affect, and trait and state anger also occur more often in patients with ischemic responses during mental stress (Burg et al. 1993; Pimple et al. 2015).

The link between depression and MSIMI is emerging as especially significant in recent studies. An analysis of the REMIT trial, including more than 300 predominantly older white men with CHD, showed that depressive symptom severity, based on the Beck Depression Inventory-II (BDI-II), predicted the occurrence of MSIMI defined primarily by measures of left ventricular dysfunction and wall motion abnormalities using echocardiography (Boyle et al. 2013). Similarly, in a smaller but more diverse sample of young patients enriched with women and minorities, who were all hospitalized for an acute myocardial infarction in the previous 6 months, depressive symptoms measured with the BDI-II were associated with severity of MSIMI assessed with myocardial perfusion imaging (Wei et al. 2014). Patients underwent single-photon emission computed tomography (SPECT) scans at rest, after mental stress (speech task), and after exercise or pharmacological stress. There was a significant positive and graded association between depressive symptom severity and a summed difference score quantifying myocardial ischemia with mental stress. After adjustment for demographic and lifestyle factors, disease severity, and medications, each 1-point increase in BDI-II score was associated with 0.14 points higher SDS; in contrast, depressive symptoms were not associated with ischemia induced by conventional methods (exercise or pharmacological stress) (Fig. 8.2). Furthermore, when somatic and cognitive depressive symptoms were examined separately, both somatic [beta=0.17; 95 % CI, 0.04, 0.30; *P*=0.01] and cognitive symptoms [beta=0.31; 95 % CI, 0.07, 0.56; *P*=0.01] were significantly associated with MSIMI. A clear dose-response association between depressive symptoms and MSIMI is illustrated when the BDI-II total score is categorized into quintiles (Fig. 8.3).

Results were consistent in a third recent study of 146 patients with stable CHD, who underwent SPECT myocardial perfusion imaging at rest and during mental stress using mental arithmetic (Burg et al. 2014). A BDI score in the depressed

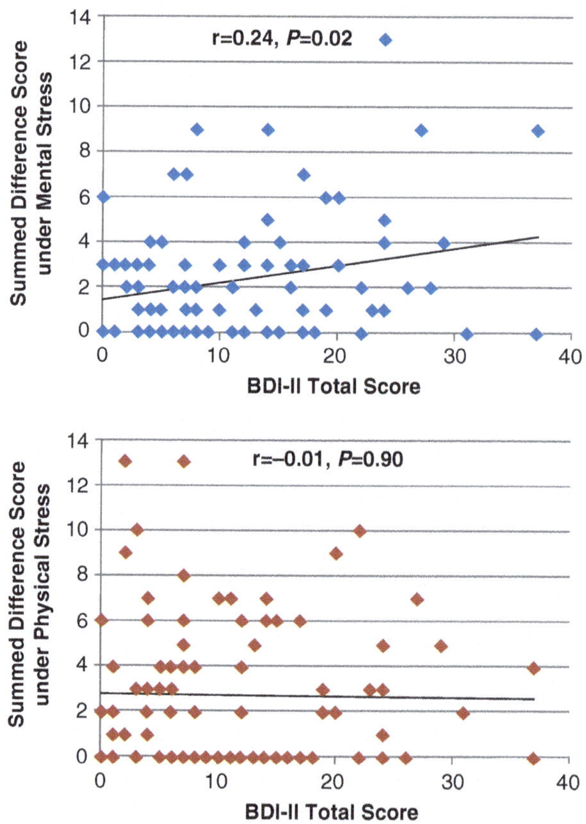

Fig. 8.2 Scatterplots of depressive symptoms (BDI-II total score) against myocardial perfusion ischemia severity (summed difference score) during mental stress (*upper* panel) and conventional stress, including exercise or pharmacological stress (*lower* panel). There was a significant correlation between depressive symptoms and ischemia severity with mental stress but not with physical stress (Wei et al. 2014)

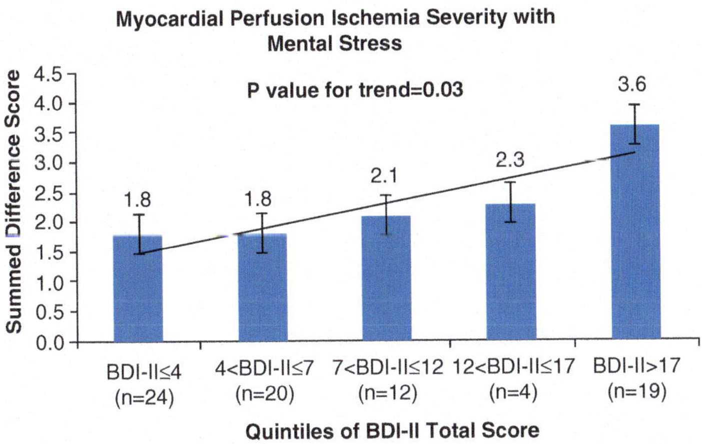

Fig. 8.3 Mean myocardial perfusion ischemia severity (summed difference score) during mental stress according to progressively higher depressive symptoms using quintiles of the BDI-II total score (Wei et al. 2014)

range was associated with an almost threefold greater odds of new or worsening impairment in myocardial perfusion comparing baseline to mental stress (odds ratio = 2.9; 95 % CI, 1.3–6.6; $P = 0.01$), which remained significant in models controlling for CHD risk factors and medications. Based on these consistent findings, depressed patients with CHD appear to be susceptible to MSIMI. It is therefore possible that at least part of the increased risk of cardiac event recurrence and mortality associated with depression may be attributable to MSIMI or the co-occurrence of MSIMI with other adverse pathophysiological processes associated with depression.

8.8 Treatment of MSIMI

Emerging evidence suggests that MSIMI is amenable to intervention with behavioral and medication approaches. Blumenthal et al. found that 31 male patients with established CHD and ambulatory or mental stress-induced myocardial ischemia, who were randomly assigned to 4 months of stress management training (1.5-h weekly class on stress management), tended to have a lower number of events over a 5-year follow-up than 26 patients randomized to exercise training (aerobic exercise three times per week), and medical costs were also lower (Blumenthal et al. 2002). This study, however, did not specifically measure the effects of treatment on MSIMI. The recent REMIT trial demonstrated that antidepressant treatment may be helpful in MSIMI. Among 127 patients with stable CHD and baseline MSIMI, 6 weeks of treatment with escitalopram, a selective serotonin reuptake inhibitor, compared with placebo, resulted in a lower rate of MSIMI (odds ratio of absence of MSIMI, 2.62 [95 % CI, 1.06–6.44]), while there was no statistically significant impact of treatment on exercise-induced ischemia (Jiang et al. 2013). The effects of escitalopram on

MSIMI were not due to changes in depression, trait anxiety, or perceived stress, for which there were no differences between groups. However, the treatment resulted in beneficial physiological responses, including a reduction in markers of platelet activity and improvements in hemodynamic responses to mental stress (heart rate and rate-pressure product). These encouraging results need replication in larger trials.

Future studies should consider more therapeutic approaches and whether the reduction in MSIMI translates into better cardiovascular outcomes in larger and more diverse patient populations. Certain cardiovascular medications, especially angiotensin-converting enzyme (ACE) inhibitors, may also be potentially useful. In a recent retrospective analysis of 218 patients with stable CHD, those using ACEI therapy displayed less than half the risk of MSIMI (assessed with SPECT myocardial perfusion imaging) but not with physical stress (Ramadan et al. 2013). This possible beneficial effect of ACEIs on MSIMI may be due to the well-established role of angiotensin II in the physiological response to stress, as well as its effects on endothelial function, and warrant further study (Saavedra et al. 2011).

8.9 Conclusions and Clinical Implications

MSIMI is a prevalent phenomenon in CHD patients, but may also occur in the preclinical phases of CHD and potentially play a role in triggering acute coronary syndromes. While larger studies are needed in more representative populations, available evidence thus far identifies MSIMI as a distinct phenomenon from ischemia induced by conventional stress testing, with unique pathophysiological mechanisms. Although few prospective studies have been conducted, all point to MSIMI as a significant independent predictor of subsequent cardiac events and mortality, with approximately a doubling of risk. There is substantial variability in the ischemic responses to mental stress; young women and depressed patients appear especially vulnerable to MSIMI. Thus, MSIMI may potentially help explain the increased risk for adverse outcomes in these subgroups and inform effective interventions. However, MSIMI has essentially been ignored by much of recent clinical research, and its applicability to cardiac care has not been assessed. Thus, currently it remains premature to advocate mental stress testing as part of the routine clinical workup of patients with suspected or established CHD. Until more data are gathered regarding its clinical applicability, mental stress testing remains a powerful means of investigation of the role of psychological stress in CHD and an effective method for elucidation of pathophysiological mechanisms linking emotional stress to cardiovascular risk.

References

Arbab-Zadeh A, Nakano M, Virmani R, Fuster V (2012) Acute coronary events. Circulation 125(9):1147–1156. doi:10.1161/CIRCULATIONAHA.111.047431

Arrighi JA, Burg M, Cohen IS, Kao AH, PfauS C-GT, Zaret BL, Soufer R (2000) Myocardial blood-flow response during mental stress in patients with coronary artery disease. Lancet 356:310–311

Arrighi JA, Burg M, Cohen IS, Soufer R (2003) Simultaneous assessment of myocardial perfusion and function during mental stress in patients with chronic coronary artery disease. J Nucl Cardiol 10:267–274

Becker LC, Pepine CJ, Bonsall R, Cohen JD, Goldberg AD, Coghlan C, Stone PH, Forman S, Knatterud G, Sheps DS, Kaufmann PG (1996) Left ventricular, peripheral vascular, and neurohumoral responses to mental stress in normal middle-aged men and women. Reference Group for the Psychophysiological Investigations of Myocardial Ischemia (PIMI) Study. Circulation 94(11):2768–2777

Bhattacharyya MR, Steptoe A (2007) Emotional triggers of acute coronary syndromes: strength of evidence, biological processes, and clinical implications. Prog Cardiovasc Dis 49(5):353–365

Blumenthal JA, Jiang W, Waugh RA, Frid DJ, Morris JJ, Coleman RE, Hanson M, Babyak M, Thyrum ET, O'Connor C (1995) Mental stress-induced ischemia in the laboratory and ambulatory ischemia during daily life. Association and hemodynamic features. Circulation 92(8):2102–2108

Blumenthal JA, Babyak M, Wei J, O'Connor C, Waugh R, Eisenstein E, Mark D, Sherwood A, Woodley PS, Irwin RJ, Reed G (2002) Usefulness of psychosocial treatment of mental stress-induced myocardial ischemia in men. Am J Cardiol 89(2):164–168

Boyle SH, Samad Z, Becker RC, Williams R, Kuhn C, Ortel TL, Kuchibhatla M, Prybol K, Rogers J, O'Connor C, Velazquez EJ, Jiang W (2013) Depressive symptoms and mental stress-induced myocardial ischemia in patients with coronary heart disease. Psychosom Med 75(9):822–831. doi:10.1097/PSY.0b013e3182a893ae

Boyle SH, Matson WR, Velazquez EJ, Samad Z, Williams RB Jr, Sharma S, Thomas B, Wilson JL, O'Connor C, Jiang W (2015) Metabolomics analysis reveals insights into biochemical mechanisms of mental stress-induced left ventricular dysfunction. Metabolomics 11(3):571–582. doi:10.1007/s11306-014-0718-y

Burg MM, Jain D, Soufer R, Kerns RD, Zaret BL (1993) Role of behavioral and psychological factors in mental stress-induced silent left ventricular dysfunction in coronary artery disease. J Am Coll Cardiol 22(2):440–448

Burg MM, Graeber B, Vashist A, Collins D, Earley C, Liu J, Lampert R, Soufer R (2009) Noninvasive detection of risk for emotion-provoked myocardial ischemia. Psychosom Med 71(1):14–20. doi:10.1097/PSY.0b013e318187c035

Burg MM, Meadows J, Shimbo D, Davidson KW, Schwartz JE, Soufer R (2014) Confluence of depression and acute psychological stress among patients with stable coronary heart disease: effects on myocardial perfusion. J Am Heart Assoc 3(6). doi:10.1161/JAHA.114.000898

Carels RA, Sherwood A, Babyak M, Gullette EC, Coleman RE, Waugh R, Jiang W, Blumenthal JA (1999) Emotional responsivity and transient myocardial ischemia. J Consult Clin Psychol 67(4):605–610

Chida Y, Steptoe A (2010) Greater cardiovascular responses to laboratory mental stress are associated with poor subsequent cardiovascular risk status: a meta-analysis of prospective evidence. Hypertension 55(4):1026–1032. doi:10.1161/HYPERTENSIONAHA.109.146621

Dakak N, Quyyumi AA, Eisenhofer G, Goldstein DS, Cannon RO 3rd (1995) Sympathetically mediated effects of mental stress on the cardiac microcirculation of patients with coronary artery disease. Am J Cardiol 76(3):125–130

Deanfield JE, Shea M, Kensett M, Horlock P, Wilson RA, de Landsheere CM, Selwyn AP (1984) Silent myocardial ischaemia due to mental stress. Lancet 2(8410):1001–1005

Ersboll M, Al Enezi F, Samad Z, Sedberry B, Boyle SH, O'Connor C, Jiang W, Velazquez EJ, Investigators R (2014) Impaired resting myocardial annular velocities are independently associated with mental stress-induced ischemia in coronary heart disease. JACC Cardiovasc Imaging 7(4):351–361. doi:10.1016/j.jcmg.2013.10.014

Flaa A, Eide IK, Kjeldsen SE, Rostrup M (2008) Sympathoadrenal stress reactivity is a predictor of future blood pressure: an 18-year follow-up study. Hypertension 52(2):336–341. doi:10.1161/HYPERTENSIONAHA.108.111625

Ghiadoni L, Donald AE, Cropley M, Mullen MJ, Oakley G, Taylor M, O'Connor G, Betteridge J, Klein N, Steptoe A, Deanfield JE (2000) Mental stress induces transient endothelial dysfunction in humans. Circulation 102(20):2473–2478

Goldberg AD, Becker LC, Bonsall R, Cohen JD, Ketterer MW, Kaufman PG, Krantz DS, Light KC, McMahon RP, Noreuil T, Pepine CJ, Raczynski J, Stone PH, Strother D, Taylor H, Sheps DS (1996) Ischemic, hemodynamic, and neurohormonal responses to mental and exercise stress. Experience from the Psychophysiological Investigations of Myocardial Ischemia Study (PIMI). Circulation 94(10):2402–2409

Gottdiener JS, Krantz DS, Howell RH, Hecht GM, Klein J, Falconer JJ, Rozanski A (1994) Induction of silent myocardial ischemia with mental stress testing: relation to the triggers of ischemia during daily life activities and to ischemic functional severity. J Am Coll Cardiol 24(7):1645–1651

Hamer M, Steptoe A (2007) Association between physical fitness, parasympathetic control, and proinflammatory responses to mental stress. Psychosom Med 69:660–666

Hamer M, Steptoe A (2012) Cortisol responses to mental stress and incident hypertension in healthy men and women. J Clin Endocrinol Metab 97(1):E29–E34. doi:10.1210/jc.2011-2132

Hamer M, Endrighi R, Venuraju SM, Lahiri A, Steptoe A (2012) Cortisol responses to mental stress and the progression of coronary artery calcification in healthy men and women. PLoS One 7(2):e31356. doi:10.1371/journal.pone.0031356

Hassan M, York KM, Li H, Li Q, Lucey DG, Fillingim RB, Sheps DS (2009) Usefulness of peripheral arterial tonometry in the detection of mental stress-induced myocardial ischemia. Clin Cardiol 32(9):E1–E6. doi:10.1002/clc.20515

Holmes SD, Krantz DS, Rogers H, Gottdiener J, Contrada RJ (2006) Mental stress and coronary artery disease: a multidisciplinary guide. Prog Cardiovasc Dis 49(2):106–122

Jain D, Burg M, Soufer R, Zaret BL (1995) Prognostic implications of mental stress-induced silent left ventricular dysfunction in patients with stable angina pectoris. Am J Cardiol 76:31–35

Jain D, Shaker SM, Burg M, Wackers FJ, Soufer R, Zaret BL (1998) Effects of mental stress on left ventricular and peripheral vascular performance in patients with coronary artery disease. J Am Coll Cardiol 31(6):1314–1322

Jiang W, Babyak M, Krantz DS, Waugh R, Coleman RE, Hanson MM, Frid DJ, McNulty S, Morris JJ, O'Connor CM, Blumenthal JA (1996) Mental-stress induced myocardial ischemia and cardiac events. JAMA 275:1651–1656

Jiang W, Samad Z, Boyle S, Becker RC, Williams R, Kuhn C, Ortel TL, Rogers J, Kuchibhatla M, O'Connor C, Velazquez EJ (2013a) Prevalence and clinical characteristics of mental stress-induced myocardial ischemia in patients with coronary heart disease. J Am Coll Cardiol 61(7):714–722. doi:10.1016/j.jacc.2012.11.037

Jiang W, Velazquez EJ, Kuchibhatla M, Samad Z, Boyle SH, Kuhn C, Becker RC, Ortel TL, Williams RB, Rogers JG, O'Connor C (2013b) Effect of escitalopram on mental stress-induced myocardial ischemia: results of the REMIT trial. JAMA 309(20):2139–2149. doi:10.1001/jama.2013.5566

Jiang W, Boyle SH, Ortel TL, Samad Z, Velazquez EJ, Harrison RW, Wilson J, Kuhn C, Williams RB, O'Connor CM, Becker RC (2015) Platelet aggregation and mental stress induced myocardial ischemia: results from the Responses of Myocardial Ischemia to Escitalopram Treatment (REMIT) study. Am Heart J 169(4):496–507, e491. doi:10.1016/j.ahj.2014.12.002

Kaplan JR, Chen H, Manuck SB (2009) The relationship between social status and atherosclerosis in male and female monkeys as revealed by meta-analysis. Am J Primatol 71(9):732–741

Kop WJ, Krantz DS, Howell RH, Ferguson MA, Papademetriou V, Lu D, Popma JJ, Quigley JF, Vernalis M, Gottdiener JS (2001) Effects of mental stress on coronary epicardial vasomotion and flow velocity in coronary artery disease: relationship with hemodynamic stress responses. J Am Coll Cardiol 37(5):1359–1366

Kop WJ, Krantz DS, Nearing BD, Gottdiener JS, Quigley JF, O'Callahan M, DelNegro AA, Friehling TD, Karasik P, Suchday S, Levine J, Verrier RL (2004) Effects of acute mental stress and exercise on T-wave alternans in patients with implantable cardioverter defibrillators and controls. Circulation 109(15):1864–1869

Krantz DS, Burg MM (2014) Current perspective on mental stress-induced myocardial ischemia. Psychosom Med 76(3):168–170. doi:10.1097/PSY.0000000000000054

Krantz DS, Helmers KF, Bairey CN, Nebel LE, Hedges SM, Rozanski A (1991) Cardiovascular reactivity and mental stress-induced myocardial ischemia in patients with coronary artery disease. Psychosom Med 53(1):1–12

Krantz DS, Santiago HT, Kop WJ, Bairey Merz CN, Rozanski A, Gottdiener JS (1999) Prognostic value of mental stress testing in coronary artery disease. Am J Cardiol 84(11):1292–1297

Kuroda T, Kuwabara Y, Watanabe S, Nakaya J, Hasegawa R, Shikama T, Matsuno K, Mikami Y, Fujii K, Saito T, Masuda Y (2000) Effect of mental stress on left ventricular ejection fraction and its relationship to the severity of coronary artery disease. Eur J Nucl Med 27(12):1760–1767

L'Abbate A, Simonetti I, Carpeggiani C, Michelassi C (1991) Coronary dynamics and mental arithmetic stress in humans. Circulation 83(4 Suppl):II94–II99

Lacy CR, Contrada RJ, Robbins ML, Tannenbaum AK, Moreyra AE, Chelton S, Kostis JB (1995) Coronary vasoconstriction induced by mental stress (simulated public speaking). Am J Cardiol 75(7):503–505

Lampert R, Joska T, Burg MM, Batsford WP, McPherson CA, Jain D (2002) Emotional and physical precipitants of ventricular arrhythmia. Circulation 106(14):1800–1805

Lampert R, Shusterman V, Burg M, McPherson C, Batsford W, Goldberg A, Soufer R (2009) Anger-induced T-wave alternans predicts future ventricular arrhythmias in patients with implantable cardioverter-defibrillators. J Am Coll Cardiol 53(9):774–778. doi:10.1016/j.jacc.2008.10.053

Lane RD, Laukes C, Marcus FI, Chesney MA, Sechrest L, Gear K, Fort CL, Priori SG, Schwartz PJ, Steptoe A (2005) Psychological stress preceding idiopathic ventricular fibrillation. Psychosom Med 67(3):359–365

Mallik S, Spertus JA, Reid KJ, Krumholz HM, Rumsfeld JS, Weintraub WS, Agarwal P, Santra M, Bidyasar S, Lichtman JH, Wenger NK, Vaccarino V (2006) Depressive symptoms after acute myocardial infarction: evidence for highest rates in younger women. Arch Int Med 166(8):876–883

Miller PF, Light KC, Bragdon EE, Ballenger MN, Herbst MC, Maixner W, Hinderliter AL, Atkinson SS, Koch GG, Sheps DS (1993) Beta-endorphin response to exercise and mental stress in patients with ischemic heart disease. J Psychosom Res 37(5):455–465

Modena MG, Corghi F, Fantini G, Mattioli G (1989) Echocardiographic monitoring of mental stress test in ischemic heart disease. Clin Cardiol 12(1):21–24

Mostofsky E, Maclure M, Sherwood JB, Tofler GH, Muller JE, Mittleman MA (2012) Risk of acute myocardial infarction after the death of a significant person in one's life: the Determinants of Myocardial Infarction Onset Study. Circulation 125(3):491–496. doi:10.1161/CIRCULATIONAHA.111.061770

Mostofsky E, Maclure M, Tofler GH, Muller JE, Mittleman MA (2013) Relation of outbursts of anger and risk of acute myocardial infarction. Am J Cardiol 112(3):343–348. doi:10.1016/j.amjcard.2013.03.035

Pepine CJ, Anderson RD, Sharaf BL, Reis SE, Smith KM, Handberg EM, Johnson BD, Sopko G, Bairey Merz CN (2010) Coronary microvascular reactivity to adenosine predicts adverse outcome in women evaluated for suspected ischemia: results from the National Heart, Lung and Blood Institute WISE (Women's Ischemia Syndrome Evaluation) Study. J Am Coll Cardiol 55(25):2825–2832

Pimple P, Shah A, Rooks C, Bremner JD, Nye J, Ibeanu I, Murrah N, Shallenberger L, Kelley M, Raggi P, Vaccarino V (2015a) Association between anger and mental stress-induced myocardial ischemia. Am Heart J 169(1):115–121 e112. doi:10.1016/j.ahj.2014.07.031

Pimple P, Shah AJ, Rooks C, Douglas Bremner J, Nye J, Ibeanu I, Raggi P, Vaccarino V (2015b) Angina and mental stress-induced myocardial ischemia. J Psychosom Res 78(5):433–437. doi:10.1016/j.jpsychores.2015.02.007

Ramachandruni S, Fillingim RB, McGorray SP, Schmalfuss CM, Cooper GR, Schofield RS, Sheps DS (2006) Mental stress provokes ischemia in coronary artery disease subjects without exercise- or adenosine-induced ischemia. J Am Coll Cardiol 47(5):987–991

Ramadan R, Quyyumi AA, Zafari AM, Binongo JN, Sheps DS (2013a) Myocardial ischemia and Angiotensin-converting enzyme inhibition: comparison of ischemia during mental and physical stress. Psychosom Med 75(9):815–821. doi:10.1097/PSY.0000000000000015

Ramadan R, Sheps D, Esteves F, Zafari AM, Bremner JD, Vaccarino V, Quyyumi AA (2013b) Myocardial ischemia during mental stress: role of coronary artery disease burden and vasomotion. J Am Heart Assoc 2(5), e000321. doi:10.1161/JAHA.113.000321
Rosengren A, Hawken S, Ounpuu S, Sliwa K, Zubaid M, Almahmeed WA, Blackett KN, Sitthi-amorn C, Sato H, Yusuf S (2004) Association of psychosocial risk factors with risk of acute myocardial infarction in 11 119 cases and 13 648 controls from 52 countries (the INTERHEART study): case-control study. Lancet 364(9438):953–962
Rozanski A, Bairey CN, Krantz DS, Friedman J, Resser KJ, Morell M, Hilton-Chalfen S, Hestrin L, Bietendorf J, Berman DS (1988) Mental stress and the induction of silent myocardial ischemia in patients with coronary artery disease. N Engl J Med 318(16):1005–1012
Saavedra JM, Sanchez-Lemus E, Benicky J (2011) Blockade of brain angiotensin II AT1 receptors ameliorates stress, anxiety, brain inflammation and ischemia: therapeutic implications. Psychoneuroendocrinology 36(1):1–18. doi:10.1016/j.psyneuen.2010.10.001
Samad Z, Boyle S, Ersboll M, Vora AN, Zhang Y, Becker RC, Williams R, Kuhn C, Ortel TL, Rogers JG, O'Connor CM, Velazquez EJ, Jiang W, REMIT Investigators R (2014) Sex differences in platelet reactivity and cardiovascular and psychological response to mental stress in patients with stable ischemic heart disease: insights from the REMIT Study. J Am Coll Cardiol 64(16):1669–1678. doi:10.1016/j.jacc.2014.04.087
Schiffer F, Hartley LH, Schulman CL, Abelmann WH (1980) Evidence for emotionally-induced coronary arterial spasm in patients with angina pectoris. Br Heart J 44(1):62–66
Sheps DS, McMahon RP, Becker L, Carney RM, Freedland KE, Cohen JD, Sheffield D, Goldberg AD, Ketterer MW, Pepine CJ, Raczynski JM, Light K, Krantz DS, Stone PH, Knatterud G, Kaufmann PG (2002) Mental stress-induced ischemia and all-cause mortality in patients with coronary artery disease: results from the Psychophysiological Investigations of Myocardial Ischemia study. Circulation 105(15):1780–1784
Shively CA, Register TC, Clarkson TB (2009) Social stress, visceral obesity, and coronary artery atherosclerosis: product of a primate adaptation. Am J Primatol 71(9):742–751. doi:10.1002/ajp.20706
Steptoe A, Kivimaki M (2013) Stress and cardiovascular disease: an update on current knowledge. Annu Rev Public Health 34:337–354. doi:10.1146/annurev-publhealth-031912-114452
Steptoe A, Fieldman G, Evans O, Perry L (1996) Cardiovascular risk and responsivity to mental stress: the influence of age, gender and risk factors. J Cardiovasc Risk 3(1):83–93
Stone PH, Krantz DS, McMahon RP, Goldberg AD, Becker LC, Chaitman BR, Taylor HA, Cohen JD, Freedland KE, Bertolet BD, Coughlan C, Pepine CJ, Kaufmann PG, Sheps DS (1999a) Relationship among mental stress-induced ischemia and ischemia during daily life and during exercise: the psychophysiologic investigations of myocardial ischemia (PIMI) Study. J Am Coll Cardiol 33(6):1477–1484
Stone PH, Krantz DS, McMahon RP, Goldberg AD, Becker LC, Chaitman BR, Taylor HA, Cohen JD, Freedland KE, Bertolet BD, Coughlan C, Pepine CJ, Kaufmann PG, Sheps DS (1999b) Relationship among mental stress-induced ischemia and ischemia during daily life and during exercise: the Psychophysiologic Investigations of Myocardial Ischemia (PIMI) study. J Am Coll Cardiol 33(6):1476–1484
Strike PC, Steptoe A (2003) Systematic review of mental stress-induced myocardial ischaemia. Eur Heart J 24(8):690–703
Thayer JF, Lane RD (2007) The role of vagal function in the risk for cardiovascular disease and mortality. Biol Psychol 74(2):224–242. doi:10.1016/j.biopsycho.2005.11.013, S0301-0511(06)00178-5 [pii]
Treiber FA, Kamarck T, Schneiderman N, Sheffield D, Kapuku G, Taylor T (2003) Cardiovascular reactivity and development of preclinical and clinical disease states. Psychosom Med 65(1):46–62
Vaccarino V, Parsons L, Every NR, Barron HV, Krumholz HM (1999) Sex-based differences in early mortality after myocardial infarction. National Registry of Myocardial Infarction 2 Participants. N Engl J Med 341(4):217–225
Vaccarino V, Shah AJ, Rooks C, Ibeanu I, Nye JA, Pimple P, Salerno A, D'Marco L, Karohl C, Bremner JD, Raggi P (2014) Sex differences in mental stress-induced myocardial ischemia in

young survivors of an acute myocardial infarction. Psychosom Med 76(3):171–180. doi:10.1097/PSY.0000000000000045

von Mering GO, Arant CB, Wessel TR, McGorray SP, Bairey Merz CN, Sharaf BL, Smith KM, Olson MB, Johnson BD, Sopko G, Handberg E, Pepine CJ, Kerensky RA (2004) Abnormal coronary vasomotion as a prognostic indicator of cardiovascular events in women: results from the National Heart, Lung, and Blood Institute-Sponsored Women's Ischemia Syndrome Evaluation (WISE). Circulation 109(6):722–725. doi:10.1161/01.CIR.0000115525.92645.16

Wei J, Pimple P, Shah AJ, Rooks C, Bremner JD, Nye JA, Ibeanu I, Murrah N, Shallenberger L, Raggi P, Vaccarino V (2014a) Depressive symptoms are associated with mental stress-induced myocardial ischemia after acute myocardial infarction. PLoS One 9(7):e102986. doi:10.1371/journal.pone.0102986

Wei J, Rooks C, Ramadan R, Shah AJ, Bremner JD, Quyyumi AA, Kutner M, Vaccarino V (2014b) Meta-analysis of mental stress-induced myocardial ischemia and subsequent cardiac events in patients with coronary artery disease. Am J Cardiol 114(2):187–192. doi:10.1016/j.amjcard.2014.04.022

Wittstein IS, Thiemann DR, Lima JAC, Baughman KL, Schulman SP, Gerstenblith G, Wu KC, Rade JJ, Bivalacqua TJ, Champion HC (2005) Neurohumoral features of myocardial stunning due to sudden emotional stress. N Engl J Med 352(6):539–548

Wong TY, Klein R, Sharrett AR, Duncan BB, Couper DJ, Tielsch JM, Klein BE, Hubbard LD (2002) Retinal arteriolar narrowing and risk of coronary heart disease in men and women. The Atherosclerosis Risk in Communities Study. JAMA 287(9):1153–1159

Yeung AC, Vekshtein VI, Krantz DS, Vita JA, Ryan TJ Jr, Ganz P, Selwyn AP (1991) The effect of atherosclerosis on the vasomotor response of coronary arteries to mental stress. N Engl J Med 325(22):1551–1556

Neuropsychological Impairment of Patients with Depression

9

Thomas Beblo

Contents

Abstract

Neuropsychological impairment is one of the most common and persistent symptoms of depressive disorders. Studies indicate impairment in the domains of executive functions, attention, and memory. However, a definite profile of these impairments has yet not been identified possibly due to the fact that the neuropsychological performance is influenced by several clinical and demographic factors, e.g., depression subtype, rumination, and age. Depression also

T. Beblo, PhD
Department of Research, Clinic of Psychiatry and Psychotherapy Bethel, Ev. Hospital Bielefeld, Remterweg 69-71, 33617 Bielefeld, Germany

Department of Psychology, University of Bielefeld, Bielefeld, Germany
e-mail: thomas.beblo@evkb.de

B.T. Baune, P.J. Tully (eds.), *Cardiovascular Diseases and Depression*,
DOI 10.1007/978-3-319-32480-7_9

further deteriorates cognitive performance of brain-damaged patients. Impairments improve with remission of the disorder but do often not reverse completely. In addition, they have an important clinical impact and are positively related to suicidality, poor treatment response, and reduced everyday functioning. Therefore, effective treatment is needed. First results raised hope that neuropsychological impairment in depression is successfully treatable with neuropsychological therapy, training of mindfulness, specific antidepressants, and new neurobiological treatments such as transcranial magnet stimulation.

9.1 Introduction

Neuropsychological impairment is one of the most common and persistent symptoms of depressive disorders. Conradi et al. (2011) demonstrated that neuropsychological impairment is present in more than 90 % of patients with major depressive disorder (MDD). In their study sample, up to 66 % of the patients still suffered from neuropsychological impairment in a 3-year course of MDD. In addition, in 44 % of the finally remitted patients, neuropsychological impairment remained present. According to the *Diagnostics and Statistical Manual of Mental Disorders, Fifth Edition* (DSM-5 American Psychiatric Association 2013) and the *International Classification of Diseases* (ICD-10 WHO 1991), neuropsychological symptoms of MDD are characterized by reduced abilities to concentrate and impaired decision-making processes. Neuropsychological research has confirmed impairment in MDD patients predominantly in the domains of attention, memory, and executive functioning. Depression also further deteriorates cognitive performance of brain-damaged patients such as patients with cerebrovascular disease.

Historically, researches attempted to characterize the profile of neuropsychological impairment in depression more precisely in order to differentiate depression from dementia and in order to make conclusions about specific neurobiological dysfunctions (Keefe 1995). These aims are still relevant but somewhat pushed into the background for different reasons. First, research could not establish a neuropsychological profile highly specific for depression making differential diagnosis on the basis of test results challenging. In addition, modern imaging methods give increasingly precise insights into the neurobiology of depression and, thus, reduce the hereof relevance of neuropsychological test results. More recently, researchers focus on factors that influence neuropsychological performance in depression. There is also hope that the discovery of endophenotypes may enable researchers to describe neuropsychological deficits in depression more precisely and specifically. In addition, clinicians and researches increasingly emphasize the clinical implications of neuropsychological deficits and the need for effective treatment strategies. First results raised hope that cognitive deficits in affective disorders are successfully treatable.

9.2 Magnitude, Profile, and Course of Neuropsychological Impairment

9.2.1 Magnitude of Neuropsychological Impairment

Estimations of the degree of neuropsychological impairment in depression indicate a statistically moderate magnitude. In a meta-analysis by Christensen et al. (1997), a deficit in neuropsychological function of, on average, −0.63 standard deviations below that of healthy controls has been reported in patients with depression. This outcome is in line with studies from our group (Beblo et al. 1999, 2010; Lahr et al. 2007). Gualtieri and Morgan (2008) reported that patients with mood disorders, on average, may exhibit mild to moderate neuropsychological impairment. However, they report that 21 % of patients with unipolar depression and 30 % of patients with bipolar disorder demonstrate severe and clinically relevant impairment (defined as test performance at least two standard deviations below normative values in at least two cognitive domains). Similar results were only found in 4 % of healthy controls.

We found that self-reports indicate much stronger neuropsychological impairment than neuropsychological tests (Lahr et al. 2007). One possible explanation of this finding relates to the essential difference between the requirements of neuropsychological test settings and the demands of everyday life. That is, the presentation of a well-circumscribed task in the highly structured context of a neuropsychological examination where all disturbing and distracting influences are excluded and where the subject's performance is continuously monitored by the examiner may enable the patient to perform almost normally. By contrast, tasks of everyday life are much less structured and frequently more complex than psychometric tests. They have often to be self-organized and self-paced and are susceptible to various kinds of external disturbances and distractions. Also, rumination might be triggered more likely in everyday life because everyday life is often characterized by situations that are related to the depressive disorder, e.g., dysfunctional family patterns. This is highly relevant because rumination is a major symptom of MDD, and rumination is known to impair cognitive performance of MDD patients (Beblo et al. 2011). However, the discrepancy between subjective cognitive complaints and neuropsychological test performance may also be explained by the patients' negatively biased self-perception and the often questioned validity of self-ratings.

9.2.2 Profile of Neuropsychological Impairment

A huge number of studies have investigated neuropsychological performance in depressed patients. Studies covering different neuropsychological domains document neuropsychological impairment in depressed patients primarily in the areas of attention, executive function, and memory (Beblo and Lautenbacher 2006). With respect to the profile of these dysfunctions, many original studies came to conflicting results, and researches came to diverging evaluations in reviews. It is to conclude that a neuropsychological profile specific for depression has yet not been established (Beblo et al. 2011; Drevets et al. 2008; Murphy et al. 2003; Porter et al. 2007).

In the domain of attention, impairments of selective attention, divided attention, and vigilance have been reported. It is still a matter of debate whether depressed patients show cognitive slowing. Christensen et al. (1997) concluded from their meta-analysis that depressed patients show impaired performance on timed tasks. However, it remains unclear whether this impairment is due to a slowing of cognitive processing or slowing of motor skills or, alternatively, has to be regarded as a consequence of increased rumination. It has also been suggested that patients with MDD primarily show deficits in "effortful tasks" (Porter et al. 2007). As compared to automatic processing, effortful processing requires increased attentional and executive resources (Hasher and Zacks 1979). However, results have been controversial.

An additional domain of impaired cognitive function in depression is related to explicit memory function and learning. There have been several attempts to interpret learning deficits as a result of impaired attention or impaired effortful processing; however, learning deficits probably go beyond attention dysfunction. Depressed patients also exhibit a decreased specificity of autobiographical memories and report rather general autobiographical memories (so-called overgeneralized autobiographical memories (Williams and Scott 1988)). These impairments seem to predict a more severe course of depression with longer and more frequent depressive episodes (Kircanski et al. 2012). Reduced autobiographical specificity seems to be related to reduced goal specificity; thus, reduced specificity is not only related to the representation of the past but also to the representation of the future (Belcher and Kangas 2014). It was shown that overgeneralized memory might be caused by executive dysfunctions, in particular deficits in cognitive control and inhibition (Kircanski et al. 2012). With respect to implicit memory and short-term memory, it remains unclear whether they are typically impaired in depression.

Recently it has been speculated that depressive patients may show the most severe impairment with respect to executive functions (Ros et al. 2013; Snyder 2013). However, many different subfunctions seem to be affected. With regard to more basic executive functions, fluency, flexibility, inhibition, and working memory (cognitive control) are impaired. With respect to word fluency, research shows that category naming (e.g., animals) is more heavily affected than letter fluency (e.g., words beginning with the letter "S" (Henry and Crawford 2005)). Several studies have also reported deficits in complex executive functions such as planning, decision-making, problem-solving, and conceptualization (Beblo and Lautenbacher 2006). Possibly, more basic impairments such as reduced flexibility contribute to these more complex dysfunctions (Cella et al. 2010; Shamay-Tsoory et al. 2009).

In addition to the reduced abilities in attention, memory, and executive function, some studies have also shown visuospatial deficits in depression. However, several researchers have suggested that these findings are less definite (Austin et al. 1992; Pálsson et al. 2000). Neuropsychological syndromes such as aphasia, apraxia, or agnosia have not been reported for depressed patients without comorbid neurological disorders.

9.2.3 Course of Neuropsychological Impairment

The reversibility of neuropsychological impairment among patients has been investigated in patients with euthymia and prospective studies. During the course of an acute episode of depression, it has been reported that cognitive deficits improve with remission of the disorder, most likely among patients with early life major depression (Maeshima et al. 2013) and early onset (Delaloye et al. 2010). However, in many cases neuropsychological deficits do not reverse completely and are, therefore, not only regarded as a state but also as a trait marker of the affective disorder. A definite profile of residual neuropsychological deficits has not been identified.

Several reasons have been discussed for persistent cognitive deficits. On the one hand, it has been suggested that neuropsychological deficits form part of residual symptoms of depression or part of a sub-threshold depression. This interpretation is in line with findings that demonstrate structural changes of the brain in depressed patients, especially in those with late-onset depression (Marano et al. 2015). It was also shown that patients with late-life depression show worse cognitive performance (Korten et al. 2014; Mackin et al. 2014). On the other hand but not necessarily in conflict with these findings, some studies indicate that neuropsychological impairments may sum up over the course of the disorder. That is neuropsychological impairment may be particularly serious not only in patients with late-onset depression but also in those who suffer from many depressive episodes during lifetime. Gorwood et al. (2008) showed in a large sample of 8,229 MDD patients that memory performance diminished by 2–3 % per previous episode of depression (calculated up to four episodes). Hasselbalch et al. (2013) found associations between the cumulative duration and number of depressive episodes and neuropsychological performance. Gorwood et al. (2008) conclude from their findings that neurotoxic effects of stress hormones (e.g., cortisol) on the hippocampus coming from stress and depression might be responsible for diminished neuropsychological performance which is exacerbated with increasing numbers of depressive episodes. This interpretation is supported by studies which have established an association between duration of the mood disorder/numbers of episodes and the degree of hippocampal damage (Mckinnon et al. 2009). These results and conclusions are also in agreement with the "kindling hypothesis" (Post 1992). This hypothesis suggests that depressive episodes become progressively independent of external triggers due to neurobiological changes as a consequence of repeated previous stressors and repeated previous episodes. However, these findings could also be interpreted in a way that a longer history of depression indicates a more severe type of depression with more prominent cognitive deficits and more pronounced neurobiological abnormalities. It is also possible that not depression itself but associated factors such as comorbid substance abuse may lead to neurotoxic effects and to a progressive decline of neuropsychological functioning in the course of the disorder (Delaloye et al. 2010).

9.3 Related Clinical and Demographic Factors

Some authors (e.g., Beblo and Herrmann (2000); Porter et al. (2007)) have suggested a more differentiated view on the relationship between depression and neuropsychological impairment by defining demographic and clinical factors that influence this relationship (Table 9.1).

9.3.1 Subtypes of Mood Disorders and Endophenotypes

It is not surprising that more severe mood disorders are associated with more severe neuropsychological deficits. For example, patients with MDD have more severe neuropsychological deficits compared to those with dysthymia (persistent depressive disorder) (Pálsson et al. 2000) and those with minor depression (Mesholam-Gately et al. 2012) but less deficits compared to bipolar patients (Burt et al. 2000). The results of other studies emphasize that differences between MDD and bipolar patients are also related to the neuropsychological profile (Taylor Tavares et al. 2007). MDD patients that additionally fulfill diagnoses of MDD subtypes with additional psychopathological symptoms (e.g., melancholic or psychotic subtype)

Table 9.1 Influencing factors for the neuropsychological performance of patients with affective disorders

Variables	Neuropsychological relevance
DSM subtypes	Deficits:
	Bipolar > unipolar
	Bipolar I > bipolar II
	Major depression > dysthymia
	Melancholia > no melancholia
	Psychotic symptoms > no psychotic symptoms
Endophenotypes	Possibly relevant
Severity/diurnal swings	More deficits in the morning, rather low associations between deficits, and severity within a certain subtype of the disorder
Processing bias	Favors processing of negative information
Experience of failure	Worse impact than for healthy subjects
Rumination	More deficits with rumination
Sleep disturbances	Negative impact
Suicidal tendencies	More (executive) deficits with suicidal tendencies
Psychiatric comorbidity	With additional alcohol abuse or anxiety > without
	Attention-deficit hyperactivity disorder, possibly relevant borderline personality disorder; cannabis use, possibly irrelevant
Age and onset	More deficits with increasing age and late onset
Motivation, education, gender, appetite/weight loss, traumatization, personality	Possibly relevant

also show poorer neuropsychological functioning (Fleming et al. 2004; Michopoulos et al. 2008). Withall et al. (2010) found for patients with melancholic compared to patients with non-melancholic subtypes of MDD not only poorer performance but also a longer time for neuropsychological recovery. Quinn et al. (2012) stated that differences between melancholia and non-melancholia go beyond a simple variation on severity and include differences of the deficit profile. With respect to bipolar patients, patients with bipolar disorder Type I demonstrated stronger neuropsychological impairment compared to patients with bipolar disorder Type II (Hsiao et al. 2009; Torrent et al. 2006).

Hasler and colleagues (2004) regard mood disorders as aggregation of various psychopathological and biological clusters. These clusters ("endophenotypes") are genetically and phenomenologically more homogenous and might act as a promising basis for the formulation of etiologically based subtypes of mood disorders with distinct neuropsychological profiles. Along these lines, Drysdale et al. (2013) suggested deficits in verbal learning and semantic verbal fluency in bipolar and MDD patients who carry a certain risk haplotype on chromosome 4.

9.3.2 Depression Severity and Diurnal Swings

Specifier of depressive disorders that requires additional psychopathological symptoms (e.g., with psychotic symptoms) represents a more severe subtype of the disorder and is related to a more severe impairment of cognitive functions as described above. In addition, some types of depression, such as melancholic subtype of MDD, are characterized by diurnal swings, with symptoms of depression reportedly worse in the morning compared to the evening. Research investigating neuropsychological function in these patients demonstrates neuropsychological profiles that reflect this diurnal pattern of depressive symptoms with poorer neuropsychological performance in the mornings compared to the evenings (Moffoot et al. 1994; Porterfield et al. 1997).

By contrast, many studies failed to find a correlation between current symptom severity within a certain diagnostic category and neuropsychological test performance (for review, see Beblo and Lautenbacher 2006; Beblo et al. 2011). Sarapas et al. (2012) found neuropsychological test performance to be associated with past average depression severity but not current depression severity indicating that more severe symptoms may have a damaging effect on cognitive functioning long term but not immediately.

9.3.3 Specific Depressive Symptoms

The observation that some subtypes of depression are related to the neuropsychological performance whereas depression severity in general is not, is in agreement with the finding that neuropsychological performance is particularly related to some symptoms. Several psychological symptoms, sleep disturbances, suicidality and appetite appear to be especially relevant.

9.3.3.1 Cognitive-Emotional Factors

Motivation Patients with depression very often report diminished drive and motivation which sometimes leads to the assumption that cognitive deficits observed in patients with depression are due to reduced motivation. Contrary to this assumption, it has been observed that patients with depression are well motivated during neuropsychological testing. Moreover, patients put themselves under pressure and wish to meet the expectations of the neuropsychologist during neuropsychological testing. In agreement with these contradicting observations, research came to conflicting results (Benitez et al. 2011; Richards and Ruff 1989; Scheurich et al. 2008). However, motivational deficits seem to be more relevant for cognitive function for day-to-day tasks rather than in an artificial neuropsychological testing environment (Lahr et al. 2007). More research is clearly needed to estimate the impact of motivation on cognitive performance in depressed patients.

Biased Processing Cognitive models of depression such as the model of Beck (1967) suggest that depressed patients show biased processing of emotional information favoring negative contents. Except for evidence from cognitive and clinical psychology, these assumptions were also confirmed by neuropsychological research. Everaert et al. (2012) pointed out that this bias occurs on different stages of information processing.

With respect to attention and working memory, Gotlib and Joormann (2010) infer from current studies that an attentional bias for negative information may primarily be evident in later stages of attentional processing. In particular, depressed patients show a reduced executive control with deficits to disengage from negative stimuli and to inhibit the elaborating and processing of negative information (Kircanski et al. 2012; Yoon et al. 2014). Apart from attentional bias toward negative information, Leppanen (2006) summarized evidence for an attentional bias away from positive emotional stimuli.

As memory performance depends on attention, it is not surprising that depressed patients also exhibit a memory bias for emotionally negative stimuli. Indeed, Koster et al. (2010) found that dysphoric subjects showed an attention bias for negative words, with the attention bias for negative words predicting free recall of negative words. This bias is more evident for explicit as compared to implicit memory and may only occur with deeper processing – similar to the domain of attention (Kircanski et al. 2012). However, Ellwart et al. (2003) speculated that results may depend on the severity of depression with severely impaired patients also demonstrating a bias for implicit processing because these patients may activate depression-related information automatically.

Rumination Rumination is a repetitive pattern of thoughts focusing on dysphoric symptoms, their causes, and consequences. A study of Beckwé et al. (2014) indicated that rumination might be induced by the diminished executive control for the processing of negative information as described above. Rumination maintains and deteriorates low mood in nonclinical samples and is related to the onset, severity, and chronicity of depression (Donaldson and Lam 2004). Apart from its destructive potential for emotional processing, rumination also affects cognitive processing in general by attracting attention (Donaldson and Lam 2004; Young et al. 2012). Indeed, several studies confirm that rumination has a negative impact on the specificity of the autobiographic memory (Crane et al. 2007), inhibition (Philippot and Brutoux 2008), cognitive flexibility (Watkins and Brown 2002), problem-solving (Donaldson and Lam 2004), and working memory (Joormann and Gotlib 2008).

Processing of Positive and Negative Feedback Roiser and Sahakian (2013) summarize findings indicating that depressive patients are hypersensitive to negative feedback and hyposensitive to positive feedback. MDD patients are more likely than healthy subjects to fail in neuropsychological tasks if they have been told or have experienced to fail in the precedent task. This effect may primarily be relevant for response accuracy (Elliott et al. 1996). It has been speculated that perceived failure triggers "ruminative" and negative thoughts about failure which interfere with task performance or, alternatively, impair motivation (Beats et al. 1996). However, Elliott et al. (1997) demonstrated that depressed patients' performance did not decreased following failure but it did not improve. By contrast, healthy subjects were able to improve their performance after having failed. Results of a recent study by Douglas et al. (2009) indicated that depressed patients may improve their performance after failure as well – but to a lesser extent than healthy participants. Furthermore, depressed patients' reaction to failure may depend on the accuracy of feedback: In a study of Murphy et al. (2003), patients with depression showed normal performance when negative feedback is accurate and informative but an impaired performance when reinforcement contingencies are misleading or ambiguous.

Integrating Models In their neuropsychological model of depression, Roiser and Sahakian (2013) summarize some of the abovementioned findings and postulate a close relationship between cognitive deficits on "standard neuropsychological" tests where emotional stimuli are emotionally neutral ("cold" cognition) and emotionally relevant cognition ("hot" cognition). From their perspective, "hot" cognition deficits such as the biased processing for negative stimuli and a deviated response to failure constitute a source for "cold" cognition deficits. In addition, Roiser and Sahakian also propose the reverse relationship between "hot" and "cold" cognition with cognitive control ("cold" cognition) being a powerful ability to regulate hot cognition processing.

Figure 9.1 shows our model of "depression-associated cognitive deficits" ("DECODE") which summarizes several relations between neuropsychological deficits ("cold cognition"), emotional cognition, and emotion-related neuropsychological performance. According to Beck (1967, 1999), depressive patients show a fundamental negatively biased view about themselves, so-called negative schemas. These schemas lead to modified reactions with respect to emotional relevant information as described above, e.g., a diminished executive control of negative information (arrow 1). The fundamental, negative schemas may also imply that depressive patients are more sensitive to negative feedback and less sensitive

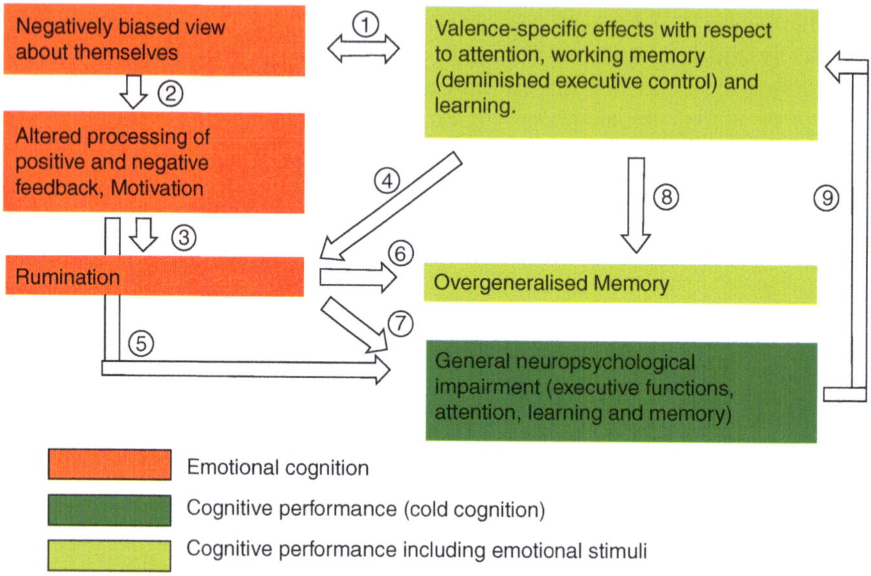

Fig. 9.1 Model of depression-associated cognitive deficits ("DECODE")

to positive feedback (arrow 2). This is also relevant for the patients' motivation as motivation depends on the expectation of reward. Negative and stressful events in general and negative feedback in particular are known to trigger rumination (arrow 3). Rumination is harder to control for those patients who show a diminished executive control of negative thoughts (arrow 4). Finally, rumination (and, maybe, reduced motivation, arrow 5) has a negative impact on autobiographical memory ("overgeneralized memory," arrow 6) and neuropsychological performance in general (even if only neutral stimuli are involved, arrow 7). In addition, overgeneralized memory may also be a more direct consequence of diminished executive control (arrow 8) as described above (Sect. 9.2.2). Finally, in accordance with Roiser and Sahakian, reverse causal relations can be assumed as well, that is, "cold cognition" (e.g., executive functions) influences the emotional neuropsychological performance (arrow 9).

9.3.3.2 Other Depression Symptoms

It has long been known that (a) depression is associated with poor sleep and that (b) poor sleep impairs cognitive functioning (Yaffe et al. 2014). Therefore, it is obvious that sleep is a relevant factor to explain neuropsychological impairment in depression. In fact, recent studies with bipolar patients support this conclusion (Merikanto et al. 2012; Volkert et al. 2015). Some studies found an association between suicidality and impaired executive function in unipolar depressed patients (Dombrovski et al. 2008; Westheide et al. 2008). Keilp et al. (2013) suggest that a reduced flexible control of attention may hinder suicidal patients to redirect thinking from hopelessness and suicidal thoughts. Keilp et al. also point at overlapping neuronal networks of executive functions and emotion regulation (dorsal and lateral prefrontal cortex, dorsal cingulated). Similarly, Richard-Devantoy et al. (2012) assumed that deficits of cognitive inhibition lead to an increased risk of suicide. Recent studies with depressed patients also suggest a positive association between cognitive functioning on the one side and weight and appetite on the other (Merikanto et al. 2012; Potter et al. 2015).

9.3.4 Demographic Factors

9.3.4.1 Age and Onset

Neuropsychological deficits associated with depression are observed in all age groups. On the basis of a comprehensive analysis of studies in this field, Baune et al. (2014) summarized that neuropsychological impairment is already evident in younger adults and adolescents.

However, the (already above mentioned) finding that neuropsychological impairment sums up over time may explain why neuropsychological impairment seems to be more severe in old patients as compared to young patients (Beblo et al. 2011). Alternatively, more prominent neuropsychological deficits in older patients may also result from a still undetected dementia of some study patients who are regarded as solely depressed (Gualtieri and Morgan 2008). In fact, the risk of developing a senile dementia of the Alzheimer's type is increased in patients with depression. Several factors may contribute to this increased risk. On the one hand, depressive disorders can be regarded as an early symptom of Alzheimer's disease. On the other hand, neurobiological changes related to depressive disorders may not only lead to a decrease of neuropsychological performance but may also increase the risk of Alzheimer's disease. Neuroendocrinological research has shown changes of the hypothalamic-pituitary-adrenal axis (HPA axis) in depressed patients as being associated with neurotoxic effects, especially in the hippocampus (Paizanis et al. 2007), predisposing to the development of Alzheimer's disease (Sotiropoulos et al. 2008). Furthermore, physical and mental activity is protective against Alzheimer's disease, most likely through the effect of an enhanced neuronal reserve based on increased neurogenesis (Mirochnic et al. 2009). This neuroprotective factor might not take effect in depression due to psychomotor-retardation. In order to explain the finding of more severe neuropsychological deficits in elder depressed patients, it has also been speculated that geriatric depression presents a distinct type of affective disorders especially for patients with late-onset depression. Known risk factors for affective disorders such as personality abnormalities, a family history of psychiatric illness, and dysfunctional past maternal relationships were found to be less relevant in late-onset MDD (Brodaty et al. 2001), whereas organic factors such as cerebrovascular disease (see Sect. 9.4) and associated structural brain abnormalities are more prominent and may cause more severe neuropsychological deficits (Laks and Engelhardt 2010).

However, it is unclear whether young and older depressed patients can be reliably distinguished by their neuropsychological profiles. For example, Porter et al. (2007) suggested a relatively stronger impairment of executive function in elderly patients. By contrast, Thomas et al. (2009) reported primarily memory deficits in older MDD patients.

9.3.4.2 Education and Gender

Education and gender have also shown to be associated with neuropsychological functioning in patients with depression (Barrett et al. 2008). Depressed patients with lower levels of education tend to perform disproportionately worse in neuropsychological testing compared to education-matched control subjects (Avila et al. 2009). It has been speculated that patients with higher levels of education are in a better position to compensate for depression-associated neuropsychological dysfunction. The relation between gender and neuropsychological performance may be moderated by personality traits. Van Den Heuvel et al. (1996) found in elderly women that depression was related to cognitive dysfunction primarily in women with a weak internal locus of control. In men, the association between depression and cognitive dysfunction was moderated by neuroticism.

9.4 Poststroke Depression and Vascular Depression

Depressive disorders and vascular diseases are closely related. With respect to cerebrovascular disease, about one third of patients with stroke develop a "poststroke depression" (PSD; Flaster et al. 2013; Robinson et al. 1984). Depression further deteriorates the cognitive performance of stroke patients (Robinson and Spalletta 2010). However, the relationship between depression and neuropsychological impairment in stroke patients is complex. First, causal relations are still a matter of debate. Given the findings in psychiatric patients with depression, it seems to be plausible that depression also worsens the cognitive performance of stroke patients. However, some findings indicate a reverse relationship, that is, neuropsychological impairment may increase the patients' risk to develop a PSD (Andersen et al. 1995). Second, the relationship between depression and neuropsychological impairment is influenced by other factors and might be particularly close for patients with left hemispheric stroke within the first year after stroke (Gabaldon et al. 2007; Hadidi et al. 2009).

Older patients with depression often show multifocal cerebrovascular lesions typically located in the white matter. This type of depression was referred to as "vascular depression" (Alexopoulos et al. 1997) and is related to increased neuropsychological impairment (Newberg et al. 2006). The appearance of depressive mood and neuropsychological impairment depends on the extent and location of the lesions (Mettenburg et al. 2012; Newberg et al. 2006). However, as with PSD the causal relations are not fully understood. Generally, both depression and neuropsychological impairment were regarded as consequences of cerebrovascular lesions, in particular of disrupted fronto-striatal pathways (Newberg et al. 2006). This interpretation is in agreement with neurobiological circuit models of depression (e.g., Drevets et al. (2008)). However, it is also possible that symptoms of depression such as rumination lead to a decreased cognitive performance (e.g., via an increase of rumination) or, alternatively, neurocognitive impairment leads to depression when patients become aware of cognitive constraints in their everyday life. This discussion is further complicated by the fact that some authors suggested the solely occurrence of executive dysfunctions to be sufficient for the diagnosis of vascular depression irrespective of the evidence of cerebrovascular lesions (Steffens and Krishnan 1998). From this point of view, the finding of an increased neuropsychological impairment in patients with vascular depression is circular.

9.5 Clinical Implications and Treatment

9.5.1 Clinical Implications

Neuropsychological deficits of depressed patients have important clinical implications. As already mentioned above, several studies indicate that these dysfunctions weaken the ability to adaptively regulate emotions and stress and, thus, finally intensify suicidal tendencies (Keilp et al. 2013; Richard-Devantoy et al. 2012). Neuropsychological impairment also has a negative impact on treatment adherence and treatment success (Martinez-Aran et al. 2009; Papakostas 2014). In addition, neuropsychological impairment of depressed patients has been associated with a reduced level of psychosocial and occupational functioning which even remained when statistical analyses controlled for further depressive symptoms. The association between neuropsychological dysfunction and psychosocial impairment has also been found among depressed patients in remission with persistent neuropsychological impairment (Baune et al. 2010) and even appears to be more prominent in patients with mood disorders than in patients with schizophrenia (Brissos et al. 2008). Given these implications, neuropsychological deficits of depressed patients lead to a vicious cycle (Fig. 9.2): Depression-associated neuropsychological impairment leads to a reduced level of psychosocial and occupational functioning. Experiences of failure in social and occupational life in its turn strengthen depression. The fatal logic of this vicious cycle gets further inflamed by the fact that treatment response is reduced in depressed patients with cognitive impairment.

These clinical implications strongly underscore the importance of the diagnosis and treatment of the patients' neuropsychological deficits. Sometimes it has been argued that depressive patients are overcharged by neuropsychological testing. While this might be true for some extremely affected patients in the very acute phase of the disorder, generally, neuropsychological testing is well tolerated (Beblo et al. 2005). With respect to therapy, it might be speculated that standard antidepressant therapy is sufficient to treat depression-related neuropsychological dysfunction. However, research shows that this assumption is only partially true as cognitive

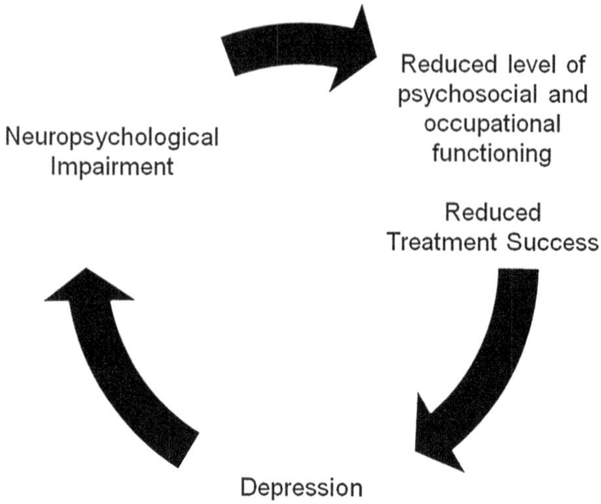

Fig. 9.2 Vicious cycle of neuropsychological impairment in depression

deficits only partially improve with clinical recovery. Therefore, an additional treatment is indicated for those patients with depression who show persistent neuropsychological impairment.

9.5.2 Treatment of Neuropsychological Impairment

At least, three different strategies have been evaluated so far. First, neuropsychological approaches that had been originally developed for brain-damaged patients (and, partially, for patients with schizophrenia) and that have been – more or less – adopted for patients with affective disorders. Studies indicate that patients profit from individual (Preiss et al. 2013) and group approaches (Naismith et al. 2010). Improvement has been documented for several cognitive domains such as memory and learning, attention, psychomotor speed, and executive function (Elgamal et al. 2007; Naismith et al. 2010; Trebo et al. 2007). While Trebo et al. (2007) also found improvements in mood and cognitive symptoms, improvements were restricted to neuropsychological functions in the Elgamal and Naismith studies (Elgamal et al. 2007; Naismith et al. 2010). Recently, some authors stress the need of therapies that are more specified for the needs of patients with affective disorders (Bowie et al. 2013; Martinez-Aran et al. 2011). In a multicenter trial with 183 patients, effects of a novel functional remediation training were analyzed (Torrent et al. 2013). Functional remediation integrates psychoeducation about neuropsychological impairment and training strategies for attention, memory, and executive functions on the base of real-life situations. In addition, social skills and stress management were also trained. With respect to their primary outcome, global psychosocial functioning, functional remediation exceeded effects of treatment as usual but not of an active control condition (psychoeducation). Deckersbach et al. (2010) developed a cognitive remediation therapy to treat residual depressive symptoms. The training focused on (1) mood management; (2) organization, planning, and time management; and (3) attention and memory. In their study, patients showed improvements in depressive symptoms, occupational and psychosocial functioning, and in executive functions. Improvements in executive functions accounted for the improvements in occupational functioning. This finding underlines the importance of neuropsychological performance for daily functions.

A second treatment approach focuses on the training of mindfulness. Historically, mindfulness is a central element of Buddhist meditation and implies to pay attention on purpose, in the present moment, and nonjudgementally to the own experience of the present moment (Kabat-Zinn 1990). In the last 30 years, the training of mindfulness has become increasingly popular for the treatment of patients with physical and mental disorders. In addition, the effects of mindfulness-based therapies have been extensively evaluated. Besides beneficial effects on well-being, it also became evident that mindfulness might improve cognitive functioning (Chiesa et al. 2011). Some studies indicate that also depressed patients may neuropsychologically profit from mindfulness-based therapies (Deckersbach et al. 2012; Ives-Deliperi et al. 2013). Positive effects on neuropsychological functioning by training of mindfulness may be moderated by different mechanisms. Since mindfulness is closely related to attention, training mindfulness may improve attention in particular and neuropsychological functions in general. In addition, cognitive deficits of patients with affective disorders are related to rumination (see above). In a sample of patients with lifetime mood disorders, mindfulness-based stress reduction (MBSR; Kabat-Zinn 1990) reduced rumination even after controlling for reductions in affective symptoms and dysfunctional beliefs (Ramel et al. 2004).

Third, several biological approaches for the treatment of depression improve cognitive functioning. Antidepressants modify neurotransmitter systems and cognitive performance. Tricyclic antidepressants (TCAs) inhibit the neurotransmitter acetylcholine and thereby may induce severe cognitive side effects, potentially leading to a delirium, particularly among elderly patients with depression. On the contrary, selective serotonin reuptake inhibitors (SSRIs) have either no or very mild anticholinergic effects. Consequently, most studies have shown that SSRIs have a substantially greater positive effect on cognitive function compared to TCAs (Peretti et al. 2000). Possibly, serotonin-norepinephrine reuptake inhibitors (SNRIs) and multimodal-acting antidepressants may have even greater positive effects (Herrera-Guzman et al. 2009; Pehrson et al. 2015). There is also some evidence that augmentation therapy may be useful approach if cognitive deficits persist after monotherapy (Keefe et al. 2014). Positive effects on cognition were also reported from relatively new neurobiological techniques such as repetitive transcranial magnetic stimulation (rTMS; e.g., Brunoni and Vanderhasselt (2014)), transcranial direct cranial stimulation (tDCS; e.g., Wolkenstein and Plewnia (2013)), or neurofeedback training

(Escolano et al. 2014). However, more research is necessary to specify these results, e.g., how to apply rTMS in order to have the best results (Nadeau et al. 2014).

Conclusions

Depression is related to neuropsychological impairment and further deteriorates cognitive performance of brain-damaged patients. However, the magnitude of these depression-related impairments is still a matter of debate as self-reports indicate much more severe deficits than neuropsychological test outcomes. Future research needs to clarify whether this discrepancy is primarily due to depressive patients' negatively biased self-perception or, alternatively, due to differences between everyday life (relevant for self-reports) and a standardized neuropsychological test setting (relevant for the application of tests). With respect to the profile of neuropsychological impairment, research demonstrated shortcomings in the domains of attention, executive functions, and declarative memory. As many factors influence the cognitive performance of depressed patients, it is not surprising that the neuropsychological profile has not been characterized more precisely. For example, more severe subtypes of depressive disorders and the presence of some depressive symptoms such as rumination or sleep disturbances are related to a generally lower cognitive performance and different neuropsychological profile. These findings indicate that the search for "the neuropsychological profile of depression" is not very promising. Instead, researches should try to specify the relationship between features of the depressive disorder on the one hand and characteristics of the neuropsychological impairment on the other.

Neuropsychological impairment of depressed patients has important clinical implications. It is related to a diminished level of social and occupational functioning as well as to reduced compliance and treatment success. Some studies even indicate an increased suicidality in those patients who are particularly affected by neuropsychological impairments. Because neuropsychological impairment often persists after psycho- and antidepressant therapy, an effective neuropsychological treatment is needed. Researchers suggested that neuropsychological therapies that had been originally developed for brain-damaged patients are also helpful for depressed patients. In the last years, it also became evident that the training of mindfulness (that always implies the training of attention) improves cognitive functioning. Because mindfulness training also reduces other symptoms of depressive disorders that are related to the cognitive performance (e.g., sleep disturbances or rumination), it might be particularly effective for depressed patients. In addition, research has shown that some biological treatment approaches such as the use of specific antidepressants, repetitive transcranial magnetic stimulation, transcranial direct cranial stimulation, or neurofeedback training have positive effects on cognitive performance. Future research has to compare the effectiveness of these different treatment approaches for depressed patients. Furthermore, it is still unclear to what extent the combination of these approaches is of additional value.

References

Alexopoulos GS, Meyers BS, Young RC et al (1997) 'Vascular depression' hypothesis. Arch Gen Psychiatry 54:915–922

American Psychiatric Association (2013) Diagnostic and statistical manual of mental disorders, (DSM-5), 5th edn. American Psychiatric Association, Washington, DC

Andersen G, Vestergaard K, Ingemann-Nielsen M et al (1995) Risk factors for post-stroke depression. Acta Psychiatr Scand 92:193–198

Austin MP, Ross M, Murray C et al (1992) Cognitive function in major depression. J Affect Disord 25:21–29

Avila R, Moscoso MA, Ribeiz S et al (2009) Influence of education and depressive symptoms on cognitive function in the elderly. Int Psychogeriatr 21:560–567

Barrett SL, Kelly C, Bell R et al (2008) Gender influences the detection of spatial working memory deficits in bipolar disorder. Bipolar Disord 10:647–654

Baune BT, Miller R, Mcafoose J et al (2010) The role of cognitive impairment in general functioning in major depression. Psychiatry Res 176:183–189

Baune BT, Fuhr M, Air T et al (2014) Neuropsychological functioning in adolescents and young adults with major depressive disorder – a review. Psychiatry Res 218:261–271

Beats BC, Sahakian BJ, Levy R (1996) Cognitive performance in tests sensitive to frontal lobe dysfunction in the elderly depressed. Psychol Med 26:591–603

Beblo T, Herrmann M (2000) Neuropsychologische Defizite bei depressiven Störungen. Fortschr Neurol Psychiatr 68:1–11

Beblo T, Lautenbacher S (2006) Neuropsychologie der Depression. Hogrefe, Göttingen

Beblo T, Baumann B, Bogerts B et al (1999) Neuropsychological correlates of major depression: a short term follow-up. Cogn Neuropsychiatr 4:333–341

Beblo T, Lahr D, Hartje W (2005) The impact of neuropsychological testing on the emotional state of patients with major depression. Z Neuropsychol 16:15–22

Beblo T, Mensebach C, Wingenfeld K et al (2010) The impact of neutral and emotionally negative distraction on memory performance and its relation to memory complaints in major depression. Psychiatry Res 178:106–111

Beblo T, Sinnamon G, Baune BT (2011) Specifying the neuropsychology of affective disorders: clinical, demographic and neurobiological factors. Neuropsychol Rev 21:337–359

Beck AT (1967) Depression: clinical, experimental and theoretical aspects. Harper and Row, New York

Beck AT, Clark DA, Alford BA (1999) Scientific foundations of cognitive theory and therapy of depression. Wiley, New York

Beckwe M, Deroost N, Koster EH et al (2014) Worrying and rumination are both associated with reduced cognitive control. Psychological Research 78:651–660

Belcher J, Kangas M (2014) Reduced goal specificity is associated with reduced memory specificity in depressed adults. Cogn Emot 28:163–171

Benitez A, Horner MD, Bachman D (2011) Intact cognition in depressed elderly veterans providing adequate effort. Arch Clin Neuropsychol: Off J Natl Acad Neuropsychol 26:184–193

Bowie CR, Gupta M, Holshausen K (2013) Cognitive remediation therapy for mood disorders: rationale, early evidence, and future directions. Can J Psychiatry 58:319–325

Brissos S, Dias VV, Carita AI et al (2008) Quality of life in bipolar type I disorder and schizophrenia in remission: clinical and neurocognitive correlates. Psychiatry Res 160:55–62

Brodaty H, Luscombe G, Parker G et al (2001) Early and late onset depression in old age: different aetiologies, same phenomenology. J Affect Disord 66:225–236

Brunoni AR, Vanderhasselt MA (2014) Working memory improvement with non-invasive brain stimulation of the dorsolateral prefrontal cortex: a systematic review and meta-analysis. Brain Cogn 86:1–9

Burt T, Prudic J, Peyser S et al (2000) Learning and memory in bipolar and unipolar major depression: effects of aging. Neuropsychiatr Neuropsychol Behav Neurol 13:246–253

Cella M, Dymond S, Cooper A (2010) Impaired flexible decision-making in major depressive disorder. J Affect Disord 124:207–210
Chiesa A, Calati R, Serretti A (2011) Does mindfulness training improve cognitive abilities? A systematic review of neuropsychological findings. Clin Psychol Rev 31:449–464
Christensen H, Griffiths K, Mackinnon A et al (1997) A quantitative review of cognitive deficits in depression and Alzheimer-type dementia. J Int Neuropsychol Soc 3:631–651
Conradi HJ, Ormel J, De Jonge P (2011) Presence of individual (residual) symptoms during depressive episodes and periods of remission: a 3-year prospective study. Psychol Med 41:1165–1174
Crane C, Barnhofer T, Visser C et al (2007) The effects of analytical and experiential rumination on autobiographical memory specificity in individuals with a history of major depression. Behav Res Ther 45:3077–3087
Deckersbach T, Nierenberg AA, Kessler R et al (2010) RESEARCH: cognitive rehabilitation for bipolar disorder: an open trial for employed patients with residual depressive symptoms. CNS Neurosci Ther 16:298–307
Deckersbach T, Holzel BK, Eisner LR et al (2012) Mindfulness-based cognitive therapy for non-remitted patients with bipolar disorder. CNS Neurosci Ther 18:133–141
Delaloye C, Moy G, De Bilbao F et al (2010) Neuroanatomical and neuropsychological features of elderly euthymic depressed patients with early- and late-onset. J Neurol Sci 299:19–23
Dombrovski AY, Butters MA, Reynolds CF 3rd et al (2008) Cognitive performance in suicidal depressed elderly: preliminary report. Am J Geriatr Psychiatry 16:109–115
Donaldson C, Lam D (2004) Rumination, mood and social problem-solving in major depression. Psychol Med 34:1309–1318
Douglas KM, Porter RJ, Frampton CM et al (2009) Abnormal response to failure in unmedicated major depression. J Affect Disord 119:92–99
Drevets WC, Price JL, Furey ML (2008) Brain structural and functional abnormalities in mood disorders: implications for neurocircuitry models of depression. Brain Struct Funct 213:93–118
Drysdale E, Knight HM, Mcintosh AM et al (2013) Cognitive endophenotypes in a family with bipolar disorder with a risk locus on chromosome 4. Bipolar Disord 15:215–222
Elgamal S, Mckinnon MC, Ramakrishnan K et al (2007) Successful computer-assisted cognitive remediation therapy in patients with unipolar depression: a proof of principle study. Psychol Med 37:1229–1238
Elliott R, Sahakian BJ, Mckay AP et al (1996) Neuropsychological impairments in unipolar depression: the influence of perceived failure on subsequent performance. Psychol Med 26:975–989
Elliott R, Sahakian BJ, Herrod JJ et al (1997) Abnormal response to negative feedback in unipolar depression: evidence for a diagnosis specific impairment. J Neurol Neurosurg Psychiatry 63:74–82
Ellwart T, Rinck M, Becker ES (2003) Selective memory and memory deficits in depressed inpatients. Depress Anxiety 17:197–206
Escolano C, Navarro-Gil M, Garcia-Campayo J et al (2014) A controlled study on the cognitive effect of alpha neurofeedback training in patients with major depressive disorder. Front Behav Neurosci 8:296
Everaert J, Koster EH, Derakshan N (2012) The combined cognitive bias hypothesis in depression. Clin Psychol Rev 32:413–424
Flaster M, Sharma A, Rao M (2013) Poststroke depression: a review emphasizing the role of prophylactic treatment and synergy with treatment for motor recovery. Top Stroke Rehabil 20:139–150
Fleming SK, Blasey C, Schatzberg AF (2004) Neuropsychological correlates of psychotic features in major depressive disorders: a review and meta-analysis. J Psychiatr Res 38:27–35
Gabaldon L, Fuentes B, Frank-Garcia A et al (2007) Poststroke depression: importance of its detection and treatment. Cerebrovasc Dis 24(Suppl 1):181–188
Gorwood P, Corruble E, Falissard B et al (2008) Toxic effects of depression on brain function: impairment of delayed recall and the cumulative length of depressive disorder in a large sample of depressed outpatients. Am J Psychiatry 165:731–739
Gotlib IH, Joormann J (2010) Cognition and depression: current status and future directions. Annu Rev Clin Psychol 6:285–312

Gualtieri CT, Morgan DW (2008) The frequency of cognitive impairment in patients with anxiety, depression, and bipolar disorder: an unaccounted source of variance in clinical trials. J Clin Psychiatr 69:1122–1130
Hadidi N, Treat-Jacobson DJ, Lindquist R (2009) Poststroke depression and functional outcome: a critical review of literature. Heart Lung: J Crit Care 38:151–162
Hasher L, Zacks RT (1979) Automatic and effortful processing in memory. J Exp Psychol Gen 108:356–388
Hasler G, Drevets WC, Manji HK et al (2004) Discovering endophenotypes for major depression. Neuropsychopharmacology 29:1765–1781
Hasselbalch B, Knorr U, Hasselbalch S et al (2013) The cumulative load of depressive illness is associated with cognitive function in the remitted state of unipolar depressive disorder. Eur Psychiatry 28:349–355
Henry J, Crawford JR (2005) A meta-analytic review of verbal fluency deficits in depression. J Clin Exp Neuropsychol 27:78–101
Herrera-Guzman I, Gudayol-Ferre E, Herrera-Guzman D et al (2009) Effects of selective serotonin reuptake and dual serotonergic-noradrenergic reuptake treatments on memory and mental processing speed in patients with major depressive disorder. J Psychiatr Res 43:855–863
Hsiao YL, Wu YS, Wu JY et al (2009) Neuropsychological functions in patients with bipolar I and bipolar II disorder. Bipolar Disord 11:547–554
Ives-Deliperi VL, Howells F, Stein DJ et al (2013) The effects of mindfulness-based cognitive therapy in patients with bipolar disorder: a controlled functional MRI investigation. J Affect Disord 150:1152–1157
Joormann J, Gotlib IH (2008) Updating the contents of working memory in depression: interference from irrelevant negative material. J Abnorm Psychol 117:182–192
Kabat-Zinn J (1990) Full catastrophe living: using the wisdom of your body and mind to face stress, pain, and illness. Delta Trade Paperbacks, New York
Keefe RS (1995) The contribution of neuropsychology to psychiatry. Am J Psychiatr 152:6–15
Keefe RS, Mcclintock SM, Roth RM et al (2014) Cognitive effects of pharmacotherapy for major depressive disorder: a systematic review. J Clin Psychiatry 75:864–876
Keilp J, Gorlyn M, Russell M et al (2013) Neuropsychological function and suicidal behavior: attention control, memory and executive dysfunction in suicide attempt. Psychol Med 43:539–551
Kircanski K, Joormann J, Gotlib IH (2012) Cognitive aspects of depression. Wiley Interdiscip Rev Cogn Sci 3:301–313
Korten N, Penninx BW, Kok RM et al (2014) Heterogeneity of late-life depression: relationship with cognitive functioning. Int Psychogeriatr 26:953–963
Koster EH, De Raedt R, Leyman L et al (2010) Mood-congruent attention and memory bias in dysphoria: exploring the coherence among information-processing biases. Behav Res Ther 48:219–225
Lahr D, Beblo T, Hartje W (2007) Cognitive performance and subjective complaints before and after remission of major depression. Cogn Neuropsychiatry 12:25–45
Laks J, Engelhardt E (2010) Peculiarities of geriatric psychiatry: a focus on aging and depression. CNS Neurosci Ther 16:374–379
Leppanen JM (2006) Emotional information processing in mood disorders: a review of behavioral and neuroimaging findings. Curr Opin Psychiatry 19:34–39
Mackin RS, Nelson JC, Delucchi KL et al (2014) Association of age at depression onset with cognitive functioning in individuals with late-life depression and executive dysfunction. Am J Geriatr Psychiatry 22:1633–1641
Maeshima H, Baba H, Nakano Y et al (2013) Time course for memory dysfunction in early-life and late-life major depression: a longitudinal study from the Juntendo university mood disorder project. J Affect Disord 151:66–70
Marano CM, Workman CI, Lyman CH et al (2015) Structural imaging in late life depression: association with mood and cognitive responses to antidepressant treatment. Am J Geriatr Psychiatr 23:6–12
Martinez-Aran A, Scott J, Colom F et al (2009) Treatment nonadherence and neurocognitive impairment in bipolar disorder. J Clin Psychiatry 70:1017–1023

Martinez-Aran A, Torrent C, Sole B et al (2011) Functional remediation for bipolar disorder. Clin Pract Epidemiol Ment Health: CP EMH 7:112–116
Mckinnon MC, Yucel K, Nazarov A et al (2009) A meta-analysis examining clinical predictors of hippocampal volume in patients with major depressive disorder. J Psychiatry Neurosci 34: 41–54
Merikanto I, Lahti T, Castaneda AE et al (2012) Influence of seasonal variation in mood and behavior on cognitive test performance among young adults. Nord J Psychiatry 66:303–310
Mesholam-Gately RI, Giuliano AJ, Zillmer EA et al (2012) Verbal learning and memory in older adults with minor and major depression. Arch Clin Neuropsychol: Off J Natl Acad Neuropsychol 27:196–207
Mettenburg JM, Benzinger TL, Shimony JS et al (2012) Diminished performance on neuropsychological testing in late life depression is correlated with microstructural white matter abnormalities. NeuroImage 60:2182–2190
Michopoulos I, Zervas IM, Pantelis C et al (2008) Neuropsychological and hypothalamic-pituitary-axis function in female patients with melancholic and non-melancholic depression. Eur Arch Psychiatry Clin Neurosci 258:217–225
Mirochnic S, Wolf S, Staufenbiel M et al (2009) Age effects on the regulation of adult hippocampal neurogenesis by physical activity and environmental enrichment in the APP23 mouse model of Alzheimer disease. Hippocampus 19:1008–1018
Moffoot AP, O'carroll RE, Bennie J et al (1994) Diurnal variation of mood and neuropsychological function in major depression with melancholia. J Affect Disord 32:257–269
Murphy FC, Michael A, Robbins TW et al (2003) Neuropsychological impairment in patients with major depressive disorder: the effects of feedback on task performance. Psychol Med 33:455–467
Nadeau SE, Bowers D, Jones TL et al (2014) Cognitive effects of treatment of depression with repetitive transcranial magnetic stimulation. Cogn Behav Neurol 27:77–87
Naismith SL, Redoblado-Hodge MA, Lewis SJ et al (2010) Cognitive training in affective disorders improves memory: a preliminary study using the NEAR approach. J Affect Disord 121:258–262
Newberg AR, Davydow DS, Lee HB (2006) Cerebrovascular disease basis of depression: post-stroke depression and vascular depression. Int Rev Psychiatry 18:433–441
Paizanis E, Hamon M, Lanfumey L (2007) Hippocampal neurogenesis, depressive disorders, and antidepressant therapy. Neural Plast 2007:73754
Pálsson S, Johansson B, Berg S et al (2000) A population study on the influence of depression on neuropsychological functioning in 85-year-olds. Acta Psychiatr Scand 101:185–193
Papakostas GI (2014) Cognitive symptoms in patients with major depressive disorder and their implications for clinical practice. J Clin Psychiatry 75:8–14
Pehrson AL, Leiser SC, Gulinello M et al (2015) Treatment of cognitive dysfunction in major depressive disorder-a review of the preclinical evidence for efficacy of selective serotonin reuptake inhibitors, serotonin-norepinephrine reuptake inhibitors and the multimodal-acting antidepressant vortioxetine. Eur J Pharmacol 753:19–31
Peretti S, Judge R, Hindmarch I (2000) Safety and tolerability considerations: tricyclic antidepressants vs. selective serotonin reuptake inhibitors. Acta Psychiatr Scand Suppl 403:17–25
Philippot P, Brutoux F (2008) Induced rumination dampens executive processes in dysphoric young adults. J Behav Ther Exp Psychiatry 39:219–227
Porter RJ, Bourke C, Gallagher P (2007) Neuropsychological impairment in major depression: its nature, origin and clinical significance. Aust N Z J Psychiatry 41:115–128
Porterfield T, Cook M, Deary IJ et al (1997) Neuropsychological function and diurnal variation in depression. J Clin Exp Neuropsychol 19:906–913
Post RM (1992) Transduction of psychosocial stress into the neurobiology of recurrent affective disorder. Am J Psychiatry 149:999–1010
Potter GG, Mcquoid DR, Steffens DC (2015) Appetite loss and neurocognitive deficits in late-life depression. Int J Geriatr Psychiatry 30:647–654
Preiss M, Shatil E, Čermáková R et al (2013) Personalized cognitive training in unipolar and bipolar disorder: a study of cognitive functioning. Front Hum Neurosci 7:108

Quinn C, Harris A, Kemp A (2012) The interdependence of subtype and severity: contributions of clinical and neuropsychological features to melancholia and non-melancholia in an outpatient sample. J Int Neuropsychol Soc 18:361–369
Ramel W, Goldin PR, Carmona PE et al (2004) The effects of mindfulness meditation on cognitive processes and affect in patients with past depression. Cogn Ther Res 28:435–455
Richard-Devantoy S, Jollant F, Kefi Z et al (2012) Deficit of cognitive inhibition in depressed elderly: a neurocognitive marker of suicidal risk. J Affect Disord 140:193–199
Richards PM, Ruff RM (1989) Motivational effects on neuropsychological functioning: comparison of depressed versus nondepressed individuals. J Consult Clin Psychol 57:396–402
Robinson RG, Spalletta G (2010) Poststroke depression: a review. Can J Psychiatry 55:341–349
Robinson RG, Kubos KL, Starr LB et al (1984) Mood disorders in stroke patients: importance of location of lesion. Brain 107:81–93
Roiser JP, Sahakian BJ (2013) Hot and cold cognition in depression. CNS Spectr 18:139–149
Ros L, Aguilar MJ, Serrano JP et al (2013) Depression affects specifically executive functioning: new evidence from older population. Int J Geriatr Psychiatry 28:327–328
Sarapas C, Shankman SA, Harrow M et al (2012) Parsing trait and state effects of depression severity on neurocognition: evidence from a 26-year longitudinal study. J Abnorm Psychol 121:830–837
Scheurich A, Fellgiebel A, Schermuly I et al (2008) Experimental evidence for a motivational origin of cognitive impairment in major depression. Psychol Med 38:237–246
Shamay-Tsoory S, Harari H, Szepsenwol O et al (2009) Neuropsychological evidence of impaired cognitive empathy in euthymic bipolar disorder. J Neuropsychiatry Clin Neurosci 21:59–67
Snyder HR (2013) Major depressive disorder is associated with broad impairments on neuropsychological measures of executive function: a meta-analysis and review. Psychol Bull 139:81–132
Sotiropoulos I, Cerqueira JJ, Catania C et al (2008) Stress and glucocorticoid footprints in the brain-the path from depression to Alzheimer's disease. Neurosci Biobehav Rev 32:1161–1173
Steffens DC, Krishnan KR (1998) Structural neuroimaging and mood disorders: recent findings, implications for classification, and future directions. Biol Psychiatry 43:705–712
Taylor Tavares JV, Clark L, Cannon DM et al (2007) Distinct profiles of neurocognitive function in unmedicated unipolar depression and bipolar II depression. Biol Psychiatry 62:917–924
Thomas AJ, Gallagher P, Robinson LJ et al (2009) A comparison of neurocognitive impairment in younger and older adults with major depression. Psychol Med 39:725–733
Torrent C, Martinez-Aran A, Daban C et al (2006) Cognitive impairment in bipolar II disorder. Br J Psychiatry 189:254–259
Torrent C, Bonnin Cdel M, Martinez-Aran A et al (2013) Efficacy of functional remediation in bipolar disorder: a multicenter randomized controlled study. Am J Psychiatry 170:852–859
Trebo E, Holzner B, Pircher M et al (2007) The effects of a computer assisted cognitive training on neuropsychological parameters, mood and dysfunctional cognitions in depressive patients. Neuropsychiatr: Klin Diagn Ther Rehabil: Organ Ges Osterreichischer Nervenarzte Psychiater 21:207–215
Van Den Heuvel N, Smits CH, Deeg DJ et al (1996) Personality: a moderator of the relation between cognitive functioning and depression in adults aged 55–85? J Affect Disord 41:229–240
Volkert J, Kopf J, Kazmaier J et al (2015) Evidence for cognitive subgroups in bipolar disorder and the influence of subclinical depression and sleep disturbances. Eur Neuropsychopharmacol J Eur Coll Neuropsychopharmacol 25:192–202
Watkins E, Brown RG (2002) Rumination and executive function in depression: an experimental study. J Neurol Neurosurg Psychiatry 72:400–402
Westheide J, Quednow BB, Kuhn KU et al (2008) Executive performance of depressed suicide attempters: the role of suicidal ideation. Eur Arch Psychiatry Clin Neurosci 258:414–421
Who (1991) ICD-10 Classification of mental and behavioral disorders with glossary and diagnostic criteria for research ICD-10: DCR-10. Churchill Livingstone, Edinburgh
Williams JM, Scott J (1988) Autobiographical memory in depression. Psychol Med 18:689–695
Withall A, Harris LM, Cumming SR (2010) A longitudinal study of cognitive function in melancholic and non-melancholic subtypes of major depressive disorder. J Affect Disord 123:150–157

Wolkenstein L, Plewnia C (2013) Amelioration of cognitive control in depression by transcranial direct current stimulation. Biol Psychiatry 73:646–651

Yaffe K, Falvey CM, Hoang T (2014) Connections between sleep and cognition in older adults. Lancet Neurol 13:1017–1028

Yoon KL, Lemoult J, Joormann J (2014) Updating emotional content in working memory: a depression-specific deficit? J Behav Ther Exp Psychiatry 45:368–374

Young KD, Erickson K, Drevets WC (2012) Differential effects of emotionally versus neutrally cued autobiographical memories on performance of a subsequent cognitive task: effects of task difficulty. Front Psychol 3:299

Neuroimaging of Risk Factors of Depression and Cardiovascular Disease

10

Nils Opel, Udo Dannlowski, and Ronny Redlich

Contents

N. Opel • R. Redlich, MA
Department of Psychiatry, University of Münster,
Albert-Schweitzer-Str. 11, 48149 Munster, Germany

U. Dannlowski, MA, MD, PhD (✉)
Department of Psychiatry, University of Münster,
Albert-Schweitzer-Str. 11, 48149 Munster, Germany

Department of Psychiatry, University of Marburg, Marburg, Germany
e-mail: dannlow@uni-muenster.de

B.T. Baune, P.J. Tully (eds.), *Cardiovascular Diseases and Depression*,
DOI 10.1007/978-3-319-32480-7_10

Abstract
Major depressive disorder (MDD) and cardiovascular disease (CVD) have been evidenced to be interconnected by a bidirectional link since MDD increases the risk of developing CVD and vice versa. However, the biological underpinnings of this relationship are poorly understood up to now. Thus, neuroimaging of shared risk factors of both disorders might shed more light on possible neurobiological implications and help to gain a broader understanding of the mechanisms behind this important clinical connection. Recent neuroimaging studies suggest a predominant involvement of alterations in neural networks of emotion regulation and reward processing in CVD, MDD, and their common risk factors. Moreover, there is evidence that functional and structural brain changes are closely related to inflammatory processes in the development of CVD and MDD. Since these alterations in brain structure and function are yet apparent in subjects at high risk but before the onset of clinically manifest disease and given the observed reversibility of these neural aberrations, neuroimaging findings point to the crucial role of preventive measures in the therapy of both disorders. Especially, therapeutic interventions at an early stage in high-risk populations should be reevaluated in the prevention of both disorders. Future research should focus on the close link between inflammatory and neural processes to provide the neurobiological basis for integrated treatment options for CVD and MDD.

10.1 Introduction

The bidirectional link between major depressive disorder (MDD) and cardiovascular disease (CVD) has been evidenced by numerous epidemiological studies (Baune et al. 2012; Charlson et al. 2011; Elderon and Whooley 2013; Thombs et al. 2006). The elevated prevalence of CVD in MDD populations and vice versa of MDD in CVD populations strongly suggests a common pathophysiological background of both conditions. However, the understanding of the biological implications underlying this shared risk constellation remains vague.

Neuroimaging studies might provide new insights into the etiological processes of this conspicuous connection. A large number of neuroimaging studies have searched to identify neurobiological markers associated with risk factors of CVD and MDD to provide the basis for enhanced preventive measures and adjusted treatment options. Thus, it might be helpful to primarily define which specific problems might indeed reasonably be assigned to neuroimaging research in this matter. Due to the genuine capabilities of describing alterations in brain structure and function in specific brain regions in patients, healthy subjects, and risk groups, it appears that foremost three main questions should be addressed by neuroimaging research:

1. Functional MRI: Is it possible to detect specific neural networks involved in the development of both CVD and MDD pointing to shared cognitive patterns?

2. Structural MRI: Is it possible to confine a chronology in the development of certain risk constellations referring to preexisting traits or state-dependent cerebral changes?
3. Treatment: In which way might neuroimaging research be able to enhance future preventive and therapeutic measures in MDD and CVD treatment?

The broad field of CVD risk factors includes a wide range of metabolic, endocrinological, social, and psychological conditions of which some have recently been connected also to affective disorders. Common risk constellations of both disorders foremost comprise stress, obesity, and lower socioeconomic status (Cohen et al. 2007; Luppino et al. 2010; Rozanski et al. 1999). In neuroimaging research, environmental stress and obesity are the most frequently investigated risk conditions for both CVD and MDD and thus might illustrate chances, potential consequences, and limitations of neuroimaging research in the evaluation of the biological underpinnings of CVD and MDD risk factors.

While the role of obesity as a risk factor of CVD might sufficiently be explained by its contribution to the pathogenesis of atherosclerosis, little is known about the mechanisms which might lead to an increased risk for affective disorders in obese subjects.

Obesity is one of the most frequently observed somatic comorbidities of MDD (de Wit et al. 2010) with an elevated prevalence not only among subjects suffering from MDD but also in high-risk populations before the onset of disease (Danese and Tan 2014). Moreover, it has been shown that obesity increases the risk of depression and vice versa pointing to a reciprocal link between depression and obesity (Luppino et al. 2010). The clinical importance of this frequent comorbidity was underlined by studies indicating that nutritional counseling and physical activity are accompanied by both weight loss and improvement of depressive symptoms in obese adolescents (Melnyk et al. 2013) and that obese and overweight MDD patients suffer from poorer treatment outcome (Kloiber et al. 2007). Given the mutual negative impact of these disorders, especially the poorer treatment outcome of obese MDD patients, further elucidation of common biological factors could be of great clinical use. A potential neurobiological connection between obesity and MDD might highlight the relevance of preventive measures against obesity and provide the basis for adjusted strategies in MDD treatment.

In contrast to obesity as a measurable somatic condition, the experience of environmental stress is primarily thought of as affecting psychological or mental states. However, as it is the case for obesity, chronic stress exerts multiple adverse effects leading to an increased risk for both somatic and psychiatric disorders (Cohen et al. 2007; Gilbert et al. 2009; Nanni et al. 2012; Rozanski et al. 1999; Steptoe and Kivimäki 2012). The stress-induced dysregulation of the hypothalamic–pituitary–adrenal axis (HPA axis) and resulting elevated levels of glucocorticoids are known to interfere with neuroplasticity, neural signaling, and diverse immunologic processes (Montoya et al. 2014; Wang et al. 2010). The adverse influence of stressful experiences seems to be dramatically increased during early life which is why childhood trauma might serve as a useful example to demonstrate the detrimental impact of environmental stress on brain structure and function (Heim et al. 2008).

10.2 Functional MRI

In the search for shared pathophysiological factors in the development of CVD and MDD, it appears reasonable to primarily focus on conditions that have been evidenced to increase the risk for both disorders. Among these shared risk factors especially stress and obesity have been shown to be decisive in the onset of both disorders by a large number of epidemiological studies (Luppino et al. 2010; Rozanski et al. 1999; Steptoe and Kivimäki 2012). Functional neuroimaging has been shown to be a valuable tool in the detection of neural alterations that might be linked to these conditions. Compared to structural imaging, functional studies benefit from the possibility of customized paradigms allowing insights into specific neural processing and therefore constitute an effective method in the elucidation of dysfunctional cognitive patterns that might contribute to an increased risk for both CVD and MDD.

10.2.1 Major Depression

In MDD, an extensive number of fMRI studies demonstrated deficits in different stages of emotion processing which are associated with neural aberrations. Clinical features of MDD like anhedonia and the predominant tendency to classify emotional stimuli as negative, sad, or adverse have been shown to be strongly associated with hyperreactivity in limbic brain regions, especially with a predominant activation of the amygdala (Sheline et al. 2001; Siegle et al. 2007; Stuhrmann et al. 2012). Besides this excess of bottom-up signaling, aberrant activation of prefrontal cortical areas has frequently been evidenced in MDD and is thought to play an important role in altered emotion regulation and control in depressed patients (Phillips et al. 2003a; Rive et al. 2013). More precisely, over-recruitment of the anterior cingulate cortex (ACC) and dorsolateral prefrontal cortex (DLPFC) during behavioral and cognitive control has been shown to be a core feature of major depressive disorder and might be interpreted as a compensation mechanism in a dysfunctional neural system (Frodl et al. 2009; Rive et al. 2013).

As another considerable aspect, dysfunctional neural processing of the reward system has frequently been linked to MDD (Zhang et al. 2013). Depressed patients were shown to exhibit altered neural response during reward processing in the nucleus accumbens, the VTA, and the cingulate cortex which suggests a major contribution of dysfunctional reward processing in the development of depressive disorder (Knutson et al. 2008; Kumar et al. 2008; Redlich et al. 2015).

10.2.2 Cardiovascular Disease

At present, the number of fMRI studies which directly investigated neural alterations in CVD is still limited. The few studies available indicate that vascular disease is associated with functional changes in hippocampal, frontal, and parietal cortical areas during executive control and memory processing much resembling neurobiological insights from dementia research and aging (Braskie et al. 2010; Chuang et al. 2014; Hayes et al. 2014).

One of the few fMRI studies which aimed to investigate emotion processing in CVD revealed greater amygdala activation and greater functional connectivity between the amygdala and the ACC during processing of angry and fearful faces to be associated with preclinical atherosclerosis (Gianaros et al. 2009). Most interestingly, a recent study of the same neuroimaging unit successfully demonstrated that greater activation of the ACC is also evident during cognitive regulation of emotion in CVD which underlines the importance of altered regulatory processing as a common feature of both CVD and MDD (Gianaros et al. 2014). However, the lack of evidence, e.g., in terms of meta-analysis of altered processing in different neural networks in CVD, makes it difficult to draw firm conclusions up to now.

10.2.3 Obesity

The rising amount of fMRI research on obesity, as a risk factor for and comorbid condition of both CVD and MDD, has allowed new insights into the neural underpinnings of the link between vascular and affective disorders.

Alterations in emotion regulation and reward processing are assumed to be among the decisive features in the development of eating disorders as well as of affective disorders, and a wealth of functional MRI studies has focused to shed more light on the neural mechanisms behind these adverse psychological conditions (Bonato and Boland 1983; García-García et al. 2014; Guerrieri et al. 2007).

Enhanced neural responsiveness to food-related reward constitutes one of the most consistent findings in fMRI research on obesity (Burger and Berner 2014; Dimitropoulos et al. 2012; Gearhardt et al. 2011). In a longitudinal study by Burger and Stice (2014), future weight gain could even be predicted by enhanced striatal responsivity during food-related reward learning (Burger and Stice 2014). Interestingly, obese individuals exhibit enhanced neural activation in areas of critical relevance for reward processing like the orbitofrontal cortex (OFC), the striatum, the insula, and the anterior cingulate cortex not only when confronted with food-related reward but also during a common monetary reward paradigm (Opel et al. 2015a). This finding suggests that adverse patterns of neural processing during reward experiences in obesity are apparent beyond the subject area food and thus might point to generalized dysfunctions in reward processing in obese individuals. Findings of associations between abnormal neural activation in reward brain regions and social decision-making in obese adolescents affirm this notion of broader dysfunctions in reward processing in obesity (Verdejo-García et al. 2014). The possibility of a generalized reward deficiency in obesity might be an important contribution in the ongoing discussion on overlapping neurobiological traits of obesity and affective disorders given the evidence for altered reward processing as an important factor in the development of MDD (Blum et al. 2014; García-García et al. 2014).

Regarding possible molecular underpinnings of dysfunctional reward processing, recent studies have pointed to the critical role of the dopaminergic system:

Genetic variation in the dopaminergic system was shown to influence striatal responsiveness to reward (Dannlowski et al. 2013; Forbes et al. 2009), and dysfunctions in dopamine pathways were demonstrated to interfere in the development of severe obesity and affective disorders and might constitute an essential link between these conditions (Blum et al. 2014; Opel et al. 2015b; Wang et al. 2009). Moreover, since D2 receptor availability was evidenced to be significantly decreased in obese subjects and since decreased striatal D2 receptor availability has been demonstrated to be positively correlated with prefrontal metabolism (Volkow et al. 2008; Wang et al. 2001), findings of prefrontal and striatal hyperreactivity might actually reflect blunted reward responsiveness in obesity as proposed by Carnell et al. (2012).

Given the pivotal role of reward deficiency in affective disorders, these findings might shed more light on possible neurobiological underpinnings which underlie the high-prevalent comorbidity of obesity and psychiatric disorders (de Wit et al. 2010).

Besides overactivation in the reward system, there is also evidence for hypoactivation in regulatory pathways during executive functions and impulse control in obesity. Batterink et al. (2010) found body mass index (BMI) scores to be negatively correlated with inhibitory control in terms of decreased medial prefrontal activation in response to food in obese individuals, and in a study by Kishinevsky et al. (2012), executive function in the prefrontal cortex during a delay discounting trial could predict subsequent weight gain in obese subjects (Kishinevsky et al. 2012). The critical role of medial prefrontal areas in obesity also finds support in results of previous fMRI studies reporting altered neural activation during impulse control and decision-making to predominantly emerge in similar brain areas (Batterink et al. 2010; Delgado-Rico et al. 2013).

10.2.4 Stress

Chronic stress is one of the best described major risk factors of CVD and MDD (Cohen et al. 2007; Gilbert et al. 2009; Nanni et al. 2012; Rozanski et al. 1999; Steptoe and Kivimäki 2012). Neuroimaging studies revealed that stress exerts multiple adverse effects on the central nervous system which are thought to contribute to the onset of somatic and psychiatric disorders. In this regard, increased activity of the amygdala represents one of the most consistent fMRI findings in subjects exposed to elevated levels of stress especially during early life in terms of childhood trauma (Dannlowski et al. 2012; Grant et al. 2011, 2014; Williams et al. 2006). Moreover, stress-related amygdala hyperreactivity seems to be associated with reduced coupling between the ventromedial prefrontal cortex and the amygdala pointing to reduced fear extinction and dysfunctional gating of adverse emotions in subjects affected by childhood trauma (Birn et al. 2014).

Most interestingly, a recent study by Muscatell et al. evidenced greater amygdala reactivity to appear even after brief periods of induced stress and that this limbic overactivation results in an increased inflammatory response (Muscatell et al. 2015). This finding is supported by the fact that hyperactivity of the amygdala is known to increase inflammatory processes through its projections to the hypothalamus and to the brainstem (Eisenberger and Cole 2012; Irwin and Cole 2011). Apparently this connection between the neural and the immune system is highly suspicious to mediate the adverse somatic effects of chronic stress and thus might be an important pathophysiological element to explain the link between psychological factors and vascular disease.

As another important aspect, early-life stress has also been associated with dysfunctions in the reward system (Dillon et al. 2009; Goff et al. 2013). Given recent findings by Montoya et al., stress-related dysfunctions in the reward system are likely to arise from cortisol-induced downregulation of neural activity in reward circuits (Montoya et al. 2014).

10.2.5 Summary of fMRI Findings

To summarize, fMRI research provides evidence for alterations in overlapping neural systems in CVD, MDD, and their shared risk factors. Neural networks involved in emotion regulation and reward processing seem to contribute to the development of both disorders and thus should be key targets in future studies investigating the bidirectional link between CVD and MDD.

Regarding the influence of environmental stress, the existing literature on fMRI findings suggests that stress might primarily contribute to the development of MDD and CVD by an imbalance of limbic hyperreactivity and lacking inhibitory bottom-down control by prefrontal brain areas. The occurrence of dysfunctions in identical brain areas like the ACC and prefrontal brain areas in subjects at an increased risk but without acute disorder might point to the relevance of aberrant emotion regulation and control as a predisposing feature of CVD and MDD. Given the fact that uncontrolled limbic hyperreactivity is thought to induce inflammatory processes, normalization of signaling in this neural circuit might represent a considerable target for future therapeutic options.

In the case of obesity, present research indicates that dysfunctions in reward-related brain circuits might be the connecting element in the pathophysiology of obesity and MDD.

The observation of generalized dysfunctions in reward-related brain circuits like the ventral striatum and medial prefrontal brain areas in obesity, chronic stress, and MDD underlines the importance of further investigation of possible clinical and neurobiological overlaps between somatic and psychopathological conditions. Since a core function of reward is to induce a subjective feeling of pleasure and positive emotion, altered responsiveness to reward and thus reinforcing stimuli might contribute to the generation and maintenance of depressive symptoms, which could reflect the higher prevalence of depression in obese participants compared to normal-weight participants (Carey et al. 2014; Luppino et al. 2010).

10.3 Structural MRI

Besides abnormalities in brain function, cardiovascular disease, depression, and obesity were shown to be associated with alterations in brain structure. While our knowledge about structural changes in patients with depression and obesity is reasonably well marked, data regarding the link between CVD and structural brain changes are still rare. Interestingly, it already appears that CVD and depression are associated with changes in brain areas that are also strongly associated with obesity and stress resilience. However, the question remains whether these common neuronal changes represent a predisposition to or a consequence of the diseases. To pursue this question, structural neuroimaging findings in both CVD and depression are first presented separately and then subsequently embedded into the context of the discussion regarding the determination of state- and trait-dependent brain changes.

10.3.1 Major Depression

Structural neuroimaging techniques have been widely used to investigate brain alterations in major depressive disorder (MDD). A wealth of structural imaging findings elucidated the role of specific brain areas in the etiopathology of affective disorders (Phillips et al. 2003a, b). Particularly, structural alterations in limbic and prefrontal cortical regions involved in emotion regulation were frequently found to be associated with MDD (Arnone et al. 2012; Cusi et al. 2012). Meta-analyses of structural MRI studies repeatedly have shown volume reductions in the hippocampus in MDD patients (Campbell et al. 2004; Hamilton et al. 2008; McKinnon et al. 2009). Additionally, alterations in prefrontal regions were also associated with MDD, particularly the ACC and medial frontal regions, including the OFC (Bora et al. 2012; Du et al. 2012; Lai 2013). More recently, studies have also shown moderate gray matter volume reductions in striatal areas (putamen and caudate nucleus) in patients with MDD compared to healthy controls, alterations which are also strongly associated with obesity (Koolschijn et al. 2009; Opel et al. 2015b; Redlich et al. 2014). There is evidence that these structural alterations are linked to clinical characteristics and course of disease, and that they are, at least partly, reversible (Abbott et al. 2014; Dukart et al. 2014; Hamilton et al. 2008; McKinnon et al. 2009).

10.3.2 Obesity

A rising amount of studies has focused on structural changes which are associated with obesity and body mass index (BMI). Neuroimaging studies revealed associations between reduced gray and white matter, as well as loss of global brain volume and BMI (Mueller et al. 2012; Ward et al. 2005). More specifically, reductions of gray matter in medial orbital parts of the prefrontal cortex, striatal areas, and the hippocampus were frequently shown in obesity (Marqués-Iturria et al. 2013; Mueller et al. 2012; Raji et al. 2010; Walther et al. 2010). Importantly, most of the studies which have recently established a link between brain volume and obesity have used cross-sectional designs. Thus, evidence of associations between changes in BMI over time and changes in brain structure is very limited. However, the present findings indicate that higher BMI is associated with greater decline in temporal, occipital (Bobb et al. 2014), and striatal gray matter volumes (Driscoll et al. 2012). Obviously, the neurostructural alterations reported in obese subjects closely resemble results in depressed patients but only few studies have investigated neurostructural correlates of both depression and obesity within the same study. A tensor-based morphometry study by Cole et al. indicated that BMI and depression might be associated with comparable changes in brain structure (Cole et al. 2013). Moreover, a recent study by Opel et al. (2015a, b) sought to clarify to which extent BMI is associated with aberrations in clinical appearance in MDD patients to shed light on potential neurobiological connections between obesity and MDD. Here, a higher BMI was associated with a highly comparable pattern of gray matter reductions in the medial prefrontal cortex, the OFC, the caudate nucleus, and the thalamus in MDD patients and healthy controls alike. Moreover, in MDD patients, BMI was associated with a more chronic course of disease, and both BMI and chronicity of disorder were related to similar morphometric anomalies in medial prefrontal areas (Opel et al. 2015b). The authors stated that a possible explanation could be dopaminergic striato-cortical pathway dysfunctions in both MDD and obesity which is suggested to be associated with the dysfunctions in reward processing, impulsivity, and regulation of eating behaviors (see also above) (Opel et al. 2015b).

10.3.3 Cardiovascular Disease

While cardiovascular dysfunction and progressive loss of cognitive brain functioning are prominent features of an aging population, surprisingly few studies have addressed the link between heart and brain. However, preliminary studies gave first insight into the link between CVD and related neurostructural brain changes, which are similar to those observed in aging and depression (Hayes et al. 2014). Structural changes in morphology of the aging brain have been independently linked to hypertension, diabetes, and hyperlipidemia (de Toledo Ferraz Alves et al. 2010). In stable coronary artery disease patients, cardiovascular disease is associated with brain atrophy in large parts of the frontal cortex, as well as hippocampal, parietal, and temporal areas (Anazodo et al. 2013). In heart failure patients, similar regional tissue changes in hippocampal and frontal cortex were found (Pan et al. 2013) as well as impaired axonal integrity including the basal forebrain, hypothalamic and limbic projections through the medial forebrain bundle (Kumar et al. 2011). A study by Woo et al. (2009) also indicated injured brain areas in patients with heart failure, reflected by reduced gray matter volumes and isolated white matter infarcts in areas that control autonomic, analgesic, emotional, and cognitive functions, including frontal areas, hippocampus, striatal, and cingulate areas (Woo et al. 2009). Older individuals with higher estimated risk of coronary artery disease tend to have decreased brain volume and cerebral blood flow (Anazodo et al. 2013; de Toledo Ferraz Alves et al. 2010). Even in older adults with no clinical diagnosis of cardiovascular disease, decline in cardiac function is associated with brain atrophy (Jefferson 2010) and white matter hyperintensities (Jefferson et al. 2007). Finally, it has also been shown that cardiovascular stiffness including end-systolic stiffness, central arterial augmentation pressure, and aortic stiffness are independently and negatively associated with gray matter volumes in healthy subjects (Katulska et al. 2014).

10.3.4 State or Trait

In summary, it can be stated that depression, CVD, and obesity go hand in hand with changes in neural structure, particularly in the hippocampal formation, prefrontal cortex, and striatal areas. These neuroanatomically overlapping findings appear to parallel the high comorbidity rates that are observed between these disorders. Moreover, it is strongly assumed that there is a bidirectional relationship between depression and CVD, as well as strong associations between depression and obesity (Baune et al. 2012; Lippi et al. 2009; Luppino et al. 2010; Pan et al. 2012). The questions remain as to whether, and to what extent, structural brain changes represent effects of current disease or long-term consequences of preexisting risk factors, like chronic stress or adversity in earlier life.

There is some evidence that differences in gray matter volume represent a variable state, while the disease is active. A large number of studies have delivered results that support the interpretation of cerebral volume reductions as a consequence of MDD. Firstly, neuroimaging studies show hippocampal volume loss to be linked to clinical characteristics and indicate progression of hippocampal volume loss in the course of disease (McKinnon et al. 2009; Sheline et al. 2003). For example, hippocampal and amygdala volume losses seem to cumulate with the number of episodes and the duration of illness, which might be explained either by repeated neurotoxic stress or by higher relapse rates in patients showing hippocampal atrophy (Lee et al. 2011; Stratmann et al. 2014). Patients who remitted during a 3-year period had less volume decline in the hippocampus, the ACC, and the prefrontal cortex compared to non-remitted patients (Frodl et al. 2008a).

Secondly, gray matter alterations seem to be at least partly reversible. In MDD, studies show that antidepressant treatment facilitates neurogenesis in the hippocampus in both nonhuman primates and rodents. In humans, a meta-analysis by Hamilton et al. (2008) reported a reliable decrease in amygdala volume in non-medicated patients with MDD, while a significantly increased amygdala volume relative to HC was found in medicated depressed patients (Hamilton et al. 2008). Moreover, recent studies investigating the effects of electroconvulsive therapy (ECT) in depressed patients have shown strong neuroplasticity effects within the hippocampus, amygdala, and subgenual cingulate gyrus, reflected by an increase in gray matter volumes after ECT in patients with MDD (Abbott et al. 2014; Dukart et al. 2014; Tendolkar et al. 2013). It is suggested that these effects could be mediated by an increased production of brain-derived neurotrophic factor (BDNF), which could promote neurogenesis and protect against volume loss in the amygdala, hippocampal, and striatal areas (Hamilton et al. 2008; Khaspekov et al. 2004; Mohapel et al. 2005). These increases in volume during treatment might constitute a surrogate parameter of neuroplasticity taking place during therapy (Abbott et al. 2014; Arnone et al. 2013; Dukart et al. 2014; Schermuly et al. 2011; Tendolkar et al. 2013). In CVD, a recent review revealed a consistent positive relationship between cardiorespiratory fitness and brain volume in cortical regions, including anterior cingulate, lateral prefrontal, and lateral parietal cortex (Hayes et al. 2013). Although there are few studies with regard to exercise trainings and neuroimaging markers reported to date, there is consistency that the physiological integrity of brain structures might be maintained by aerobic training (Hayes et al. 2014). Poor physical and cardiorespiratory fitness is further associated with reduced structural integrity of the brain in heart failure and morphological brain changes, including white matter lesions (Hayes et al. 2014; Sen et al. 2012). The reversibility of therapy-induced structural changes suggests that structural alterations are caused by the disease. This conclusion is further supported by studies showing associations between severity of disease and the extent of structural changes.

However, a variety of findings (and facts) indicate that some structural changes might be apparent before the onset of diseases. First, hippocampal size is known to be highly heritable, and several reports on the influence of genetic variations on shape alterations in the hippocampus support the hypothesis that hippocampal volume reductions are a predisposing trait of MDD (Frodl et al. 2008b, 2010; Stein et al. 2012). Second, healthy individuals at familial risk of depression (i.e., with a positive family history for MDD) also show morphometric anomalies, even if they do not have any history of depression or CVD (Amico et al. 2011; Chen et al. 2010). In the case of obesity, the little available data also suggest that healthy individuals at risk for weight gain show structural differences in brain regions and that brain structure predicts the risk for obesity (Smucny et al. 2012). A study by Yau et al. (2014) showed that adolescents with uncomplicated obesity already exhibit subtle neurostructural alterations that exist before the onset of clinically significant obesity (Yau et al. 2014). This notion is further supported by findings that overall brain volume is associated with future BMI (Yokum et al. 2012). However, further metabolic dysregulation, such as marked fasting hyperinsulinemia or fasting hyperglycemia, might be necessary to cause serious structural damage (Yau et al. 2014).

Third, recent data suggests that volume loss in gray matter might appropriately be characterized as a function of early-life stress rather than depression. Structural alterations are reported only in those depressed patients who have experienced maltreatment, but not in those who do not have any history of adversity (Opel et al. 2014). This finding is further supported by studies reporting that even healthy adults who have experienced maltreatment during childhood show reduced hippocampal gray matter volumes (Dannlowski et al. 2012).

These observations lead to the assumption that neurostructural alterations might already be present before the onset of disease and that early-life adversity and chronic stress appear to be a crucial mechanism for brain atrophic alterations. Chronic stress leads to, inter alia, neuroinflammation and HPA axis hyperactivity, both of which are not only strongly associated with MDD and CVD (Baune et al. 2012; Dantzer et al. 2010; Lamers et al. 2013; Miller et al. 2009) but also with obesity (Lucassen and Cizza 2012; Vicennati et al. 2014). It has been postulated that obesity may be considered as a maladaptation to stress, thus indirectly leading to hyperactivation of the HPA axis and higher-than-normal cortisol levels (Lucassen and Cizza 2012). In addition to CVD, depression is also significantly associated with several major cardiovascular risk factors, including obesity and diabetes (Skala et al. 2006). A systemic immune activation and HPA axis hyperactivity are suggestive of the biological mechanism which links CVD and depression (Baune et al. 2012). Excessive stress exposure like childhood maltreatment leads to a chronic HPA axis hyperactivity, which might trigger neurotoxic effects of cortisol and possibly neuroinflammation, which in turn might cause damage to brain structure and function (Frodl and O'Keane 2013). Remarkably, recent evidence suggests that smaller hippocampal volumes indeed partially control the effect of early-life adversity on the development of MDD during longitudinal follow-up (Rao et al. 2010). Accordingly, hippocampal aberrations could be hypothesized to act as a connecting element in the development of severe psychopathology in maltreated individuals (Opel et al. 2014). Taken together, one might speculate that changes in hippocampal structure during brain development may have effects on HPA axis functioning later in life, resulting in alterations of cortisol feedback regulation and, thus, higher cortisol levels, which could exert negative effects on brain structure and functioning, eventually leading to higher vulnerability to diseases like depression or CVD (Frodl and O'Keane 2013).

This summary suggests that brain structural alterations might be characterized as a function of both a preexisting trait risk factor and a state of disease. A potential mechanism might be preferably mediated by stress, although the underpinnings of these associations are likely to be of much greater complexity. Nevertheless, it appears exigent to investigate the structural impact of both early-life stress and current disease status in longitudinal studies, in patients diagnosed with CVD, depression, obesity, or any combination of the three, carefully screened for comorbidities.

10.4 Treatment

The overall conclusion of neuroimaging research indicates that CVD, depression, and obesity are associated with neuroanatomically similar functional and structural aberrations. The underlying mechanisms are poorly understood, but it is likely that stress is one of the most decisive mediators. Stress-associated changes, such as a hyperactive HPA axis and neuroinflammation, might lead to brain changes, which in turn may mediate and facilitate the onset of comorbid diseases. This leads to several implications for the therapy of CVD and depression.

Firstly, an enhancement of general stress resilience, including actively coping with stress, optimism, cognitive reappraisal, positive reframing, and increasing social support, is desirable, since studies suggest that brain volume loss is acquired by stressful life experiences, and might therefore constitute a trait-like risk factor. Increased stress resilience might mitigate these effects, to the extent of prevention before onset. It has been shown that resilience is mediated by adaptive changes in several neural circuits that involve numerous neurobiological and molecular pathways. These changes shape the functioning of neural circuits that regulate reward, fear, and processing of emotion, which are thought to mediate successful coping with stress (Feder et al. 2009).

Secondly, extensive multidisciplinary screening and treatment appears exigent. Several studies have shown that brain volume alterations are at least partly reversible. In MDD, volume increase in affected brain areas has been shown during ECT and antidepressant treatment (Abbott et al. 2014; Arnone et al. 2013; Dukart et al. 2014; Schermuly et al. 2011; Tendolkar et al. 2013).

Also it has been shown that normalization of aberrant amygdala function can be achieved by the use of antidepressant medication in MDD (Sheline et al. 2001). Since amygdala hyperactivation is thought to contribute to the maintenance of inflammatory processes, recovery of physiological limbic signaling via therapeutic intervention should be evaluated in the prevention of vascular and psychiatric disorders (Eisenberger and Cole 2012; Muscatell et al. 2015).

In CVD, brain structure and functioning consistently benefit from aerobic training, and disease-related effects typically appear to be reversible through moderate aerobic programs (Anazodo et al. 2013; Hayes et al. 2014). Moreover, physical activity per se has been repeatedly associated with generally improved cognitive function and reversal of cortical decline (Anazodo et al. 2013; Colcombe et al. 2006; Erickson et al. 2009, 2011).

The overall coordination of health-care providers is fundamental for patients with combined medical and mental health diagnoses. In particular, patients with CVD who have a comorbid depression should be carefully monitored for adherence to their medical care and for drug efficacy with respect to their cardiovascular and mental health (Lippi et al. 2009). Furthermore, the importance of measures addressing BMI normalization and prevention of weight gain during in-patient treatment should be reconsidered, since obesity constitutes a common risk factor for both depression and CVD. In addition to standard clinical practices, the positive benefits of maintaining a healthy lifestyle and dietary modification are indicated (e.g., to improve glycemic control, triglycerides, and protein intake and to lower insulin levels) (Brand-Miller et al. 2009; Lippi et al. 2009). Finally, aerobic training and exercises should be urgently considered, for both reducing cardiovascular risk and countering depression (Singh et al. 2005) by maintaining physiological neuronal function and structure and stress resilience. In the future, neuroimaging might serve as valuable tool in the detection of high-risk subjects before the onset of clinically manifest disorder and thus contribute to the allocation of intensified preventive measures. Moreover, given the reversibility of neural alterations, the use of structural and functional MRI during therapeutic progress might be an important approach to gain a better understanding of the neurobiological effects of different therapeutic strategies.

Conclusion

Neuroimaging research has evidenced the involvement of alterations in overlapping neural systems in CVD, MDD, and their common risk factors. Neural networks of emotion regulation and reward processing seem to be among the primarily affected brain circuits in the development of both disorders. Since alterations in brain structure and function are apparent in subjects at high risk but before the onset of clinically manifest disease and given the reversibility of these neural aberrations, neuroimaging findings point to the crucial role of therapeutic intervention in high-risk populations at an early stage in the prevention of both disorders. Future research should aim to confine the relationship between inflammatory and neural processes which might provide the neurobiological basis for integrated treatment options for CVD and MDD.

References

Abbott CC, Jones T, Lemke NT, Gallegos P, McClintock SM, Mayer AR, Bustillo J, Calhoun VD (2014) Hippocampal structural and functional changes associated with electroconvulsive therapy response. Transl Psychiatry 4:e483. doi:10.1038/tp.2014.124

Amico F, Meisenzahl EM, Koutsouleris NN, Reiser M, Möller H-JH-J, Frodl T (2011) Structural MRI correlates for vulnerability and resilience to major depressive disorder. J Psychiatry Neurosci 36:15–22. doi:10.1503/jpn.090186

Anazodo UC, Shoemaker JK, Suskin N, St Lawrence KS (2013) An investigation of changes in regional gray matter volume in cardiovascular disease patients, pre and post cardiovascular rehabilitation. Neuroimage 3:388–395. doi:10.1016/j.nicl.2013.09.011

Arnone D, McIntosh AM, Ebmeier KP, Munafò MR, Anderson IM (2012) Magnetic resonance imaging studies in unipolar depression: systematic review and meta-regression analyses. Eur Neuropsychopharmacol 22:1–16. doi:10.1016/j.euroneuro.2011.05.003

Arnone D, McKie S, Elliott R, Juhasz G, Thomas EJ, Downey D, Williams S, Deakin JFW, Anderson IM (2013) State-dependent changes in hippocampal grey matter in depression. Mol Psychiatry 18:1265–1272. doi:10.1038/mp.2012.150

Batterink L, Yokum S, Stice E (2010) Body mass correlates inversely with inhibitory control in response to food among adolescent girls: an fMRI study. Neuroimage 52:1696–1703. doi:10.1016/j.neuroimage.2010.05.059

Baune BT, Stuart M, Gilmour a, Wersching H, Heindel W, Arolt V, Berger K (2012) The relationship between subtypes of depression and cardiovascular disease: a systematic review of biological models. Transl Psychiatry 2:e92. doi:10.1038/tp.2012.18

Birn RM, Patriat R, Phillips ML, Germain A, Herringa RJ (2014) Childhood maltreatment and combat posttraumatic stress differentially predict fear-related fronto-subcortical connectivity. Depress Anxiety 31:880–892. doi:10.1002/da.22291

Blum K, Thanos PK, Gold MS (2014) Dopamine and glucose, obesity, and reward deficiency syndrome. Front Psychol 5:919. doi:10.3389/fpsyg.2014.00919

Bobb JF, Schwartz BS, Davatzikos C, Caffo B (2014) Cross-sectional and longitudinal association of body mass index and brain volume. Hum Brain Mapp 35:75–88. doi:10.1002/hbm.22159

Bonato DP, Boland FJ (1983) Delay of gratification in obese children. Addict Behav 8:71–74. doi:10.1016/0306-4603(83)90059-X
Bora E, Fornito A, Pantelis C, Yücel M (2012) Gray matter abnormalities in major depressive disorder: a meta-analysis of voxel based morphometry studies. J Affect Disord 138:9–18
Brand-Miller J, Dickinson S, Barclay A, Allman-Farinelli M (2009) Glycemic index, glycemic load, and thrombogenesis. Semin Thromb Hemost 35:111–118. doi:10.1055/s-0029-1214154
Braskie MN, Small GW, Bookheimer SY (2010) Vascular health risks and fMRI activation during a memory task in older adults. Neurobiol Aging 31:1532–1542. doi:10.1016/j.neurobiolaging.2008.08.016
Burger KS, Berner LA (2014) A functional neuroimaging review of obesity, appetitive hormones and ingestive behavior. Physiol Behav. doi:10.1016/j.physbeh.2014.04.025
Burger KS, Stice E (2014) Greater striatopallidal adaptive coding during cue-reward learning and food reward habituation predict future weight gain. Neuroimage 99:122–128. doi:10.1016/j.neuroimage.2014.05.066
Campbell S, Marriott M, Nahmias C, MacQueen GM (2004) Lower hippocampal volume in patients suffering from depression: a meta-analysis. Am J Psychiatry 161:598–607
Carey M, Small H, Yoong SL, Boyes A, Bisquera A, Sanson-Fisher R (2014) Prevalence of comorbid depression and obesity in general practice: a cross-sectional survey. Br J Gen Pract 64:e122–e127. doi:10.3399/bjgp14X677482
Carnell S, Gibson C, Benson L, Ochner CN, Geliebter A (2012) Neuroimaging and obesity: current knowledge and future directions. Obes Rev 13:43–56. doi:10.1111/j.1467-789X.2011.00927.x
Charlson FJ, Stapelberg NJC, Baxter AJ, Whiteford HA (2011) Should global burden of disease estimates include depression as a risk factor for coronary heart disease? BMC Med 9:47. doi:10.1186/1741-7015-9-47
Chen MC, Hamilton JP, Gotlib IH (2010) Decreased hippocampal volume in healthy girls at risk of depression. Arch Gen Psychiatry 67:270–276. doi:10.1001/archgenpsychiatry.2009.202
Chuang Y-F, Eldreth D, Erickson KI, Varma V, Harris G, Fried LP, Rebok GW, Tanner EK, Carlson MC (2014) Cardiovascular risks and brain function: a functional magnetic resonance imaging study of executive function in older adults. Neurobiol Aging 35:1396–1403. doi:10.1016/j.neurobiolaging.2013.12.008
Cohen S, Janicki-Deverts D, Miller GE (2007) Psychological stress and disease. JAMA 298:1685–1687. doi:10.1001/jama.298.14.1685
Colcombe SJ, Erickson KI, Scalf PE, Kim JS, Prakash R, McAuley E, Elavsky S, Marquez DX, Hu L, Kramer AF (2006) Aerobic exercise training increases brain volume in aging humans. J Gerontol 61:1166–1170
Cole JH, Boyle CP, Simmons A, Cohen-Woods S, Rivera M, McGuffin P, Thompson PM, Fu CHY (2013) Body mass index, but not FTO genotype or major depressive disorder, influences brain structure. Neuroscience 252:109–117
Cusi AM, Nazarov A, Holshausen K, Macqueen GM, McKinnon MC (2012) Systematic review of the neural basis of social cognition in patients with mood disorders. J Psychiatry Neurosci 37:154–169. doi:10.1503/jpn.100179
Danese a, Tan M (2014) Childhood maltreatment and obesity: systematic review and meta-analysis. Mol Psychiatry 19:544–554. doi:10.1038/mp.2013.54
Dannlowski U, Stuhrmann A, Beutelmann V, Zwanzger P, Lenzen T, Grotegerd D, Domschke K, Hohoff C, Ohrmann P, Bauer J, Lindner C, Postert C, Konrad C, Arolt V, Heindel W, Suslow T, Kugel H (2012) Limbic scars: long-term consequences of childhood maltreatment revealed by functional and structural magnetic resonance imaging. Biol Psychiatry 71:286–293. doi:10.1016/j.biopsych.2011.10.021
Dannlowski U, Domschke K, Birosova E, Lawford B, Young R, Voisey J, Morris CP, Suslow T, Konrad C, Kugel H, Ohrmann P, Bauer J, Schöning S, Zavorotnyy M, Diemer J, Arolt V, Baune BT, Zwanzger P (2013) Dopamine D3 receptor gene variation: impact on electroconvulsive therapy response and ventral striatum responsiveness in depression. Int J Neuropsychopharmacol 16:1443–1459. doi:10.1017/S1461145711001659

Dantzer R, Connor JCO, Freund GG, Johnson RW, Kelley KW (2010) From inflammation to sickness and depression: when the immune system subjugates the brain. Nat Rev Neurosci 9:46–56. doi:10.1038/nrn2297.From
De Toledo Ferraz Alves TC, Ferreira LK, Wajngarten M, Busatto GF (2010) Cardiac disorders as risk factors for Alzheimer's disease. J Alzheimers Dis 20:749–763. doi:10.3233/JAD-2010-091561
De Wit L, Luppino F, van Straten A, Penninx B, Zitman F, Cuijpers P (2010) Depression and obesity: a meta-analysis of community-based studies. Psychiatry Res 178:230–235. doi:10.1016/j.psychres.2009.04.015
Delgado-Rico E, Soriano-Mas C, Verdejo-Román J, Río-Valle JS, Verdejo-García A (2013) Decreased insular and increased midbrain activations during decision-making under risk in adolescents with excess weight. Obesity (Silver Spring) 21:1662–1668. doi:10.1002/oby.20375
Dillon DG, Holmes AJ, Birk JL, Brooks N, Lyons-Ruth K, Pizzagalli DA (2009) Childhood adversity is associated with left basal ganglia dysfunction during reward anticipation in adulthood. Biol Psychiatry 66:206–213. doi:10.1016/j.biopsych.2009.02.019
Dimitropoulos A, Tkach J, Ho A, Kennedy J (2012) Greater corticolimbic activation to high-calorie food cues after eating in obese vs. normal-weight adults. Appetite 58:303–312. doi:10.1016/j.appet.2011.10.014
Driscoll I, Beydoun M a, An Y, Davatzikos C, Ferrucci L, Zonderman AB, Resnick SM (2012) Midlife obesity and trajectories of brain volume changes in older adults. Hum Brain Mapp 33:2204–2210. doi:10.1002/hbm.21353
Du MY, Wu QZ, Yue Q, Li J, Liao Y, Kuang WH, Huang XQ, Chan RCK, Mechelli A, Gong QY (2012) Voxelwise meta-analysis of gray matter reduction in major depressive disorder. Prog Neuropsychopharmacol Biol Psychiatry 36:11–16. doi:10.1016/j.pnpbp.2011.09.014
Dukart J, Regen F, Kherif F, Colla M, Bajbouj M, Heuser I (2014) Electroconvulsive therapy-induced brain plasticity determines therapeutic outcome in mood disorders. PNAS 111:1156–1161. doi:10.1073/pnas.1321399111
Eisenberger NI, Cole SW (2012) Social neuroscience and health: neurophysiological mechanisms linking social ties with physical health. Nat Neurosci 15:669–674. doi:10.1038/nn.3086
Elderon L, Whooley MA (2013) Depression and cardiovascular disease. Prog Cardiovasc Dis 55:511–23. doi:10.1016/j.pcad.2013.03.010
Erickson KI, Prakash RS, Voss MW, Chaddock L, Hu L, Morris KS, White SM, Wójcicki TR, McAuley E, Kramer AF (2009) Aerobic fitness is associated with hippocampal volume in elderly humans. Hippocampus 19:1030–1039. doi:10.1002/hipo.20547
Erickson KI, Voss MW, Prakash RS, Basak C, Szabo A, Chaddock L, Kim JS, Heo S, Alves H, White SM, Wojcicki TR, Mailey E, Vieira VJ, Martin SA, Pence BD, Woods JA, McAuley E, Kramer AF (2011) Exercise training increases size of hippocampus and improves memory. Proc Natl Acad Sci U S A 108:3017–3022. doi:10.1073/pnas.1015950108
Feder A, Nestler EJ, Charney DS (2009) Psychobiology and molecular genetics of resilience. Nat Rev Neurosci 10:446–457. doi:10.1038/nrn2649
Forbes EE, Brown SM, Kimak M, Ferrell RE, Manuck SB, Hariri AR (2009) Genetic variation in components of dopamine neurotransmission impacts ventral striatal reactivity associated with impulsivity. Mol Psychiatry 14:60–70. doi:10.1038/sj.mp.4002086
Frodl T, O'Keane V (2013) How does the brain deal with cumulative stress? A review with focus on developmental stress, HPA axis function and hippocampal structure in humans. Neurobiol Dis 52:24–37. doi:10.1016/j.nbd.2012.03.012
Frodl T, Koutsouleris N, Bottlender R, Born C, Jäger M, Scupin I, Reiser M, Möller H-J, Meisenzahl EM (2008a) Depression-related variation in brain morphology over 3 years: effects of stress? Arch Gen Psychiatry 65:1156–1165. doi:10.1001/archpsyc.65.10.1156
Frodl T, Koutsouleris NN, Bottlender R, Born C, Jäger M, Mörgenthaler M, Scheuerecker J, Zill P, Baghai T, Schüle C, Rupprecht R, Bondy B, Reiser M, Möller H-JH-J, Meisenzahl EM (2008b) Reduced gray matter brain volumes are associated with variants of the serotonin transporter gene in major depression. Mol Psychiatry 13:1093–1101. doi:10.1038/mp.2008.62

Frodl T, Scheuerecker J, Albrecht J, Kleemann AM, Müller-Schunk S, Koutsouleris N, Möller H-J, Brückmann H, Wiesmann M, Meisenzahl E (2009) Neuronal correlates of emotional processing in patients with major depression. World J Biol Psychiatry 10:202–208
Frodl T, Reinhold E, Koutsouleris NN, Donohoe G, Bondy B, Reiser M, Möller H-J, Meisenzahl EM (2010) Childhood stress, serotonin transporter gene and brain structures in major depression. Neuropsychopharmacology 35:1383–1390. doi:10.1038/npp.2010.8
García-García I, Horstmann A, Jurado MA, Garolera M, Chaudhry SJ, Margulies DS, Villringer A, Neumann J (2014) Reward processing in obesity, substance addiction and non-substance addiction. Obes Rev. doi:10.1111/obr.12221
Gearhardt AN, Yokum S, Orr PT, Stice E, Corbin WR, Brownell KD (2011) Neural correlates of food addiction. Arch Gen Psychiatry 68:808–816. doi:10.1001/archgenpsychiatry.2011.32
Gianaros PJ, Hariri AR, Sheu LK, Muldoon MF, Sutton-Tyrrell K, Manuck SB (2009) Preclinical atherosclerosis covaries with individual differences in reactivity and functional connectivity of the amygdala. Biol Psychiatry 65:943–950. doi:10.1016/j.biopsych.2008.10.007
Gianaros PJ, Marsland AL, Kuan DC-H, Schirda BL, Jennings JR, Sheu LK, Hariri AR, Gross JJ, Manuck SB (2014) An inflammatory pathway links atherosclerotic cardiovascular disease risk to neural activity evoked by the cognitive regulation of emotion. Biol Psychiatry 75:738–745. doi:10.1016/j.biopsych.2013.10.012
Gilbert R, Widom CS, Browne K, Fergusson D, Webb E, Janson S (2009) Burden and consequences of child maltreatment in high-income countries. Lancet 373:68–81. doi:10.1016/S0140-6736(08)61706-7
Goff B, Gee DG, Telzer EH, Humphreys KL, Gabard-Durnam L, Flannery J, Tottenham N (2013) Reduced nucleus accumbens reactivity and adolescent depression following early-life stress. Neuroscience 249:129–138. doi:10.1016/j.neuroscience.2012.12.010
Grant MM, Cannistraci C, Hollon SD, Gore JC, Shelton RC (2011) Childhood trauma history differentiates amygdala response to sad faces within MDD. J Psychiatr Res. doi:10.1016/j.jpsychires.2010.12.004
Grant MM, White D, Hadley J, Hutcheson N, Shelton R, Sreenivasan K, Deshpande G (2014) Early life trauma and directional brain connectivity within major depression. Hum Brain Mapp 35:4815–4826. doi:10.1002/hbm.22514
Guerrieri R, Nederkoorn C, Stankiewicz K, Alberts H, Geschwind N, Martijn C, Jansen A (2007) The influence of trait and induced state impulsivity on food intake in normal-weight healthy women. Appetite 49:66–73. doi:10.1016/j.appet.2006.11.008
Hamilton JP, Siemer M, Gotlib IH (2008) Amygdala volume in major depressive disorder: a meta-analysis of magnetic resonance imaging studies. Mol Psychiatry 13:993–1000. doi:10.1038/mp.2008.57
Hayes SM, Hayes JP, Cadden M, Verfaellie M (2013) A review of cardiorespiratory fitness-related neuroplasticity in the aging brain. Front Aging Neurosci 5:31. doi:10.3389/fnagi.2013.00031
Hayes SMM, Alosco MLL, Forman DEE (2014) The effects of aerobic exercise on cognitive and neural decline in aging and cardiovascular disease. Curr Geriatr Rep 3:282–290. doi:10.1007/s13670-014-0101-x
Heim CM, Newport DJ, Mletzko TC, Miller AH, Nemeroff CB (2008) The link between childhood trauma and depression: insights from HPA axis studies in humans. Psychoneuroendocrinology 33:693–710. doi:10.1016/j.psyneuen.2008.03.008
Irwin MR, Cole SW (2011) Reciprocal regulation of the neural and innate immune systems. Nat Rev Immunol 11:625–632. doi:10.1038/nri3042
Jefferson AL (2010) Cardiac output as a potential risk factor for abnormal brain aging. J Alzheimers Dis 20:813–821. doi:10.3233/JAD-2010-100081.Cardiac
Jefferson AL, Tate DF, Poppas A, Brickman AM, Paul RH, Gunstad J, Cohen R a (2007) Lower cardiac output is associated with greater white matter hyperintensities in older adults with cardiovascular disease. J Am Geriatr Soc 55:1044–1048. doi:10.1111/j.1532-5415.2007.01226.x
Katulska K, Wykrętowicz M, Minczykowski A, Krauze T, Milewska A, Piskorski J, Marciniak R, Stajgis M, Wysocki H, Guzik P, Wykrętowicz A (2014) Gray matter volume in relation to cardio-vascular stiffness. J Neurol Sci 343:100–104. doi:10.1016/j.jns.2014.05.044

Khaspekov LG, Brenz Verca MS, Frumkina LE, Hermann H, Marsicano G, Lutz B (2004) Involvement of brain-derived neurotrophic factor in cannabinoid receptor-dependent protection against excitotoxicity. Eur J Neurosci 19:1691–1698. doi:10.1111/j.1460-9568.2004.03285.x

Kishinevsky FI, Cox JE, Murdaugh DL, Stoeckel LE, Cook EW, Weller RE (2012) fMRI reactivity on a delay discounting task predicts weight gain in obese women. Appetite 58:582–592. doi:10.1016/j.appet.2011.11.029

Kloiber S, Ising M, Reppermund S, Horstmann S, Dose T, Majer M, Zihl J, Pfister H, Unschuld PG, Holsboer F, Lucae S (2007) Overweight and obesity affect treatment response in major depression. Biol Psychiatry 62:321–326. doi:10.1016/j.biopsych.2006.10.001

Knutson B, Bhanji JP, Cooney RE, Atlas LY, Gotlib IH (2008) Neural responses to monetary incentives in major depression. Biol Psychiatry 63:686–692. doi:10.1016/j.biopsych.2007.07.023

Koolschijn PCMP, van Haren NEM, Lensvelt-Mulders GJLM, Hulshoff Pol HE, Kahn RS (2009) Brain volume abnormalities in major depressive disorder: a meta-analysis of magnetic resonance imaging studies. Hum Brain Mapp 30:3719–3735. doi:10.1002/hbm.20801

Kumar P, Waiter G, Ahearn T, Milders M, Reid I, Steele JD (2008) Abnormal temporal difference reward-learning signals in major depression. Brain 131:2084–2093. doi:10.1093/brain/awn136

Kumar R, Woo MA, Macey PM, Fonarow GC, Hamilton MA, Harper RM (2011) Brain axonal and myelin evaluation in heart failure. J Neurol Sci 307:106–113. doi:10.1016/j.jns.2011.04.028

Lai CH (2013) Gray matter volume in major depressive disorder: a meta-analysis of voxel-based morphometry studies. Psychiatry Res 211:37–46. doi:10.1016/j.pscychresns.2012.06.006

Lamers F, Vogelzangs N, Merikangas KR, de Jonge P, Beekman ATF, Penninx BWJH (2013) Evidence for a differential role of HPA-axis function, inflammation and metabolic syndrome in melancholic versus atypical depression. Mol Psychiatry 18:692–699. doi:10.1038/mp.2012.144

Lee H-Y, Tae WS, Yoon H-K, Lee B-T, Paik J-W, Son K-R, Oh Y-W, Lee M-S, Ham B-J (2011) Demonstration of decreased gray matter concentration in the midbrain encompassing the dorsal raphe nucleus and the limbic subcortical regions in major depressive disorder: an optimized voxel-based morphometry study. J Affect Disord 133:128–136. doi:10.1016/j.jad.2011.04.006

Lippi G, Montagnana M, Favaloro EJ, Franchini M (2009) Mental depression and cardiovascular disease: a multifaceted, bidirectional association. Semin Thromb Hemost 35:325–336. doi:10.1055/s-0029-1222611

Lucassen EA, Cizza G (2012) The hypothalamic-pituitary-adrenal axis, obesity, and chronic stress exposure: sleep and the HPA axis in obesity. Curr Obes Rep 1:208–215. doi:10.1007/s13679-012-0028-5

Luppino F, de Wit LM, Bouvy PF, Stijnen T, Cuijpers P, Penninx B, Zitman FG (2010) Overweight, obesity, and depression. Arch Gen Psychiatry 67:220–229. doi:10.1001/archgenpsychiatry.2010.2

Marqués-Iturria I, Pueyo R, Garolera M, Segura B, Junqué C, García-García I, José Sender-Palacios M, Vernet-Vernet M, Narberhaus A, Ariza M, Jurado MA (2013) Frontal cortical thinning and subcortical volume reductions in early adulthood obesity. Psychiatry Res 214:109–115

McKinnon MCM, Yucel K, Nazarov A, MacQueen GM (2009) A meta-analysis examining clinical predictors of hippocampal volume in patients with major depressive disorder. J Psychiatry Neurosci 34:41–54

Melnyk BM, Jacobson D, Kelly S, Belyea M, Shaibi G, Small L, O'Haver J, Marsiglia FF (2013) Promoting healthy lifestyles in high school adolescents: a randomized controlled trial. Am J Prev Med 45:407–415. doi:10.1016/j.amepre.2013.05.013

Miller AH, Maletic V, Raison CL (2009) Inflammation and its discontents: the role of cytokines in the pathophysiology of major depression. Biol Psychiatry 65:732–741. doi:10.1016/j.biopsych.2008.11.029

Mohapel P, Frielingsdorf H, Häggblad J, Zachrisson O, Brundin P (2005) Platelet-derived growth factor (PDGF-BB) and brain-derived neurotrophic factor (BDNF) induce striatal neurogenesis in adult rats with 6-hydroxydopamine lesions. Neuroscience 132:767–776. doi:10.1016/j.neuroscience.2004.11.056

Montoya ER, Bos PA, Terburg D, Rosenberger LA, van Honk J (2014) Cortisol administration induces global down-regulation of the brain's reward circuitry. Psychoneuroendocrinology 47:31–42. doi:10.1016/j.psyneuen.2014.04.022

Mueller K, Sacher J, Arelin K, Holiga S, Kratzsch J, Villringer A, Schroeter ML (2012) Overweight and obesity are associated with neuronal injury in the human cerebellum and hippocampus in young adults: a combined MRI, serum marker and gene expression study. Transl Psychiatr 2:e200. doi:10.1038/tp.2012.121

Muscatell KA, Dedovic K, Slavich GM, Jarcho MR, Breen EC, Bower JE, Irwin MR, Eisenberger NI (2015) Greater amygdala activity and dorsomedial prefrontal-amygdala coupling are associated with enhanced inflammatory responses to stress. Brain Behav Immun 43:46–53. doi:10.1016/j.bbi.2014.06.201

Nanni V, Uher R, Ph D, Danese A (2012) Childhood maltreatment predicts unfavorable course of illness and treatment outcome in depression: a meta-analysis. Am J Psychiatry 169:141–151

Opel N, Redlich R, Zwanzger P, Grotegerd D, Arolt V, Heindel W, Konrad C, Kugel H, Dannlowski U (2014) Hippocampal atrophy in major depression: a function of childhood maltreatment rather than diagnosis? Neuropsychopharmacology 39:2723–2731. doi:10.1038/npp.2014.145

Opel N, Redlich R, Grotegerd D, Dohm K, Haupenthal C, Heindel W, Kugel H, Arolt V, Dannlowski U (2015a) Enhanced neural responsiveness to reward associated with obesity in the absence of food-related stimuli. Hum Brain Mapp. 36:2330–2337. doi:10.1002/hbm.22773

Opel N, Redlich R, Grotegerd D, Dohm K, Heindel W, Kugel H, Arolt V, Dannlowski U (2015b) Obesity and major depression: body-mass index (BMI) is associated with a severe course of disease and specific neurostructural alterations. Psychoneuroendocrinology 51:219–226. doi:10.1016/j.psyneuen.2014.10.001

Pan A, Sun Q, Czernichow S, Kivimaki M, Okereke OI, Lucas M, Manson JE, Ascherio A, Hu FB (2012) Bidirectional association between depression and obesity in middle-aged and older women. Int J Obes 36:595–602. doi:10.1038/ijo.2011.111

Pan A, Kumar R, Macey PM, Fonarow GC, Harper RM, Woo MA (2013) Visual assessment of brain magnetic resonance imaging detects injury to cognitive regulatory sites in patients with heart failure. J Card Fail 19:94–100. doi:10.1016/j.cardfail.2012.12.001

Phillips ML, Drevets WC, Rauch SL, Lane R (2003a) Neurobiology of emotion perception II: implications for major psychiatric disorders. Biol Psychiatry 54:515–528. doi:10.1016/S0006-3223(03)00171-9

Phillips ML, Drevets WC, Rauch SL, Lane R (2003b) Neurobiology of emotion perception I: the neural basis of normal emotion perception. Biol Psychiatry 54:504–514. doi:10.1016/S0006-3223(03)00168-9

Raji CA, Ho AJ, Parikshak NN, Becker JT, Lopez OL, Kuller LH, Hua X, Leow AD, Toga AW, Thompson PM (2010) Brain structure and obesity. Hum Brain Mapp 31:353–364. doi:10.1002/hbm.20870

Rao U, Chen L-A, Bidesi AS, Shad MU, Thomas MA, Hammen CL (2010) Hippocampal changes associated with early-life adversity and vulnerability to depression. Biol Psychiatry 67:357–364. doi:10.1016/j.biopsych.2009.10.017

Redlich R, Almeida JJR, Grotegerd D, Opel N, Kugel H, Heindel W, Arolt V, Phillips ML, Dannlowski U (2014) Brain morphometric biomarkers distinguishing unipolar and bipolar depression. JAMA Psychiatr 71:1222. doi:10.1001/jamapsychiatry.2014.1100

Redlich R, Dohm K, Grotegerd D, Opel N, Zwitserlood P, Heindel W, Arolt V, Kugel H, Dannlowski U (2015) Reward processing in unipolar and bipolar depression: a functional MRI study. Neuropsychopharmacology. doi:10.1038/npp.2015.110

Rive MM, van Rooijen G, Veltman DJ, Phillips ML, Schene AH, Ruhé HG (2013) Neural correlates of dysfunctional emotion regulation in major depressive disorder. A systematic review of neuroimaging studies. Neurosci Biobehav Rev. doi:10.1016/j.neubiorev.2013.07.018

Rozanski A, Blumenthal JA, Kaplan J (1999) Impact of psychological factors on the pathogenesis of cardiovascular disease and implications for therapy. Circulation 99:2192–2217. doi:10.1161/01.CIR.99.16.2192

Schermuly I, Wolf D, Lieb K, Stoeter P, Fellgiebel A (2011) State dependent posterior hippocampal volume increases in patients with major depressive disorder. J Affect Disord 135:405–409. doi:10.1016/j.jad.2011.07.017

Sen A, Gider P, Cavalieri M, Freudenberger P, Farzi A, Schallert M, Reichmann F, Watzinger N, Zweiker R, Schmidt R, Schmidt H (2012) Association of cardiorespiratory fitness and morphological brain changes in the elderly: results of the Austrian Stroke Prevention Study. Neurodegener Dis 10:135–137. doi:10.1159/000334760

Sheline YI, Barch DM, Donnelly JM, Ollinger JM, Snyder AZ, Mintun MA (2001) Increased amygdala response to masked emotional faces in depressed subjects resolves with antidepressant treatment: an fMRI study. Biol Psychiatry 50:651–658. doi:10.1016/S0006-3223(01)01263-X

Sheline YI, Gado MH, Kraemer HC (2003) Untreated depression and hippocampal volume loss. Am J Psychiatry 160:1516–1518

Siegle GJ, Thompson WK, Carter CS, Steinhauer SR, Thase ME (2007) Increased amygdala and decreased dorsolateral prefrontal BOLD responses in unipolar depression: related and independent features. Biol Psychiatry 61:198–209. doi:10.1016/j.biopsych.2006.05.048

Singh NA, Stavrinos TM, Scarbek Y, Galambos G, Liber C, Fiatarone Singh MA (2005) A randomized controlled trial of high versus low intensity weight training versus general practitioner care for clinical depression in older adults. J Gerontol 60:768–776

Skala JA, Freedland KE, Carney RM (2006) Coronary heart disease and depression: a review of recent mechanistic research. Can J Psychiatry 51:738–745

Smucny J, Cornier M-A, Eichman LC, Thomas E a, Bechtell JL, Tregellas JR (2012) Brain structure predicts risk for obesity. Appetite 59:859–865. doi:10.1016/j.appet.2012.08.027

Steptoe A, Kivimäki M (2012) Stress and cardiovascular disease. Nat Rev Cardiol 9:360–370. doi:10.1038/nrcardio.2012.45

Stratmann M, Konrad C, Kugel H, Krug A, Schöning S, Ohrmann P, Uhlmann C, Postert C, Suslow T, Heindel W, Arolt V, Kircher T, Dannlowski U (2014) Insular and hippocampal gray matter volume reductions in patients with major depressive disorder. PLoS One 9:e102692. doi:10.1371/journal.pone.0102692

Stuhrmann A, Dohm K, Kugel H, Zwanzger P, Redlich R, Grotegerd D, Rauch AV, Arolt V, Heindel W, Suslow T, Zwitserlood P, Dannlowski U (2012) Mood-congruent amygdala responses to subliminally presented facial expressions in major depression: associations with anhedonia. J Psychiatry Neurosci 38:249–258

Tendolkar I, van Beek M, van Oostrom I, Mulder M, Janzing J, Voshaar RO, van Eijndhoven P (2013) Electroconvulsive therapy increases hippocampal and amygdala volume in therapy refractory depression: a longitudinal pilot study. Psychiatry Res 214:197–203. doi:10.1016/j.pscychresns.2013.09.004

Thombs BD, Bass EB, Ford DE, Stewart KJ, Tsilidis KK, Patel U, Fauerbach JA, Bush DE, Ziegelstein RC (2006) Prevalence of depression in survivors of acute myocardial infarction. J Gen Intern Med 21:30–38. doi:10.1111/j.1525-1497.2005.00269.x

Verdejo-García A, Verdejo-Román J, Rio-Valle JS, Lacomba JA, Lagos FM, Soriano-Mas C (2014) Dysfunctional involvement of emotion and reward brain regions on social decision making in excess weight adolescents. Hum Brain Mapp. doi:10.1002/hbm.22625

Vicennati V, Garelli S, Rinaldi E, Di Dalmazi G, Pagotto U, Pasquali R (2014) Cross-talk between adipose tissue and the HPA axis in obesity and overt hypercortisolemic states. Horm Mol Biol Clin Investig 17:63–77. doi:10.1515/hmbci-2013-0068

Volkow ND, Wang G-J, Telang F, Fowler JS, Thanos PK, Logan J, Alexoff D, Ding Y-S, Wong C, Ma Y, Pradhan K (2008) Low dopamine striatal D2 receptors are associated with prefrontal metabolism in obese subjects: possible contributing factors. Neuroimage 42:1537–1543. doi:10.1016/j.neuroimage.2008.06.002

Walther K, Birdsill AC, Glisky EL, Ryan L (2010) Structural brain differences and cognitive functioning related to body mass index in older females. Hum Brain Mapp 31:1052–1064. doi:10.1002/hbm.20916

Wang G-J, Volkow ND, Logan J, Pappas NR, Wong CT, Zhu W, Netusll N, Fowler JS (2001) Brain dopamine and obesity. Lancet 357:354–357. doi:10.1016/S0140-6736(00)03643-6

Wang G-J, Volkow ND, Thanos PK, Fowler JS (2009) Imaging of brain dopamine pathways: implications for understanding obesity. J Addict Med 3:8–18. doi:10.1097/ADM.0b013e31819a86f7. Imaging

Wang Y-C, Huang C-C, Hsu K-S (2010) The role of growth retardation in lasting effects of neonatal dexamethasone treatment on hippocampal synaptic function. PLoS One 5:e12806. doi:10.1371/journal.pone.0012806

Ward MA, Carlsson CM, Trivedi MA, Sager MA, Johnson SC (2005) The effect of body mass index on global brain volume in middle-aged adults: a cross sectional study. BMC Neurol 5:23. doi:10.1186/1471-2377-5-23

Williams LM, Kemp AH, Felmingham K, Barton M, Olivieri G, Peduto A, Gordon E, Bryant RA (2006) Trauma modulates amygdala and medial prefrontal responses to consciously attended fear. Neuroimage 29:347–357. doi:10.1016/j.neuroimage.2005.03.047

Woo MA, Kumar R, Macey PM, Fonarow GC, Harper RM (2009) Brain injury in autonomic, emotional, and cognitive regulatory areas in patients with heart failure. J Card Fail 15:214–223. doi:10.1016/j.cardfail.2008.10.020

Yau PL, Kang EH, Javier DC, Convit A (2014) Preliminary evidence of cognitive and brain abnormalities in uncomplicated adolescent obesity. Obesity 22:1865–1871. doi:10.1002/oby.20801

Yokum S, Ng J, Stice E (2012) Relation of regional gray and white matter volumes to current BMI and future increases in BMI: a prospective MRI study. Int J Obes (Lond) 36:656–664. doi:10.1038/ijo.2011.175

Zhang W-N, Chang S-H, Guo L-Y, Zhang K-L, Wang J (2013) The neural correlates of reward-related processing in major depressive disorder: a meta-analysis of functional magnetic resonance imaging studies. J Affect Disord 151:531–539. doi:10.1016/j.jad.2013.06.039

Zubicaray GI, Deary IJ, Donohoe G, de Geus EJC, Espeseth T, Fernández G, Glahn DC, Grabe HJ, Hardy J, Hulshoff Pol HE, Jenkinson M, Kahn RS, McDonald C, McIntosh AM, McMahon FJ, McMahon KL, Meyer-Lindenberg A, Morris DW, Müller-Myhsok B, Nichols TE, Ophoff RA, Paus T, Pausova Z, Penninx BWJH, Potkin SG, Sämann PG, Saykin AJ, Schumann G, Smoller JW, Wardlaw JM, Weale ME, Martin NG, Franke B, Wright MJ, Thompson PM (2012) Identification of common variants associated with human hippocampal and intracranial volumes. Nat Genet 44:552–561. doi:10.1038/ng.2250

Heart Rate Variability, Affective Disorders and Health

11

A.H. Kemp

Contents

Abstract

Resting-state heart rate variability (HRV) may have important functional significance for social approach behaviour, emotion regulation and psychological flexibility in the face of stressors. It may also reflect the functioning of important physiological processes including vagal regulation over a variety of allostatic systems and multisystemic adaptations to maintain homeostasis. Research on the effects of the affective disorders on HRV therefore has important implications for the health and wellbeing of patients. Studies have demonstrated that HRV is reduced in otherwise healthy patients with these disorders, especially major depression and generalised anxiety disorder, and that the behavioural features of these disorders (e.g. smoking, physical inactivity) do not fully explain the observed HRV reductions. Vagal impairment may underpin many of the observed symptoms in affective disorders including flattened affect, attenuated facial expressions and lack of emotional prosody. It may also contribute to a pathophysiological 'wear and tear' effect on the body leading to

A.H. Kemp
Department of Psychology, Swansea University,
Swansea, United Kingdom
e-mail: a.h.kemp@swansea.ac.uk

B.T. Baune, P.J. Tully (eds.), *Cardiovascular Diseases and Depression*,
DOI 10.1007/978-3-319-32480-7_11

increased morbidity and mortality. Health behaviours such as a healthy diet, physical exercise and even meditation may have an important role to play in appropriate psychiatric care of patients with affective disorders because these interventions facilitate increases in HRV, which reflect enhanced vagal function that may lead to subsequent improvements in mental and physical health. Further study is needed to determine whether simple health behaviours are able to ameliorate the reductions in HRV associated with use of antidepressant medications. Research is also needed on possible moderators and mediators of vagal impairment, and its improvement, in the affective disorders.

11.1 Introduction

Heart rate variability (or HRV) – a non-invasive marker of health and wellbeing – reflects activity in the vagus nerve, the primary nerve in the parasympathetic nervous system. While mental and physical health are generally investigated independently, research has demonstrated robust bidirectional relationships between the two, highlighting the implications of one for the other. For instance, a meta-review on 20 different mental disorders in over 1.7 million patients reported that all mental disorders have an increased risk of all-cause mortality, relative to the general population. Strikingly, all disorders were associated with substantial reductions in life expectancy (7–24 years), an effect similar to or greater than that for heavy smoking (8–10 years) (Chesney et al. 2014). Together with colleagues, I recently demonstrated that comorbid MDD and anxiety disorders ($n=434$) are associated with a threefold increase in coronary heart disease (CHD), while MDD alone ($n=170$) was associated with a twofold increase (Kemp et al. 2015b). Studies have also demonstrated that positive psychological wellbeing is associated with reduced mortality in healthy individuals in studies with follow-ups of up to 10 years (Chida and Steptoe 2008) (see also Steptoe et al. (2015)). A meta-analysis (Chida and Steptoe 2008) on 35 studies in initially healthy populations revealed that wellbeing is associated with reduced all-cause mortality (19 % reduction in hazard ratio) and cardiovascular mortality (29 % reduction). Together, these studies highlight a robust relationship between mental and physical health. It is possible that HRV provides a candidate marker for the mechanism that links mental and physical health (see Kemp and Quintana (2013) for a recent review).

HRV indexes the beat-to-beat variability in heart rate measured by the electrocardiogram, and although different measures may reflect distinct physiological mechanisms, all measures predominantly reflect vagal nerve activity (Reyes Del Paso et al. 2013). I now turn my attention to the varied psychological and physiological functions indexed by HRV. This discussion helps to highlight the implications of alterations in vagal function and provides an important foundation for interpreting the findings of studies on HRV in affective disorders, discussed in the following section. Finally, I provide some recommendations for future studies in this exciting area of research.

11.2 The Vagus: Psychological and Physiological Associations

The vagus has been described as the most important nerve in the human body (Tracey 2007). Vagal function may underpin a variety of important psychological and physiological functions including emotion recognition (Quintana et al. 2012) and its regulation (Smith et al. 2011), cognitive flexibility (Verkuil et al. 2010), control over inflammatory processes (Wang et al. 2003), regulation of the hypothalamic-pituitary-adrenal (HPA) axis (Porges 2011), glucose metabolism (Pocai et al. 2005; Wang et al. 2008) and neurotrophic processes (Follesa et al. 2007). Vagal function is also understood to play an important role in the communication of changes in the gastrointestinal tract to the central nervous system (Bravo et al. 2011). While phasic decreases in vagal activity are normal responses to environmental challenge or stress (Hanson et al. 2013; Kemp et al. 2014b), phasic increases facilitate emotion regulation (Geisler et al. 2010; Smith et al. 2011) and social engagement (Kok and Fredrickson 2010; Kemp et al. 2012b; Geisler et al. 2013). A properly functioning vagus nerve may underpin psychophysiological flexibility (Thayer et al. 2009), psychological wellbeing (Kok and Fredrickson 2010; Kok et al. 2013), cardiovascular health (Hillebrand et al. 2013) and even survival in critical illness including cancer (Giese-Davis et al. 2015) and trauma (Riordan et al. 2009). By contrast, its impairment is associated with psychophysiological rigidity (Thayer et al. 2009), dysregulation of a variety of allostatic systems (Thayer and Sternberg 2006), increased morbidity and risk for mortality (Thayer et al. 2010; Kemp and Quintana 2013). Vagal dysfunction may also manifest as flattened affect, poor eye gaze, attenuated facial expressions, lack of prosody and hyperacusis (Porges 2011), core symptoms of the affective disorders (Fig. 11.1).

There is now considerable evidence demonstrating that the affective disorders are associated with a chronic low-grade inflammatory response (see Berk et al. (2013) for review) increasing risk for a host of disorders and disease associated with ageing (see Kiecolt-Glaser et al. (2002) for review). The vagus is known to play an important regulatory role over these inflammatory processes, a neural mechanism known as the cholinergic anti-inflammatory reflex (Tracey 2002, 2007; Huston and Tracey 2010; Tracey and Pavlov 2012). This reflex is a neural mechanism regulated by the vagus nerve that controls metabolic homeostasis and innate immune responses. It is involved in the detection of cytokines and pathogen-derived products by the afferent (sensory) vagus nerve and the regulation and control of cytokine release by the efferent (motor) vagus nerve. Regulation of inflammatory processes is achieved through the binding of acetylcholine to nAChRα7 expressed on macrophages in the periphery and microglia in the brain (Cheyuo et al. 2011). Reduced vagal function leads to elevated systemic inflammation (Pavlov and Tracey 2012), triggering hepatic synthesis of C-reactive protein (Jarczok et al. 2014), increasing risk for cardiovascular disease morbidity and mortality (Casas et al. 2008).

More broadly, the vagus is considered to play a key regulatory role in a variety of allostatic systems including inflammatory processes, the hypothalamic-pituitary-adrenal axis and glucose metabolism (Thayer and Sternberg 2006). Allostasis is a

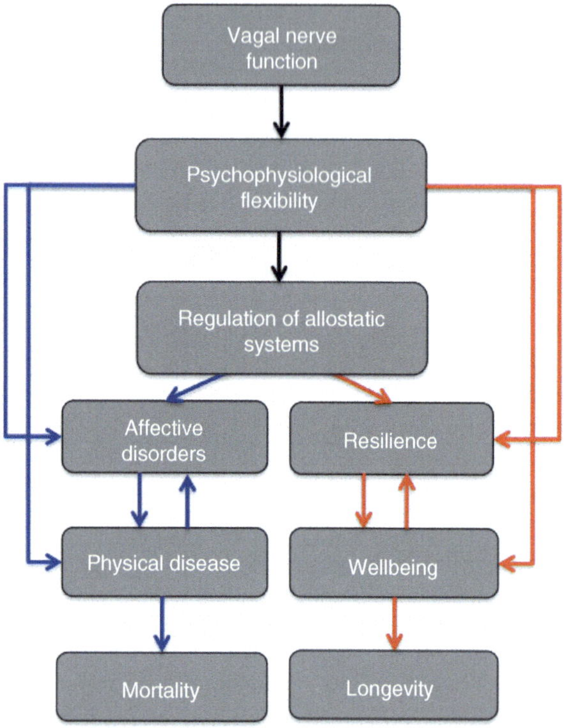

Fig. 11.1 A simplified model for the associations between vagal function, the affective disorders and health. A properly functioning vagus nerve underpins psychophysiological flexibility to environmental challenge, homeostatic regulation over a variety of allostatic systems, resilience, wellbeing and longevity. By contrast, its impairment leads to psychophysiological rigidity, allostatic load, affective disorders, physical disease and mortality. The model explicitly acknowledges the bidirectional associations between the affective disorders (resilience) and physical disease (wellbeing)

term that describes the multisystemic adaptations to maintain homeostasis, allowing the body to cope with environmental challenges (McEwen 1998). The affective disorders are characterised by patterns of pathophysiology associated with a 'wear and tear' effect on the human body or 'allostatic load' (McEwen 1998). Preserved vagal function is therefore critical to antagonising these pathologic processes (Cheyuo et al. 2011) and may underpin many of the benefits of simple health interventions such as dietary improvements and physical activity, which include better regulation of pro-inflammatory conditions and induction of growth factor cascades (Cotman et al. 2007; Gomez-Pinilla 2008a, b).

This extensive set of observations and associated theoretical foundations highlight the broad utility of HRV measurement leading to sustained research interest in HRV by researchers from multiple disciplines. I now turn my attention to the findings reported by studies that have investigated the impact of affective disorders on HRV.

11.3 Affective Disorders and HRV

The study of HRV in affective disorders has captured the attention of researchers for more than two decades. In one of the first studies on this topic (Carney et al. 1988), depressed patients with coronary artery disease were found to have a higher heart rate relative to nondepressed patients with coronary artery disease, independent of age, smoking and beta-blocker medication. Depressed patients also had reduced heart rate variability, although this association fell short of statistical significance. The HRV measure reported in this study was the standard deviation of the mean R-R intervals over consecutive 5-min intervals, extracted from 24-h ambulatory ECG recordings. The standard deviation of normal-to-normal R-R intervals (SDNN) is a commonly reported, time-domain measure, reflecting all of the cyclic components responsible for variability. SDNN is often reported in studies on long-term HRV recordings and has been demonstrated to be a robust predictor of adverse cardiovascular events and mortality (Hillebrand et al. 2013; Huikuri and Stein 2013).

Reliable and valid measures of heart rate and its variability may also be obtained from shorter recordings under standardised and controlled conditions (Task Force of the European Society of Cardiology the North American Society of Pacing Electrophysiology 1996). An early study (Thayer et al. 1996) on patients with generalised anxiety disorder (GAD) reported that patients display lower high-frequency heart rate variability (HF-HRV), relative to non-anxious control participants, concluding that GAD and its cardinal feature – worry – may be associated with reduced vagal activity. This study was based on HRV measures extracted from short-term ECG recordings (3.5 min). Short-term recordings may also predict coronary heart disease and mortality (Dekker et al. 2000; Carnethon et al. 2002). The most commonly reported measures of HRV reported from short-term recordings include the root mean square of successive differences (RMSSD) and HF-HRV, which are time- and frequency-domain measures, respectively. While the two are highly correlated, the former is less affected by changes in breathing frequency (Penttilä et al. 2001; Saboul et al. 2013), highlighting the utility of RMSSD during ambulatory recordings and research on patients with high levels of anxiety in particular (e.g. Wilhelm et al. 2001) (see also Carnevali et al. (2013)).

Recent research has concentrated on whether HRV is reduced in the mood and anxiety disorders or, instead, whether these reductions are driven by medications that are prescribed for these conditions (Kemp et al. 2011a, b; Licht et al. 2011a, b; Kemp 2011, 2012; Brunoni et al. 2012). Contradictory findings have been reported in the literature, the reasons for which may include small, heterogeneous and medicated samples. Meta-analysis is an important quantitative technique that allows objective conclusions to be drawn from individual studies, which may be affected by low study power. Meta-analysis overcomes this limitation by drawing conclusions on the basis of summary statistics calculated from multiple individual studies and allows for the heterogeneity of contributing studies to be systematically examined. Our recent meta-analyses on resting-state HRV in major depressive disorder (MDD) (Kemp et al. 2010) and anxiety disorders (Chalmers et al. 2014) were an explicit attempt to draw objective conclusions from a contradictory body of previously published studies.

Our first meta-analysis ($N = 1080$) on patients with MDD (Kemp et al. 2010) was conducted to determine whether unmedicated depressed patients display HRV reductions across time-, frequency- and non-linear domains. We also focused on otherwise healthy patients with depression because cardiovascular disease may have led to overestimations of the association between depression and resting-state

HRV. An earlier study (Licht et al. 2008) based on the large Netherlands Study of Depression and Anxiety (NESDA) cohort ($N=2373$) had concluded that while lowered HRV was observed in depression, this finding was mainly driven by the effect of antidepressants. Our meta-analysis (Kemp et al. 2010) indicated that HRV was lower in unmedicated depressed patients ($n=673$), relative to healthy controls ($n=407$), with effect sizes ranging from small (based on time- and frequency-domain HRV measures) to large (non-linear measures). Depression severity was also observed to correlate negatively with HRV ($r=-0.35$, $p<0.001$). We speculated that somatic symptoms, commonly observed in patients with severe depression, might have contributed to this finding. We recently supported this possibility in a study on patients with melancholia (Kemp et al. 2014c), a subtype of depression characterised by somatic symptoms, cognitive impairment and reduced responsiveness to the environment. (This more recent study is discussed further below.) In our earlier meta-analysis (Kemp et al. 2010), we also reported that tricyclic antidepressants – but not other classes of antidepressants – were associated with substantial HRV reductions, findings associated with a large effect size. While our meta-analysis confirmed the well-known adverse effects of tricyclic antidepressants (Glassman et al. 1993), our findings in unmedicated patients also demonstrated that antidepressant medications do not necessarily drive the HRV findings that have been observed in samples with affective disorders, an argument that has now been made by several groups of researchers (e.g. Licht et al. 2009; O'Regan et al. 2014).

Our more recent meta-analysis on anxiety disorders ($N=4380$) (Chalmers et al. 2014) was also conducted because prior studies had reported inconsistent findings, again, highlighting the need for objective meta-analysis. An earlier study on the anxiety disorders, also on the NESDA cohort ($N=2095$), had concluded that the effects of antidepressant medications drove lowered HRV in these patients. By contrast, our more recent meta-analysis (Chalmers et al. 2014) on anxiety disorders ($n=2086$) observed that lower HRV is observed in patients with anxiety disorders (based on HF-HRV and time-domain measures) and that these findings were associated with a small-to-moderate effect size. Critically, medication use and medical comorbidity did not impact on these findings. Inspection of specific anxiety disorders also indicated that patients with panic disorder ($n=447$), post-traumatic stress disorder ($n=192$), generalised anxiety disorder ($n=68$) and social anxiety disorder ($n=90$) all displayed moderate reductions in HF-HRV, relative to controls. Patients with specific phobias ($n=61$) displayed reductions in time-domain measures of HRV, although these findings were associated with a small effect size. Only obsessive-compulsive disorder was not associated with significant reductions in HRV, null findings that could have been due to a relatively small sample size ($n=40$). Unfortunately, no meta-analysis could be conducted on specific treatments for anxiety disorders due to the small number of studies investigating this issue, highlighting the need for further research in this area.

It is important to point out here that MDD and anxiety are frequently comorbid conditions: MDD has high comorbidities with the whole range of anxiety disorders (Goldberg and Fawcett 2012). Correlations range from 0.62 for generalised anxiety disorder, 0.52 for agoraphobia and social phobia, 0.48 for panic disorder to 0.42 for obsessive-compulsive disorder (Goldberg and Fawcett 2012). The close relationship between MDD and generalised anxiety disorder in particular is thought to relate to shared symptoms – especially negative affect – and genetic risk factors (Goldberg and Fawcett 2012). My colleagues and I have now published multiple studies in independent samples (Kemp et al. 2012a, 2014a) demonstrating that GAD patients may display the most robust reductions in HRV. Lowered HRV in GAD patients may relate to their inability to disengage from threat detection, even in the absence of any real threat (Thayer and Lane 2000; Kemp et al. 2012a), a behavioural characteristic that may be underpinned by prolonged prefrontal inactivity, disinhibition of the central nucleus of the amygdala and activation of medullary cardioacceleratory circuits (Thayer et al. 2009; Kemp et al. 2012a).

In the largest independent cohort to date ($N = 15{,}105$), we reported (Kemp et al. 2014a) that the use of antidepressant medications was associated with substantial decreases in HRV, while only GAD was observed to display robust, albeit small, reductions in vagal activity after controlling for multiple confounding variables, including medication use. This study employed propensity score matching procedures, a technique that involves estimating the difference between groups after accounting for covariates that predict group membership. This propensity score technique has several advantages over traditional analytical techniques such as analysis of covariance (ANCOVA) and multiple regression analysis including reduced bias by accounting for the effects of covariates without reference to the outcome variable (HRV) and the opportunity to analyse data with some of the advantages of a randomised controlled design (McCaffrey et al. 2013). This technique is particularly helpful when researchers have access to a large sample of participants and seek answers to research questions that have previously led researchers to draw contradictory conclusions. Although participants with comorbid depression and anxiety disorders were not found to display lowered HRV, many of the factors adversely affecting HRV had already been controlled using propensity score weighting and matching techniques (Kemp et al. 2014a). We concluded, therefore, that comprehensive cardiovascular risk reduction strategies are still needed in such patients to minimise subsequent morbidity and mortality in these patients (Nemeroff and Goldschmidt-Clermont 2012).

Studies have also examined HRV in the bipolar spectrum disorders (BSDs) (see Outhred et al. (2014) for review), a cluster of disorders characterised by extreme changes in mood involving depression and (hypo)mania (Malhi et al. 2012). HRV appears to be decreased in both the manic (Henry et al. 2010; Chang et al. 2014) and depressive phases (Lee et al. 2012; Chang et al. 2015) of the illness, although contradictory findings have again been reported, with other studies reporting that mania is associated with higher, not lower HRV (Gruber et al. 2008, 2011). For instance, a study on young adults categorised into high relative to low mania risk groups displayed elevated positive emotion and tonic vagal function at rest and during presentation of positive, negative and neutral films (Gruber et al. 2008). While this study was conducted on a non-patient population, a more recent study by the same authors reported that patients with bipolar disorder ($n = 23$) display smaller decreases in RSA – as determined by the peak-valley method – during emotion-eliciting films, compared to non-clinical controls ($n = 24$) (Gruber et al. 2011). Critically, this study further reported that 'BD participants exhibited greater increases in RSA [during film stimuli] from already higher RSA levels' collected during a resting baseline period relative to controls. These contradictory findings in BD highlight the importance of continued work in this area.

Research has also begun to compare HRV across multiple psychiatric disorders. In this regard, a study (Moon et al. 2013) compared resting-state measures of HRV collected from patients with schizophrenia, bipolar disorder, post-traumatic disorder and MDD. This study observed robust decreases in patients with bipolar disorder across a variety of HRV measures. Significant reductions in high-frequency HRV (HF-HRV) were also observed in schizophrenia, post-traumatic stress disorder and MDD relative to controls. However the authors (Moon et al. 2013) did not find any differences across the disorders. More recent work (Alvares et al. 2016) suggests that the most pronounced HRV reductions may be observed in physically healthy patients with psychotic disorders. A major limitation of this study was that patient groups were being treated with a variety of medications, which as discussed above, may impact on HRV (Kemp et al. 2010, 2014a; Licht et al. 2010). Another limitation of this study (Moon et al. 2013) was that groups differed on age, a major confounding variable (Voss et al. 2012, 2015), which again makes it difficult to draw robust conclusions.

Recently, other researchers reported that HRV may help to distinguish bipolar II depression from unipolar major depressive disorder (Chang et al. 2015). Patients with bipolar were reported to display lower mean R-R intervals, variance (total HRV), low-frequency (LF)-HRV and high-frequency (HF-)HRV but higher LF/HF ratio compared to those with major depression. In comparison with controls, the authors reported that bipolar patients display cardiac sympathetic excitation – based on a larger LF/HF ratio – in combination with reciprocal vagal impairment, while patients with unipolar depression display only vagal impairment. These authors concluded that the additional findings for the LF/HF ratio – which the authors argued to reflect sympathetic nervous system activity – may be used to aid differential diagnosis of bipolar depression. This conclusion, however, is incorrect for at least two reasons (see discussion in Kemp (2015)). Firstly, this conclusion assumes that LF component of HRV is an index of sympathetic cardiac control and that the LF/HF ratio reflects an index of autonomic balance, yet HRV – especially that during the resting state – predominantly reflects activity in the parasympathetic nervous system rather than the sympathetic nervous system (Reyes Del Paso et al. 2013) (see also Goldstein et al. (2011)). Secondly, this study did not take into consideration the heterogeneity of major depression. For instance, we have reported that patients with melancholic depression – but not those with non-melancholic depression – display HRV decreases relative to controls (Kemp et al. 2014c), findings associated with a moderate effect size. While the large group of unipolar depressed patients in Chang's study was comprised of 130 patients with melancholic features, they did not compare patients with melancholia to those with bipolar.

In addition to generally lowered HRV in patients with affective disorders, studies have also observed HRV reductions during their remission (Kemp et al. 2010; Chang et al. 2013; Brunoni et al. 2013; Braeken et al. 2013). These findings suggest that vagal impairment may actually persist despite successful treatment, perhaps providing a psychophysiological mechanism for the observation that asymptomatic individuals are more vulnerable to future episodes, a phenomenon known as 'kindling' (Post 1992). We recently demonstrated that unmedicated women ($n=22$) with a history of – but not current – anxiety disorders display decreases in HRV (Braeken et al. 2013). These findings indicate that patients with prior affective disorders may still display lowered HRV, even in unmedicated individuals. Strikingly, we also observed that the 2–4-month-old offspring of these pregnant women with a past history affective disorders also display low HRV relative to children from the women without such history. Furthermore, these HRV decreases at 2–4 months of age also predicted fearful behaviour at 9–10 months of age, pointing to possible underlying mechanisms of future psychopathology. In another recent study, we argued that HRV reductions may reflect a trait marker of MDD ($n=93$ following treatment) (Brunoni et al. 2013). This study demonstrated that HRV did not change following treatment with either a non-pharmacological (transcranial direct current stimulation) or pharmacological (sertraline) intervention, nor was HRV observed to increase with clinical response to either treatment. Another study, however, on unmedicated individuals with a diagnosis of MDD earlier in life ($n=470$) (Chang et al. 2013) observed that autonomic dysregulation was observed only in those remitted patients with a history of suicidal ideation ($n=237$), while HRV otherwise appeared to resolve in individuals with fully remitted MDD.

In summary, studies have shown that the affective disorders generally display impairment in vagal function indicated by HRV reductions (see Table 11.1 for summary of key, recent studies). It should be noted that while decreases in HRV are generally indicative of autonomic dysfunction (Thayer et al. 2010), higher values may also reflect an unhealthy, highly irregular heart rate pattern in cardiac patients (Huikuri and Stein 2013). However, it is unlikely that this finding is relevant to patients with affective disorders for several reasons. Firstly, reduced HRV is observed in *otherwise healthy* patients with affective disorders (e.g. Kemp et al. 2010, 2012a). Secondly, these concerns relate more to older individuals who are increasingly likely to display abnormal cardiac rhythms. As HRV reductions are observed in otherwise healthy patients with affective disorders, these changes may reflect an early, upstream, marker of dysfunction that subsequently leads to an inflammatory cascade increasing risk for morbidity and mortality (Tracey 2002, 2007; Thayer and Sternberg 2010; Huston and Tracey 2010; Tracey and Pavlov 2012; Kemp and Quintana 2013). It is suggested therefore that lower HRV may provide an early marker of ill health in otherwise healthy patients with affective disorders that precedes established risk factors for medical illness. Further study is needed to determine whether particular disorders display greater reductions than others (recent evidence suggests that otherwise healthy patients with psychotic disorders may display the greatest reductions, Alvares et al. 2016), in addition to research on the various pathways through which these reductions may contribute to physical ill health. I now turn our attention to some of the methodological considerations facing researchers using HRV in their research activities.

11.3.1 Future Directions

The extant research on the impact of affective disorders on HRV has largely focused on whether or not there is an effect, rather than when, or how an effect appears. This focus

Table 11.1 Brief summary of major recent findings from studies on HRV in affective disorders[1,2]

Finding	Comment	Reference
HRV is reduced in otherwise healthy patients with major depressive disorder (MDD) (n=673) relative to healthy controls (n=407). Tricyclic medications (TCAs) decreased HRV (n=32), although serotonin reuptake inhibitors (n=92) had no significant impact on HRV, despite patient response to treatment	These findings were obtained from meta-analysis on a body of previously reported contradictory findings (N=1080). For MDD, small effect sizes were observed for time- and frequency-domain measures, while a large effect size was observed for non-linear domain measures. For TCAs, a large effect size was observed. This study was the first to conclusively demonstrate that HRV is reduced in MDD in otherwise healthy patients and that these effects are not due to medication	Kemp et al. (2010)
HRV was reduced in MDD (n=73) relative to controls (n=94), and patients with comorbid generalised anxiety disorder (GAD) (n=24) displayed the most robust reductions	This study (N=167) focused on the impact of anxiety comorbidity in patients with MDD. All patients were unmedicated and otherwise healthy, yet HRV reductions were still observed, providing important evidence that medications alone are not the only reason for driving HRV reductions, as has been argued now by several research groups	Kemp et al. (2012a)
HRV is reduced in patients with generalised anxiety disorder (GAD) only (n=1183). HRV is also reduced in users of antidepressants. Findings were greatest for users of tricyclic antidepressants (n=84) and the serotonin and noradrenaline reuptake inhibitors (n=52), followed by other antidepressants (n=75) and the selective serotonin reuptake inhibitors (n=356)	These findings were obtained from the largest cohort study conducted to date (N=15,105) on the impact of common mental disorders and antidepressants. This study also used an underused analytical technique known as propensity score analysis, which has advantages over traditional regression-based techniques to control for confounding variables. This study demonstrated that while the effects of antidepressant treatments are the most robust, patients with generalised anxiety disorder display significant, albeit small, reductions in HRV	Kemp et al. (2014a)
HRV is reduced in MDD patients with melancholia (n=40) – but not non-melancholia (n=32)	This study (N=166) was conducted to follow up on the American Journal of Psychiatry (AJP) observation (above) that HRV was not reduced in MDD. The findings reported in Frontiers in Psychology were based on the sample used in the above 2012 PLOS ONE study. However, this sample was an independent sample to those used for the AJP publication. Findings highlight the importance of investigating heterogeneity in MDD. The HRV reductions observed in melancholia relative to controls were associated with moderate effect size	Kemp et al. (2014b)

Table 11.1 (continued)

Finding	Comment	Reference
HRV is reduced in MDD patients ($n=120$), and these findings were not ameliorated by either sertraline or transcranial direct current stimulation (tDCS)	This study ($N=240$) replicated the previously reported – albeit contradictory – findings of HRV reductions in HRV. This study further reported that HRV was still reduced following treatment with either sertraline or tDCS in both those that responded and did not respond to treatment. Based on these findings, it was concluded that HRV reductions may reflect a trait marker of MDD and that these reductions are not due to antidepressant medications. HRV reductions were associated with a small-to-moderate effect size	Brunoni et al. (2013)
HRV is reduced in women with a past history ($n=22$) – but not current – anxiety disorder relative to those without a history of psychopathology ($n=34$). HRV was also reduced in the offspring of women with a past anxiety disorder ($n=16$), relative to the offspring of women without a history of psychopathology ($n=28$). In all children, low HRV at 2–4 months of age were associated with a higher chance of fearful behaviour at 9–10 months	Participants in this study consisted of 56 women during their first trimester and their offspring (15 male, 29 female). Women had a history of an anxiety disorder ($n=22$) or no psychopathology ($n=34$). This study is unique because it not only demonstrates that past anxiety disorder is associated with HRV reductions, but that the offspring of the women with a past anxiety disorder also displayed HRV reductions. Finally, the associations between offspring HRV and future fearful behaviour have important implications for future psychopathology of the offspring	Braeken et al. (2013)
HRV is reduced in the anxiety disorders including those diagnosed with panic disorder ($n=447$), post-traumatic stress disorder ($n=192$), generalised anxiety disorder ($n=68$), social anxiety disorder ($n=90$) and specific phobias ($n=61$)	These findings were obtained from meta-analysis on a body of previously reported contradictory findings ($N=4380$). Moderate effect sizes were observed for patients with panic disorder, post-traumatic stress disorder, generalised anxiety disorder and social anxiety disorder, while a small effect size was observed for patients with specific phobias. No meta-analysis could be conducted on specific treatments for anxiety disorders due to the small number of studies investigating this issue	Chalmers et al. (2014)

[1]Studies contributing to the main conclusions drawn in the book chapter are included in this table

[2]The studies included in this table focus on major depressive disorder (*MDD*) and the anxiety disorders. While considerable debate has concentrated on whether HRV reductions are driven by the disorder versus antidepressant treatment, the most recent studies (summarised in this table) demonstrate that HRV is reduced in unmedicated patients with affective disorders. HRV reductions appear to be greatest for patients with generalised anxiety disorder (*GAD*), a finding that may relate to the inability of patients to disengage from threat detection, even in the absence of any real threat. These findings have important implications for the health of patients with anxiety disorders and especially those with GAD

may in part have led to some of the contradictory and discrepant findings reported in the literature. For instance, a study involving 22-h ambulatory monitoring (Schwerdtfeger and Friedrich-Mai 2009) demonstrated that while depression is associated with reduced time-domain HRV (RMSSD) when participants are alone, social interactions (with partner, family or friends) may ameliorate this effect. These findings are important as laboratory-based recordings involve social interaction with experimenters, which may inadvertently ameliorate differences between depressed participants and controls. Social connectedness is associated with increased HRV (Kok and Fredrickson 2010), and Porges' polyvagal theory (Porges 2011) provides a theoretical basis for such findings, which may also be apparent in psychiatric populations, particularly depressed individuals. It is possible that further examination of group differences under multiple conditions including resting state, stressor and recovery from stressor may help to elucidate more robust effects in affective disorders.

Researchers also need to give consideration to what might moderate HRV reductions in order to better clarify the conditions under which effects may or may not be observed. It is possible, for instance, that the effect sizes of the disorders are larger than have been reported but that the effects have been suppressed by not taking into consideration particular moderating factors. In addition to the above example in regard to social engagement, certain clinical characteristics and their amelioration may also moderate observed findings. For example, specific subtypes of depression (e.g. melancholia) or symptoms of a depressive episode or the anxiety disorders (e.g. somatic symptoms) may have stronger effects on vagal activity. This particular issue was examined in a recently published report conducted in our laboratory, with findings indicating that patients with melancholia display more robust reductions in resting-state HRV, relative to controls, than those patients without melancholic symptoms (Kemp et al. 2014c).

Another potential moderator that needs to be investigated in studies on affective disorders is the impact of ethnic differences. Recent work has demonstrated large ethnicity effects on HRV demonstrating that African Americans have higher HRV than individuals with a white European background (Hill et al. 2015). These findings are consistent with findings from the National Comorbidity Survey Replication indicating that 'Blacks' have a lower lifetime risk of mood and anxiety disorders and that this lower lifetime risk begins in childhood (i.e. prior to the age of 10) (Breslau et al. 2006). Curiously, however, African Americans also have higher mortality rates from coronary heart disease and stroke (Keenan and Shaw 2011), a surprising finding considering that increased HRV is usually associated with reduced, not increased risk for cardiovascular disease, a phenomenon the authors (Hill et al. 2015) labelled as a cardiovascular 'conundrum'. These findings highlight a need for further research to better understand the moderating and mediating mechanisms underpinning not only decreases in HRV in psychiatric disorders, but also in the downstream causal pathways that lead to increased morbidity and mortality.

In regard to the causal pathways from psychiatric illness to morbidity and mortality, researchers still need to determine what might be major mediators of downstream adverse effects (i.e. physical disease and mortality) in otherwise healthy patients with psychiatric illness. Research methodologists argue that 'we better understand some phenomenon when we can answer not only whether X affects Y, but also how X exerts its effect on Y, and when X affects Y and when it does not…' (Hayes 2013). In this regard, 'the how question relates to the underlying psychological, cognitive, or biological process that causally links X to Y, whereas the "when" question pertains to the boundary conditions of the causal association…' (Hayes 2013). Researchers need to move beyond questions like 'is there an effect?' to questions such as 'when do effects appear?' (moderation), 'how do effects arise?' (mediation) and 'how strong are these effects?' (effect size) (Cumming 2012; Hayes 2013). In doing so, researchers will gain better understanding of the causal pathways involved and clarify whether, how and when these effects (HRV reductions) lead to morbidity and mortality. Longitudinal studies also play an important role in finding the right answers to these questions.

Another important question relates to the effects of different types of treatment – particularly non-pharmacological treatments – on HRV and how to ameliorate the adverse effects of antidepressant medications (Licht et al. 2010; Kemp et al. 2014a). Even the most commonly prescribed class of antidepressants, the selective serotonin reuptake inhibitors (SSRIs), appear to have adverse effects on HRV (Licht et al. 2010) (but see Kemp et al. (2011b)). These considerations have important implications for future research on HRV in psychiatry and psychology, raising the question as to whether or not regular physical activity – a health behaviour with powerful beneficial effects on the autonomic nervous system – is able to increase HRV in participants using antidepressant medications. Given that antidepressant drugs alone do not seem to protect patients from cardiovascular disease (CVD) (Whang et al. 2009; Hamer et al. 2011; Kemp et al. 2015a), longitudinal studies are needed to evaluate the impact of exercise in patients receiving long-term antidepressant treatment.

In summary, while researchers have generated a significant body of research on which our understanding of the relationship between HRV and affective disorders has improved, much research examining causal pathways linking HRV, psychiatric disorders and cardiovascular risk remains to be done.

Conclusions

Previous studies investigating the association between affective disorders and HRV have largely been correlational in nature. Therefore, it remains unclear whether psychiatric disorders adversely affect HRV or whether reductions in HRV precede the manifestation of the disorder. It is proposed here that the relationship between mood and HRV is a bidirectional one. Higher baseline levels of HRV are associated with increased positive emotions and social connectedness over a 9-week period (Kok and Fredrickson 2010). Importantly, this study also showed that increases in positive emotions and connectedness predicted increases in HRV, independent of baseline levels. The authors concluded that results supported 'an upward spiral relationship of reciprocal causality' whereby HRV and psychological wellbeing reciprocally and prospectively predict each other. This reciprocal relationship may also apply to the affective disorders such that HRV and intense negative emotions reciprocally and prospectively predict each other in a 'downward' spiral relationship.

The vagus nerve clearly plays an important role in the affective disorders. Through its interconnections with other cranial nerves, it underpins a host of symptoms such as flattened facial affect and lack of prosody (Porges 2011). A poorly functioning cholinergic anti-inflammatory reflex (Tracey 2002) – underpinned by the vagus – contributes to the chronic low-grade inflammation characteristic of depression and other psychiatric disorders (Berk et al. 2013) subsequently contributing to physical ill health over the longer term. As the vagus nerve plays a critical role in the regulation of inflammatory processes (Tracey 2002) and other allostatic systems (Thayer and Sternberg 2006), vagal function – indexed by HRV – is an important factor underpinning individual differences in morbidity and mortality from a host of conditions and disorders.

Acknowledgements This chapter includes a partial republication of an earlier chapter published as Kemp and Quintana (in press). Content is republished here with the kind permission from Taylor & Francis.

References

Alvares GA, Quintana DS, Hickie IB, Guastella AJ (2016) Autonomic nervous system dysfunction in psychiatric disorders and the impact of psychotropic medications: a systematic review and meta-analysis. J Psychiatry Neurosci 41(2):89–104

Berk M, Williams LJ, Jacka FN et al (2013) So depression is an inflammatory disease, but where does the inflammation come from? BMC Med 11:1. doi:10.1186/1741-7015-11-200

Braeken MAKA, Kemp AH, Outhred T et al (2013) Pregnant mothers with resolved anxiety disorders and their offspring have reduced heart rate variability: implications for the health of children. PLoS One 8:e83186. doi:10.1371/journal.pone.0083186

Bravo JA, Forsythe P, Chew MV et al (2011) Ingestion of lactobacillus strain regulates emotional behavior and central GABA receptor expression in a mouse via the vagus nerve. Proc Natl Acad Sci U S A 108:16050–16055. doi:10.1073/pnas.1102999108

Breslau J, Aguilar-Gaxiola S, Kendler KS et al (2006) Specifying race-ethnic differences in risk for psychiatric disorder in a USA national sample. Psychol Med 36:57–68. doi:10.1017/S0033291705006161

Brunoni AR, Lotufo PA, Benseñor IM (2012) Are antidepressants good for the soul but bad for the matter? Using noninvasive brain stimulation to detangle depression/antidepressants effects on heart rate variability and cardiovascular risk. Biol Psychiatry 71:e27–e28. doi:10.1016/j.biopsych.2011.08.026, author reply e29–30

Brunoni AR, Kemp AH, Dantas EM et al (2013) Heart rate variability is a trait marker of major depressive disorder: evidence from the sertraline vs. electric current therapy to treat depression clinical study. Int J Neuropsychopharm 16:1937–1949. doi:10.1017/S1461145713000497

Carnethon MR, Liao D, Evans GW et al (2002) Does the cardiac autonomic response to postural change predict incident coronary heart disease and mortality? The atherosclerosis risk in communities study. Am J Epidemiol 155:48–56

Carnevali L, Sgoifo A, Trombini M et al (2013) Different patterns of respiration in rat lines selectively bred for high or low anxiety. PLoS One 8:e64519. doi:10.1371/journal.pone.0064519

Carney RM, Rich MW, teVelde A et al (1988) The relationship between heart rate, heart rate variability and depression in patients with coronary artery disease. J Psychosom Res 32:159–164. doi:10.1016/0022-3999(88)90050-5

Casas JP, Shah T, Hingorani AD et al (2008) C-reactive protein and coronary heart disease: a critical review. J Intern Med 264:295–314. doi:10.1111/j.1365-2796.2008.02015.x

Chalmers JA, Quintana DS, Abbott MJ-A, Kemp AH (2014) Anxiety disorders are associated with reduced heart rate variability: a meta-analysis. Front Psychiatry 5:80. doi:10.3389/fpsyt.2014.00080

Chang HA, Chang CC, Chen CL et al (2013) Heart rate variability in patients with fully remitted major depressive disorder. Acta Neuropsychiatr. doi:10.1111/j.1601-5215.2012.00658.x

Chang H-A, Chang C-C, Tzeng NS et al (2014) Heart rate variability in unmedicated patients with bipolar disorder in the manic phase. Psychiatry Clin Neurosci 68:674–682. doi:10.1111/pcn.12178

Chang H-A, Chang C-C, Kuo TBJ, Huang S-Y (2015) Distinguishing bipolar II depression from unipolar major depressive disorder: differences in heart rate variability. World J of Biol Psychiatry 1–10. doi:10.3109/15622975.2015.1017606

Chesney E, Goodwin GM, Fazel S (2014) Risks of all-cause and suicide mortality in mental disorders: a meta-review. World Psychiatry 13:153–160. doi:10.1002/wps.20128

Cheyuo C, Jacob A, Wu R et al (2011) The parasympathetic nervous system in the quest for stroke therapeutics. J Cereb Blood Flow Metab 31:1187–1195. doi:10.1038/jcbfm.2011.24

Chida Y, Steptoe A (2008) Positive psychological well-being and mortality: a quantitative review of prospective observational studies. Psychosom Med 70:741–756. doi:10.1097/PSY.0b013e31818105ba

Cotman CW, Berchtold NC, Christie L-A (2007) Exercise builds brain health: key roles of growth factor cascades and inflammation. Trends Neurosci 30:464–472. doi:10.1016/j.tins.2007.06.011

Cumming G (2012) Understanding the new statistics. Routledge, New York

Dekker JM, Crow RS, Folsom AR et al (2000) Low heart rate variability in a 2-minute rhythm strip predicts risk of coronary heart disease and mortality from several causes: the ARIC study. Atherosclerosis risk in communities. Circulation 102:1239–1244

Follesa P, Biggio F, Gorini G et al (2007) Vagus nerve stimulation increases norepinephrine concentration and the gene expression of BDNF and bFGF in the rat brain. Brain Res 1179:28–34. doi:10.1016/j.brainres.2007.08.045

Geisler FCM, Vennewald N, Kubiak T, Weber H (2010) The impact of heart rate variability on subjective well-being is mediated by emotion regulation. Personal Individ Differ 49:723–728. doi:10.1016/j.paid.2010.06.015

Geisler FCM, Kubiak T, Siewert K, Weber H (2013) Cardiac vagal tone is associated with social engagement and self-regulation. Biol Psychol 93:279–286. doi:10.1016/j.biopsycho.2013.02.013

Giese-Davis J, Wilhelm FH, Tamagawa R, et al (2015) Higher vagal activity as related to survival in patients with advanced breast cancer. Psychosom Med 1. doi:10.1097/PSY.0000000000000167

Glassman AH, Roose SP, Bigger JT (1993) The safety of tricyclic antidepressants in cardiac patients. Risk-benefit reconsidered. JAMA 269:2673–2675

Goldberg D, Fawcett J (2012) The importance of anxiety in both major depression and bipolar disorder. Depress Anxiety 29:471–478. doi:10.1002/da.21939

Goldstein DS, Bentho O, Park M-Y, Sharabi Y (2011) Low-frequency power of heart rate variability is not a measure of cardiac sympathetic tone but may be a measure of modulation of cardiac autonomic outflows by baroreflexes. Exp Physiol 96:1255–1261. doi:10.1113/expphysiol.2010.056259

Gomez-Pinilla F (2008a) The influences of diet and exercise on mental health through hormesis. Ageing Res Rev 7:49–62. doi:10.1016/j.arr.2007.04.003

Gomez-Pinilla F (2008b) Brain foods: the effects of nutrients on brain function. Nat Rev Neurosci 9:568–578. doi:10.1038/nrn2421

Gruber J, Johnson SL, Oveis C, Keltner D (2008) Risk for mania and positive emotional responding: too much of a good thing? Emotion 8:23–33. doi:10.1037/1528-3542.8.1.23

Gruber J, Harvey AG, Purcell A (2011) What goes up can come down? A preliminary investigation of emotion reactivity and emotion recovery in bipolar disorder. J Affect Disord 133:457–466. doi:10.1016/j.jad.2011.05.009

Hamer M, David Batty G, Seldenrijk A, Kivimaki M (2011) Antidepressant medication use and future risk of cardiovascular disease: the Scottish Health Survey. Eur Heart J 32:437–442. doi:10.1093/eurheartj/ehq438

Hanson CS, Outhred T, Brunoni AR, et al (2013) The impact of escitalopram on vagally mediated cardiovascular function to stress and the moderating effects of vigorous physical activity: a randomized controlled treatment study in healthy participants. Front Physiol 1–11. doi:10.3389/fphys.2013.00259/abstract

Hayes AF (2013) The Guilford press, pp 1–527

Henry BL, Minassian A, Paulus MP et al (2010) Heart rate variability in bipolar mania and schizophrenia. J Psychiatr Res 44:168–176. doi:10.1016/j.jpsychires.2009.07.011

Hill LK, Hu DD, Koenig J et al (2015) Ethnic differences in resting heart rate variability: a systematic review and meta-analysis. Psychosom Med 77:16–25. doi:10.1097/PSY.0000000000000133

Hillebrand S, Gast KB, de Mutsert R et al (2013) Heart rate variability and first cardiovascular event in populations without known cardiovascular disease: meta-analysis and dose-response meta-regression. Europace 15:742–749. doi:10.1093/europace/eus341

Huikuri HV, Stein PK (2013) Heart rate variability in risk stratification of cardiac patients. Prog Cardiovasc Dis 56:153–159. doi:10.1016/j.pcad.2013.07.003

Huston JM, Tracey KJ (2010) The pulse of inflammation: heart rate variability, the cholinergic anti-inflammatory pathway and implications for therapy. J Intern Med 269:45–53. doi:10.1111/j.1365-2796.2010.02321.x

Jarczok MN, Koenig J, Mauss D et al (2014) Lower heart rate variability predicts increased level of C-reactive protein 4 years later in healthy, nonsmoking adults. J Intern Med 276:667–671. doi:10.1111/joim.12295

Keenan NL, Shaw KM (2011) Coronary heart disease and stroke deaths – United States, 2006

Kemp AH (2011) Depression, antidepressant treatment and the cardiovascular system. Acta Neuropsychiatr 23:82–83. doi:10.1111/j.1601-5215.2011.00535.x

Kemp AH (2012) Reply to: are antidepressants good for the soul but bad for the matter? Using noninvasive brain stimulation to detangle depression/antidepressants effects on heart rate variability and cardiovascular risk. Biol Psychiatry 71:e29–e30. doi:10.1016/j.biopsych.2011.11.002

Kemp AH (2015) Distinguishing bipolar from unipolar disorders on the basis of heart rate variability. World J Biol Psychiatry 1–2. doi:10.3109/15622975.2015.1073857

Kemp AH, Quintana DS. (in press) Heart rate variability in psychiatric disorders, methodological considerations and recommendations for future research. In Jelinek J, Cornforth D, Khandoker AH (Eds). ECG Time Series Variability Analysis: Engineering and Medicine. Boca Raton, CRC Press

Kemp AH, Quintana DS (2013) The relationship between mental and physical health: insights from the study of heart rate variability. Int J Psychophysiol 89:288–296. doi:10.1016/j.ijpsycho.2013.06.018

Kemp AH, Quintana DS, Gray MA et al (2010) Impact of depression and antidepressant treatment on heart rate variability: a review and meta-analysis. Biol Psychiatry 67:1067–1074. doi:10.1016/j.biopsych.2009.12.012

Kemp AH, Quintana DS, Gray MA (2011a) Is heart rate variability reduced in depression without cardiovascular disease? Biol Psychiatry 69:e3–e4. doi:10.1016/j.biopsych.2010.07.030

Kemp AH, Quintana DS, Malhi GS (2011b) Effects of serotonin reuptake inhibitors on heart rate variability: methodological issues, medical comorbidity, and clinical relevance. Biol Psychiatry 69:e25–e26. doi:10.1016/j.biopsych.2010.10.035, author reply e27–8

Kemp AH, Quintana DS, Felmingham KL et al (2012a) Depression, comorbid anxiety disorders, and heart rate variability in physically healthy, unmedicated patients: implications for cardiovascular risk. PLoS One 7:e30777. doi:10.1371/journal.pone.0030777.t002

Kemp AH, Quintana DS, Kuhnert R-L et al (2012b) Oxytocin increases heart rate variability in humans at rest: implications for social approach-related motivation and capacity for social engagement. PLoS One 7:e44014. doi:10.1371/journal.pone.0044014

Kemp AH, Brunoni AR, Santos IS et al (2014a) Effects of depression, anxiety, comorbidity, and antidepressants on resting-state heart rate and its variability: an ELSA-Brasil cohort baseline study. Am J Psychiatry. doi:10.1176/appi.ajp.2014.13121605

Kemp AH, Outhred T, Saunders S et al (2014b) Impact of escitalopram on vagally mediated cardiovascular function in healthy participants: implications for understanding differential age-

related, treatment emergent effects. Psychopharmacology (Berl) 231:2281–2290. doi:10.1007/s00213-013-3374-4
Kemp AH, Quintana DS, Quinn CR et al (2014c) Major depressive disorder with melancholia displays robust alterations in resting state heart rate and its variability: implications for future morbidity and mortality. Front Psychol 5:1387. doi:10.3389/fpsyg.2014.01387
Kemp AH, Brunoni AR, Bittencourt MS et al (2015a) The association between antidepressant medications and coronary heart disease in Brazil: a cross-sectional analysis on the Brazilian longitudinal study of adult health (ELSA-Brazil). Front Public Health 3:9. doi:10.3389/fpubh.2015.00009
Kemp AH, Brunoni AR, Nunes MA et al (2015b) The association between mood and anxiety disorders, and coronary heart disease in Brazil: a cross-sectional analysis on the Brazilian longitudinal study of adult health (ELSA-Brasil). Front Psychol. doi:10.3389/fpsyg.2015.00187
Kiecolt-Glaser JK, McGuire L, Robles TF, Glaser R (2002) Emotions, morbidity, and mortality: new perspectives from psychoneuroimmunology. Annu Rev Psychol 53:83–107. doi:10.1146/annurev.psych.53.100901.135217
Kok BE, Fredrickson BL (2010) Upward spirals of the heart: autonomic flexibility, as indexed by vagal tone, reciprocally and prospectively predicts positive emotions and social connectedness. Biol Psychol 85:432–436. doi:10.1016/j.biopsycho.2010.09.005
Kok BE, Coffey KA, Cohn MA et al (2013) How positive emotions build physical health: perceived positive social connections account for the upward spiral between positive emotions and vagal tone. Psychol Sci: J Am Psychol Soc/APS 24:1123–1132. doi:10.1177/0956797612470827
Lee J-S, Kim B, Hong Y, Joo YH (2012) Heart rate variability in the subsyndromal depressive phase of bipolar disorder. Psychiatry Clin Neurosci 66:361–366. doi:10.1111/j.1440-1819.2012.02335.x
Licht CMM, de Geus EJC, Zitman FG, Hoogendijk WJG, van Dyck R, Penninx BWJH (2008) Association between major depressive disorder and heart rate variability in the Netherlands Study of Depression and Anxiety (NESDA). Arch Gen Psychiatry 65(12):1358–1367, http://doi.org/10.1001/archpsyc.65.12.1358
Licht CMM, de Geus EJC, van Dyck R, Penninx BWJH (2009) Association between anxiety disorders and heart rate variability in The Netherlands Study of Depression and Anxiety (NESDA). Psychosom Med 71:508–518. doi:10.1097/PSY.0b013e3181a292a6
Licht CMM, de Geus EJC, van Dyck R, Penninx BWJH (2010) Longitudinal evidence for unfavorable effects of antidepressants on heart rate variability. Biol Psychiatry 68:861–868. doi:10.1016/j.biopsych.2010.06.032
Licht CMM, Penninx BW, de Geus EJC (2011a) To include or not to include? A response to the meta-analysis of heart rate variability and depression. Biol Psychiatry 69:e1. doi:10.1016/j.biopsych.2010.06.034, author reply e3–4
Licht CMM, Penninx BWJH, Geus EJC de (2011b) Reply to: effects of serotonin reuptake inhibitors on heart rate variability: methodological issues, medical comorbidity, and clinical relevance. BPS 1–2. doi:10.1016/j.biopsych.2010.12.039
Malhi GS, Bargh DM, Cashman E et al (2012) The clinical management of bipolar disorder complexity using a stratified model. Bipolar Disord 14(Suppl 2):66–89. doi:10.1111/j.1399-5618.2012.00993.x
McCaffrey D, Griffin BA, Almirall D et al (2013) A tutorial on propensity score estimation for multiple treatments using generalized boosted models. Stat Med 32:3388–3414. doi:10.1002/sim.5753
McEwen BS (1998) Stress, adaptation, and disease: allostasis and allostatic load. Ann N Y Acad Sci 840:33–44. doi:10.1111/j.1749-6632.1998.tb09546.x
Moon E, Lee S-H, Kim D-H, Hwang B (2013) Comparative study of heart rate variability in patients with schizophrenia, bipolar disorder, post-traumatic stress disorder, or major depressive disorder. Clin Psychopharmacol Neurosci 11:137–143. doi:10.9758/cpn.2013.11.3.137
Nemeroff C, Goldschmidt-Clermont PJ (2012) Heartache and heartbreak – the link between depression and cardiovascular disease. Nat Rev Cardiol 9:526–539. doi:10.1038/nrcardio.2012.91

O'Regan C, Kenny RA, Cronin H, et al (2014) Antidepressants strongly influence the relationship between depression and heart rate variability: findings from The Irish Longitudinal Study on Ageing (TILDA). Psychol Med 1–14. doi:10.1017/S0033291714001767

Outhred T, Kemp AH, Malhi G (2014) Physiological correlates of bipolar spectrum disorders and their treatment. Curr Top Behav Neurosci 1–56. doi:10.1007/7854_2014_297

Pavlov VA, Tracey KJ (2012) The vagus nerve and the inflammatory reflex—linking immunity and metabolism: abstract. Nat Rev Endocrinol

Penttilä J, Helminen A, Jartti T et al (2001) Time domain, geometrical and frequency domain analysis of cardiac vagal outflow: effects of various respiratory patterns. Clin Physiol 21:365–376. doi:10.1046/j.1365-2281.2001.00337.x

Pocai A, Obici S, Schwartz GJ, Rossetti L (2005) A brain-liver circuit regulates glucose homeostasis. Cell Metab 1:53–61. doi:10.1016/j.cmet.2004.11.001

Porges SW (2011) The polyvagal theory: neurophysiological foundations of emotions, attachment, communication, and self-regulation, 1st edn. W. W. Norton & Company, New York

Post RM (1992) Transduction of psychosocial stress into the neurobiology of recurrent affective disorder. Am J Psychiatry 149:999–1010

Quintana DS, Guastella AJ, Outhred T et al (2012) Heart rate variability is associated with emotion recognition: direct evidence for a relationship between the autonomic nervous system and social cognition. Int J Psychophysiol 86:168–172. doi:10.1016/j.ijpsycho.2012.08.012

Reyes Del Paso GA, Langewitz W, Mulder LJM et al (2013) The utility of low frequency heart rate variability as an index of sympathetic cardiac tone: a review with emphasis on a reanalysis of previous studies. Psychophysiology 50:477–487. doi:10.1111/psyp.12027

Riordan WP, Norris PR, Jenkins JM, Morris JA (2009) Early loss of heart rate complexity predicts mortality regardless of mechanism, anatomic location, or severity of injury in 2178 trauma patients. J Surg Res 156:283–289. doi:10.1016/j.jss.2009.03.086

Saboul D, Pialoux V, Hautier C (2013) The impact of breathing on HRV measurements: implications for the longitudinal follow-up of athletes. Eur J Sport Sci 13:534–542. doi:10.1080/17461391.2013.767947

Schwerdtfeger A, Friedrich-Mai P (2009) Social interaction moderates the relationship between depressive mood and heart rate variability: evidence from an ambulatory monitoring study. Health Psychol 28:501–509. doi:10.1037/a0014664

Smith TW, Cribbet MR, Nealey-Moore JB et al (2011) Matters of the variable heart: respiratory sinus arrhythmia response to marital interaction and associations with marital quality. J Pers Soc Psychol 100:103–119. doi:10.1037/a0021136

Steptoe A, Deaton A, Stone AA (2015) Subjective wellbeing, health, and ageing. Lancet 385:640–648. doi:10.1016/S0140-6736(13)61489-0

Task Force of the European Society of Cardiology the North American Society of Pacing Electrophysiology (1996) Heart rate variability: standards of measurement, physiological interpretation, and clinical use. Circulation 93(5):1043–1065

Thayer J, Lane RD (2000) A model of neurovisceral integration in emotion regulation and dysregulation. J Affect Disord 61:201–216

Thayer J, Sternberg E (2006) Beyond heart rate variability: vagal regulation of allostatic systems. Ann N Y Acad Sci 1088:361–372. doi:10.1196/annals.1366.014

Thayer J, Sternberg EM (2010) Neural aspects of immunomodulation: focus on the vagus nerve. Brain Behav Immun 24:1223–1228. doi:10.1016/j.bbi.2010.07.247

Thayer J, Friedman BH, Borkovec TD (1996) Autonomic characteristics of generalized anxiety disorder and worry. Biol Psychiatry 39:255–266. doi:10.1016/0006-3223(95)00136-0

Thayer J, Hansen AL, Saus-Rose E, Johnsen BH (2009) Heart rate variability, prefrontal neural function, and cognitive performance: the neurovisceral integration perspective on self-regulation, adaptation, and health. Ann Behav Med 37:141–153. doi:10.1007/s12160-009-9101-z

Thayer J, Yamamoto SS, Brosschot JF (2010) The relationship of autonomic imbalance, heart rate variability and cardiovascular disease risk factors. Int J Cardiol 141:122–131. doi:10.1016/j.ijcard.2009.09.543

Tracey KJ (2002) The inflammatory reflex. Nature 420:853–859. doi:10.1038/nature01321
Tracey KJ (2007) Physiology and immunology of the cholinergic antiinflammatory pathway. J Clin Invest 117:289–296. doi:10.1172/JCI30555
Tracey KJ, Pavlov VA (2012) The vagus nerve and the inflammatory reflex – linking immunity and metabolism. Nat Rev Endocrinol 8:743–754. doi:10.1038/nrendo.2012.189
Verkuil B, Brosschot J, Gebhardt W, Thayer J (2010) When worries make you sick: a review of perseverative cognition, the default stress response and somatic health. JEP 1:87–118. doi:10.5127/jep.009110
Voss A, Heitmann A, Schroeder R, Peters A, Perz S (2012) Short-Term Heart Rate Variability—Age Dependence in Healthy Subjects. Physiological Measurement 33(8):1289–1311. doi:10.1088/0967-3334/33/8/1289
Voss A, Schroeder R, Heitmann A, Peters A, Perz S (2015) Short-Term Heart Rate Variability—Influence of Gender and Age in Healthy Subjects. Edited by Adrian V Hernandez. PLoS ONE 10(3):e0118308. doi:10.1371/journal.pone.0118308
Wang H, Yu M, Ochani M et al (2003) Nicotinic acetylcholine receptor alpha7 subunit is an essential regulator of inflammation. Nature 421:384–388. doi:10.1038/nature01339
Wang P, Caspi L, Lam C, et al (2008) Upper intestinal lipids trigger a gut–brain–liver axis to regulate glucose production
Whang W, Kubzansky LD, Kawachi I et al (2009) Depression and risk of sudden cardiac death and coronary heart disease in women. J Am Coll Cardiol 53:950–958. doi:10.1016/j.jacc.2008.10.060
Wilhelm FH, Trabert W, Roth WT (2001) Physiologic instability in panic disorder and generalized anxiety disorder. Biol Psychiatry 49:596–605. doi:10.1016/S0006-3223(00)01000-3

Arterial Stiffness in the Depression and Cardiovascular Comorbidity

12

Evelyn Smith and Joel Singer

Contents

Abstract

Arterial stiffness is a process of vascular ageing, and it is a consequence of arteriosclerosis. In this chapter we describe how arterial stiffness is measured, and we evaluate the evidence on how arterial stiffness independently exacerbates both cardiovascular disease and depression and in turn how depression predicts arterial stiffness. The association between arterial stiffness and cardiovascular disease is well established, and so is the association between arterial stiffness and depression. Arterial stiffness may be one of several vascular processes that mediate the hypothesised bidirectional relationship between depression and cardiovascular disease. The importance of assessing arterial stiffness as a measure of cardiovascular disease, especially if it is comorbid with depression, is discussed.

E. Smith (✉)
Clinical and Health Psychology Research Initiative, School of Social Sciences and Psychology, Western Sydney University, Bankstown, NSW, Australia
e-mail: evelyn.smith@unsw.edu.au

J. Singer
School of Psychiatry, University of New South Wales, Sydney, NSW 2052, Australia

B.T. Baune, P.J. Tully (eds.), *Cardiovascular Diseases and Depression*,
DOI 10.1007/978-3-319-32480-7_12

Arterial stiffness is a process of vascular ageing, caused by structural and cellular change within vessel walls (Nichols et al. 2011). With age, haemodynamic factors such as repetitive cyclic stress and extrinsic factors such as hormone, salt and glucose levels combine to damage the tunica media of blood vessels, causing the fragmentation of elastin and a decline in the elastin/collagen ratio (Nichols et al. 2011). This lessens the elasticity of large arteries and decreases their ability to stretch during systole to absorb the pulsatile energy from each heartbeat. In turn, increased systolic pressure and higher flow pulsations are transmitted down the vascular tree into the microvasculature of end organs (Zieman et al. 2005; O'Rourke and Hashimoto 2007).

12.1 How to Measure Arterial Stiffness?

While there are many methods by which to measure arterial stiffness, carotid-femoral pulse wave velocity (CF-PWV) is seen to be the most clinically relevant. This is due to its quantification of pulse waves in the aortic and aorto-iliac pathways which are responsible for the majority of the pathophysiological effects of arterial stiffness (Laurent et al. 2006). CF-PWV is measured by placing subjects in a supine position with three ECG monitoring electrodes placed on their chest to allow ECG synchronisation. A high-fidelity tonometer is then placed sequentially over the right carotid and femoral pulses and gently pressed down until a steady waveform is achieved. Using ECG synchronisation and the formula $C\text{-}F\text{-PWV} = \Delta D/\Delta t$, CF-PWV in m/s is calculated. Distance between recording sites (ΔD) is measured via the surface distance, and time (Δt) is measured between the feet of the two waveforms.

Some limitations associated with PWV measurement have been noted. The femoral pressure waveform may be difficult to record accurately in patients with metabolic syndrome, obesity, diabetes and peripheral artery disease. Further, in the presence of aortic, iliac or proximal femoral stenosis, the pressure wave may be attenuated and delayed (Van Bortel al. 2002).

Another accepted measure of arterial stiffening is central augmentation index, which is the ratio of augmentation pressure to pulse pressure. However central augmentation index has been criticised as an ineffective measure of arterial stiffness among older adults (Fantin et al. 2007).

12.2 Arterial Stiffness and Cardiovascular Disease

The association between arterial stiffness and cardiovascular disease is well established, with arterial stiffness shown to be an independent predictor of coronary disease and stroke (Mattace-Raso et al. 2006) and predictive of cardiovascular and total mortality (Lacolley et al. 2008). Additionally, adding PWV to the standard array of cardiovascular risk factors measured by clinicians improves the prediction of cardiovascular disease (Mitchell et al. 2010). A meta-analysis of 17 longitudinal studies that evaluated PWV and followed over 15,000 individuals for an average of 7.7 years found that the predicted risk of total and cardiovascular mortality was twice as high among individuals with high PWV compared to those with low PWV (Vlachopoulos et al. 2010). The predictive power of PWV was even greater for individuals with high cardiovascular risk factors at baseline (Vlachopoulos et al. 2010). The prognostic importance of CF-PWV in cardiovascular disease is probably attributed to the adverse haemodynamic effects of aortic stiffening with increased systolic load and decreased myocardial perfusion pressure (Cecelja and Chowienczyk 2012), in combination with higher levels of inflammation in arterial stiffness (Pasceri et al. 2000; Willerson and Ridker 2004).

12.3 Arterial Stiffness and Depression

Depression has repeatedly been found to be associated with arterial stiffness when measured by PWV (Tiemeier et al. 2003; Seldenrijk et al. 2011; Poongothai et al. 2015). Persistent depression has also been linked to significantly greater increases in PWV velocity over a 3-year period, compared to nondepressed individuals (Satoh et al. 2015). Increased arterial stiffness as measured by higher PWV has been found to be associated with more severe depressive symptoms (Dietz and Matthews 2011) and a greater likelihood of diagnosed depression, even after controlling for atherosclerosis (Tiemeier 2003).

Decreased arterial stiffness has also been found to be associated with timely and effective antidepressant treatment among highly depressed women (Oulis et al. 2010). Women presenting with a current severe major depressive episode experienced higher PWV compared to healthy controls before antidepressant treatment. However, this difference decreased over the course of treatment, and arterial stiffness became comparable across groups at treatment completion. Moreover, full responders exhibited significantly greater vascular improvement than partial responders, and the magnitude of their arterial stiffness amelioration was strongly associated with the magnitude of their clinical improvement (Oulis et al. 2010). The interaction between antidepressant drug therapy and arterial stiffness is less clear among older adults. In a sample of adults aged 70 years or older with newly diagnosed depression, duloxetine but not escitalopram significantly increased PWV after 12 months of treatment. The drug-specific effect remained after controlling for cardiovascular risk factors (Scuteri et al. 2013).

Arterial stiffness may also be more strongly associated with particular subtypes of depression. One study found arterial stiffness to be associated with prolonged depression, but not episodic depression (Satoh et al. 2015). Further research utilising standardised operational definitions and measurements of depression is needed to elucidate this point. Past studies examining depression and arterial stiffness have defined depression in a multitude of ways, with some utilising categorical DSM definitions of depressive disorders such as dysthymia and major depressive disorder, and others looking rather at depressive symptoms on a linear scale as defined by various depression measures.

Arterial stiffness has also been shown to be associated with other psychopathologies that share clinical features with depression. Depressive and anxiety disorders are highly overlapping, heterogeneous conditions that both have been associated with an increased risk of cardiovascular disease. Investigations of the relationship between arterial stiffness and both depression and anxiety have found mixed results. In one study, both depressed and anxious subjects experienced increased arterial stiffness as measured by central augmentation index. Subjects with lifetime comorbidity or higher severity or duration of depressive or anxiety symptoms showed an increased augmentation index, a manifestation of early wave reflection because of arterial stiffness (Seldenrijk et al. 2011). In contrast, another study investigating the relationship between arterial stiffness and depression and anxiety sensitivity found that increased arterial stiffness was associated with greater fearfulness and anxiety sensitivity only. No relationship between depression sensitivity and arterial stiffness was found (Seldenrijk et al. 2013). However, this study measured arterial stiffness by the heart rate-normalised central augmentation index and carotid M-mode ultrasound, both less than recommended measures.

Depressive symptoms are also common among individuals diagnosed with bipolar disorder. Among a sample of bipolar adults, participants over the age of 32 had greater arterial stiffness than would be expected based on age-based population norms. Younger individuals with bipolar did not differ significantly from the norm based on arterial stiffness (Sohdi et al. 2012).

Further, several other studies have found arterial stiffness to be associated with other psychosocial factors associated with depression. For example, increased arterial stiffness was associated with experiences of childhood trauma, recently experienced stressful events, general negative life events and job stress (Bomhof-Roordink et al. 2015). Arterial stiffness was also associated with anxious attachment in adolescents (Midei and Matthews 2009).

It may indeed be that arterial stiffness is not associated with depression itself but rather other psychosocial stressors or traits that are themselves often highly correlated with depression. Hence, more research is necessary to determine if arterial stiffness is only associated with certain subtypes or features of depression before clarity regarding the mechanisms underlying the association between depression and arterial stiffness can be obtained.

In any case, the mechanism underlying the association between arterial stiffness and depression remains speculative (Tiemeier 2003; Paranthaman et al. 2010; Dietz and Matthews 2011; Seldenrijk et al. 2011; Satoh et al. 2015). It is possible that arterial stiffness impacts on depression via changes in brain structure. In fact, the effect of arterial stiffness on the brain is well established. Structurally, arterial stiffness has been associated with white matter hyperintensities, cerebral lacunar infarction and cortical brain atrophy (Bateman et al. 2008; Henry-Feugeas et al. 2009; Nichols et al. 2011). It is hypothesised that increased flow pulsations through the carotid and vertebral arteries extend deep into the microvasculature of the brain leading to vascular rupture and subsequent micro-haemorrhages, endothelial denudation and thrombotic obstruction (O'Rourke 2007; Henskens et al. 2008). Damage to cerebral microvessels is then followed by oedema, haemorrhage and finally inflammation as part of the reparative process, all of which lead to structural change (Henry-Feugeas 2009; Nichols et al. 2011). Functionally speaking, arterial stiffness has also been repeatedly shown to be associated with decreased levels of cognitive function and dementia (Singer et al. 2014).

12.4 How Depression May Predict Arterial Stiffness

While the exact mechanism underlying the relationship between depression and arterial stiffness remains unclear, associations have been found between depression and several physiological processes that have the potential to increase arterial stiffness such as inflammation and cortisol secretion. In particular, depression has been shown to increase inflammatory markers such as C-reactive protein. Inflammation may lead to endothelial dysfunction by limiting the bioavailability of nitric oxide through the inhibition of nitric oxide synthase (Venugopal et al. 2002; Brydon et al. 2009; Hansel et al. 2010; Satoh et al. 2015). This in turn leads to increased vascular tone and arterial stiffening.

Depression may also lead to arterial stiffness via its effect on neuroendocrine function. Depression has been shown to be associated with hypothalamic-pituitary-adrenal axis hyperactivity, characterised by increased secretion of cortisol from the adrenal gland (Midei and Matthews 2009; Baune et al. 2012). Cortisol causes increased sympathetic activity, which increases resting systolic blood pressure and heart rate, both of which are known risk factors for arterial stiffness (Lehmann et al. 1993; Sutton-Tyrrell et al. 2005). Cortisol is also known to cause abdominal fat accumulation, resulting in visceral obesity which itself has been shown to be a predictor of both arterial stiffness and cardiovascular disease (Midei and Matthews 2009; Gottsater et al. 2015). Depression can also be associated with poor diet and lack of physical activity, both of which can lead to abdominal obesity, hyperglycaemia, dyslipidaemia and chronic inflammation, which are all predictors of arterial stiffness (Gottsater et al. 2015; Park and Lakatta 2012).

The neuroimaging findings of neurological small vessel disease associated with arterial stiffness have also been shown to be associated with unipolar depression in the elderly (Herrmann et al. 2008; Fujishima et al. 2014; van Uden et al. 2015) and bipolar depression in paediatric subjects (Serafini et al. 2014).

12.5 Arterial Stiffness, Cardiovascular Disease and Depression

Arterial stiffness is one of several vascular processes that have been proposed to mediate the hypothesised bidirectional relationship between depression and cardiovascular disease (Baune et al. 2012). The relationships between arterial stiffness, cardiovascular disease and depression seem to be interactive. In other words, it seems that they exacerbate each other. Again it is speculated that arterial stiffness may be one of the mediators of depression leading to cardiovascular disease, with prolonged depression being shown to significantly accelerate arterial stiffening (Satoh et al. 2015). From a clinical standpoint, treatment modalities that reduce arterial stiffness may have a role in either prevention or treatment of depression and cardiovascular disease. Proposed pharmacological approaches to reducing arterial stiffness include traditional antihypertensives such as beta-blockers and calcium channel blockers, as well as novel agents designed to target advanced glycation end products and prevent them from binding with arterial collagen and causing stiffening (McEniery 2006). However, before the efficacy of any of these modalities can be investigated, further research is required in order to gain a greater clarity regarding the role of arterial stiffness in mediating the bidirectional relationship between cardiovascular disease and depression.

Conclusion

As described in a previous chapter, depression can exacerbate cardiovascular disease, and cardiovascular disease can exacerbate depression. Arterial stiffness is associated with both depression and cardiovascular disease and may mediate the bidirectional relationship of these constructs. Higher arterial stiffness exacerbates cardiovascular diseases. We speculate that arterial stiffness also impacts on the brain and exacerbates depression, and depression may lead to arterial stiffness via its effect on neuroendocrine function. Reducing arterial stiffness could impact both depression and cardiovascular disease, and treatment strategies could focus on this in the future.

References

Bateman GA, Levi CR et al (2008) The venous manifestations of pulse wave encephalopathy: windkessel dysfunction in normal aging and senile dementia. Neuroradiology 50(6):491–497

Baune BT, Stuart M et al (2012) The relationship between subtypes of depression and cardiovascular disease: a systematic review of biological models. Transl Psychiatry 2:e92

Bomhof-Roordink H, Seldenrijk A et al (2015) Associations between life stress and subclinical cardiovascular disease are partly mediated by depressive and anxiety symptoms. J Psychosom Res 78(4):332–339

Brydon L, Walker C et al (2009) Synergistic effects of psychological and immune stressors on inflammatory cytokine and sickness responses in humans. Brain Behav Immun 23(2):217–224

Cecelja M, Chowienczyk P (2012) Role of arterial stiffness in cardiovascular disease. JRSM Cardiovasc Dis 1(4)

Dietz LJ, Matthews KA (2011) Depressive symptoms and subclinical markers of cardiovascular disease in adolescents. J Adolesc Health: Off Publ Soc Adolesc Med 48(6):579–584

Fantin F, Mattocks A et al (2007) Is augmentation index a good measure of vascular stiffness in the elderly? Age and Ageing 36(1):43–48

Fujishima M, Maikusa N et al (2014) Mild cognitive impairment, poor episodic memory, and late-life depression are associated with cerebral cortical thinning and increased white matter hyperintensities. Front Aging Neurosci 6:306

Gottsater M, Ostling G et al (2015) Non-hemodynamic predictors of arterial stiffness after 17 years of follow-up: the Malmo diet and cancer study. J Hypertens 33(5):957–965

Hansel A, Hong S et al (2010) Inflammation as a psychophysiological biomarker in chronic psychosocial stress. Neurosci Biobehav Rev 35(1):115–121
Henry-Feugeas MC (2009) Intracranial MR dynamics in clinically diagnosed Alzheimer's disease: the emerging concept of "pulse wave encephalopathy". Curr Alzheimer Res 6(6):488–502
Henry-Feugeas MC, Roy C et al (2009) Leukoaraiosis and pulse-wave encephalopathy: observations with phase-contrast MRI in mild cognitive impairment. J Neuroradiol 36(4):212–218
Henskens LHG, Kroon AA et al (2008) Increased aortic pulse wave velocity is associated with silent cerebral small-vessel disease in hypertensive patients. Hypertension 52(6):1120–1126
Herrmann LL, Le Masurier M et al (2008) White matter hyperintensities in late life depression: a systematic review. J Neurol Neurosurg Psychiatry 79(6):619–624
Lacolley P, Challande P et al (2008) Genetics and pathophysiology of arterial stiffness. Cardiovasc Res 81(4):637–648
Lehmann ED, Hopkins KD et al (1993) Aortic compliance measurements using Doppler ultrasound: in vivo biochemical correlates. Ultrasound Med Biol 19(9):683–710
Laurent S, Cockcroft J et al (2006) Expert consensus document on arterial stiffness: methodological issues and clinical applications. Eur Heart J 27, 2588–2605
Mattace-Raso FU, van der Cammen TJ et al (2006) Arterial stiffness and risk of coronary heart disease and stroke: the Rotterdam Study. Circulation 7;113(5):657–663
McEniery C (2006) Novel therapeutic strategies for reducing arterial stiffness. Br J Pharmacol 148(7):881–883
Midei AJ, Matthews KA (2009) Social relationships and negative emotional traits are associated with central adiposity and arterial stiffness in healthy adolescents. Health Psychol: Off J Div Health Psychol Am Psychol Assoc 28(3):347–353
Mitchell GF, Hwang SJ et al (2010) Arterial stiffness and cardiovascular events: the Framingham Heart Study. Circulation 121(4):505–511
Nichols W, O'Rourke M et al (2011) McDonald's blood flow in arteries. Arnold, London
O'Rourke MF, Hashimoto J (2007) Mechanical factors in arterial aging. J Am Coll Cardiol 50(1):1–13
O'Rourke MF (2007) Arterial aging: pathophysiological principles. Vasc Med 12(4):329–341
Oulis P, Kouzoupis A et al (2010) Reversal of increased arterial stiffness in severely depressed women after 6-week antidepressant treatment. J Affect Disord, 122(1-2):164–166
Paranthaman R, Greenstein AS et al (2010) Vascular function in older adults with depressive disorder. Biol Psychiatry 68(2):133–139
Park S, Lakatta EG (2012) Role of inflammation in the pathogenesis of arterial stiffness. Yonsei Med J 53(2):258–261
Pasceri V, Willerson JT, Yeh ET (2000) Direct proinflammatory effect of C-reactive protein on human endothelial cells. Circulation 102(18):2165–8
Poongothai S, Pradeepa R et al (2015) Association of depression with common carotid artery intima media thickness and augmentation index in a large Urban South Indian population- The Chennai Urban Rural Epidemiology Study. Indian Journ End Met 19(1):136–142
Satoh H, Fujii S et al (2015) Persistent depression is a significant risk factor for the development of arteriosclerosis in middle-aged Japanese male subjects. Hypertens Res: Off J Jpn Soc Hypertens 38(1):84–88
Seldenrijk A, van Hout HP et al (2011) Depression, anxiety, and arterial stiffness. Biol Psychiatry 69(8):795–803
Seldenrijk A, van Hout HP et al (2013) Sensitivity to depression or anxiety and subclinical cardiovascular disease. J Affect Disord 146(1):126–131
Serafini G, Pompili M et al (2014) Brain changes in early-onset bipolar and unipolar depressive disorders: a systematic review in children and adolescents. Eur Child Adolesc Psychiatry 23(11):1023–1041
Scuteri A, Modestino A et al (2013) Depression treatment selectively modifies arterial stiffness in older participants. J Gerontol A Biol Sci Med Sci 68(6):719–725

Singer J, Trollor JN et al (2014) Arterial stiffness, the brain and cognition: a systematic review. Ageing Res Rev 15:16–27

Sohdi SK, Linder J et al (2012) Evidence for accelerated vascular aging in bipolar disorder. J Psychosom Res 73(3):175–179

Sutton-Tyrrell K, Najjar SS et al (2005) Elevated aortic pulse wave velocity, a marker of arterial stiffness, predicts cardiovascular events in well-functioning older adults. Circulation 111(25):3384–3390

Tiemeier H, Bretler M, van Popele N, Hofman A, Witeman J (2003) Late-life depression is associated with arterial stiffness: a population-based study. J Am Geriatr Soc 51:1105–1110

Van Bortel LM, Duprez D et al (2002) Clinical applications of arterial stiffness, Task Force III: recommendations for user procedures. Am J Hypertens (5):445–452

van Uden IW, Tuladhar AM et al (2015) White matter integrity and depressive symptoms in cerebral small vessel disease: the RUN DMC study. Am J Geriatr Psychiatry 23(5):525–535

Venugopal SK, Devaraj S et al (2002) Demonstration that C-reactive protein decreases eNOS expression and bioactivity in human aortic endothelial cells. Circulation 106(12):1439–1441

Vlachopoulos C, Aznaouridis K, Stefanadis C (2010) Prediction of cardiovascular events and all-cause mortality with arterial stiffness: a systematic review and meta-analysis. J Am Coll Cardiol 55:1318–1327

Willerson JT, Ridker PM (2004) Inflammation as a cardiovascular risk factor. Circulation 109(21 Suppl 1):II2–10

Zieman SJ, Melenovsky V et al (2005) Mechanisms, pathophysiology, and therapy of arterial stiffness. Arterioscler Thromb Vasc Biol 25(5):932–943

Depression and Markers of Arteriosclerosis: Cross-Sectional Analyses of the Baseline Examination of the BiDirect Cohort Study

13

Maren Nagel and Hans-Werner Hense

Contents

Abstract

The prospective BiDirect study was set up to uncover the potential bidirectional links between depression and arteriosclerosis, with a focus on markers of early and subclinical arteriosclerosis.

The BiDirect cohort is composed of three different samples: a subsample of patients with clinically manifest depression, a cohort of patients after an acute cardiovascular event, and a reference group that was drawn from the general population. All study participants underwent interviews, anthropometric measurements, and measurements of blood pressure, ankle-brachial index (ABI), pulse wave velocity (PWV), augmentation index, body impedance, and carotid intima-media thickness (IMT). Composite, unweighted scores were created as

M. Nagel, MD • H.-W. Hense, MD (✉)
Institute of Epidemiology and Social Medicine, Medical Faculty, Westfälische Wilhelms University, Albert-Schweitzer-Campus 1 D3, 48149 Münster, Germany
e-mail: hense@uni-muenster.de; http://campus.uni-muenster.de/epi_start.html

B.T. Baune, P.J. Tully (eds.), *Cardiovascular Diseases and Depression*,
DOI 10.1007/978-3-319-32480-7_13

summary measures to assess the burden of subclinical arteriosclerosis in the different subsamples. The BiDirect baseline examination lasted from May 2010 to June 2013. Cross-sectional analyses of the baseline examination revealed significantly increased measures for body and fat mass, but lower levels of blood pressure in the depressive cohort. Single indicators of subclinical arteriosclerosis (ankle-brachial index (ABI), pulse wave velocity (PWV), intima-media thickness (IMT), and carotid plaque) as well as an unweighted composite score of these markers showed no differences between the depression and the reference cohort at baseline. However, when the presence of adverse lifestyle factors, such as smoking and overweight, was additionally taken into consideration, the depressive cohort showed a raised propensity to arteriosclerosis, especially among those younger than 50 years. Expectedly, the cohort with clinically manifest cardiovascular disease showed consistently the highest values and scores of arteriosclerosis.

13.1 Background of the BiDirect Study

Cardiovascular diseases as well as depression are among the most frequent and most impairing diseases worldwide. Both are common causes for the frequent contacts with ambulatory and hospital services and for long-term utilization of health care (Mathers and Loncar 2006). The scope of cardiovascular disease encompasses a variety of arteriosclerotic diseases of the heart and the entire vascular system that occur as the sequel of pathophysiologic changes in the arterial vessel walls. The arteriosclerotic alterations develop over a lifetime and are accelerated by certain lifestyles and in the presence of concomitant risk factors. The frequently observed concurrent increase of inflammatory markers in the blood seems to suggest that chronic inflammatory processes are centrally involved in these processes (Libby 2012; Libby et al. 2011). Considering the frequency of cardiovascular diseases in the population, ischemic heart disease and cerebrovascular disease are among the leading causes of death in the world (Mathers and Loncar 2006). In Germany, chronic ischemic heart disease and acute myocardial infarction were the two most common causes of death in 2012 (Deutscher 2013).

Clinically manifest depression is characterized by symptoms, such as feelings of sadness or emptiness, reduced interest in formerly enjoyed activities, sleep disturbances, loss of energy, weight changes, difficulties concentrating or making decisions, and in suicidal thoughts or intentions (Diagnostic and statistical manual of mental disorders 2000). Therefore, depression has severe consequences for a patient, because it is a highly impairing disease, frequently causing repeated periods of health professionals' support, assistance in everyday life, and possibly also limitations in pursuing a professional career. Psychiatric conditions, predominantly unipolar depression, are the most important causes of disability in high-income countries as well as in middle- and low-income countries (Mathers and Loncar 2006). The prevalence of current depressive symptoms in German adults aged 18–79 years is as high as 8.1 %, and the lifetime prevalence of a diagnosed depression is as high as 11.6 %; it is also known that women have a considerably higher lifetime prevalence than men (Busch et al. 2013).

The relationship between depression and arteriosclerosis has been investigated in the past. Most of the studies supported the hypothesis that the two diseases are related, but various aspects and mechanisms of the association still remain unexplained (Nicholson et al. 2006). Etiological studies examined whether people who suffer from depression had a higher risk of developing cardiovascular disease. Reviews and meta-analyses supported the hypothesis that depression or depressive symptoms increased the risk of coronary heart disease (Nicholson et al. 2006; Rugulies 2002; Wulsin and Singal 2003; Wulsin et al. 2005; Van den Oord et al. 2013; Van der Kooy et al. 2007). If survived, myocardial infarction and stroke often result in severe changes in the personal life of a patient, mostly due to a lack of autonomy in everyday life or the inability to pursue a former profession, which in turn leads to a need for social support, both in personal as well as in financial terms. Prognostic studies confirmed that patients after a myocardial infarction had a higher prevalence of depression than the general population. Most of these studies also examined if patients had a different clinical outcome depending on whether they developed a post-myocardial depression or not. Meta-analyses addressing this question found an increased risk of cardiac or all-cause mortality for patients who developed depression after the coronary event (Nicholson et al. 2006; Meijer et al. 2011; Barth et al. 2004). Thus, the association between the two diseases seems to work in both directions.

The proposed mechanisms of the association include biological, psychophysiological, and behavioral explanations (Barth et al. 2004; De Jonge et al. 2010; Gehi et al. 2010; Grippo and Johnson 2009). Among the behavioral explanations, physical inactivity and fatigue with resulting elevated classical cardiac risk factors as well as an elevated percentage of smokers among patients with depression have been emphasized (Rugulies 2002). Given the spectrum of symptoms in patients with depression, differential effects of these proposed mechanisms in patients with different subtypes of depression are likely. In addition, whether the proposed factors act directly, indirectly (i.e., by increasing classical risk factors), or by using a common pathway remains to be further explained and investigated (Barth et al. 2004).

The BiDirect study was designed to uncover links between depression and arteriosclerosis in a longitudinal and bidirectional manner. Three different cohorts were sampled from well-defined populations involving one cohort of patients with clinically diagnosed depression, one cohort of patients with clinically manifest coronary heart disease, and a reference sample from the general population. We compared, in a cross-sectional perspective, the baseline characteristics in the three cohorts with a specific focus on indicators of subclinical arteriosclerosis that represent early vascular alterations that have not yet resulted in a clinical manifestation.

13.2 Methods

13.2.1 The Sample of the BiDirect Study

The BiDirect study is a prospective cohort study. In total, the data of 2.181 individuals, aged 35–65 years, who participated in the baseline examinations between May 2010 and June 2013, were included for the present report. The sample of patients with depression was recruited in six psychiatric and psychosomatic hospitals and departments in the city of Münster and its vicinity and in two psychiatric practices in Münster; however, outpatients were included only if they had been hospitalized due to depression within the 12 months prior to inclusion in the study. Eligibility criteria were current hospital admittance or ambulatory treatment due to acute depression and ability to understand German language. Excluded were patients admitted under the regulation of compulsory admission using the Mental Health Act. Patients with dementia, drug and/or alcohol addiction, and eating disorders were also excluded. The subsample of patients with coronary heart disease was recruited in four cardiology and rehabilitation departments and institutions of Münster and in regional centers. Eligibility criteria were acute myocardial infarction, acute coronary syndrome, or treatment of cardiac disease due to myocardial infarction during the previous 3 months. Excluded were patients with heart diseases other than myocardial infarction or acute coronary syndrome. The participants in this cohort were asked for study consent during the acute hospitalization period; they were then contacted 2–6 months later for an appointment in the study center. The reference group consisted of a random sample of residents drawn from the residents' registration office of the city of Münster. All participants had to be able to tolerate an approximately 3.5-h examination (Teismann et al. 2014).

13.2.2 Interview and Assessment of Risk Factor Levels and Burden of Subclinical Arteriosclerosis

The baseline examination consisted of an interview and self-administered questionnaire, anthropometric and medical measurements including the assessment of subclinical arteriosclerosis, psychiatric interviews and diagnostic tools for the assessment of cognitive functioning, and an MRI of the brain. Also blood samples were drawn from participants for future research. The methods of psychiatric interviews, the diagnostic tools for the assessment of cognitive functioning, the MRI, and the blood samples are not the topic of the present analysis and have been described elsewhere (Teismann et al. 2014).

The computer-assisted personal interview was performed by trained study nurses obtaining information about sociodemographic factors, medical history, medication, diagnoses, health-care utilization, and risk factors. Participants of the reference group and the cardiovascular cohort underwent a shortened, computer-based version of the Mini International Neuropsychiatric Interview, German Version 5.0.0. Only if there were signs for depression in this interview, a shortened version of the

Hamilton Questionnaire and of the Inventory of Depressive Symptomatology was administered by a psychologist. Participants of the depression cohort underwent both interviews conducted by psychologists.

The participant's height and weight as well as hip and waist circumferences were measured in a standardized fashion. We estimated body fat and lean body mass using the Bioelectrical Impedance Analyzer, BIA 2000-S, and the software Nutri Plus.

Systolic and diastolic blood pressure (BP), ankle-brachial index (ABI), pulse wave velocity (PWV), and augmentation index (AIX) were determined by using the Vascular Explorer of the Enverdis Company (Jena, Germany). Blood pressure was measured once in supine position on both arms after at least 5 min of rest, and the mean values from both arms were used for the analyses. The ankle-brachial index was calculated as the ratio of the systolic blood pressure of the ankle and the brachial systolic blood pressure. Systolic BP was determined with the Vascular Explorer using occlusion pressures on arms and legs detected by plethysmographic sensors on fingers and toes.

Pulse wave velocity and augmentation index were used as parameters of arterial stiffness and markers of subclinical arteriosclerosis. Measurements were performed with the Vascular Explorer, with the plethysmographic sensors attached to fingers and toes recording the participant's pressure curves. The augmentation index was calculated as another parameter of vascular stiffness reflecting the central aortic augmentation, that is, the difference between the maximum of the retrograde pulse wave (P2) and the pressure maximum of the anterograde pulse (P1), divided by P1; P1 and P2 are discernible components of the recorded pressure curve.

The carotid intima-media thickness (IMT) was determined by ultrasound as a surrogate marker of arteriosclerotic changes of the vascular system. It was measured by trained study nurses with a Siemens ACUSON X 300 ultrasound device, a high resolution B-mode system operating at a frequency of 10 MHz. The IMT was measured on both sides in the far walls of the common carotid artery within 1 cm of the bulb proximal to the carotid bifurcation. The IMT measurement was carried offline in a semiautomated fashion. A plaque was defined as a focal thickening of the IMT by more than 50 % of the IMT value surrounding this enlargement.

13.2.3 Categorization of Interview and Measurement Variables

Many of the interview data and the measurements were obtained on a continuous scale and were transformed into categories for further analyses. Smokers were divided into never smokers, ex-smokers, and current smokers. The body mass index (BMI) was used as both a continuous variable and categorized as obesity (BMI $\geq$30 kg/m^2). The fat mass index (FMI in kg/m^2) was pathological for men if $\geq$8.2 and for women if $\geq$11.8 (Schutz et al. 2002). The waist circumference was normal for women if $\leq$88 cm and for men if $\leq$102 cm (Lean et al. 1995). Blood pressure values were classified as hypertensive, if the systolic mean value of the right and left measurement was 140 mmHg or higher and/or the diastolic mean value was 90 mmHg or higher (Clement et al. 2013). Also, the category hypertension was attributed, if a participant was on antihypertensive medication ("actual hypertension") as reported in the interview. The ankle-brachial index (ABI) was classified as pathological if ABI was <0.9 for men or <0.85 for women on at least one side (Huxley et al. 2014; Aboyans et al. 2007; Smith et al. 2003). The pulse wave velocity (PWV) was classified as pathological in case of values greater or equal to 10 m/s (Clement et al. 2013). The mean values of the right and left intima-media thickness (IMT) were grouped as pathological if values of 0.9 mm and above were measured (Clement et al. 2013). Plaques were considered as present if a plaque was detected on at least one side.

13.2.4 Statistical Analyses

In the descriptive analysis, the continuous data were analyzed mainly as a comparison between the cohort of the patients with depression and the reference group; the cohort of patients with coronary heart disease served mainly as an "internal calibration" group to validate the arteriosclerotic markers. We used t-tests for the comparison of crude values and linear regression models for covariate-adjusted comparisons. Categorical variables were compared using chi-square test statistics and logistic regression for multivariable adjusted comparisons.

We created two scores that were composed of single markers to obtain summary estimates for the different levels of arteriosclerotic burden in the different cohorts: The score of subclinical arteriosclerosis (SSA) consisted of four variables that were dichotomized, based on the categorizations explained above, as normal (0 points) or pathological (1 point): ankle-brachial index, intima-media thickness, plaque in the common carotid arteries, and pulse wave velocity. The individual SSA was the unweighted sum of the 4-point values and ranged from a minimum of 0 points to a maximum of 4 points. In addition, a score of subclinical arteriosclerosis and lifestyle (SSA_LS) was created. SSA_LS was created by adding to the SSA data on never smoking (yes = 1 point), elevated waist circumference, and raised FMI as measures of nutrition and physical activity. A maximum of 7 points was possible for the SSA_LS score. As the score distributions were skewed, we compared adjusted geometric mean values. They were obtained taking the natural logarithm of the scores, adjusting the log scores to age and gender in linear regression models, and finally taking the antilogarithm of these values. All analyses were carried out with SAS 9.3 for Windows.

The BiDirect study was approved by the Ethics Committee of the Medical Faculty of the University of Münster.

13.3 Results

There were 997 participants in the depression cohort, and the number of participants in the reference group was $N = 841$; the coronary cohort consisted of 343 patients. The cohort of patients with depression was significantly younger (mean age 49.8 ± 7.3 years) than the reference sample (52.8 ± 8.1 years, $p < 0.001$), and the proportion of women (59.4 vs. 50.8 %, resp., $p<0.001$) was higher. The group of coronary patients was the oldest (54.9±6.6 years) and consisted of 85.7 % male patients. To account for these major differences, the following data are reported as age-/gender-adjusted values throughout.

Table 13.1 contains the adjusted baseline characteristics of the three study cohorts. Of note, even after taking the differences in age and gender into account, the average BMI and FMI as well as the waist circumferences were significantly higher in patients of the depression cohort as compared to the reference group; interestingly, the anthropometric values of the depressives were even higher than those for the coronary patients. By contrast, blood pressure as well as the pulse wave velocity and the augmentation index were all lower in depressive patients as compared to the reference. The average ABI and IMT were, however, very similar between these groups. Since the systolic and diastolic blood pressure, the PWV, and the AIX may be affected by the use of antihypertensive medication, additional adjustments were made by taking into account the use of antihypertensive medication (Table 13.2). Despite some differences in the antihypertensive treatment status, the results remained largely unaffected.

The prevalence of current smoking was significantly higher among patients with depression than in the reference sample (Table 13.3). Surprisingly, the presence of carotid plaques was highest in the reference group, while there were no major differences with regard to the (low) prevalence of peripheral artery disease.

To summarize the measurement results, two types of scores were created, one indicating the burden of subclinical arteriosclerosis (SSA) and one the burden of subclinical arteriosclerosis plus an adverse lifestyle (SSA_LS). Figure 13.1 reveals that the burden of subclinical arteriosclerosis, as assessed by the crude SSA in terms of the presence of pathological values of IMT and PWV and the presence of PAD or carotid plaques, was low in all three cohorts.

Table 13.1 Mean values of continuous measurement variables, adjusted for age and gender

	Cohort			
	Depression	Reference	*p*-value	Coronary
BMI [kg/m^2]	28.90	26.71	<0.0001	28.19
FMI [kg/m^2]	9.63	8.20	<0.0001	9.07
Waist [cm]	98.07	91.76	<0.0001	95.62
Systolic BP [mmHg]	133.0	135.7	<0.0001	129.4
Diastolic BP [mmHg]	82.1	84.3	<0.0001	79.5
ABI	1.11	1.11	*0.3953*	1.09
PWV [m/s]	7.74	7.93	0.0015	7.68
AIX% (75 bpm)	22.28	25.59	<0.0001	30.53
IMT [mm]	0.69	0.69	*0.9593*	0.72

BiDirect study, baseline examination
BMI body mass index, *FMI* fat mass index, *BP* blood pressure, *ABI* ankle-brachial index, *PWV* pulse wave velocity, *AIX% (75 bpm)* augmentation index in percent, calibrated to heart rate of 75 beat per minute, *IMT* intima-media thickness

Table 13.2 Mean values for blood pressure, adjusted for age, gender, and antihypertensive medication

	Cohort			
	Depression	Reference	*p*-value	Coronary
Proportion taking antihypertensive medication	30.0 %	25.1 %		94.7 %
Systolic BP [mmHg]	133.3	136.5	<0.0001	136.5
Diastolic [mmHg] BP	82.2	84.6	<0.0001	78.5
PWV [m/s]	7.75	7.95	0.0006	7.61
AIX% (75 bpm)	22.36	25.84	<0.0001	29.60

BiDirect study, baseline examination

PWV pulse wave velocity, *AIX% (75 bpm)* augmentation index in percent, calibrated to heart rate of 75 beat per minute

Table 13.3 Prevalence (in percent) of smoking, peripheral artery disease, and plaques

	Cohort			
	Depression	Reference	*p*-value	Coronary
Ex-smokers	25.6	37.6	<0.001	64.1
Current smokers	44.3	21.1	<0.001	17.2
PAD	2.6	1.7	0.17	3.5
Plaques	2.6	5.6	0.005	4.7

BiDirect study, baseline examination

PAD peripheral artery disease

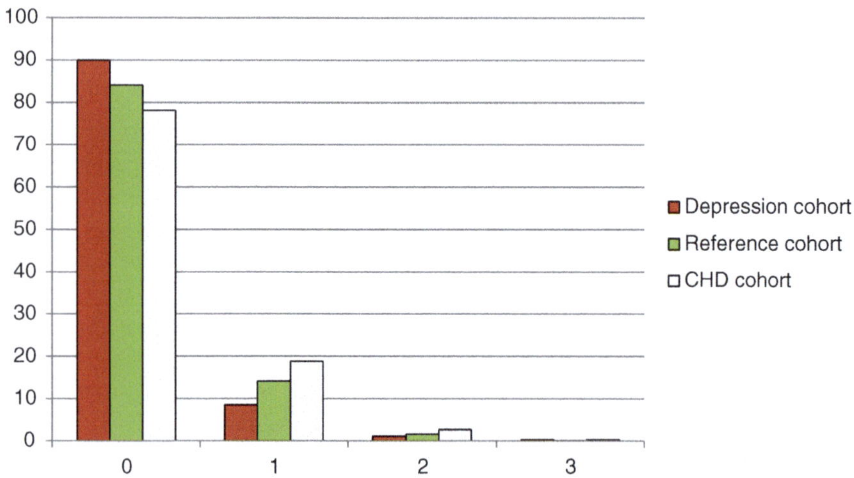

Fig. 13.1 Relative frequencies of unadjusted SSA (score for subclinical arteriosclerosis) in the three cohorts. BiDirect study, baseline examination

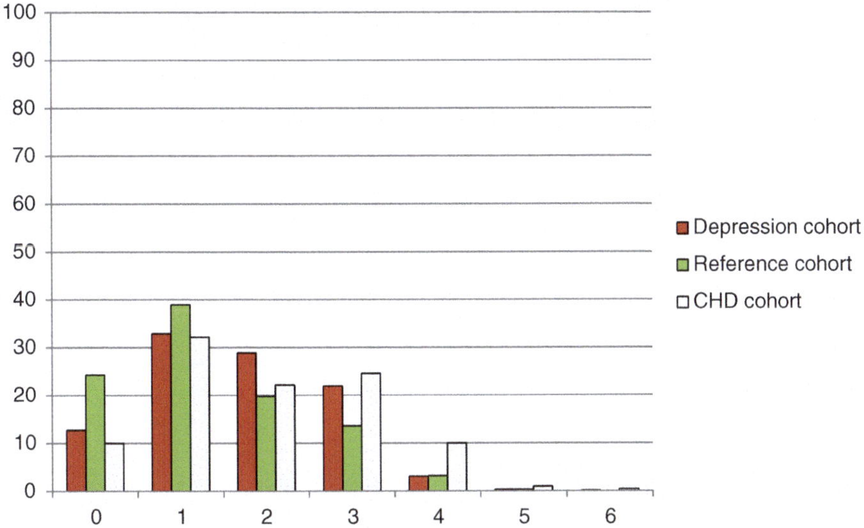

Fig. 13.2 Relative frequencies of unadjusted SSA_LS (score for subclinical arteriosclerosis plus adverse lifestyle) in the three cohorts. BiDirect study, baseline examination

Table 13.4 Geometric mean values of SSA and SSA_LS, adjusted for age and sex

	Cohort			
	Depression	Reference	*p*-value	Cardiovascular
SSA	0.14	0.14	0.18	0.15
SSA, <50 years	0.11	0.11	0.60	0.12
SSA, ≥50 years	0.15	0.16	0.28	0.17
SSA_LS	1.61	0.97	<.0.001	2.36
SSA_LS, <50 years	1.49	0.67	<0.001	2.08
SSA_LS, ≥50 years	1.61	1.26	0.003	2.64

BiDirect study, baseline examination
SSA score for subclinical arteriosclerosis, *SSA_LS* score for subclinical arteriosclerosis plus adverse lifestyle

By contrast, the SSA_LS was more broadly distributed in the study population and showed generally a higher prevalence of raised score values among the cohort with depression as compared to the reference group (Fig. 13.2). While the adjusted geometric means of the SSA revealed no statistically significant differences between the study cohorts, the adjusted geometric means of the SSA_LS showed highly significant differences between the depression cohort and the reference group. As expected, the cardiovascular cohort showed consistently the highest score values across study groups (Table 13.4).

In a sensitivity analysis, we stratified the adjusted geometric mean scores by age. Score values were generally higher in those 50 years and older. Nevertheless, the SSA continued to be nonsignificant in both strata of age. Likewise, the significant differences observed between the depression cohort and the reference group for the overall SSA_LS were maintained both in the younger and in the older age groups. There was, however, a tendency that the contrast was more pronounced in the young (1.49 among those with depression and 0.67 among the referents, $p<0.001$) than in the older (1.61 vs. 1.26, resp., $p=0.003$; Table 13.4).

13.4 Discussion

This cross-sectional study investigated the baseline distributions of cardiovascular risk factors and the prevalence of clinical and subclinical arteriosclerotic alterations across three subsamples consisting of depression, of cardiovascular disease, and of a reference group who will be followed as part of the prospective BiDirect study over the next years. These three cohorts were markedly different in terms of age and gender, in that participants from the cardiovascular cohort were considerably older than those in the depression cohort and in the reference group. The proportion of males was also significantly higher in the cardiovascular cohort. This contrasted significantly with the depression cohort, where females were more common, while the male-to-female ratio was almost even in the reference cohort. These pronounced differences required that all comparisons in this study were adjusted for age and gender. We found that adjusted mean values for BMI, FMI, and waist circumference were significantly higher in the depression cohort when compared to the reference group. Likewise, adverse health behaviors, such as smoking, were more prevalent among the depressive cohort. By contrast, the systolic and diastolic blood pressure values were lower in the depression cohort even after adjustment for age, gender, and antihypertensive medication. In addition, the adjusted PWV and AIX were also lower, while indicators of subclinical arteriosclerosis, like IMT and ABI, showed no differences with the reference group after multivariate adjustments. In fact, plaques in the common carotid artery were even significantly less prevalent. We attempted to integrate the results of single independent measurements into unweighted score values that were derived by attributing point values to abnormal measurement results or risk conditions and by summing up these point values without assigning specific weights to any of the individual measurements. For the SSA, representing mostly subclinical arteriosclerotic changes, the presence of a score value >0 was very uncommon at baseline, and only about 20 % of the coronary cohort had a raised SSA. When adding aspects of lifestyle and health behavior, this pattern changed. The depression group displayed considerably higher scores in the SSA_LS than the reference group, possibly indicating that the present adverse conditions harbor the prospect of a raised probability of arteriosclerosis in the future.

Previous reports mostly examined the association between depression and clinical cardiovascular end points, such as myocardial infarction or cardiac and/or all-cause mortality rather than atherosclerotic changes. These studies mostly found that patients with depression had an increased risk of nonfatal and fatal cardiovascular events (Nicholson et al. 2006; Rugulies 2002). Similarly, the prognosis of preexisting CHD was also adversely affected (Nicholson et al. 2006; Meijer et al. 2011). In

2014, an American Heart Association Scientific Statement on "Depression as a Risk Factor for Poor Prognosis among Patients with Acute Coronary Syndrome" came to the conclusion that "...the American Heart Association should elevate depression to the status of a risk factor for adverse medical outcomes in patients with acute coronary syndrome" (Lichtman et al. 2014).

However, the mechanisms behind these associations are still not clearly understood and seem to be of a rather complex and potentially bidirectional nature. The BiDirect study aimed at elucidating whether earlier stages in the development of disease are already identifiable in patients with depressive disorders and – vice versa – whether depression occurs more frequently in patients after an acute cardiovascular event. As BiDirect is a population-based epidemiological cohort study, the diagnostic tools and instruments had to be safe, reliable, noninvasive, and not too time-consuming. Therefore, the measurement of blood pressure, ABI, PWV, and AIX with plethysmographic methods and the measurement of IMT and the detection of plaques in the common carotid artery by ultrasonography were used to assess early signs of arteriosclerosis. This was complemented with anthropometric measurements such as body weight and height, waist circumference, and body composition by impedance analysis.

BMI and obesity as part of the metabolic syndrome are established risk factor for cardiovascular disease (WHO | 10 facts on obesity). There have been reports of a reciprocal relationship between obesity and depression (Luppino et al. 2010). As there is an ongoing debate, whether the FMI might be a better predictor of the metabolic syndrome than the BMI and whether abdominal obesity rather than general obesity is a better prognostic factor, we included all these parameters in our analyses (Liu et al. 2013). We observed that the age- and gender-adjusted means for BMI, FMI, and waist circumference were all significantly higher in the depression cohort as compared to the reference group. This risk constellation was compounded by the higher percentage of current smokers in the depression cohort. These data are in line with results of other large population-based studies (Wulsin et al. 2005; Niranjan et al. 2012).

Numerous clinical studies have examined the relationship between depression and hypertension. In their analysis of the prospective CARDIA study, Davidson et al. concluded that participants with depressive symptoms were at high risk of developing hypertension (Davidson et al. 2000). A recent meta-analysis of nine prospective studies with a mean follow-up of 9.6 years found a relative risk of RR = 1.45 for participants with depression to develop hypertension (Meng et al. 2012). Other reports from prospective studies seem to support these associations (Nabi et al. 2011). By contrast, the prospective MESA study did *not* find an increased risk of incident hypertension (RR 1.02) among participants with baseline depressive symptoms (Delaney et al. 2010), and the Norwegian HUNT Study even showed that symptoms of anxiety and depression were associated with a *de*crease in blood pressure (Hildrum et al. 2011). This was also confirmed in a recent report about a British birth cohort, in which the authors concluded that "a cumulative effect of symptoms of anxiety and depression across adulthood results in lower systolic blood pressure in late middle age that is not explained by life style factors and antihypertensive treatment" (Tikhonoff et al. 2014). The evidence on an association of depression and hypertension thus seems surprisingly inconclusive. In the baseline examination of BiDirect, the systolic and diastolic blood pressures were clearly lower in the depression cohort than in the reference group. Of note, the cardiovascular cohort displayed the lowest values indicating the highly prevalent utilization of antihypertensive medication which was far less common in the other two cohorts. Of note, however, after additionally controlling for antihypertensive medication, the differences in systolic and diastolic blood pressure remained. For one thing, this result might indicate a truly inverse association of depression and blood pressure for which some pathophysiological explanations have been suggested (Hildrum et al. 2011; Tikhonoff et al. 2014). On the other hand, our finding may have resulted from insufficient adjustments, especially with regard to medication. We did not, for example, take into account the type and dosage of antidepressive treatment. Depending on the active component of the medication, differing effects on blood pressure appear conceivable.

In recent years, indices of arterial stiffness have been increasingly used to assess cardiovascular risk (Laurent et al. 2006; Van Bortel et al. 2012). The 2013 European Society of Hypertension – European Society of Cardiology Guidelines for the Management of Hypertension – lists high values of PWV as a marker for target-organ damage (Clement et al. 2013; Van Bortel et al. 2012). By contrast, the prognostic validity of the augmentation index AIX has been controversially discussed (Wang et al. 2010; Izzo and Mitchell 2007). Association studies with depression were few and often small (Seldenrijk et al. 2011; Dietz and Matthews 2011). Our analysis revealed lower unadjusted values of PWV and AIX in the depression cohort even after adjustment for antihypertensive medication, age, and gender. Since, in particular, the impact of different antihypertensive medications on measures of arterial stiffness may be diverse (Baulmann et al. 2010; Ong et al. 2011), residual confounding may have arisen from non-differential adjustments for antihypertensive drugs as a group.

The ABI is a noninvasive tool to assess peripheral artery disease (PAD) of the lower extremity. It has been shown that the ABI is an indicator of atherosclerosis at other vascular sites and can serve as a prognostic marker for cardiovascular events and functional impairment, even in the absence of symptoms of PAD (Aboyans et al. 2012). Previous cross-sectional and longitudinal studies on the association of depression and ABI did not find a clear association between low ABI/PAD and depression (Tiemeier et al. 2004; Newson et al. 2010). Likewise, our cross-sectional analyses did not demonstrate a clear association between depression and adjusted ABI and PAD. Of note, the numbers of prevalent PAD cases were very low in our study, which may have limited the statistical power to find such an association.

The IMT is a surrogate marker of subclinical arteriosclerosis (Van den Oord et al. 2013; Lorenz et al. 2007). Some previous studies that examined the association between depression and IMT reported no association (Ohira et al. 2012; Elovainio et al. 2005; Rice et al. 2009), while others found positive associations (Stewart et al. 2007). In this study, there was no significant association between depression and age- and gender-adjusted IMT.

In order to integrate these singular observations into measures of arteriosclerotic burden and risk, scores were created that should help to summarize the manifold results in a more structured manner. These scores are intended as a tool that facilitates comparisons of the burden of arteriosclerosis at the beginning of the prospective follow-up and of the changes in this burden over time in the different cohorts. The scores presented here are unweighted, thus attributing the same weight to each single item. The study by Newson et al. examined whether a composite score, created from four extra-coronary measures, increased the risk of incident depression or depressive symptoms (Newson et al. 2010). To our knowledge, no other studies used such an approach. In our cross-sectional analysis of the BiDirect baseline data, the adjusted geometric mean SSA – representing the sum of dichotomized subclinical measurements of ABI, IMT, PWV, and plaques – was very similar in the depression and in the reference group. Sensitivity analyses, stratifying the results by age under and over 50 years, did not change this finding. Thus, at the outset of the prospective BiDirect study, there was no clear difference between patients with depression and their referent counterparts with regard to the burden of subclinical arteriosclerosis. By contrast, the SSA_LS which additionally took into account matters of health behavior and lifestyle including smoking, body circumference, and body composition showed significantly higher scores in the depression group, irrespective of age. This seems to indicate that, while the burden of prevalent arteriosclerotic changes is still similar, patients with depression carry a higher risk of future incident arteriosclerotic events based on the pattern of their individual risk constellations. In perspective, it appears meaningful to utilize information of the SSA_LS as a predictor variable in prospective cohort analyses, while the SSA may be used to assess incident changes of subclinical disease in addition to incident clinical manifestations.

13.5 Limitations and Strengths

The most important limitation of this analysis is its cross-sectional design precluding any causal inferences. Also, alternative or optional methods of quantifying arteriosclerosis are conceivable, such as aortic calcification via X-ray or coronary calcification via electron-beam computed tomographic scan, which were not performed in BiDirect but in other studies such as the Rotterdam Study (Newson et al. 2010). However, the inclusion of X-ray-based examinations was dismissed to avoid inappropriate radiation exposure in the study groups, and the measurement of aortic calcification was not feasible in our study setting. Clearly, a strength of the study is its size, the well-characterized groups of patients and comparison groups, the standardized and reliable measurement of risk factors and markers of arteriosclerosis, and – in due time – the availability of longitudinal data.

Conclusion

In conclusion, we did not find a higher arteriosclerotic burden within the depression in comparison to the reference group. Residual confounding cannot be ruled out as a possible explanation. Considering lifestyle factors and anthropometric measurements, there was definitive evidence for a raised cardiovascular risk within the depressive cohort.

References

Aboyans V et al (2007) Intrinsic contribution of gender and ethnicity to normal ankle-brachial index values: the Multi-Ethnic Study of Atherosclerosis (MESA). J Vasc Surg 45:319–327

Aboyans V et al (2012) Measurement and interpretation of the ankle-brachial index a scientific statement from the American Heart Association. Circulation 126:2890–2909

Barth J, Schumacher M, Herrmann-Lingen C (2004) Depression as a risk factor for mortality in patients with coronary heart disease: a meta-analysis. Psychosom Med 66:802–813

Baulmann J et al (2010) Arterial stiffness and pulse wave analysis. Dtsch Med Wochenschr 135(Suppl 1):S4–S14

Busch MA, Maske UE, Ryl L, Schlack R, Hapke U (2013) Prävalenz von depressiver Symptomatik und diagnostizierter Depression bei Erwachsenen in Deutschland: Ergebnisse der Studie zur Gesundheit Erwachsener in Deutschland (DEGS1). Bundesgesundheitsbl Gesundheitsforsch Gesundheitsschutz 56:733–739

Clement DL et al, with Mancia G et al, ESH Scientific Council, Redon J et al, ESC Committee for Practice Guidelines (CPG), Zamorano JL et al, Document Reviewers (2013) 2013 ESH/ESC guidelines for the management of arterial hypertension: the Task Force for the management of arterial hypertension of the European Society of Hypertension (ESH) and of the European Society of Cardiology (ESC). Eur Heart J 34: 2159–2219

Davidson K, Jonas BS, Dixon KE, Markovitz JH (2000) Do depression symptoms predict early hypertension incidence in young adults in the cardia study? Arch Intern Med 160:1495–1500

De Jonge P et al (2010) Psychophysiological biomarkers explaining the association between depression and prognosis in coronary artery patients: a critical review of the literature. Neurosci Biobehav Rev 35:84–90

Delaney JAC et al (2010) Baseline depressive symptoms are not associated with clinically important levels of incident hypertension during two years of follow-up the multi-ethnic study of atherosclerosis. Hypertension 55:408–414

Deutscher Herzbericht (2013) Deutsche Herzstiftung (Hg.), Frankfurt

Dietz LJ, Matthews KA (2011) Depressive symptoms and subclinical markers of cardiovascular disease in adolescents. J Adolesc Health Off Publ Soc Adolesc Med 48:579–584

Elovainio M et al (2005) Depressive symptoms and carotid artery intima-media thickness in young adults: the Cardiovascular Risk in Young Finns Study. Psychosom Med 2005(67):561–567

Gehi A et al (2010) Depression and platelet activation in outpatients with stable coronary heart disease: findings from the Heart and Soul Study. Psychiatry Res 175:200–204

Grippo AJ, Johnson AK (2009) Stress, depression and cardiovascular dysregulation: a review of neurobiological mechanisms and the integration of research from preclinical disease models: review. Stress Int J Biol Stress 12:1–21

Hildrum B, Romild U, Holmen J (2011) Anxiety and depression lowers blood pressure: 22-year follow-up of the population based HUNT study, Norway. BMC Public Health 11:601

Huxley RR et al (2014) A comparative analysis of risk factors for stroke in blacks and whites: the atherosclerosis risk in communities study. Ethn Health 19:601–616

Izzo JL Jr, Mitchell GF (2007) Aging and arterial structure-function relations. Adv Cardiol 44:19–34

Laurent S et al, on behalf of the European Network for Non-invasive Investigation of Large Arteries (2006) Expert consensus document on arterial stiffness: methodological issues and clinical applications. Eur. Heart J 27:2588–2605

Lean MEJ, Han TS, Morrison CE (1995) Waist circumference as a measure for indicating need for weight management. BMJ 311:158–161

Libby P (2012) Inflammation in atherosclerosis. Arterioscler Thromb Vasc Biol 32:2045–2051

Libby P, Ridker PM, Hansson GK (2011) Progress and challenges in translating the biology of atherosclerosis. Nature 473:317–325

Lichtman JH et al (2014) Depression as a risk factor for poor prognosis among patients with acute coronary syndrome: systematic review and recommendations a scientific statement from the American Heart Association. Circulation 129:1350–1369

Liu P, Ma F, Lou H, Liu Y (2013) The utility of fat mass index vs. body mass index and percentage of body fat in the screening of metabolic syndrome. BMC Public Health 13:629

Lorenz MW, Markus HS, Bots ML, Rosvall M, Sitzer M (2007) Prediction of clinical cardiovascular events with carotid intima-media thickness: a systematic review and meta-analysis. Circulation 115:459–467

Luppino FS et al (2010) Overweight, obesity, and depression: a systematic review and meta-analysis of longitudinal studies. Arch Gen Psychiatry 67:220–229

Mathers CD, Loncar D (2006) Projections of global mortality and burden of disease from 2002 to 2030. PLoS Med 3:e442

Meijer A et al (2011) Prognostic association of depression following myocardial infarction with mortality and cardiovascular events: a meta-analysis of 25 years of research. Gen Hosp Psychiatry 33:203–216

Meng L, Chen D, Yang Y, Zheng Y, Hui R (2012) Depression increases the risk of hypertension incidence: a meta-analysis of prospective cohort studies. J Hypertens 30:842–851

Nabi H et al (2011) Trajectories of depressive episodes and hypertension over 24 years the Whitehall II prospective cohort study. Hypertension 57:710–716

Newson RS et al (2010) Atherosclerosis and incident depression in late life. Arch Gen Psychiatry 67:1144–1151

Nicholson A, Kuper H, Hemingway H (2006) Depression as an aetiologic and prognostic factor in coronary heart disease: a meta-analysis of 6362 events among 146 538 participants in 54 observational studies. Eur Heart J 27:2763–2774

Niranjan A, Corujo A, Ziegelstein RC, Nwulia E (2012) Depression and heart disease in US adults. Gen Hosp Psychiatry 34:254–261

Ohira T et al (2012) Associations of anger, anxiety, and depressive symptoms with carotid arterial wall thickness: the multi-ethnic study of atherosclerosis. Psychosom Med 74:517–525

Ong K-T et al (2011) Aortic stiffness is reduced beyond blood pressure lowering by short-term and long-term antihypertensive treatment: a meta-analysis of individual data in 294 patients. J Hypertens 2011(29):1034–1042

Rice SC, Zonderman AB, Metter EJ, Najjar SS, Waldstein SR (2009) Absence of relation between depressive symptoms and carotid intimal medial thickness in the Baltimore Longitudinal Study of Aging. Psychosom Med 71:70–76

Rugulies R (2002) Depression as a predictor for coronary heart disease a review and meta-analysis. Am J Prev Med 23:51–61

Sass H, Wittchen H-U, Zaudig M (1996) Diagnostic and statistical manual psychischer Störungen - DSM-IV. Deutsche Bearbeitung u. Einleitung von Sass H, Wittchen H-U, Zaudig M Göttingen: Hogrefe

Schutz Y, Kyle UG, Pichard C (2002) Fat-free mass index and fat mass index percentiles in Caucasians aged 18–98 y. Int J Obes 26:953–960

Seldenrijk A et al (2011) Depression, anxiety, and arterial stiffness. Biol Psychiatry 69:795–803

Smith FB, Lee AJ, Price JF, van Wijk MCW, Fowkes FGR (2003) Changes in ankle brachial index in symptomatic and asymptomatic subjects in the general population. J Vasc Surg 38:1323–1330

Stewart JC, Janicki DL, Muldoon MF, Sutton-Tyrrell K, Kamarck TW (2007) Negative emotions and 3-year progression of subclinical atherosclerosis. Arch Gen Psychiatry 64:225–233

Teismann H et al (2014) Establishing the bidirectional relationship between depression and subclinical arteriosclerosis-rationale, design, and characteristics of the BiDirect study. BMC Psychiatry 14:174

Tiemeier H et al (2004) Relationship between atherosclerosis and late-life depression: the Rotterdam study. Arch Gen Psychiatry 61:369–376

Tikhonoff V et al (2014) Symptoms of anxiety and depression across adulthood and blood pressure in late middle age: the 1946 British birth cohort. J Hypertens 32:1590–1598

Van Bortel LM et al (2012) Expert consensus document on the measurement of aortic stiffness in daily practice using carotid-femoral pulse wave velocity. J Hypertens 30:445–448

Van den Oord SCH et al (2013) Carotid intima-media thickness for cardiovascular risk assessment: systematic review and meta-analysis. Atherosclerosis 228:1–11
Van der Kooy K et al (2007) Depression and the risk for cardiovascular diseases: systematic review and meta-analysis. Int J Geriatr Psychiatry 22:613–626
Wang K-L et al (2010) Wave reflection and arterial stiffness in the prediction of 15-year all-cause and cardiovascular mortalities a community-based study. Hypertension 55:799–805
WHO | 10 facts on obesity. At: http://www.who.int/features/factfiles/obesity/facts/en/
Wulsin LR, Singal BM (2003) Do depressive symptoms increase the risk for the onset of coronary disease? A systematic quantitative review. Psychosom Med 65:201–210
Wulsin LR et al (2005) Depressive symptoms, coronary heart disease, and overall mortality in the Framingham Heart study. Psychosom Med 67:697–702

Metabolic-Inflammation Aspects of Depression and Cardiovascular Disease

14

Joshua D. Rosenblat, Ron Kakar, and Roger S. McIntyre

Contents

J.D. Rosenblat • R.S. McIntyre, MD, FRCPC (✉)
Mood Disorder Psychopharmacology Unit, University Health Network,
399 Bathurst Street, MP 9-325, Toronto, ON M5T 2S8, Canada

Department of Psychiatry and Pharmacology, University of Toronto,
399 Bathurst Street, MP 9-325, Toronto, ON M5T 2S8, Canada
e-mail: roger.mcintyre@uhn.ca

R. Kakar
Mood Disorder Psychopharmacology Unit, University Health Network,
399 Bathurst Street, MP 9-325, Toronto, ON M5T 2S8, Canada

Department of Psychiatry and Pharmacology, University of Toronto,
399 Bathurst Street, MP 9-325, Toronto, ON M5T 2S8, Canada

Department of Psychiatry, Western University, London and Windsor, ON, Canada

B.T. Baune, P.J. Tully (eds.), *Cardiovascular Diseases and Depression*,
DOI 10.1007/978-3-319-32480-7_14

Abstract
Major depressive disorder (MDD) and cardiovascular disease (CVD) are prevalent and chronic diseases with high rates of morbidity and mortality. A bidirectional interaction appears to exist between MDD and CVD as epidemiological studies have revealed a strong association. Given the poor prognosis of patients with comorbid CVD and MDD, there is great need for an improved understanding of the mechanisms subserving their interaction. The objective of the current chapter is to explore metabolic-inflammatory aspects of the interaction between MDD and CVD. Inflammation and metabolic dysfunction have been proposed as key substrates with converging pathways of pathogenesis subserving the interaction between CVD and MDD. Metabolic dysfunction may induce inflammation through the release of inflammatory cytokines from visceral adipose tissue, producing a chronic, low-grade inflammatory state. Inflammation may also induce metabolic dysfunction through activation of the hypothalamic-pituitary-adrenal (HPA) axis and increasing insulin resistance. Inflammation and metabolic dysfunction independently and synergistically contribute to the etiology and pathophysiology of both CVD and MDD. For CVD, the metabolic-inflammatory pathway is a key player in atherosclerotic plaque formation and propagation. For MDD, inflammation and metabolic dysfunction induce monoamine alterations, microglial activation, impaired neuroplasticity, and impaired brain connectivity ultimately leading to mood and cognitive dysfunction. A further understanding of metabolic-inflammatory aspects may therefore lead to improved preventative and therapeutic strategies for comorbid CVD and MDD. Repurposing of anti-inflammatory and antidiabetic agents may be used in the future in the treatment of MDD; however, currently there is insufficient evidence for routine use.

14.1 Introduction

Major depressive disorder (MDD) and cardiovascular disease (CVD) are prevalent and chronic diseases with high rates of morbidity and mortality (Kessler et al. 2003, 2006; Go et al. 2013). For decades, investigators have attempted to understand the underlying pathophysiology of both of these diseases independently. Epidemiological observations showing an association between CVD and MDD have alerted investigators to the potential existence of shared etiological and pathophysiological substrates between MDD and CVD (Fenton and Stover 2006).

Metabolic and inflammatory dysfunction have emerged as key processes underlying the etiology and pathophysiology of disease onset and progression of both MDD and CVD (Fenton and Stover 2006; Rosenblat et al. 2014; Mansur et al. 2014, 2015; Gans 2006; Ghattas et al. 2013; Libby et al. 2009). Moreover, metabolic and inflammatory dysfunction has become increasingly recognized to be two sides of the same coin, as the two processes are intimately connected (Mathieu et al. 2008, 2010).

The objective of the current chapter is therefore to summarize the bidirectional interaction between inflammation and metabolic dysfunction as it relates to CVD and MDD. A discussion of therapeutic implications and proposed future direction of research will subsequently ensue. The current topic is highly relevant and timely with the worldwide increasing rates of obesity, diabetes, CVD, and MDD (Andrade et al. 2003; Kessler et al. 2003, 2006; Danaci et al. 2009) requiring an improved understanding of the pathophysiology of these disorders that may lead to improved therapeutic and preventative strategies.

14.2 Co-prevalence of Cardiovascular Disease and Depression

An increased prevalence of MDD in CVD patients has been repeatedly shown by observational studies; a diagnosis of MDD is present in approximately one in five patients with CVD, as compared to approximately one in ten in the general population (Thombs et al. 2006; Elderon and Whooley 2013). Moreover, the interaction appears to be bidirectional as MDD has been associated with poorer outcomes for coronary heart disease (CHD) even after controlling for traditional CVD risk factors (Thombs et al. 2006; Elderon and Whooley 2013). Indeed, MDD or the presence of depressive symptoms has been associated with increased CHD in healthy individuals as well as increased secondary events in CHD patients (Barth et al. 2004).

The INTERHEART study evaluating modifiable risk factors for myocardial infarction (MI) in over 25,000 individuals from 52 different countries found psychosocial factors, including MDD and depressive symptoms, to be significant risk factors similar to or greater than several traditional risk factors such as diabetes, obesity, smoking and hypertension (Yusuf et al. 2004). Taking into consideration this reproducible finding, the 2010 Global Burden of Disease Study officially recognized MDD as a risk factor of CHD (Charlson et al. 2011).

In addition to being associated with increased risk and poorer outcomes in CHD patients, MDD has also been associated with poorer outcomes for heart failure, peripheral arterial disease, and stroke patients (Pan et al. 2011; Rutledge et al. 2006; Grenon et al. 2012). Taken together, several large epidemiological studies have shown a strong and bidirectional interaction between MDD and CVD (Thombs et al. 2006; Elderon and Whooley 2013). Investigations to understand the mechanisms subserving this interaction have been, and continue to be, an active area of research for psychiatrist and cardiologist alike. The metabolic-inflammatory pathway has been of increasing interest in this area of study.

14.3 Metabolic Dysfunction Promotes Inflammation

Visceral adiposity (e.g., central obesity), a key feature of metabolic dysfunction, is a significant and independent risk factor for both MDD and CVD (Mansur et al. 2014, 2015; Mathieu et al. 2008, 2010). Visceral adipose tissue is fundamentally different from subcutaneous adipose tissue. As such, visceral adiposity is often regarded as harmful ectopic adipose tissue and a source of chronic low-grade inflammation, increasing the production of pro-inflammatory cytokines including IL-6, TNF-α, and C-reactive protein (CRP) (Mathieu et al. 2008, 2010). Subcutaneous adipose tissue serves as a "metabolic sink" to prevent accumulation of visceral adipose tissue; however, under certain genetic (e.g., polygenic risk factors for central obesity) and environmental (e.g., sedentary lifestyle and poor diet) condition, high volumes of dysfunctional visceral adipose tissue may accumulate (Mathieu et al. 2008, 2010).

Perturbation of adipocyte development and maturation is central to the formation of dysfunctional, pro-inflammatory visceral adipocytes (Unger 2005). In normal physiologic conditions, pre-adipocytes will differentiate into mature adipocytes and aid in homeostasis (Spalding et al. 2008). Conversely, in the context of chronic positive energy balance (e.g., greater caloric intake then expenditure), adipocytes undergo hypertrophy and have increased triglyceride stores (Unger 2005; Spalding et al. 2008). The lypolytic rate is therefore increased leading to increased production of leptin (pro-inflammatory) and decreased production of adiponectin (anti-inflammatory), thereby signaling the release of inflammatory cytokines (Unger 2005; Spalding et al. 2008). Further, adipocyte hypertrophy promotes macrophage infiltration of adipose tissue (Spalding et al. 2008). The resultant cross talk between macrophages and adipocytes promotes further release of pro-inflammatory cytokines and adipokines (Mathieu et al. 2010). Increased density of macrophages in adipose tissue is also associated with insulin resistance. Mechanistically, the resultant increase in TNF-α production decreases the systemic production of GLUT-4, PPAR-γ, and adiponectin, thereby decreasing insulin sensitivity and glucose uptake.

Hypertrophied adipocytes also produce higher levels of free fatty acids (FFAs) that potently activate Toll-like receptor-4 (TLR-4), leading to increased TNF-α production through the NF-κβ pathway (Nguyen et al. 2007). Toll-like receptors are responsible for the recognition of both pathogenic antigens and endogenous antigens, thus serving as a potential pathway to promote inflammation with the presence of endogenous antigens of interest. Therefore, the increased production of FFAs by hypertrophied adipocytes may chronically activate TLR-4, producing increased levels of TNF-α (Nguyen et al. 2007). Increased levels of TNF-α further activate lipolysis leading to a feed-forward loop with the increased production of FFAs (Nguyen et al. 2007; Unger 2005; Spalding et al. 2008). TNF-α also increases the production of IL-6 and macrophage chemoattractant protein-1 (MCP-1), a potent chemokine that signals further recruitment of macrophages into the adipose tissue, further perpetuating the pro-inflammatory cascade (Lyngso et al. 2002). As well, the increased production of IL-6 produced in visceral adipose tissue travels directly to the liver via the portal system, promoting the hepatic production of CRP (Abeywardena et al. 2009).

Taken together, visceral adipose tissue, through a variety of feed-forward pathways, induces and maintains a chronic, systemic low-grade inflammatory state. Visceral adipocytes are hyperlipolytic, thereby increasing the production of pro-inflammatory cytokines (IL-6, TNF-α, and CRP) and adipokines. A chronic positive energy balance promotes the dysfunctional development of visceral hypertrophied adipocytes that recruit macrophages, which synergistically increase the production of pro-inflammatory signals (Mathieu et al. 2010).

14.4 Inflammation Promotes Metabolic Dysfunction

The interaction between inflammation and metabolic dysfunction appears to be bidirectional in nature (Mathieu et al. 2010). As discussed, metabolic dysfunction appears to be a potent activator of the inflammatory system as accumulation of visceral adipose tissue induces the production of TNF-α, IL-6, and CRP. Furthermore, inflammation may promote dysfunctional metabolic pathways, most notably through derangement of the hypothalamic-pituitary-adrenal (HPA) axis (Beishuizen and Thijs 2003; Grinevich et al. 2001; Silverman et al. 2004; Turnbull and Rivier 1999).

Pro-inflammatory cytokines, such as IL-1, IL-6, TNF-α, and interferon (IFN), activate the HPA axis, increasing levels of corticotrophin releasing hormone (CRH), adrenocorticotropic hormone (ACTH), and cortisol as part of the generalized stress response induced by inflammation (Beishuizen and Thijs 2003; Grinevich et al. 2001; Silverman et al. 2004; Turnbull and Rivier 1999; Brydon et al. 2009; McQuade and Young 2000; Murphy 1991; Pace and Miller 2009; Reichenberg et al. 2001). This process normally serves as an important physiologic negative feedback loop during an acute inflammatory event, such as during an acute infection (Abbas et al. 2012). Conversely, chronic inflammation, as seen in inflammatory disorders (e.g., autoimmune disease, CVD, central obesity, etc.), may lead to the pathologic continuous activation of the HPA axis; the chronic production of inflammatory cytokines may thus lead to the chronic production of elevated levels of glucocorticoids (Miller et al. 2007, 2009, 2013).

Additionally, inflammatory cytokines decrease the synthesis, translocation, and binding of glucocorticoid receptors (Pace and Miller 2009). This decrease in glucocorticoid receptors has two important downstream effects: (1) cortisol has a decreased ability to inhibit CRH production by the hypothalamus, thereby allowing for continued HPA over-activity, and (2) the systemic anti-inflammatory effects of cortisol are blunted (Pace and Miller 2009; Raison and Miller 2003; Grinevich et al. 2001). Therefore, in the case of a chronic inflammatory state, the HPA axis is continually overactive leading to chronic hypercortisolemia. Hypercortisolemia is a potent trigger of metabolic dysfunction, leading to obesity, hypercholesterolemia, hyperglycemia, and insulin resistance (Kahn and Joslin 2005).

Inflammation may induce metabolic dysfunction through several other pathways (e.g., in addition to HPA dysregulation). Notably, inflammatory cytokines may directly induce insulin resistance via decreasing the production of GLUT-4, PPAR-γ, and adiponectin, thereby decreasing insulin sensitivity and glucose uptake (Mathieu et al. 2010). Inflammation may also induce metabolic dysfunction through the overactivation (hyperthyroidism) or destruction (hypothyroidism) of the thyroid gland (Boutzios and Kaltsas 2000).

Taken together, a clear bidirectional interaction exists between metabolic dysfunction and inflammation (Boutzios and Kaltsas 2000; Mathieu et al. 2010). Metabolic dysfunction leading to central obesity and insulin resistance promotes a feed-forward loop of FFA production, cytokine production, and macrophage recruitment leading to a chronic low-grade inflammatory state. Chronic inflammation (caused by metabolic dysfunction or other causes of chronic inflammation) promotes metabolic dysfunction through the production of cytokines and overactivation of the HPA axis leading to chronic hypercortisolemia, a potent cause of obesity, hyperglycemia, and insulin resistance. The role of microRNA is likely also important in the converging pathways of metabolic dysfunction and inflammation; however, further research is required to understand microRNA-mediated mechanisms (Olivieri et al. 2013).

14.5 The Inflammatory-Metabolic Pathway Promotes CVD

The effect of inflammation and metabolic dysfunction on CVD has been well established for many years and has been extensively reviewed elsewhere (Libby et al. 2009; Mathieu et al. 2008, 2010; Van Gaal et al. 2006; Matsuzawa 2006; Poirier et al. 2006). Therefore, the evidence and pathways for CVD secondary to metabolic and inflammatory dysfunction will only be briefly discussed.

Metabolic dysfunction has been shown to directly affect several traditional risk factors of CVD including cholesterol profiles, blood glucose levels, and blood pressure. Vascular dysfunction is therefore induced in coronary, cerebral, and peripheral arteries through the formation and propagation of atherosclerotic plaques in the presence of these risk factors (Libby et al. 2009; Van Gaal et al. 2006; Wang et al. 2014).

Inflammation has also been shown to be a key substrate in atherosclerotic plaque formation and propagation. Innate immunity plays a role through the action of monocytes and macrophages. Essential to this process is the release of chemokines that attract monocytes into the arterial intima. Subsequently, monocytes mature into macrophages and multiply, promoting the release of inflammatory cytokines and the formation of atherosclerotic plaques (Libby et al. 2009).

Adaptive immunity also plays a pivotal role in plaque formation. Dendritic cells populate atherosclerotic plaques and surrounding lymph nodes, presenting antigens to T cells promoting an inflammatory response and propagation of the plaque. NKT cells may also be activated by lipid antigens presented by CD1 molecules on antigen presenting cells leading to further release of inflammatory cytokines (Libby et al. 2009; Tupin et al. 2004).

The improved understanding of inflammation as a mediator of CVD has also proven to be clinically beneficial (Libby et al. 2009; Van Gaal et al. 2006). Indeed, measurement of CRP as a marker of inflammation has proven to be a strong predictor of prognosis and guide of therapeutic choices. As shown by the PROVE-IT (TIMI-22) trial, CRP less than 2 mg/L along with cholesterol profile was predictive of statin treatment benefit (Ridker et al. 2005). Further, the JUPITER trial showed significant benefits to statin therapy for patients previously classified as "low risk" (e.g., Framingham Risk Score less than 10 %) with CRP greater than 2 mg/dL (Ridker et al. 2009). Of note, the benefit for this group of "inflamed" patients (e.g., patients with hsCRP >2) was so large that the trial was stopped prematurely as a 44 % reduction in vascular events was observed, making withholding of statin therapy from the placebo group unethical.

Taken together, inflammation and metabolic dysfunction both independently and synergistically promote CVD through several pathways. They are both also predictive of prognosis and treatment response (Libby et al. 2009; Van Gaal et al. 2006; Wang et al. 2014).

14.6 Inflammation Promotes Mood Dysfunction

Inflammatory dysregulation has been increasingly recognized as a mechanism subserving the etiology and pathophysiology of MDD and several other psychiatric and neuropsychiatric disorders (Rosenblat et al. 2014; McNamara and Lotrich 2012). Inflammation was first recognized as a potential pathogenic factor in mental illness by Julius Wagner-Jauregg of the University of Vienna in 1887, affording him the opportunity to be the only psychiatrist to ever win a Nobel Prize in 1927 (Raju 1998). The study of inflammation (or "fever" as previously described) and MDD was largely abandoned for decades with the advent of monoaminergic antidepressants, which provided the satisfactory serotonin hypothesis, thus blunting the investigation of other potential pathogenic pathways (Lopez-Munoz and Alamo 2009). The role of inflammation in mood symptoms was revisited with the observation that the psychological and psychomotor symptomatology of acutely medically ill patients was similar to that of MDD patients (e.g., sick patients had lethargy, decreased motivation, decreased socializing, depressed mood, anxiety, loss of appetite, sleep disturbances, hyperalgesia, reduction in self-care, and impaired concentration and attention) a phenomenon later referred to as "sickness behavior" (Kent et al. 1992; Hart 1988).

"Sickness behavior" has also been observed in chronic medical illness, most notably inflammatory disorders (Rosenblat et al. 2014). Further, MDD has been associated with elevated rates of inflammatory medical comorbidities and vice versa (Rosenblat et al. 2014; McNamara and Lotrich 2012; Miller et al. 2009). Autoimmune diseases serve as a prototypic group of disorders known to induce a pro-inflammatory state and thus would be expected to be associated with MDD via the inflammatory-mood pathway. Indeed, several autoimmune disorders including psoriasis, rheumatoid arthritis (RA), inflammatory bowel disease (IBD), and systemic lupus erythematosus (SLE) have been strongly associated with MDD with increased frequency of mood episode during inflammatory flare-ups (Weigle and McBane 2013; Covic et al. 2012; Frol et al. 2013; Liu et al. 2012b; Mok et al. 2012; Nicassio et al. 2012; Sato et al. 2013; Palagini et al. 2013; Graff et al. 2009; Walker et al. 2011). Of note, even more benign inflammatory conditions such as asthma and allergies have been shown to have an elevated prevalence of MDD (Ahmedani et al. 2013;

Loerbroks et al. 2012; Nathan 2007; Peltzer and Phaswana-Mafuya 2013; Sharma et al. 2013; Wilczynska-Kwiatek et al. 2009).

As previously discussed, CVD, obesity and diabetes have also been recognized as inflammatory disorders (Soczynska et al. 2011; McElroy and Keck 2012; McElroy et al. 2004; Morriss and Mohammed 2005). Indeed, elevated rates of these conditions as well are found in the MDD population and vice versa indicative of a potential bidirectional interaction (Mansur et al. 2014; McIntyre et al. 2013; Soczynska et al. 2011). Taken together, the association between MDD and inflammatory comorbidities suggests a potential bidirectional interaction between MDD and inflammatory dysregulation; however, this observation alone does not prove causation or aid in understanding the directionality of the interaction. In support of a causative interaction, however, are preliminary reports showing the ability of anti-inflammatory treatment of autoimmune disorders to decrease symptomatology in this group (Krishnan et al. 2007; Tyring et al. 2006). For example, anti-inflammatory treatments (specifically anti-TNF-alpha agents) of psoriasis have been shown to decrease depression scores independent of psoriasis severity (Krishnan et al. 2007; Tyring et al. 2006).

To further establish causation, rather than simply an observed association, preclinical and clinical studies have assessed mood symptoms in response to an induced inflammatory state. In preclinical models, numerous studies have induced an inflammatory state by administering lipopolysaccharide (LPS) and/or IL-1 (Dunn et al. 2005). These animal studies have reproducibly demonstrated the induction of depressive symptomatology, including lethargy, anorexia, decreased interest in exploring, decreased sexual activity, and increased sleep (reviewed by Dunn et al. 2005).

Clinically, in the treatment of hepatitis C, IFN is often used to boost the immune system to aid in the defense against the viral infection (Liang and Ghany 2013). After initiation of IFN therapy, 25–80 % (depending on the dose) of individuals developed a MDE (Alavi et al. 2012; Birerdinc et al. 2012; Raison et al. 2005; Udina et al. 2012). Cancer patients have also been observed to develop depressive symptoms after administration of immune boosting therapies including IFN and IL-2 (Capuron et al. 2000, 2001, 2002, 2003, 2004; Eller et al. 2009).

In healthy individuals, inflammation has also been induced through administration of LPS, vaccinations, endotoxins, IFN, and IL-2. Reproducibly, symptoms of decreased mood, anxiety, appetite changes, and impaired memory and attention in the absence of fever or physical symptoms have been demonstrated in healthy volunteers (Reichenberg et al. 2001; Wright et al. 2005; Brydon et al. 2009; Strike et al. 2004; Grigoleit et al. 2011). A dose response has also been demonstrated with LPS revealing that an increase in LPS dose (and subsequent measured increase in serum inflammatory cytokines) was associated with increased depressive symptomatology (Grigoleit et al. 2011).

The interaction between MDD and inflammatory dysfunction has been further established by studies investigating the profile of inflammatory cytokine levels both peripherally (in blood serum) and centrally (in cerebral spinal fluid (CSF)). Elevated levels of pro-inflammatory cytokines including but not limited to prostaglandin E2

(PGE2), CRP, TNF-α, IL-1β, IL-2, IL-6, and MCP-1 have been repeatedly shown peripherally and centrally in MDD (Danner et al. 2003; Dowlati et al. 2010; Felger and Lotrich 2013; Miller et al. 2013; Ford and Erlinger 2004; Kling et al. 2007; Kop et al. 2002; Lanquillon et al. 2000; Lieb et al. 1983; Linnoila et al. 1983; Zorrilla et al. 2001; Young et al. 2014). In a recent meta-analysis, 29 studies were identified evaluating cytokine levels in MDD (Liu et al. 2012a). The most significantly elevated cytokines in MDD serum, when compared to healthy controls, were IL-6, TNF-α, and soluble interleukin-2 receptors (sIL-2R) (Liu et al. 2012a).

Another question of debate has been whether cytokine levels are chronically elevated in MDD or only during acute mood episode. The debate has continued as some investigators have suggested that pro-inflammatory cytokines are only present during major depressive episodes (MDE) while others have shown continued elevation during periods of remission (Young et al. 2014; Miller et al. 2009). Of note, in a meta-analysis evaluating cytokine levels after antidepressant treatments, resolution of depressive symptoms was associated with reduced levels of IL-1β and possibly IL-6; however, TNF-α remained elevated (Hannestad et al. 2011).

Further analysis of cytokine studies has also revealed that it is likely a subpopulation of MDD that has elevation of inflammatory cytokines, suggesting that inflammation is likely a pathogenic factor only in a subset of MDD cases (Miller et al. 2009; Raison and Miller 2013; Raison et al. 2013). This important observation has immense implications for the use of cytokines as biomarkers in future studies and treatment interventions. Indeed, Raison et al. (2013) found anti-TNF-α therapy to only have antidepressant effects for a subgroup of patients with an elevated CRP indicative of an inflammatory state (Raison et al. 2013). Therefore, future studies of anti-inflammatory agents for antidepressant use may require the use of inflammatory biomarkers to allow for valid results including only the treatment group of interest (e.g., a subgroup of "inflammatory depression").

Inflammatory cytokines have also been found to be key signaling molecules in the inflammatory-mood pathway, rather than only serving as "innocent bystanders" of inflammation (Young et al. 2014; Miller et al. 2009, 2013). Indeed, cytokines play an active role in the pathogenic mechanism by which inflammation may interact with mood alteration, inducing and propagating neuroinflammation and promoting the signaling cascade subserving the inflammatory-mood pathway to be described in turn (Boutzios and Kaltsas 2000; Dantzer et al. 2008; Dowlati et al. 2010).

Pro-inflammatory cytokines including, but not limited to TNF-α, IL-2, IL-6, and IFN have been shown to directly alter monoamine levels, serving as a potential mechanism for mood alteration. Specifically, IL-2 and IFN directly increase the enzymatic activity of indolamine 2,3-dioxygenase (IDO) that in turn catalyzes the breakdown of tryptophan-to-tryptophan catabolites (TRYCATs), namely, kynurenine, kynurenic acid, and quinolinic acid (Dunn et al. 2005; Rosenblat et al. 2014). This reaction may lead to mood symptoms through two separate pathways: (1) through depletion of tryptophan, production of serotonin is decreased, a well-established feature of MDD pathophysiology (Arango et al. 2002; Barton et al. 2008; Rosa-Neto et al. 2004; Vaswani et al. 2003) and (2) TRYCATs also have direct and independent depressogenic and anxiogenic effects (Maes et al. 2011).

Pro-inflammatory cytokines IL-6 and TNF-α modulate monoamine levels through a separate pathway by increasing the breakdown of serotonin to 5-hydroxyindoleacetic acid (5-HIAA) (Wang and Dunn 1998; Zhang et al. 2001). Taken together, pro-inflammatory cytokines may induce mood symptoms by promoting the depletion of tryptophan, the breakdown of serotonin, and the production of TRYCATs.

Pro-inflammatory cytokines TNF-α and IL-1β also activate microglial cells centrally, the macrophages of the central nervous system (Harry and Kraft 2012; Kraft and Harry 2011). Activated macrophages also release TNF-α to increase neuroinflammation and activate other macrophages locally (Frick et al. 2013). Under physiologic conditions, microglia play an essential role in neuroplasticity and synaptic pruning (Kraft and Harry 2011). Activated microglia facilitate destruction of unused synapses to allow for increased capacity of synapses and circuits more frequently used, leading to increased functional connectivity of key brain circuitry (Harry and Kraft 2012). However, when microglia become pathologically overactive, microglia may lead to oxidative and nitrosative stress, over-pruning, and induction of neuronal damage. The net effect of microglial over-activation would therefore be neurodegeneration, aberrant neuronal apoptosis, and impaired neuroplasticity leading to dysfunctional neural circuits resulting in impaired function at the level of cognition, mood, and behavior (Frick et al. 2013; Ekdahl 2012; Harry and Kraft 2012; Rosenblat et al. 2014). The over-activation of microglia may also prevent neurogenesis and new synapse formation, thus further limiting neuroplasticity and the ability for the brain to adapt effectively.

Of note, current evidence suggests that while microglia may play an important role in the pathogenesis of MDD, idiopathic microglia activation does not appear to be the first step in the cascade (Frick et al. 2013). The over-activation of microglia and resultant downward spiral may be initiated from increased levels of pro-inflammatory cytokines peripherally which may traverse the blood-brain barrier (BBB) and over-activate microglia inappropriately. Once activated, the microglia may release more cytokines and further activate other microglia in a feed-forward loop in the absence of adequate anti-inflammatory signaling (Stertz et al. 2013; Frick et al. 2013).

Given that the microglia hypothesis suggests that overactive microglia impact the structure and function of brain regions subserving affective symptoms, several imaging studies have been conducted with the hypothesis that inflammation would be associated with decreased volume and functional connectivity in key brain regions. Indeed, several investigators have found inflammation to be associated with structural and functional brain changes, such as lateral ventricular enlargement, alterations in subgenual cingulate activity, and decreased mesolimbic connectivity, all of which have also been implicated in the pathogenesis of mood disorders (Harrison et al. 2009; Kempton et al. 2011; Miller et al. 2013).

Recently, the strongest evidence for aberrant microglial activation in MDD was reported by Setiawan et al. (2015) showing increased microglial activation in the anterior cingulate cortex (ACC), prefrontal cortex (PFC), and insula in patients with a current MDE compared to healthy controls. This study was the first to use positron emission tomography (PET) imaging to show increased translocator protein density measured by distribution volume (TSPO VT), a marker of activated microglia, in MDD (Setiawan et al. 2015). Prior to this study, there was often question of the validity of correlating peripheral serum or even central CSF cytokine levels to presumed microglial activation in key brain regions. Identifying over-activation of microglia in the ACC, PFC, and insula, key brain regions for mood and cognition, certainly adds validity to the microglial hypothesis of mood disorders. While this study was a preliminary report (MDD patients $n=20$, healthy controls $n=20$) requiring replication, the results greatly add to the assumptions often made when describing the inflammatory-mood hypothesis.

Another inflammatory pathway to consider is the HPA axis. As previously discussed, pro-inflammatory cytokines potently increase HPA activity. Therefore, continued production of inflammatory cytokines may lead to continued production of cortisol, a potent mood-altering steroid implicated in the production of "sickness behavior" (Murphy 1991). Cortisol may also alter monoamine levels through increasing hepatic tryptophan 2,3-dioxygenase (TDO) activity, thereby increasing the breakdown of tryptophan to TRYCATs (Hoes and Sijben 1981; Maes et al. 2011).

14.7 Metabolic Dysfunction Promotes Mood Dysfunction

Metabolic dysfunction has a bidirectional interaction with MDD; a strong correlation between insulin resistance, obesity, and MDD has been well established (Kan et al. 2013; Kaidanovich-Beilin et al. 2012; Barnard et al. 2006). Epidemiological data is particularly strong for showing an association between MDD and type II diabetes mellitus (T2DM) (Kan et al. 2013; Kaidanovich-Beilin et al. 2012; Barnard et al. 2006). Indeed, the risk of developing MDD is increased after the onset of T2DM or impaired glucose tolerance (IGT) (Knol et al. 2006; Mezuk et al. 2008). Moreover, the presence of MDEs increases the risk of developing T2DM later in life (Knol et al. 2006; Mezuk et al. 2008). Comorbid MDD is also associated with an early onset of T2DM (e.g., on average 5 years earlier), worse prognosis, poor glycemic control, and lower adherence to medical and lifestyle management plans (Kan et al. 2013; Lustman et al. 2000; de Groot et al. 2001).

Several mechanisms have been investigated which may subserve this interaction (Kaidanovich-Beilin et al. 2012). As discussed, metabolic dysfunction may directly induce, and be induced by, inflammatory dysfunction. Therefore, metabolic dysfunction may induce mood symptoms through the previously described inflammatory-mood pathway. Other etiological and pathophysiological factors of interest are the effects of shared psychosocial risk factors, the presence of microangiopathic changes, and the development of CNS insulin resistance converging on the common pathway of impaired neuroplasticity leading to depressive symptomatology (Kaidanovich-Beilin et al. 2012).

Epidemiological studies provide evidence for low socioeconomic status (SES), early childhood adversity, medical comorbidities, addiction, and psychiatric comorbidities as being common risk factors for obesity, T2DM, and MDD (Zhou et al.

2010; Dallman et al. 2003; Teegarden and Bale 2007; Anderson et al. 2001; Everson et al. 2002; Talbot and Nouwen 2000). Therefore, one potential explanation for the observed association may be common psychosocial etiologic factors (Kaidanovich-Beilin et al. 2012). Indeed, certain life circumstances may predispose individuals to the development of obesity, insulin resistance, and MDD. While these psychosocial risk factors may certainly account for part of the observed association, controlling for these factors reveals that they do not account for the entire observed effect (de Groot et al. 2001; Kan et al. 2013; Lustman et al. 2000; Mezuk et al. 2008; Vancampfort et al. 2013). Biological metabolic-neuronal mechanisms, particularly the effect of CNS insulin resistance, metabolic inflammation, and the effect of microangiopathic changes, may certainly play an independent and synergistic role in the etiology and pathophysiology of comorbid MDD, obesity, and insulin resistance (Kaidanovich-Beilin et al. 2012).

Diabetes is strongly associated with both microvascular (nephropathy, neuropathy, retinopathy) and macrovascular (stroke, myocardial infarction) complications (Kahn and Joslin 2005). Diabetes and MDD are also associated with microangiopathic changes in the brain, independent of large vessel disease (Bourdel-Marchasson et al. 2010; Nelson et al. 2009). Microangiopathic changes may induce depressive symptoms through multiple mechanisms. Decreased blood flow to key brain regions subserving mood and cognition (e.g., the amygdala, hippocampus, anterior cingulate cortex, and prefrontal cortex) may directly impair neuronal function in these regions leading to affective and cognitive dysfunction, key features of MDD (Bourdel-Marchasson et al. 2010; Nelson et al. 2009; Direk et al. 2012). Microangiopathic changes also increase inflammation and thus may induce depressive symptoms through the previously described mechanisms (Li et al. 2014). Therefore, microangiopathic changes may be one mechanism facilitating the interaction between metabolic dysfunction, CVD, and MDD.

The effects of insulin in the brain have also been of great interest. With the discovery of insulin receptors in numerous brain regions, the previous understanding that insulin had no effect on the brain has now been abolished (Banks et al. 2012; Bingham et al. 2002; Craft and Watson 2004). Insulin receptors have been identified in the hypothalamus, cerebral cortex, olfactory bulb, substantia nigra, basal ganglia, hippocampus, and amygdala (Banks et al. 2012). To enter the central nervous system (CNS), insulin produced in the pancreas is transported across the BBB via a saturable, receptor-mediated process (Woods et al. 2003). Once in the CNS, insulin acts as a trophic factor, facilitating glucose uptake in specific regions as well as promoting neurogenesis and neuroplasticity (McIntyre et al. 2008; Banks et al. 2012).

Type 2 diabetes mellitus is characterized by hyperglycemia, insulin resistance with compensatory hyperinsulinemia, and subsequent pancreatic decompensation causing a relative hypoinsulinemia in later stages (Kahn and Joslin 2005). Chronic hyperinsulinemia may downregulate the transport of insulin across the BBB (Woods et al. 2003). Consequentially, CNS insulin levels may be decreased. As previously discussed, CNS insulin is an important trophic factor promoting neuroplasticity in key brain regions. Therefore, in the setting of T2DM, CNS insulin level may be decreased secondary to BBB receptor downregulation.

While the majority of glucose uptake in the brain is insulin independent, certain regions also have insulin dependent glucose uptake (McNay et al. 2010; McNay and Recknagel 2011; Henneberg and Hoyer 1994; Hoyer et al. 1996; Bingham et al. 2002). In the presence of insulin resistance and decreased CNS insulin, there may be decreased uptake in these regions. Notably, in the context of MDD, Glut4 receptors in the hippocampus, amygdala, and prefrontal cortex may have decreased glucose uptake secondary to insulin resistance and thus impaired function in these regions (Reagan 2005). Indeed, in animal models of insulin resistance, decreased glucose uptake in the hippocampus has been observed (Winocur and Greenwood 2005; Winocur et al. 2005).

In addition to facilitating the uptake of glucose, CNS insulin serves as a direct trophic factor via the phosphoinositide-3 kinase (PI3) pathways, promoting the production and release of several growth factors including brain-derived neurotrophic factor (BDNF) and vascular endothelial growth factor (VEGF) (Rodgers and Theibert 2002; Scheid and Woodgett 2003), thereby promoting neuronal survival, synaptogenesis, and dendritic arborization (McIntyre et al. 2008). Similarly, long-term potentiation cascades, important for learning, memory, and adaptability, are promoted by insulin (Skeberdis et al. 2001; van der Heide et al. 2005).

In summary, insulin acts as a growth factor and mediator of glucose uptake in key brain regions subserving affective and cognitive functioning. In the setting of insulin resistance and decreased CNS insulin levels, decreased glucose uptake and decreased growth factor signaling ultimately lead to impaired neurogenesis and neuroplasticity, a key pathophysiological mechanisms of MDD (Kaidanovich-Beilin et al. 2012).

14.8 Therapeutic and Preventative Implications

Understanding the metabolic-inflammatory pathways subserving the pathophysiology of MDD and CVD may provide insight into novel therapeutic and preventative strategies. Several strategies are simple and may be readily implemented, while others are more theoretical, requiring more research before reaching clinical application.

Improved screening practice is one simple intervention. Given the high co-prevalence of MDD and CVD, screening for MDD in the CVD population and vice versa are merited and, in the presence of signs of metabolic and/or inflammatory dysfunction, provide even greater merit for improved screening in such patients. Improved screening may result in early detection and treatment and thus improved outcomes for both CVD and MDD.

From a cardiovascular health perspective, exercise and a healthy diet have long been emphasized (Topp et al. 2004). Applying the same vigor to encouraging MDD patients to pursue physical activity may greatly improve outcomes as exercise has been repeatedly shown to have a positive effect on mood and cognition in MDD (Baldwin 2010; Beavers et al. 2010; Carek et al. 2011; Conn 2010a, b; Cooney et al. 2013; Fenton and Stover 2006). Similarly, with metabolic dysfunction and T2DM in specific, lifestyle modification has long been a part of first-line therapy with clear effects on cognition and mood (Nolan et al. 2011; Fiocco et al. 2013; Anderson-Hanley et al. 2012). Therefore, lifestyle modification should be emphasized from a mental health perspective, rather than only for its cardiovascular benefits.

Novel treatments targeting the metabolic-inflammatory pathway may yield improved MDD and CVD outcomes in the future; however, further research is still required in this area prior to making clinical recommendations. Repurposing of antidiabetic and anti-inflammatory agents in the treatment of MDD has been of particular interest (Rosenblat et al. 2014; Mansur et al. 2015; McIntyre et al. 2007, 2008, 2013; McIntyre 2014).

Several antidiabetic agents have become of interest as novel treatments of MDD (Kaidanovich-Beilin et al. 2012; McIntyre et al. 2007, 2008, 2013). Increasing insulin sensitivity centrally may allow for increased effects of insulin on the brain, increasing glucose uptake, neurogenesis and neuroplasticity through the previously described mechanisms. As previously discussed, CNS insulin plays a key role in brain function. Therefore, intranasal insulin is currently being investigated in MDD for its affect on mood and cognition (clinicaltrials.gov – NCT00570050, trial completed, results pending). The antidiabetic agents thiazolidinediones (TZDs) and incretins have also been of interest; however, further studies are required (Seaquist et al. 2013; McIntyre et al. 2007, 2013).

Anti-inflammatory agents have also become of great interest in the novel treatment of MDD. In a recent meta-analysis, Kohler et al. (2014) identified 14 trials assessing the efficacy of anti-inflammatory agents on MDD. They found that anti-inflammatory agents decreased depressive symptoms while not increasing the risk of adverse events. Included in the analysis were cytokine inhibitors and NSAIDS. Of the agents assessed, celecoxib had the greatest effect (Kohler et al. 2014). Of note, excluded from the meta-analysis were omega-3 polyunsaturated fatty acids (O-3 PUFAs). In a separate meta-analysis of nineteen clinical trials, O-3 PUFAs were shown to have a significant anti-inflammatory and anti-depressive effect and were extremely well tolerated when used adjunctively to standard therapy for MDD (McNamara and Strawn 2013; Su et al. 2013; Grosso et al. 2014).

Taken together, several novel treatments targeting the metabolic-inflammatory pathway are currently being investigated in the treatment of MDD. Future research is still needed in this area prior to the routine clinical usage of these novel agents. Currently, simple strategies that may have great benefit include improved screening and increased physical activity in CVD and MDD patients.

Conclusion

Metabolic and inflammatory dysfunctions are two intimately connected processes with convergent pathways. The metabolic-inflammatory pathway is a key substrate subserving the well-established association between CVD and MDD. The metabolic-inflammatory pathways potently increase CVD risk through a variety of mechanisms. Similarly, metabolic and inflammatory dysfunction independently and synergistically increases risk of developing and perpetuating MDD. Given the currently high and ever-increasing prevalence, morbidity, and mortality of CVD and MDD, understanding their pathophysiology is highly relevant.

Further understanding the metabolic-inflammatory-mood pathway may provide insight to future treatments and preventative strategies for comorbid CVD and MDD. Improved screening and increased physical activity are two methods that may be implemented as preventative strategies. Anti-inflammatory and antidiabetic medications may be repurposed as novel treatments of MDD and CVD through targeting the metabolic-inflammatory pathway; however, further research is still needed to elucidate efficacy and tolerability in this patient population prior to clinical recommendation.

References

Abbas AK, Lichtman AH, Pillai S (2012) Cellular and molecular immunology. Elsevier Saunders, Philadelphia

Abeywardena MY, Leifert WR, Warnes KE, Varghese JN, Head RJ (2009) Cardiovascular biology of interleukin-6. Curr Pharm Des 15:1809–1821

Ahmedani BK, Peterson EL, Wells KE, Williams LK (2013) Examining the relationship between depression and asthma exacerbations in a prospective follow-up study. Psychosom Med 75:305–310

Alavi M, Grebely J, Matthews GV, Petoumenos K, Yeung B, Day C, Lloyd AR, Van Beek I, Kaldor JM, Hellard M, Dore GJ, Haber PS, ATAHC Study Group (2012) Effect of pegylated interferon-alpha-2a treatment on mental health during recent hepatitis C virus infection. J Gastroenterol Hepatol 27:957–965

Anderson RJ, Freedland KE, Clouse RE, Lustman PJ (2001) The prevalence of comorbid depression in adults with diabetes: a meta-analysis. Diabetes Care 24:1069–1078

Anderson-Hanley C, Arciero PJ, Westen SC, Nimon J, Zimmerman E (2012) Neuropsychological benefits of stationary bike exercise and a cybercycle exergame for older adults with diabetes: an exploratory analysis. J Diabetes Sci Technol 6:849–857

Andrade L, Caraveo-Anduaga JJ, Berglund P, Bijl RV, De Graaf R, Vollebergh W, Dragomirecka E, Kohn R, Keller M, Kessler RC, Kawakami N, Kilic C, Offord D, Ustun TB, Wittchen HU (2003) The epidemiology of major depressive episodes: results from the International Consortium of Psychiatric Epidemiology (ICPE) Surveys. Int J Methods Psychiatr Res 12:3–21

Arango V, Underwood MD, Mann JJ (2002) Serotonin brain circuits involved in major depression and suicide. Prog Brain Res 136:443–453

Baldwin RC (2010) Preventing late-life depression: a clinical update. Int Psychogeriatr/IPA 22:1216–1224

Banks WA, Owen JB, Erickson MA (2012) Insulin in the brain: there and back again. Pharmacol Ther 136:82–93

Barnard KD, Skinner TC, Peveler R (2006) The prevalence of co-morbid depression in adults with Type 1 diabetes: systematic literature review. Diabet Med: J Br Diab Assoc 23:445–448

Barth J, Schumacher M, Herrmann-Lingen C (2004) Depression as a risk factor for mortality in patients with coronary heart disease: a meta-analysis. Psychosom Med 66:802–813

Barton DA, Esler MD, Dawood T, Lambert EA, Haikerwal D, Brenchley C, Socratous F, Hastings J, Guo L, Wiesner G, Kaye DM, Bayles R, Schlaich MP, Lambert GW (2008) Elevated brain serotonin turnover in patients with depression: effect of genotype and therapy. Arch Gen Psychiatry 65:38–46

Beavers KM, Brinkley TE, Nicklas BJ (2010) Effect of exercise training on chronic inflammation. Clin Chim Acta; Int J Clin Chem 411:785–793

Beishuizen A, Thijs LG (2003) Endotoxin and the hypothalamo-pituitary-adrenal (HPA) axis. J Endotoxin Res 9:3–24

Bingham EM, Hopkins D, Smith D, Pernet A, Hallett W, Reed L, Marsden PK, Amiel SA (2002) The role of insulin in human brain glucose metabolism: an 18fluoro-deoxyglucose positron emission tomography study. Diabetes 51:3384–3390

Birerdinc A, Afendy A, Stepanova M, Younossi I, Baranova A, Younossi ZM (2012) Gene expression profiles associated with depression in patients with chronic hepatitis C (CH-C). Brain Behav 2:525–531

Bourdel-Marchasson I, Mouries A, Helmer C (2010) Hyperglycaemia, microangiopathy, diabetes and dementia risk. Diabetes Metab 36(Suppl 3):S112–S118

Boutzios G, Kaltsas G (2000) Immune system effects on the endocrine system. In: De Groot LJ, Beck-Peccoz P, Chrousos G, Dungan K, Grossman A, Hershman JM, Koch C, Mclachlan R, New M, Rebar R, Singer F, Vinik A, Weickert MO (eds) Endotext. South Dartmouth. http://www.ncbi.nlm.nih.gov/pubmed/25905362

Brydon L, Walker C, Wawrzyniak A, Whitehead D, Okamura H, Yajima J, Tsuda A, Steptoe A (2009) Synergistic effects of psychological and immune stressors on inflammatory cytokine and sickness responses in humans. Brain Behav Immun 23:217–224

Capuron L, Ravaud A, Dantzer R (2000) Early depressive symptoms in cancer patients receiving interleukin 2 and/or interferon alfa-2b therapy. J Clin Oncol: Off J Am Soc Clin Oncol 18:2143–2151

Capuron L, Ravaud A, Gualde N, Bosmans E, Dantzer R, Maes M, Neveu PJ (2001) Association between immune activation and early depressive symptoms in cancer patients treated with interleukin-2-based therapy. Psychoneuroendocrinology 26:797–808

Capuron L, Ravaud A, Neveu PJ, Miller AH, Maes M, Dantzer R (2002) Association between decreased serum tryptophan concentrations and depressive symptoms in cancer patients undergoing cytokine therapy. Mol Psychiatry 7:468–473

Capuron L, Neurauter G, Musselman DL, Lawson DH, Nemeroff CB, Fuchs D, Miller AH (2003) Interferon-alpha-induced changes in tryptophan metabolism. Relationship to depression and paroxetine treatment. Biol Psychiatry 54:906–914

Capuron L, Ravaud A, Miller AH, Dantzer R (2004) Baseline mood and psychosocial characteristics of patients developing depressive symptoms during interleukin-2 and/or interferon-alpha cancer therapy. Brain Behav Immun 18:205–213

Carek PJ, Laibstain SE, Carek SM (2011) Exercise for the treatment of depression and anxiety. Int J Psychiatry Med 41:15–28

Charlson FJ, Stapelberg NJ, Baxter AJ, Whiteford HA (2011) Should global burden of disease estimates include depression as a risk factor for coronary heart disease? BMC Med 9:47

Conn VS (2010a) Anxiety outcomes after physical activity interventions: meta-analysis findings. Nurs Res 59:224–231

Conn VS (2010b) Depressive symptom outcomes of physical activity interventions: meta-analysis findings. Ann Behav Med: Publ Soc Behav Med 39:128–138

Cooney GM, Dwan K, Greig CA, Lawlor DA, Rimer J, Waugh FR, McMurdo M, Mead GE (2013) Exercise for depression. Cochrane Database Syst Rev 9:CD004366

Covic T, Cumming SR, Pallant JF, Manolios N, Emery P, Conaghan PG, Tennant A (2012) Depression and anxiety in patients with rheumatoid arthritis: prevalence rates based on a comparison of the Depression, Anxiety and Stress Scale (DASS) and the hospital, Anxiety and Depression Scale (HADS). BMC Psychiatry 12:6. doi:10.1186/1471-244X-12-6

Craft S, Watson GS (2004) Insulin and neurodegenerative disease: shared and specific mechanisms. Lancet Neurol 3:169–178

Dallman MF, Pecoraro N, Akana SF, La Fleur SE, Gomez F, Houshyar H, Bell ME, Bhatnagar S, Laugero KD, Manalo S (2003) Chronic stress and obesity: a new view of "comfort food". Proc Natl Acad Sci U S A 100:11696–11701

Danaei G, Ding EL, Mozaffarian D, Taylor B, Rehm J, Murray CJ, Ezzati M (2009) The preventable causes of death in the United States: comparative risk assessment of dietary, lifestyle, and metabolic risk factors. PLoS Med 6:e1000058

Danner M, Kasl SV, Abramson JL, Vaccarino V (2003) Association between depression and elevated C-reactive protein. Psychosom Med 65:347–356
Dantzer R, O'Connor JC, Freund GG, Johnson RW, Kelley KW (2008) From inflammation to sickness and depression: when the immune system subjugates the brain. Nat Rev Neurosci 9:46–56
de Groot M, Anderson R, Freedland KE, Clouse RE, Lustman PJ (2001) Association of depression and diabetes complications: a meta-analysis. Psychosom Med 63:619–630
Direk N, Koudstaal PJ, Hofman A, Ikram MA, Hoogendijk WJ, Tiemeier H (2012) Cerebral hemodynamics and incident depression: the Rotterdam Study. Biol Psychiatry 72:318–323
Dowlati Y, Herrmann N, Swardfager W, Liu H, Sham L, Reim EK, Lanctot KL (2010) A meta-analysis of cytokines in major depression. Biol Psychiatry 67:446–457
Dunn AJ, Swiergiel AH, de Beaurepaire R (2005) Cytokines as mediators of depression: what can we learn from animal studies? Neurosci Biobehav Rev 29:891–909
Ekdahl CT (2012) Microglial activation – tuning and pruning adult neurogenesis. Front Pharmacol 3:41
Elderon L, Whooley MA (2013) Depression and cardiovascular disease. Prog Cardiovasc Dis 55:511–523
Eller T, Vasar V, Shlik J, Maron E (2009) The role of IL-2 and soluble IL-2R in depression and antidepressant response. Curr Opin Investig Drugs (London, England: 2000) 10:638–643
Everson SA, Maty SC, Lynch JW, Kaplan GA (2002) Epidemiologic evidence for the relation between socioeconomic status and depression, obesity, and diabetes. J Psychosom Res 53:891–895
Felger JC, Lotrich FE (2013) Inflammatory cytokines in depression: neurobiological mechanisms and therapeutic implications. Neuroscience 246:199–229
Fenton WS, Stover ES (2006) Mood disorders: cardiovascular and diabetes comorbidity. Curr Opin Psychiatry 19:421–427
Fiocco AJ, Scarcello S, Marzolini S, Chan A, Oh P, Proulx G, Greenwood C (2013) The effects of an exercise and lifestyle intervention program on cardiovascular, metabolic factors and cognitive performance in middle-aged adults with type II diabetes: a pilot study. Can J Diabet 37:214–219
Ford DE, Erlinger TP (2004) Depression and C-reactive protein in US adults: data from the Third National Health and Nutrition Examination Survey. Arch Intern Med 164:1010–1014
Frick LR, Williams K, Pittenger C (2013) Microglial dysregulation in psychiatric disease. Clin Dev Immunol 2013:608654
Frol AB, Vasquez A, Getahun Y, Pacheco M, Khan DA, Brown ES (2013) A comparison of clinician-rated neuropsychological and self-rated cognitive assessments in patients with asthma and rheumatologic disorders. Allergy Asthma Proc: Off J Reg State Allergy Soc 34:170–175
Gans RO (2006) The metabolic syndrome, depression, and cardiovascular disease: interrelated conditions that share pathophysiologic mechanisms. Med Clin North Am 90:573–591
Ghattas A, Griffiths HR, Devitt A, Lip GY, Shantsila E (2013) Monocytes in coronary artery disease and atherosclerosis: where are we now? J Am Coll Cardiol 62:1541–1551
Go AS, Mozaffarian D, Roger VL, Benjamin EJ, Berry JD, Borden WB, Bravata DM, Dai S, Ford ES, Fox CS, Franco S, Fullerton HJ, Gillespie C, Hailpern SM, Heit JA, Howard VJ, Huffman MD, Kissela BM, Kittner SJ, Lackland DT, Lichtman JH, Lisabeth LD, Magid D, Marcus GM, Marelli A, Matchar DB, McGuire DK, Mohler ER, Moy CS, Mussolino ME, Nichol G, Paynter NP, Schreiner PJ, Sorlie PD, Stein J, Turan TN, Virani SS, Wong ND, Woo D, Turner MB, American Heart Association Statistics Committee, Stroke Statistics Subcommittee (2013) Heart disease and stroke statistics – 2013 update: a report from the American Heart Association. Circulation 127:e6–e245
Graff LA, Walker JR, Bernstein CN (2009) Depression and anxiety in inflammatory bowel disease: a review of comorbidity and management. Inflamm Bowel Dis 15:1105–1118
Grenon SM, Hiramoto J, Smolderen KG, Vittinghoff E, Whooley MA, Cohen BE (2012) Association between depression and peripheral artery disease: insights from the heart and soul study. J Am Heart Assoc 1:e002667

Grigoleit JS, Kullmann JS, Wolf OT, Hammes F, Wegner A, Jablonowski S, Engler H, Gizewski E, Oberbeck R, Schedlowski M (2011) Dose-dependent effects of endotoxin on neurobehavioral functions in humans. PLoS One 6:e28330

Grinevich V, Ma XM, Herman JP, Jezova D, Akmayev I, Aguilera G (2001) Effect of repeated lipopolysaccharide administration on tissue cytokine expression and hypothalamic-pituitary-adrenal axis activity in rats. J Neuroendocrinol 13:711–723

Grosso G, Pajak A, Marventano S, Castellano S, Galvano F, Bucolo C, Drago F, Caraci F (2014) Role of omega-3 fatty acids in the treatment of depressive disorders: a comprehensive meta-analysis of randomized clinical trials. PLoS One 9:e96905

Hannestad J, DellaGioia N, Bloch M (2011) The effect of antidepressant medication treatment on serum levels of inflammatory cytokines: a meta-analysis. Neuropsychopharmacology 36:2452–2459

Harrison NA, Brydon L, Walker C, Gray MA, Steptoe A, Critchley HD (2009) Inflammation causes mood changes through alterations in subgenual cingulate activity and mesolimbic connectivity. Biol Psychiatry 66:407–414

Harry GJ, Kraft AD (2012) Microglia in the developing brain: a potential target with lifetime effects. Neurotoxicology 33:191–206

Hart BL (1988) Biological basis of the behavior of sick animals. Neurosci Biobehav Rev 12:123–137

Henneberg N, Hoyer S (1994) Short-term or long-term intracerebroventricular (i.c.v.) infusion of insulin exhibits a discrete anabolic effect on cerebral energy metabolism in the rat. Neurosci Lett 175:153–156

Hoes MJ, Sijben N (1981) The clinical significance of disordered renal excretion of xanthurenic acid in depressive patients. Psychopharmacology (Berl) 75:346–349

Hoyer S, Henneberg N, Knapp S, Lannert H, Martin E (1996) Brain glucose metabolism is controlled by amplification and desensitization of the neuronal insulin receptor. Ann N Y Acad Sci 777:374–379

Kahn CR, Joslin EP (2005) Joslin's diabetes mellitus. Lippincott Williams & Willkins, Philadelphia

Kaidanovich-Beilin O, Cha DS, McIntyre RS (2012) Crosstalk between metabolic and neuropsychiatric disorders. F1000 Biol Rep 4:14–14, Epub 2012 Jul 2

Kan C, Silva N, Golden SH, Rajala U, Timonen M, Stahl D, Ismail K (2013) A systematic review and meta-analysis of the association between depression and insulin resistance. Diabetes Care 36:480–489

Kempton MJ, Salvador Z, Munafo MR, Geddes JR, Simmons A, Frangou S, Williams SC (2011) Structural neuroimaging studies in major depressive disorder. Meta-analysis and comparison with bipolar disorder. Arch Gen Psychiatry 68:675–690

Kent S, Bluthe RM, Kelley KW, Dantzer R (1992) Sickness behavior as a new target for drug development. Trends Pharmacol Sci 13:24–28

Kessler RC, Berglund P, Demler O, Jin R, Koretz D, Merikangas KR, Rush AJ, Walters EE, Wang PS, National Comorbidity Survey, R (2003) The epidemiology of major depressive disorder: results from the National Comorbidity Survey Replication (NCS-R). JAMA 289:3095–3105

Kessler RC, Akiskal HS, Ames M, Birnbaum H, Greenberg P, Hirschfeld RM, Jin R, Merikangas KR, Simon GE, Wang PS (2006) Prevalence and effects of mood disorders on work performance in a nationally representative sample of U.S. workers. Am J Psychiatry 163:1561–1568

Kling MA, Alesci S, Csako G, Costello R, Luckenbaugh DA, Bonne O, Duncko R, Drevets WC, Manji HK, Charney DS, Gold PW, Neumeister A (2007) Sustained low-grade pro-inflammatory state in unmedicated, remitted women with major depressive disorder as evidenced by elevated serum levels of the acute phase proteins C-reactive protein and serum amyloid A. Biol Psychiatry 62:309–313

Knol MJ, Twisk JW, Beekman AT, Heine RJ, Snoek FJ, Pouwer F (2006) Depression as a risk factor for the onset of type 2 diabetes mellitus. A meta-analysis. Diabetologia 49:837–845

Kohler O, Benros ME, Nordentoft M, Farkouh ME, Iyengar RL, Mors O, Krogh J (2014) Effect of anti-inflammatory treatment on depression, depressive symptoms, and adverse effects: a systematic review and meta-analysis of randomized clinical trials. JAMA Psychiatry 71:1381

Kop WJ, Gottdiener JS, Tangen CM, Fried LP, McBurnie MA, Walston J, Newman A, Hirsch C, Tracy RP (2002) Inflammation and coagulation factors in persons > 65 years of age with symptoms of depression but without evidence of myocardial ischemia. Am J Cardiol 89:419–424
Kraft AD, Harry GJ (2011) Features of microglia and neuroinflammation relevant to environmental exposure and neurotoxicity. Int J Environ Res Public Health 8:2980–3018
Krishnan R, Cella D, Leonardi C, Papp K, Gottlieb AB, Dunn M, Chiou CF, Patel V, Jahreis A (2007) Effects of etanercept therapy on fatigue and symptoms of depression in subjects treated for moderate to severe plaque psoriasis for up to 96 weeks. Br J Dermatol 157:1275–1277
Lanquillon S, Krieg JC, Bening-Abu-Shach U, Vedder H (2000) Cytokine production and treatment response in major depressive disorder. Neuropsychopharm: Off Publ Am Coll Neuropsychopharm 22:370–379
Li W, Ling S, Yang Y, Hu Z, Davies H, Fang M (2014) Systematic hypothesis for post-stroke depression caused inflammation and neurotransmission and resultant on possible treatments. Neuro Endocrinol Lett 35:104–109
Liang TJ, Ghany MG (2013) Current and future therapies for hepatitis C virus infection. N Engl J Med 368:1907–1917
Libby P, Ridker PM, Hansson GK, Leducq Transatlantic Network on, A (2009) Inflammation in atherosclerosis: from pathophysiology to practice. J Am Coll Cardiol 54:2129–2138
Lieb J, Karmali R, Horrobin D (1983) Elevated levels of prostaglandin E2 and thromboxane B2 in depression. Prostaglandins Leukot Med 10:361–367
Linnoila M, Whorton AR, Rubinow DR, Cowdry RW, Ninan PT, Waters RN (1983) CSF prostaglandin levels in depressed and schizophrenic patients. Arch Gen Psychiatry 40:405–406
Liu Y, Ho RC, Mak A (2012a) Interleukin (IL)-6, tumour necrosis factor alpha (TNF-alpha) and soluble interleukin-2 receptors (sIL-2R) are elevated in patients with major depressive disorder: a meta-analysis and meta-regression. J Affect Disord 139:230–239
Liu Y, Ho RC, Mak A (2012b) The role of interleukin (IL)-17 in anxiety and depression of patients with rheumatoid arthritis. Int J Rheum Dis 15:183–187
Loerbroks A, Herr RM, Subramanian S, Bosch JA (2012) The association of asthma and wheezing with major depressive episodes: an analysis of 245 727 women and men from 57 countries. Int J Epidemiol 41:1436–1444
Lopez-Munoz F, Alamo C (2009) Monoaminergic neurotransmission: the history of the discovery of antidepressants from 1950s until today. Curr Pharm Des 15:1563–1586
Lustman PJ, Anderson RJ, Freedland KE, de Groot M, Carney RM, Clouse RE (2000) Depression and poor glycemic control: a meta-analytic review of the literature. Diabetes Care 23:934–942
Lyngso D, Simonsen L, Bulow J (2002) Metabolic effects of interleukin-6 in human splanchnic and adipose tissue. J Physiol 543:379–386
Maes M, Leonard BE, Myint AM, Kubera M, Verkerk R (2011) The new '5-HT' hypothesis of depression: cell-mediated immune activation induces indoleamine 2,3-dioxygenase, which leads to lower plasma tryptophan and an increased synthesis of detrimental tryptophan catabolites (TRYCATs), both of which contribute to the onset of depression. Prog Neuropsychopharmacol Biol Psychiatry 35:702–721
Mansur RB, Cha DS, Woldeyohannes HO, Soczynska JK, Zugman A, Brietzke E, McIntyre RS (2014) Diabetes mellitus and disturbances in brain connectivity: a bidirectional relationship? Neuromolecular Med 16:658
Mansur RB, Brietzke E, McIntyre RS (2015) Is there a "metabolic-mood syndrome"? A review of the relationship between obesity and mood disorders. Neurosci Biobehav Rev 52:89
Mathieu P, Pibarot P, Larose E, Poirier P, Marette A, Despres JP (2008) Visceral obesity and the heart. Int J Biochem Cell Biol 40:821–836
Mathieu P, Lemieux I, Despres JP (2010) Obesity, inflammation, and cardiovascular risk. Clin Pharmacol Ther 87:407–416
Matsuzawa Y (2006) Therapy insight: adipocytokines in metabolic syndrome and related cardiovascular disease. Nat Clin Pract Cardiovasc Med 3:35–42

McElroy SL, Keck PE Jr (2012) Obesity in bipolar disorder: an overview. Curr Psychiatry Rep 14:650–658

McElroy SL, Kotwal R, Malhotra S, Nelson EB, Keck PE, Nemeroff CB (2004) Are mood disorders and obesity related? A review for the mental health professional. J Clin Psychiatry 65:634–651, quiz 730

McIntyre RS (2014) A vision for drug discovery and development: novel targets and multilateral partnerships. Adv Ther 31:245–246

McIntyre RS, Soczynska JK, Woldeyohannes HO, Lewis GF, Leiter LA, MacQueen GM, Miranda A, Fulgosi D, Konarski JZ, Kennedy SH (2007) Thiazolidinediones: novel treatments for cognitive deficits in mood disorders? Expert Opin Pharmacother 8:1615–1628

McIntyre RS, Vagic D, Swartz SA, Soczynska JK, Woldeyohannes HO, Voruganti LP, Konarski JZ (2008) Insulin, insulin-like growth factors and incretins: neural homeostatic regulators and treatment opportunities. CNS Drugs 22:443–453

McIntyre RS, Powell AM, Kaidanovich-Beilin O, Soczynska JK, Alsuwaidan M, Woldeyohannes HO, Kim AS, Gallaugher LA (2013) The neuroprotective effects of GLP-1: possible treatments for cognitive deficits in individuals with mood disorders. Behav Brain Res 237:164–171

McNamara RK, Lotrich FE (2012) Elevated immune-inflammatory signaling in mood disorders: a new therapeutic target? Expert Rev Neurother 12:1143–1161

McNamara RK, Strawn JR (2013) Role of long-chain omega-3 fatty acids in psychiatric practice. PharmaNutrition 1:41–49

McNay EC, Recknagel AK (2011) Brain insulin signaling: a key component of cognitive processes and a potential basis for cognitive impairment in type 2 diabetes. Neurobiol Learn Mem 96:432–442

McNay EC, Ong CT, McCrimmon RJ, Cresswell J, Bogan JS, Sherwin RS (2010) Hippocampal memory processes are modulated by insulin and high-fat-induced insulin resistance. Neurobiol Learn Mem 93:546–553

McQuade R, Young AH (2000) Future therapeutic targets in mood disorders: the glucocorticoid receptor. Br J Psychiatry: J Ment Sci 177:390–395

Mezuk B, Eaton WW, Albrecht S, Golden SH (2008) Depression and type 2 diabetes over the lifespan: a meta-analysis. Diabetes Care 31:2383–2390

Miller GE, Chen E, Zhou ES (2007) If it goes up, must it come down? Chronic stress and the hypothalamic-pituitary-adrenocortical axis in humans. Psychol Bull 133:25–45

Miller AH, Maletic V, Raison CL (2009) Inflammation and its discontents: the role of cytokines in the pathophysiology of major depression. Biol Psychiatry 65:732–741

Miller AH, Haroon E, Raison CL, Felger JC (2013) Cytokine targets in the brain: impact on neurotransmitters and neurocircuits. Depress Anxiety 30:297–306

Mok CC, Lok EY, Cheung EF (2012) Concurrent psychiatric disorders are associated with significantly poorer quality of life in patients with rheumatoid arthritis. Scand J Rheumatol 41:253–259

Morriss R, Mohammed FA (2005) Metabolism, lifestyle and bipolar affective disorder. J Psychopharmacol (Oxford, England) 19:94–101

Murphy BE (1991) Steroids and depression. J Steroid Biochem Mol Biol 38:537–559

Nathan RA (2007) The burden of allergic rhinitis. Allergy Asthma Proc: Off J Reg State Allergy Soc 28:3–9

Nelson PT, Smith CD, Abner EA, Schmitt FA, Scheff SW, Davis GJ, Keller JN, Jicha GA, Davis D, Wang-Xia W, Hartman A, Katz DG, Markesbery WR (2009) Human cerebral neuropathology of Type 2 diabetes mellitus. Biochim Biophys Acta 1792:454–469

Nguyen MT, Favelyukis S, Nguyen AK, Reichart D, Scott PA, Jenn A, Liu-Bryan R, Glass CK, Neels JG, Olefsky JM (2007) A subpopulation of macrophages infiltrates hypertrophic adipose tissue and is activated by free fatty acids via Toll-like receptors 2 and 4 and JNK-dependent pathways. J Biol Chem 282:35279–35292

Nicassio PM, Ormseth SR, Custodio MK, Irwin MR, Olmstead R, Weisman MH (2012) A multidimensional model of fatigue in patients with rheumatoid arthritis. J Rheumatol 39:1807–1813

Nolan CJ, Damm P, Prentki M (2011) Type 2 diabetes across generations: from pathophysiology to prevention and management. Lancet 378:169–181

Olivieri F, Rippo MR, Procopio AD, Fazioli F (2013) Circulating inflamma-miRs in aging and age-related diseases. Front Genet 4:121

Pace TW, Miller AH (2009) Cytokines and glucocorticoid receptor signaling. Relevance to major depression. Ann N Y Acad Sci 1179:86–105

Palagini L, Mosca M, Tani C, Gemignani A, Mauri M, Bombardieri S (2013) Depression and systemic lupus erythematosus: a systematic review. Lupus 22:409–416

Pan A, Sun Q, Okereke OI, Rexrode KM, Hu FB (2011) Depression and risk of stroke morbidity and mortality: a meta-analysis and systematic review. JAMA 306:1241–1249

Peltzer K, Phaswana-Mafuya N (2013) Depression and associated factors in older adults in South Africa. Glob Health Action 6:1–9

Poirier P, Giles TD, Bray GA, Hong Y, Stern JS, Pi-Sunyer FX, Eckel RH, American Heart Association, Obesity Committee of the Council on Nutrition, Physical Activity, and Metabolism (2006) Obesity and cardiovascular disease: pathophysiology, evaluation, and effect of weight loss: an update of the 1997 American Heart Association Scientific Statement on Obesity and Heart Disease from the Obesity Committee of the Council on Nutrition, Physical Activity, and Metabolism. Circulation 113:898–918

Raison CL, Miller AH (2003) When not enough is too much: the role of insufficient glucocorticoid signaling in the pathophysiology of stress-related disorders. Am J Psychiatry 160:1554–1565

Raison CL, Miller AH (2013) Malaise, melancholia and madness: the evolutionary legacy of an inflammatory bias. Brain Behav Immun 31:1–8

Raison CL, Broadwell SD, Borisov AS, Manatunga AK, Capuron L, Woolwine BJ, Jacobson IM, Nemeroff CB, Miller AH (2005) Depressive symptoms and viral clearance in patients receiving interferon-alpha and ribavirin for hepatitis C. Brain Behav Immun 19:23–27

Raison CL, Rutherford RE, Woolwine BJ, Shuo C, Schettler P, Drake DF, Haroon E, Miller AH (2013) A randomized controlled trial of the tumor necrosis factor antagonist infliximab for treatment-resistant depression: the role of baseline inflammatory biomarkers. JAMA Psychiatry 70:31–41

Raju TN (1998) The Nobel chronicles. 1927: Julius Wagner-Jauregg (1857–1940). Lancet 352:1714

Reagan LP (2005) Neuronal insulin signal transduction mechanisms in diabetes phenotypes. Neurobiol Aging 26(Suppl 1):56–59

Reichenberg A, Yirmiya R, Schuld A, Kraus T, Haack M, Morag A, Pollmacher T (2001) Cytokine-associated emotional and cognitive disturbances in humans. Arch Gen Psychiatry 58:445–452

Ridker PM, Morrow DA, Rose LM, Rifai N, Cannon CP, Braunwald E (2005) Relative efficacy of atorvastatin 80 mg and pravastatin 40 mg in achieving the dual goals of low-density lipoprotein cholesterol <70 mg/dl and C-reactive protein <2 mg/l: an analysis of the PROVE-IT TIMI-22 trial. J Am Coll Cardiol 45:1644–1648

Ridker PM, Danielson E, Fonseca FA, Genest J, Gotto AM Jr, Kastelein JJ, Koenig W, Libby P, Lorenzatti AJ, Macfadyen JG, Nordestgaard BG, Shepherd J, Willerson JT, Glynn RJ, JUPITER Trial Study Group (2009) Reduction in C-reactive protein and LDL cholesterol and cardiovascular event rates after initiation of rosuvastatin: a prospective study of the JUPITER trial. Lancet 373:1175–1182

Rodgers EE, Theibert AB (2002) Functions of PI 3-kinase in development of the nervous system. Int J Dev Neurosci: Official J Int Soc Dev Neurosci 20:187–197

Rosa-Neto P, Diksic M, Okazawa H, Leyton M, Ghadirian N, Mzengeza S, Nakai A, Debonnel G, Blier P, Benkelfat C (2004) Measurement of brain regional alpha-[11C]methyl-L-tryptophan trapping as a measure of serotonin synthesis in medication-free patients with major depression. Arch Gen Psychiatry 61:556–563

Rosenblat JD, Cha DS, Mansur RB, McIntyre RS (2014) Inflamed moods: a review of the interactions between inflammation and mood disorders. Prog Neuropsychopharmacol Biol Psychiatry 53:23–34

Rutledge T, Reis VA, Linke SE, Greenberg BH, Mills PJ (2006) Depression in heart failure a meta-analytic review of prevalence, intervention effects, and associations with clinical outcomes. J Am Coll Cardiol 48:1527–1537

Sato E, Nishimura K, Nakajima A, Okamoto H, Shinozaki M, Inoue E, Taniguchi A, Momohara S, Yamanaka H (2013) Major depressive disorder in patients with rheumatoid arthritis. Mod Rheumatol/Jpn Rheum Assoc 23:237–244

Scheid MP, Woodgett JR (2003) Unravelling the activation mechanisms of protein kinase B/Akt. FEBS Lett 546:108–112

Seaquist ER, Miller ME, Fonseca V, Ismail-Beigi F, Launer LJ, Punthakee Z, Sood A (2013) Effect of thiazolidinediones and insulin on cognitive outcomes in ACCORD-MIND. J Diabetes Complications 27:485–491

Setiawan E, Wilson AA, Mizrahi R, Rusjan PM, Miler L, Rajkowska G, Suridjan I, Kennedy JL, Rekkas PV, Houle S, Meyer JH (2015) Role of translocator protein density, a marker of neuroinflammation, in the brain during major depressive episodes. JAMA Psychiatry 72:268–275

Sharma BB, Singh S, Sharma VK, Choudhary M, Singh V, Lane S, Lepping P, Krishna M, Copeland J (2013) Psychiatric morbidity in chronic respiratory disorders in an Indian service using GMHAT/PC. Gen Hosp Psychiatry 35:39–44

Silverman MN, Miller AH, Biron CA, Pearce BD (2004) Characterization of an interleukin-6- and adrenocorticotropin-dependent, immune-to-adrenal pathway during viral infection. Endocrinology 145:3580–3589

Skeberdis VA, Lan J, Zheng X, Zukin RS, Bennett MV (2001) Insulin promotes rapid delivery of N-methyl-D- aspartate receptors to the cell surface by exocytosis. Proc Natl Acad Sci U S A 98:3561–3566

Soczynska JK, Kennedy SH, Woldeyohannes HO, Liauw SS, Alsuwaidan M, Yim CY, McIntyre RS (2011) Mood disorders and obesity: understanding inflammation as a pathophysiological nexus. Neuromolecular Med 13:93–116

Spalding KL, Arner E, Westermark PO, Bernard S, Buchholz BA, Bergmann O, Blomqvist L, Hoffstedt J, Naslund E, Britton T, Concha H, Hassan M, Ryden M, Frisen J, Arner P (2008) Dynamics of fat cell turnover in humans. Nature 453:783–787

Stertz L, Magalhaes PV, Kapczinski F (2013) Is bipolar disorder an inflammatory condition? The relevance of microglial activation. Curr Opin Psychiatry 26:19–26

Strike PC, Wardle J, Steptoe A (2004) Mild acute inflammatory stimulation induces transient negative mood. J Psychosom Res 57:189–194

Su KP, Wang SM, Pae CU (2013) Omega-3 polyunsaturated fatty acids for major depressive disorder. Expert Opin Investig Drugs 22:1519

Talbot F, Nouwen A (2000) A review of the relationship between depression and diabetes in adults: is there a link? Diabetes Care 23:1556–1562

Teegarden SL, Bale TL (2007) Decreases in dietary preference produce increased emotionality and risk for dietary relapse. Biol Psychiatry 61:1021–1029

Thombs BD, Bass EB, Ford DE, Stewart KJ, Tsilidis KK, Patel U, Fauerbach JA, Bush DE, Ziegelstein RC (2006) Prevalence of depression in survivors of acute myocardial infarction. J Gen Intern Med 21:30–38

Topp R, Fahlman M, Boardley D (2004) Healthy aging: health promotion and disease prevention. Nurs Clin North Am 39:411–422

Tupin E, Nicoletti A, Elhage R, Rudling M, Ljunggren HG, Hansson GK, Berne GP (2004) CD1d-dependent activation of NKT cells aggravates atherosclerosis. J Exp Med 199:417–422

Turnbull AV, Rivier CL (1999) Regulation of the hypothalamic-pituitary-adrenal axis by cytokines: actions and mechanisms of action. Physiol Rev 79:1–71

Tyring S, Gottlieb A, Papp K, Gordon K, Leonardi C, Wang A, Lalla D, Woolley M, Jahreis A, Zitnik R, Cella D, Krishnan R (2006) Etanercept and clinical outcomes, fatigue, and depression in psoriasis: double-blind placebo-controlled randomised phase III trial. Lancet 367:29–35

Udina M, Castellvi P, Moreno-Espana J, Navines R, Valdes M, Forns X, Langohr K, Sola R, Vieta E, Martin-Santos R (2012) Interferon-induced depression in chronic hepatitis C: a systematic review and meta-analysis. J Clin Psychiatry 73:1128–1138

Unger RH (2005) Longevity, lipotoxicity and leptin: the adipocyte defense against feasting and famine. Biochimie 87:57–64

van der Heide LP, Kamal A, Artola A, Gispen WH, Ramakers GM (2005) Insulin modulates hippocampal activity-dependent synaptic plasticity in a N-methyl-d-aspartate receptor and phosphatidyl-inositol-3-kinase-dependent manner. J Neurochem 94:1158–1166

Van Gaal LF, Mertens IL, De Block CE (2006) Mechanisms linking obesity with cardiovascular disease. Nature 444:875–880

Vancampfort D, Correll CU, Wampers M, Sienaert P, Mitchell AJ, De Herdt A, Probst M, Scheewe TW, De Hert M (2013) Metabolic syndrome and metabolic abnormalities in patients with major depressive disorder: a meta-analysis of prevalences and moderating variables. Psychol Med 44(10):2017–2028. doi: 10.1017/S0033291713002778. http://www.ncbi.nlm.nih.gov/pubmed/?term=24262678

Vaswani M, Linda FK, Ramesh S (2003) Role of selective serotonin reuptake inhibitors in psychiatric disorders: a comprehensive review. Prog Neuropsychopharmacol Biol Psychiatry 27:85–102

Walker JR, Graff LA, Dutz JP, Bernstein CN (2011) Psychiatric disorders in patients with immune-mediated inflammatory diseases: prevalence, association with disease activity, and overall patient well-being. J Rheumatol Suppl 88:31–35

Wang J, Dunn AJ (1998) Mouse interleukin-6 stimulates the HPA axis and increases brain tryptophan and serotonin metabolism. Neurochem Int 33:143–154

Wang M, Jiang L, Monticone RE, Lakatta EG (2014) Proinflammation: the key to arterial aging. Trends Endocrinol Metab 25:72–79

Weigle N, McBane S (2013) Psoriasis. Am Fam Physician 87:626–633

Wilczynska-Kwiatek A, Bargiel-Matusiewicz K, Lapinski L (2009) Asthma, allergy, mood disorders, and nutrition. Eur J Med Res 14(Suppl 4):248–254

Winocur G, Greenwood CE (2005) Studies of the effects of high fat diets on cognitive function in a rat model. Neurobiol Aging 26(Suppl 1):46–49

Winocur G, Greenwood CE, Piroli GG, Grillo CA, Reznikov LR, Reagan LP, McEwen BS (2005) Memory impairment in obese Zucker rats: an investigation of cognitive function in an animal model of insulin resistance and obesity. Behav Neurosci 119:1389–1395

Woods SC, Seeley RJ, Baskin DG, Schwartz MW (2003) Insulin and the blood-brain barrier. Curr Pharm Des 9:795–800

Wright CE, Strike PC, Brydon L, Steptoe A (2005) Acute inflammation and negative mood: mediation by cytokine activation. Brain Behav Immun 19:345–350

Young JJ, Bruno D, Pomara N (2014) A review of the relationship between proinflammatory cytokines and major depressive disorder. J Affect Disord 169:15–20

Yusuf S, Hawken S, Ounpuu S, Dans T, Avezum A, Lanas F, McQueen M, Budaj A, Pais P, Varigos J, Lisheng L, Investigators IS (2004) Effect of potentially modifiable risk factors associated with myocardial infarction in 52 countries (the INTERHEART study): case-control study. Lancet 364:937–952

Zhang J, Terreni L, De Simoni MG, Dunn AJ (2001) Peripheral interleukin-6 administration increases extracellular concentrations of serotonin and the evoked release of serotonin in the rat striatum. Neurochem Int 38:303–308

Zhou H, Lu W, Shi Y, Bai F, Chang J, Yuan Y, Teng G, Zhang Z (2010) Impairments in cognition and resting-state connectivity of the hippocampus in elderly subjects with type 2 diabetes. Neurosci Lett 473:5–10

Zorrilla EP, Luborsky L, McKay JR, Rosenthal R, Houldin A, Tax A, McCorkle R, Seligman DA, Schmidt K (2001) The relationship of depression and stressors to immunological assays: a meta-analytic review. Brain Behav Immun 15:199–226

Genetic Overlap Between Depression and Cardiometabolic Disorders

15

Azmeraw T. Amare, Klaus Oliver Schubert, and Bernhard T. Baune

Contents

Abstract

Depression and major cardiometabolic disorders (in this chapter, cardiometabolic disorders refer to the cardiovascular diseases, metabolic disorders, and associated risk factors) are highly heritable, i.e., they are caused by a combination of genetic and environmental factors. Moreover, there are genetic co-heritabilities (genetic correlations) in these disorders suggesting the influence of common genes and shared biological pathways between them. Several candidate gene studies performed so far have identified risk-associated genes for depression, cardiovascular, and/or metabolic diseases. Besides, meta-analysis of genome-wide association (meta-GWA) studies reported a number of single nucleotide polymorphisms (SNPs) and candidate genes for the cardiometabolic disorders. Compared to the cardiometabolic disorders, the meta-GWA studies of depression have had limited success due to the heterogeneity of the disorder and lack of statistical power (sample size) to detect the associations. The first successfully replicated meta-GWA study for depression was published in July 2015.

A.T. Amare (✉) • K.O. Schubert • B.T. Baune
Discipline of Psychiatry, University of Adelaide, Adelaide, Australia
e-mail: azmeraw.amare@adelaide.edu.au

B.T. Baune, P.J. Tully (eds.), *Cardiovascular Diseases and Depression*,
DOI 10.1007/978-3-319-32480-7_15

In this chapter, we present an appraisal and analysis of pleiotropic genes (pleiotropy occurs when a genetic region influences more than two phenotypes, disorders in this case) and shared biological pathways underlying the association of depression and the cardiometabolic diseases. These genes are shared between depression and (a) metabolic disorders (type 2 diabetes), (b) cardiovascular disorders (coronary artery diseases, hypertension), and (c) associated risk factors (blood pressure, obesity (body mass index), plasma lipid levels (high-density lipoprotein, low-density lipoprotein, triglycerides, total cholesterol), insulin and glucose-related traits (fasting glucose, fasting insulin, fasting proinsulin, insulin resistance-HOMA-IR, beta-cell function-HOMA-β, and glycated hemoglobin A1C- HbA1C).

Generally speaking, pleiotropic genes and shared biological mechanisms could explain part of the comorbidity between depression and cardiometabolic disorders. Genetic polymorphisms within the genes: *MTHFR*, *CACNA1D*, *CACNB2*, *GNAS*, *ADRB1*, *NCAN*, *REST*, *FTO*, *POMC*, *BDNF*, *CREB*, *ITIH4*, *LEP*, *GSK3B*, *SLC18A1*, *TLR4*, *APOE*, *CRY2*, *HTR1A*, *ADRA2A*, *MTNR1B*, and *IGF1* are associated with both depression and cardiometabolic disorders. These genes belong to biologically relevant signaling pathways that are potentiality important in the relationship between depression and cardiometabolic diseases. The pathways include: *corticotrophin-releasing hormone signaling*, *AMPK signaling*, *cAMP-mediated and G-protein-coupled receptor signaling*, *axonal guidance signaling*, and *serotonin and dopamine receptor signaling*. A better understanding of these genes and related pathways will enhance knowledge as to why patients suffer from multiple diseases at a time and how multi-morbidities influence pharmacological treatment response.

15.1 Introduction

15.1.1 The Comorbidity of Depression and Cardiometabolic Diseases

In the last century, improvements in public health, nutrition, education, living conditions, and medicine have led to an increase in life expectancy. However, unhealthy lifestyle and population aging have increased the prevalence of chronic long-term disorders such as cardiovascular and metabolic diseases and psychiatric disorders. Major depressive disorder (MDD), coronary artery diseases, type 2 diabetes, and hypertension are the major sources of disability, morbidity, and mortality (Murray et al. 2015; Whiteford et al. 2013).

Currently, the co-occurrence (comorbidity) of depression with cardiometabolic diseases is a burden facing the health-care systems worldwide (Barnett et al. 2012; Murray et al. 2015; Whiteford et al. 2013). It is also a challenge for psychosomatic medicine, as the relationship of the diseases is not clearly understood. Several clinical and epidemiological studies that investigated the relationship between depression and cardiometabolic disorders concluded that the epidemiological relationship is reciprocal in that depression may lead to cardiometabolic disease or it may result from cardiometabolic disorders (Chauvet-Gélinier et al. 2013; Plante 2005). The prevalence of MDD among patients with cardiometabolic diseases is high, with a complex multidirectional relationship between them (Barnett et al. 2012; Golden et al. 2008; Huffman et al. 2013) (Fig. 15.1). For instance, 20–40% of patients with cardiovascular diseases meet the criteria for major depression (Celano and Huffman 2011; Huffman et al. 2013), and the risk of developing MDD among cardiometabolic disease patients is also substantial: 15–25% in type 2 diabetes (Mezuk et al. 2008; Nouwen et al. 2010), 17–27% in coronary artery disease (Rudisch and Nemeroff 2003), and 21.7–32.3% in hypertension (Li et al. 2015). Conversely, depressed individuals have 37–60% increased risk of developing type 2 diabetes (Knol et al. 2006; Mezuk et al. 2008) and 30–64% risk for coronary artery diseases (Gan et al. 2014; Rugulies 2002) compared to nondepressed individuals. One explanation for this association could be the presence of pleiotropic (common) genes and shared biological pathways that function as a hub encoding for proteins that connect the disorders; additionally, a gene-environment interaction that affects multiple phenotypes may exist. Possible common biological mechanisms underlying depression and cardiometabolic disease comorbidity have been proposed, including altered circadian rhythms (Zelinski et al. 2014), abnormal hypothalamic-pituitary-adrenal axis (HPA axis) function (Rosmond and Björntorp 2000), imbalanced neurotransmitters (Szczepanska-Sadowska et al. 2010), and inflammation (Kemp et al. 2010). However, further genetic and molecular studies are urgently required to fully understand the underlying mechanisms linking these disorders.

15.1.2 Common Genes Shared Between Depression and Cardiometabolic Disorders

15.1.2.1 Twin Studies

Depression and cardiometabolic disorders are heritable and they are caused by a combination of genetic and environmental factors. Genetic factors contribute to 31–42% in MDD (Sullivan et al. 2000), 30–60% in coronary artery diseases (Marenberg et al. 1994), 26–69% in type 2 diabetes (Almgren et al. 2011; Poulsen et al. 1999), 24–37% in blood pressure (hypertension) (Van Rijn et al. 2007), 35–48% in heart rate variability (Kupper et al. 2004), 40–70% in obesity (body mass index) (Willyard 2014), and 58–66% in the level of serum lipids (Knoblauch et al. 1997). Moreover, there are fairly high genetic co-heritabilities (genetic correlations) between depression and the different cardiometabolic disorders suggesting the influence of pleiotropic genes and shared biological pathways within them. For instance, the genetic correlation of depression with hypertension is estimated to be 19%, and between depression and heart disease is about 42% (Scherrer et al. 2003). The genetic correlation between depressive symptoms and plasma lipid levels ranges from 10% to 31%(Lopez-Leon et al. 2010), and 12% of the genetic

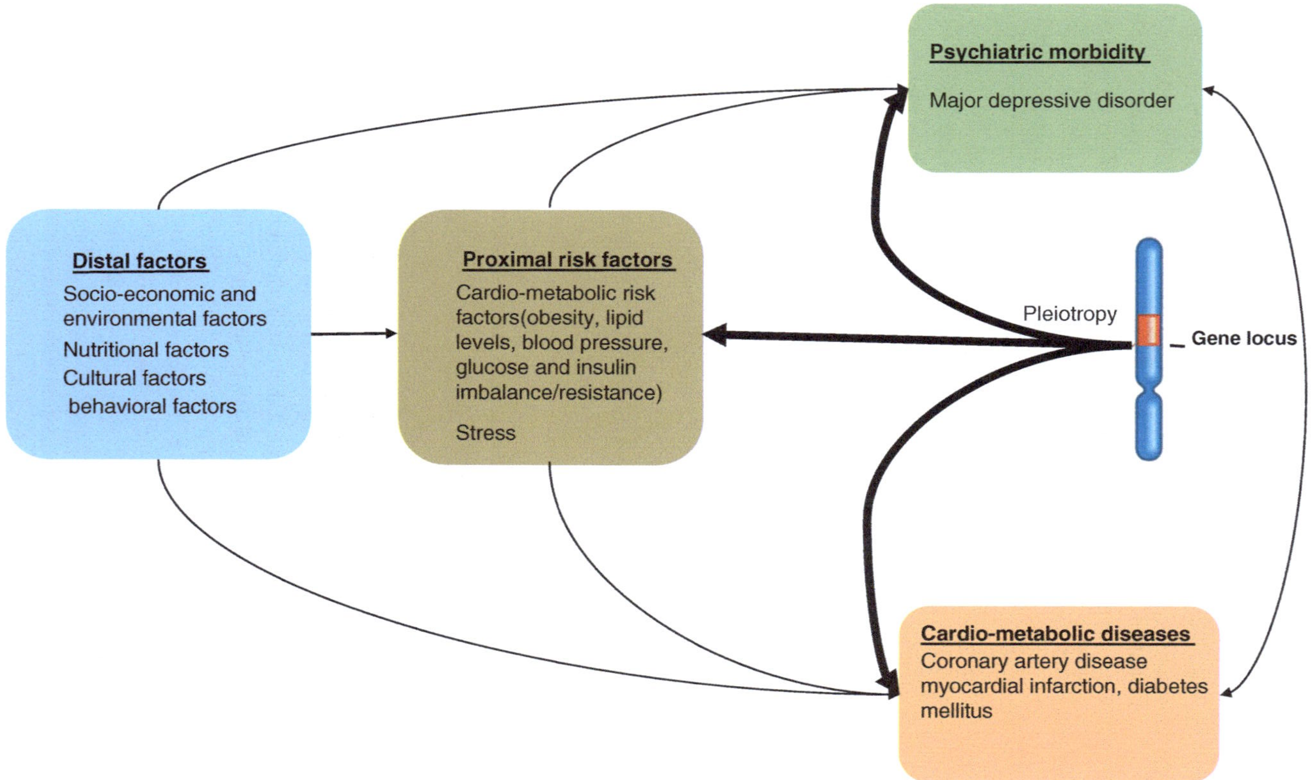

Fig. 15.1 Shows the comorbidity between major depressive and cardiometabolic disorders. It also demonstrates how a genetic locus (pleiotropic region) could affect the different disease conditions simultaneously

component for depression is shared with obesity (Afari et al. 2010). Su et al. (2010) also found a significant inverse genetic correlation of 21–24 % between depressive symptoms and heart rate variability (Su et al. 2010). Two main genetic research approaches have been applied to investigate the specific genetic components related to depression and the cardiometabolic disorders: candidate gene studies and genome-wide association studies (GWAS).

15.1.2.2 Candidate Gene and Genome-Wide Association Studies

In the last decade, a substantial amount of univariate (single disease) meta-analyses of genome-wide association (meta-GWA) and candidate gene studies has been published. Indeed, the meta-GWA and candidate gene studies have successfully identified a considerable list of candidate genes for major depressive disorder (CONVERGE Consortium 2015; Flint and Kendler 2014; Lohoff 2010), coronary artery diseases (Nikpay et al. 2015), type 2 diabetes (Dupuis et al. 2010; Gaulton et al. 2015; Ng et al. 2014), hypertension (Lu et al. 2015), obesity (Locke et al. 2015), plasma lipid level (Willer et al. 2013), insulin- and glucose-related traits (Dupuis et al. 2010; Hwang et al. 2015; Manning et al. 2012; Scott et al. 2012; Soranzo et al. 2010), and blood pressure (Lu et al. 2015; Ehret et al. 2011). Although the studies were entirely focused on a single phenotype approach (single disease), genes appear to influence multiple disorders simultaneously. A genetic pathway involving these genes might actually function as a hub to link depression and the cardiometabolic diseases or vice versa.

Since the formal introduction of the term "pleiotropy" by the German geneticist Ludwig Plate in 1910 (Stearns 2010), pleiotropic genes have been investigated. For instance, a recent analysis of SNPs and genes from the NHGRI GWAS catalogue (Welter et al. 2014) has showed as 16.9 % genes and 4.6 % SNPs have pleiotropic effects on complex diseases (Sivakumaran et al. 2011). In this chapter of the book, we provide a brief overview of the pleiotropic genes obtained through a systematic literature review of genome-wide association and candidate gene studies in PubMed (MEDLINE database) and from the National Human Genome Research Institute (NHGRI) GWAS catalogue (Welter et al. 2014). We also explored the shared biological pathways that link depression and cardiometabolic disorders.

Understanding of the common genetic pathways of depression and cardiometabolic diseases may provide new insights and novel ways for the diagnosis and treatment of both diseases. The list of pleiotropic genes shared between depression and cardiometabolic disorders is provided in Table 15.1. We named these candidate genes, the cardiometabolic-depressive disorder (CMD) genes. The genes are *MTHFR*, *CACNA1D*, *CACNB2*, *GNAS*, *ADRB1*, *NCAN*, *REST*, *FTO*, *POMC*, *BDNF*, *CREB*, *ITIH4*, *LEP*, *GSK3B*, *SLC18A1*, *TLR4*, *APOE*, *CRY2*, *HTR1A*, *ADRA2A*, *MTNR1B*, and *IGF1* (Table 15.1, Fig. 15.2). The genes belong to biological pathways important in the hypothesis of both cardiometabolic diseases and mood disorders. We analyzed and visualized the functional relationship between the genes associated with coronary artery disease, hypertension, type 2 diabetes, major depressive disorder, and bipolar disorder through the use of QIAGEN's Ingenuity®

Table 15.1 Pleiotropic genes shared between depression and the cardiometabolic disorders

Pleiotropic genes	Polymorphisms associated with	
	Cardiometabolic disorders	Depression (description)
MTHFR	Blood pressure (Newton-Cheh et al. 2009; Wain et al. 2011)	*MTHFR* C677T was associated with depression (Kelly et al. 2004; Lewis et al. 2006; Wu et al. 2013). The interaction between the *MTHFR* gene polymorphism and childhood trauma increased the risk for depressive disorder (Lok et al. 2013)
CACNA1D	Blood pressure and hypertension (Lu et al. 2015)	Calcium channel genes (*CACNA1B*, *CACNA1C*, *CACNA1D*, and *CACNG2*) contribute to psychiatric disorders including MDD (Smoller 2013)
GNAS	Blood pressure and hypertension (Ehret et al. 2011; Wain et al. 2011)	SNPs in the *GNAS* gene influence antidepressant treatment response (Klenke and Siffert 2011)
ADRB1	Blood pressure (Wain et al. 2011)	Gly389 polymorphism of the beta(1)-adrenergic receptor gene might lead to better response to antidepressants in patients with major depression (Zill et al. 2003)
CACNB2	Blood pressure and cardiovascular disease risk (Levy et al. 2009; Ehret et al. 2011; Wain et al. 2011)	Polymorphisms in the *CACNB2* gene were implicated in MDD (Smoller 2013)
REST	Coronary artery disease (Nikpay et al. 2015)	Reduced expression of the *REST* gene in MDD patients at depressive state (Otsuki et al. 2010) and sex-specific alteration in the expression of the *REST* gene was revealed in the brain of women with MDD (Goswami et al. 2010)
LEP	Type 2 diabetes (Hara et al. 2014)	Polymorphisms in the leptin gene, decreased leptin gene expression, and leptin deficiency in serum were suggested as risk factors for resistance to antidepressant therapy in depressed patients (Kloiber et al. 2013). A significant reduction of the mRNA expression was found in the brain of suicidal patients (Eikelis et al. 2006)
POMC	Obesity (BMI) (Berndt et al. 2013; Speliotes et al. 2010)	Genetic variants in the *POMC* gene were involved in treatment response to selective serotonin reuptake inhibitors (SSRIs), escitalopram or mirtazapine, in MDD patients (Chang et al. 2015)
ITIH4	Obesity (BMI) (Wen et al. 2014)	A candidate gene study has confirmed the association of genetic variants in the *ITIH3* and *ITIH4* genes and suicidal attempt (Finseth et al. 2014). The ITIH4 protein level was upregulated during depressive state (Schmidt et al. 2011)
FTO	Obesity (BMI) (Berndt et al. 2013; Locke et al. 2015)	The *FTO* gene variants were associated with depression (Samaan et al. 2013). Also, they were involved in the mechanism underlying the association between mood disorders and obesity (Rivera et al. 2011)
	Type 2 diabetes (Mahajan et al. 2014)	
	Plasma lipid level (Willer et al. 2013)	

Table 15.1 (continued)

Pleiotropic genes	Polymorphisms associated with	
	Cardiometabolic disorders	Depression (description)
CREB1	Obesity (BMI) (Locke et al. 2015)	Variations in the *CREB1* gene were associated with sex-specific MDD risk (women) (Zubenko et al. 2003) and antidepressant treatment resistance in MDD patients (Serretti et al. 2011). Genetic variation in the *CREB1* gene and its interaction with *BDNF* variants predicted response to the SSRIs (paroxetine) (Murphy et al. 2013)
BDNF	Obesity (BMI) (Locke et al. 2015; Speliotes et al. 2010)	The Val66Met polymorphism in the *BDNF* gene was associated with depressive disorder (Herbert et al. 2012; Yang et al. 2010; Zhang et al. 2010) and suicidal behavior in depressed patients (Sarchiapone et al. 2008). It was also associated with SSRI (escitalopram) response in depressed patients (El-Hage et al. 2014). Moreover, a significantly decreased expression of the *BDNF* gene was observed in the lymphocytes and platelets of depressed patients (Pandey et al. 2010). Treatment-responsive depressive patients have also shown decreased mRNA levels of the *BDNF* gene (Hong et al. 2014)
TLR4	Obesity (BMI) (Locke et al. 2015)	The mRNA levels of the *TLR3* and *TLR4* genes were increased in depressed suicidal patients (Pandey et al. 2014). *TLR4* gene expression was related to severity of major depression (Hung et al. 2014)
NCAN	Plasma lipid level (Willer et al. 2008)	The *NCAN* genotype is associated with limbic gray matter alterations in depressed subjects (Dannlowski et al. 2015)
GSK3B	Plasma lipid level (Willer et al. 2013)	Higher *GSK3B* gene activity was observed in MDD patients with severe depressive episode (Diniz et al. 2011). Polymorphisms in this gene were implicated in MDD (Saus et al. 2010). The *GSK3B* gene is a target gene for several mood stabilizers including lithium (Iwahashi et al. 2014; Mitjans et al. 2015)
APOE		Genetic variation at the *APOE* gene contributed to depressive symptoms (Yen et al. 2007)
SLC18A1	Plasma lipid level (Ko et al. 2014; Kooner et al. 2008)	Variations in the *SLC18A1* gene showed a suggestive association with MDD (Shyn et al. 2011). Lithium ions modulate the expression of *SLC18A1* gene in rats brain (Cordeiro et al. 2002)
ADRA2A	Fasting glucose and type 2 diabetes (Dupuis et al. 2010)	*ADRA2A* gene polymorphisms were associated with sex-specific MDD (Haefner et al. 2008), predicted antidepressant treatment outcome in MDD (Kato et al. 2015), and modified the effect of antidepressants (better improvement) (Wakeno et al. 2008). However, they increased suicidal ideation during antidepressant treatment (Perroud et al. 2009)

(continued)

Table 15.1 (continued)

Pleiotropic genes	Polymorphisms associated with	
	Cardiometabolic disorders	Depression (description)
CRY2	Glucose-/insulin-related traits (Dupuis et al. 2010; Manning et al. 2012)	Polymorphisms in the *CRY2* gene were significantly associated with MDD (Lavebratt et al. 2010; Soria et al. 2010)
MTNR1B	Plasma glucose level (Bouatia-Naji et al. 2009; Chambers et al. 2009; Dupuis et al. 2010), type 2 diabetes (Voight et al. 2010)	The significance of the *MTNR1B* gene polymorphism was reported for recurrent MDD. A SNP within this gene increased mRNA level in MDD patients (Gałecka et al. 2011)
IGF1	Fasting insulin, fasting glucose, glucose homeostasis (Dupuis et al. 2010; Manning et al. 2012)	Elevated levels of IGF-I were significantly associated with MDD and antidepressant treatment response (Kopczak et al. 2015). A long-term deficiency of IGF-1 in adult mice induced depressive behavior (Mitschelen et al. 2011)
HTR1A	Fasting insulin and insulin resistance (Zheng et al. 2013)	Genetic variants in the *HTR1A* gene were related to MDD (Kishi et al. 2013) and with antidepressant treatment response in MDD (Baune et al. 2008; Kato et al. 2009; Lemonde et al. 2004; Suzuki et al. 2004). A significant decrease in *HTR1A* mRNA levels in the brain of patients with MDD was found (López-Figueroa et al. 2004)

BMI body mass index, *SNP* single nucleotide polymorphism, *MDD* major depressive disorder

Variant Analysis™ software (www.qiagen.com/ingenuity) from QIAGEN Redwood City (Fig. 15.2). This analysis implicates the following top canonical (molecular) pathways as potentially shared mechanisms of depression and cardiometabolic disorders pathophysiology: corticotrophin-releasing hormone signaling (*BDNF*, *CREB1*, *GNAS*, *POMC*), AMPK signaling (*ADRA2A*, *ADRB1*, *CREB1*,*GNAS*, *LEP*), cAMP-mediated and G-protein-coupled receptor signaling (*ADRA2A*, *ADRB1*, *CREB1*, *GNAS*, *HTR1A*), axonal guidance signaling (*BDNF*, *GNAS*, *GSK3B*, *IGF1*); serotonin and dopamine receptor signaling (*GNAS*, *HTR1A*, *SLC18A1*), and cardiac hypertrophy signaling (*ADRA2A*, *ADRB1*, *CACNA1D*, *CREB1*, *GNAS*, *GSK3B*, *IGF1*).

The following section gives a brief overview of the top molecular pathways and the overrepresented CMD genes within them.

15.1.2.3 Shared Biological Pathway and Gene Network

Corticotrophin-Releasing Hormone (CRH) Signaling

The CRH-signaling pathway comprises the corticotrophin-releasing hormone, CRH receptors (CRHR1, CRHR2), and other CRH-related peptides. The CRH signaling is the principal regulator of the hypothalamic-pituitary-adrenal (HPA) axis, which is well-known to control the body's adaptation to stress. Genes that stimulate the CRH pathway can increase the risk of developing both depression and cardiometabolic

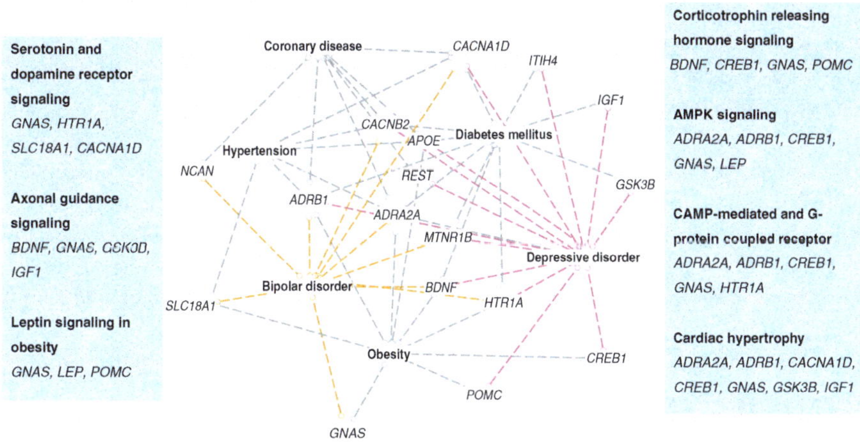

Fig. 15.2 Shows a network of genes, as indicated by the *dashed lines*, shared between cardiometabolic diseases/risk factors and mood disorders, highlighting CMD genes that were related to bipolar disorder (*orange*) and depression (*red*). Implicated signaling pathways and overrepresented CMD genes are shown in the right and left side of the figure. *AMPK* 5′ adenosine monophosphate-activated protein kinase, *cAMP* cyclic adenosine 3′,5′-monophosphate

diseases through their influence on the immune system (inflammation), sleep homeostasis, and the HPA axis.

Among the CMD genes, brain-derived neurotrophic factor (*BDNF*), cAMP-responsive element binding protein 1 (*CREB1*), GNAS complex locus (*GNAS*), and proopiomelanocortin (*POMC*) genes are involved into the corticotropin-releasing hormone signaling pathway (Fig. 15.2).

***BDNF* gene** The brain-derived neurotrophic factor (*BDNF*) gene, one of the most studied genes for depression, encodes the brain-derived neurotrophic factor that promotes the survival of nerve cells by regulating their growth, differentiation, and maintenance (Jeanneteau et al. 2012). The BDNF protein is active at the connections between nerve cells (synapses), in which cell-to-cell communication takes place. It might be possible that the *BDNF* gene alters the risk of depression and cardiometabolic disorders as it regulates both neuronal functions and somatic functions such as eating, drinking, and body weight.

Polymorphisms in the *BDNF* gene were associated with obesity (Locke et al. 2015), depressive disorder (Zhang et al. 2010; Zou et al. 2010), suicidal behavior in depressed patients (Sarchiapone et al. 2008), and treatment response to SSRIs (El-Hage et al. 2014). A decreased expression of the *BDNF* gene was shown in depressed patients (Pandey et al. 2010) and patients who were responsive to antidepressants (Hong et al. 2014) (Table 15.1).

***CREB1* gene** It encodes a transcription factor that binds to the cAMP-responsive element and induces transcription of genes in response to hormonal stimulation of the cAMP pathway. Polymorphisms in the *CREB1* gene were implicated in obesity (Locke et al. 2015), major depression (Liu et al. 2010), treatment resistance in MDD (Serretti et al. 2011), antidepressant treatment response in geriatric population (Murphy et al. 2013), sex-specific (women) mood disorders (Maher et al. 2010; Zubenko et al. 2003), and suicide in mood disorder patients (Antypa et al. 2015) (Table 15.1).

GNAS **gene** It encodes the stimulatory alpha subunit of the guanine nucleotide-binding protein (G protein) complex. The G protein made with the subunit produced from the *GNAS* gene helps to stimulate the activity of adenylate cyclase enzyme, an enzyme involved in controlling the production of hormones that help to regulate the activity of endocrine glands such as the thyroid, pituitary gland, ovaries and testes (gonads), and adrenal glands. Genetic variants in the *GNAS* gene were associated with blood pressure and hypertension (Ehret et al. 2011) and may influence antidepressant treatment response (Klenke and Siffert 2011) (Table 15.1).

POMC **gene** The other important CMD gene in the CRH pathway is the *POMC* gene that encodes the proopiomelanocortin (POMC). The POMC is primarily produced in the pituitary gland. It is then cut (cleaved) into as many as ten biologically active peptides involved in normal steroidogenesis, pain control, energy homeostasis, and immune modulation. The adrenocorticotropin (ACTH), β-lipotropin (β-LPH), β-endorphin, and three similar peptides called alpha-, beta-, and gamma-melanocyte-stimulating hormones (α, β, and γ-MSH) are all cleaved from the POMC protein. These proteins bind to other proteins in the body to trigger signaling pathways that control vital functions. For example, the binding of:

(a) ACTH to melanocortin 2 receptor (MC2R) stimulates the production and release of cortisol hormone that helps to regulate blood sugar levels, protects the body from the effect of stress, and suppresses inflammation.
(b) β-endorphin to opioid receptors in the brain stimulates signaling for pain relief.
(c) β-MSH or α-MSH peptide to the melanocortin 4 receptor (MC4R) helps to regulate weight and the body energy balance.
(d) γ-MSH to melanocortin 3 receptor (MC3R) and signaling stimulated by this interaction regulate the amount of sodium in the body.

Altogether, these interactions have a significant role in the cardiovascular and metabolic system and the well-functioning of our brain. Polymorphisms in the *POMC* gene were associated with obesity (BMI) (Berndt et al. 2013; Speliotes et al. 2010) and treatment response to antidepressants in patients with MDD (Chang et al. 2015) (Table 15.1).

Adenosine Monophosphate-Activated Protein Kinase (AMPK) Signaling Pathways

The AMPK pathway inhibits or induces ATP-consuming pathways that generate ATP as needed. It promotes glucose uptake and it is activated by stimuli like inflammation, metabolic poisoning, exercise, hypoxia, ischemia, heat shock, and neuronal necrosis. The CMD genes in the AMPK pathway were the adrenoceptor alpha-2A

(*ADRA2A*), adrenoceptor beta 1(*ADRB1*), leptin (*LEP*), cAMP-responsive element binding protein 1(*CREB1*), and GNAS complex locus (*GNAS*) genes.

ADRA2A **gene** It encodes the alpha-2-adrenergic receptors, which has a crucial role in the regulation of neurotransmitter release from sympathetic nerves and adrenergic neurons in the central nervous system. The receptors are required for normal presynaptic control of neurotransmitter release from sympathetic nerves in the heart and from central noradrenergic neuronsa (Pruitt et al. 2012). Genetic variants in the *ADRA2A* gene were associated with fasting glucose and type 2 diabetes (Dupuis et al. 2010), MDD (Haefner et al. 2008), antidepressant treatment response in major MDD (Kato et al. 2015), and increase suicidal ideation during antidepressant treatment (Perroud et al. 2009). The *ADRA2A* gene is highly expressed in the rats' brain with lithium treatment (Cuffí et al. 2010) (Table 15.1).

ADRB1 **gene** It encodes the adrenergic beta 1 receptor that mediates the physiological effects of the epinephrine hormone and the neurotransmitter norepinephrine (Pruitt et al. 2012). Polymorphisms in the *ADRB1* gene were associated with blood pressure (Wain et al. 2011) and better and faster response to antidepressant treatment in MDD patients (Zill et al. 2003) (Table 15.1).

LEP **gene** It encodes a protein secreted by adipocytes and later acts through the leptin receptor. The protein regulates body weight and maintains the constancy of the adipose mass. It is also involved in several endocrine functions, the regulation of immune and inflammatory responses, angiogenesis, and wound healing (Pruitt et al. 2012). Mutations in the leptin gene could cause type 2 diabetes (Hara et al. 2014). Leptin gene mRNA expression in the brain was significantly reduced in MDD and suicidal patients (Eikelis et al. 2006). Decreased leptin gene expression and leptin deficiency in serum were risk factors for resistance to antidepressant therapy in depressed patients (Kloiber et al. 2013) (Table 15.1).

Axonal Guidance Signaling

This pathway is related to neuronal connections formed by the extension of axons, which migrate to reach their synaptic targets. The brain-derived neurotrophic factor (*BDNF*), GNAS complex locus (*GNAS*), glycogen synthase kinase 3 beta (*GSK3B*), and insulin-like growth factor 1(*IGF1*) are among the CMD genes involved in this pathway (Fig. 15.2).

GSK3B **gene** It encodes the serine-threonine kinase protein that is involved in energy metabolism, neuronal cell development, and body pattern formation (Pruitt et al. 2012). Genetic variants in the *GSK3B* gene were implicated for the lipid level (plasma high-density lipoprotein) (Willer et al. 2013) and in unipolar depression (Saus et al. 2010), and higher *GSK3B* activity was observed in patients with severe depressive episode (Diniz et al. 2011). The *GSK3B* is a target gene for several mood stabilizers (Iwahashi et al. 2014; Mitjans et al. 2015) (Table 15.1).

IGF1 **gene** It encodes the insulin-like growth factor protein, which is structurally and functionally related to insulin (Pruitt et al. 2012). Defects in this gene were associated with plasma level of glycemic traits: fasting insulin, fasting glucose, and glucose homeostasis (Dupuis et al. 2010). The *IGF1* gene is highly expressed in the brain (Fernandez and Torres-Alemán 2012). Elevated levels of IGF-I are significantly associated with major depression and antidepressant treatment response (Kopczak et al. 2015). A long-term deficiency of circulating IGF-1 in adult mice induced depressive behaviors suggesting the association between low brain levels of IGF-1 and increased risk for depression (Mitschelen et al. 2011) (Table 15.1).

Serotonin and Dopamine Receptor Signaling

Serotonin signaling is an important modulator of several physiological processes including the regulation of appetite, mood, sleep, body temperature, and metabolism. Serotonin functions via receptors known as the 5-hydroxytryptamine (5-HT) receptors and it is released at the synapse of the presynaptic neuron where it binds to its receptor on the postsynaptic neuron (Raote et al. 2007). Monoamine oxidase catalyzes the oxidative deamination of serotonin (5-HT) to 5-hydroxyindoleacetic acid, which is translocated to cerebrospinal fluid.

Dopamine is a neurotransmitter that serves as a chemical messenger in the nervous system. Its signaling plays important roles in brain processes, emotion, positive reinforcement, motivation and movement, and in the periphery as a modulator of renal, cardiovascular, and the endocrine systems. It is then enzymatically degraded by catechol-O-methyl transferase (COMT) and monoamine oxidase (MAO) to homovanillic acid which enters the cerebrospinal fluid.

The solute carrier family 18 (vesicular monoamine transporter), member 1 (*SLC18A1*), 5-hydroxytryptamine (serotonin) receptor 1A (*HTR1A*), *GNAS*, and the calcium voltage-gated channel subunit alpha-1D (*CACNA1D*) genes are involved in the serotonin and dopamine receptor signaling pathways (Fig. 15.2).

SLC18A1 **gene** This gene encodes for the vesicular monoamine transporter that transports for monoamines and acetylcholine. The appropriate function of this protein is essential to the proper activity of the monoaminergic systems that are involved in several human neuropsychiatric disorders (Peter et al. 1993; Pruitt et al. 2012). Variations in the *SLC18A1* gene were associated with plasma lipid level (Willer et al. 2013) and a suggestive association was reported for MDD (Shyn et al. 2011). Lithium ions modulate the expression of *SLC18A1* gene in the rats' brain (Cordeiro et al. 2002) (Table 15.1).

HTR1A **gene** It encodes a receptor for 5-hydroxytryptamine (serotonin), and it belongs to the 5-hydroxytryptamine receptor subfamily (Pruitt et al. 2012). Dysregulation of the serotonergic neurotransmission has been suggested to contribute for the pathogenesis of MDD and it is implicated in the action of SSRIs. Functional genetic variants in the *HTR1A* gene were associated fasting insulin and insulin resistance (Zheng et al. 2013), depressive disorder, and treatment response in major depression (Baune et al. 2008; Kato et al. 2009; Lemonde et al. 2004; Suzuki et al.

2004). Postsynaptic 5-HT1A receptor binding is reduced in women with postpartum depression (Moses-Kolko et al. 2008). The interaction between polymorphisms of the *HTR1A* gene with negative life stressors accounts for current major depressive episodes and depressive symptoms (Kim et al. 2011a). A significant decrease in *HTR1A* mRNA levels in the brain of MDD patients was also found (López-Figueroa et al. 2004) (Table 15.1).

***CACNA1D* gene** It encodes the alpha-1D subunit of the calcium channels. Voltage-dependent calcium channel proteins mediate the entry of calcium ions into excitable cells and are also involved in a variety of calcium-dependent processes, including hormone or neurotransmitter release and gene expression. Calcium channels are multi-subunit complexes composed of alpha-1, beta, alpha-2, delta, and gamma subunits. The calcium channels activity is directed by the pore-forming alpha-1 subunit, while the others function as auxiliary subunits (Pruitt et al. 2012). Polymorphisms of this gene were associated with blood pressure and hypertension (Lu et al. 2015). Genetic variants in the calcium channel genes (*CACNA1B*, *CACNA1C*, *CACNA1D*, and *CACNG2*) contribute to psychiatric disorders including MDD (Smoller 2013).

Cardiac Hypertrophy Signaling

The *ADRA2A*, *ADRB1*, *CACNA1D*, *CREB1*, *GNAS*, *GSK3B*, and *IGF1* were the CMD genes that encode the components of the cardiac hypertrophy signaling pathway (Fig. 15.2).

Other Genes

Other CMD genes that play a significant role in the pathophysiology of both cardiometabolic diseases and depression were the *MTHFR*, *REST*, *CACNB2*, *NCAN*, *ITIH4*, *TLR4*, *CRY2*, *MTNR1B*, *FTO* and *APOE* genes. Single nucleotide polymorphisms of these genes were reported for blood pressure- *MTHFR* (Newton-Cheh et al. 2009; Wain et al. 2011), *CACNB2* (Ehret et al. 2011), *ADRB1* (Wain et al. 2011), coronary artery diseases- *REST* (Nikpay et al. 2015; Ehret et al. 2011), lipid levels- *APOE* (Kim et al. 2011b; Willer et al. 2013), *FTO* (Willer et al. 2013), *NCAN* (Willer et al. 2008), obesity- *FTO* (Locke et al. 2015), *ITIH4* (Locke et al. 2015; Wen et al. 2014), *TLR4* (Locke et al. 2015), type 2 diabetes- *FTO* (Mahajan et al. 2014), *MTNR1B* (Voight et al. 2010)), glucose- or insulin-related traits- *CRY2* (Dupuis et al. 2010; Manning et al. 2012), *MTNR1B* (Bouatia-Naji et al. 2009; Dupuis et al. 2010), and also with depression- *MTHFR* (Kelly et al. 2004; Lewis et al. 2006; Wu et al. 2013), *CACNB2*, *CRY2* (Soria et al. 2010), *FTO* (Samaan et al. 2013), *TLR4* (Liu et al. 2014), and *MTNR1B* (Gałecka et al. 2011) genes. An interaction of the *MTHFR* gene variant with childhood adversities increased the risk of depression (Lok et al. 2013). Gene expression analysis studies also found a significant reduction in the expression of *REST* gene (Otsuki et al. 2010) and an overexpression of the *TLR4* gene (Pandey et al. 2014) in MDD patients. The *CRY2* locus increases vulnerability for depression through the mechanisms of action that involve dysregulation of *CRY2* gene expression (Lavebratt et al. 2010). Gałecka et al. (2011)

reported the significance of the melatonin receptor gene expression in recurrent MDD (Gałecka et al. 2011). The *NCAN* genotype is associated with limbic gray matter alterations in depressed subjects (Dannlowski et al. 2015). A candidate gene study confirmed the association of genetic variants in the *ITIH3* and *ITIH4* genes and suicidal behavior (Finseth et al. 2014). The ITIH4 protein level was upregulated during depressive state (Schmidt et al. 2011) (Table 15.1, Fig. 15.2).

15.2 Implications for the Treatment and Prevention of Comorbid Depression and Cardiometabolic Disorders

Knowledge of genetic risk variants and associated molecular pathways that are shared between MDD and cardiometabolic disorders could have several important implications for future research and clinical practice. It is expected that increasing sample size and consequently increasing power will identify many more of these variants in the near future.

Firstly, the identification of shared molecular pathways, implicated in disease susceptibility, supports a growing evidence base for cross-diagnostic treatment paradigms. For example, there is now some preliminary evidence for the role of aspirin, statins, and insulin-sensitizing agents such as pioglitazone in the prevention or treatment augmentation of MDD, although such effects may be restricted to certain patient groups (Eyre and Baune 2015; Glaus et al. 2015; Hu et al. 2015; Kohler et al. 2014; Parsaik et al. 2014; Pasco et al. 2010; Williams et al. 2016). Similarly, shared molecular pathways could help to explain recent findings of reduced cardiovascular mortality (Acharya et al. 2013) or improved diabetic control (Brieler et al. 2016) in MDD patients treated with SSRIs. Secondly, further exploration of overlapping molecular pathophysiology has the potential to unveil novel targets for drug development and may give clues for the repurposing of other existing medications.

Thirdly, cardiometabolic disorders are thought to increase the risk of poor response to standard treatments in MDD (Woo et al. 2016) and bipolar disorder (Calkin et al. 2015). Genetic profiling for cardiometabolic vulnerability may identify poor treatment responders at an early stage, thereby reducing the costs of ineffective exposure to medicines for the individual and for society. Early identification of at-risk individuals would also guide practitioner's treatment recommendations, which may involve alternative somatic (e.g., electroconvulsive therapy, repetitive transcranial magnetic stimulation, ketamine) or specific psychological therapies as first- or second-line treatments.

Fourthly, studying the mechanisms of pleiotropic genes and shared pathways of depression and somatic disorders could help untangle the clinical and genetic heterogeneity that characterizes these illnesses. It is possible that a "cardiometabolic" endophenotype exists among mood disorder patients that may be identifiable, for example, through the development of specific polygenic risk scores (PGRS) (Samaan et al. 2015; Wray et al. 2014) or associated blood protein biomarkers. Working toward personalized care that allows for precise diagnostic, treatment, and prevention strategies, research could then focus on genetically stratified patient cohorts instead of the very diverse patient pool currently diagnosed with MDD. There is a growing consensus that such stratification approaches have the potential to substantially improve the quality of mental health research and mental health care over the coming decades (Schumann et al. 2014).

15.3 Summary and Conclusion

Altogether, earlier genetic studies suggest the involvement of pleiotropic genes in the comorbidity between depression and cardiometabolic diseases. While our appraisal provides some insight into common mechanisms and the role of pleiotropic genes, in-depth understanding of how these genes (and possibly others) mediate the association between depression and cardiometabolic diseases requires future comprehensive cross-disorder research in large-scale genetic studies. This will enable us to better understand why patients suffer from multiple diseases at a time and how multi-morbidities influence pharmacological treatment response to diseases.

Acknowledgments Azmeraw T.Amare would like to acknowledge the University of Adelaide for the PhD scholarship support through the Adelaide Scholarship International (ASI) program.

Azmeraw T.Amare has also been a student of Professor Harold Snieder, Professor Ute Bültmann, and Dr. Catharina A. Hartman, all from the University Medical Center Groningen (UMCG), the University of Groningen in the Netherlands and he acknowledges the input during their mentorship.

References

Acharya T, Acharya S, Tringali S et al (2013) Association of antidepressant and atypical antipsychotic use with cardiovascular events and mortality in a veteran population. Pharmacotherapy 33:1053–1061

Afari N, Noonan C, Goldberg J et al (2010) Depression and obesity: do shared genes explain the relationship? Depress Anxiety 27:799–806

Almgren P, Lehtovirta M, Isomaa B et al (2011) Heritability and familiality of type 2 diabetes and related quantitative traits in the Botnia Study. Diabetologia 54:2811–2819

Antypa N, Souery D, Tomasini M et al (2015) Clinical and genetic factors associated with suicide in mood disorder patients. Eur Arch Psychiatry Clin Neurosci 266(2):181–193

Barnett K, Mercer SW, Norbury M et al (2012) Epidemiology of multimorbidity and implications for health care, research, and medical education: a cross-sectional study. Lancet 380:37–43

Baune BT, Hohoff C, Roehrs T et al (2008) Serotonin receptor 1A–1019C/G variant: impact on antidepressant pharmacoresponse in melancholic depression? Neurosci Lett 436:111–115

Berndt SI, Gustafsson S, Mägi R et al (2013) Genome-wide meta-analysis identifies 11 new loci for anthropometric traits and provides insights into genetic architecture. Nat Genet 45:501–512

Bouatia-Naji N, Bonnefond A, Cavalcanti-Proenca C et al (2009) A variant near MTNR1B is associated with increased fasting plasma glucose levels and type 2 diabetes risk. Nat Genet 41:89–94

Brieler JA, Lustman PJ, Scherrer JF et al (2016) Antidepressant medication use and glycaemic control in co-morbid type 2 diabetes and depression. Fam Pract 33:30–36

Calkin CV, Ruzickova M, Uher R et al (2015) Insulin resistance and outcome in bipolar disorder. Br J Psychiatry 206:52–57

Celano CM, Huffman JC (2011) Depression and cardiac disease: a review. Cardiol Rev 19:130–142

Chambers JC, Weihua Z, Zabaneh D et al (2009) Common genetic variation near melatonin receptor MTNR1B contributes to raised plasma glucose and increased risk of type 2 diabetes among Indian Asians and European Caucasians. Diabetes 58:2703–2708

Chang HS, Won ES, Lee HY et al (2015) The association of proopiomelanocortin polymorphisms with the risk of major depressive disorder and the response to antidepressants via interactions with stressful life events. J Neural Transm 122:59–68

Chauvet-Gélinier JC, Trojak B, Vergès-Patois B et al (2013) Review on depression and coronary heart disease. Arch Cardiovasc Dis 106:103–110

CONVERGE Consortium (2015) Sparse whole-genome sequencing identifies two loci for major depressive disorder. Nature 523:588

Cordeiro ML, Gundersen CB, Umbach JA (2002) Lithium ions modulate the expression of VMAT2 in rat brain. Brain Res 953:189–194

Cuffí ML, Artells R, Navarro A et al (2010) Regulation of α_2-adrenoceptor gene expression by chronic lithium treatment in rat brain. Methods Find Exp Clin Pharmacol 32:721–725

Dannlowski U, Kugel H, Grotegerd D et al (2015) NCAN cross-disorder risk variant is associated with limbic gray matter deficits in healthy subjects and major depression. Neuropsychopharmacol Off Publ Am Coll Neuropsychopharmacol 40:2510–2516

Diniz BS, Talib LL, Joaquim HPG et al (2011) Platelet GSK3B activity in patients with late-life depression: marker of depressive episode severity and cognitive impairment? World J Biol Psychiatry Off J World Fed Soc Biol Psychiatry 12:216–222

Dupuis JJ, Langenberg C, Prokopenko I et al (2010) New genetic loci implicated in fasting glucose homeostasis and their impact on type 2 diabetes risk. Nat Genet 42:105–116

Ehret GB, Munroe PB et al (2011) Genetic variants in novel pathways influence blood pressure and cardiovascular disease risk. Nature 478:103–109

Eikelis N, Esler M, Barton D et al (2006) Reduced brain leptin in patients with major depressive disorder and in suicide victims. Mol Psychiatry 11:800–801

El-Hage W, Vourc'h P, Gaillard P et al (2014) The BDNF Val66Met polymorphism is associated with escitalopram response in depressed patients. Psychopharmacology (Berl) 232: 575–581

Eyre HA, Baune BT (2015) Anti-inflammatory intervention in depression. JAMA Psychiatry 72:511

Fernandez AM, Torres-Alemán I (2012) The many faces of insulin-like peptide signalling in the brain. Nat Rev Neurosci 13:225–239

Finseth PI, Sønderby IE, Djurovic S et al (2014) Association analysis between suicidal behaviour and candidate genes of bipolar disorder and schizophrenia. J Affect Disord 163:110–114

Flint J, Kendler KS (2014) The genetics of major depression. Neuron 81:484–503

Gałecka E, Szemraj J, Florkowski A et al (2011) Single nucleotide polymorphisms and mRNA expression for melatonin MT2 receptor in depression. Psychiatry Res 189:472–474

Gan Y, Gong Y, Tong X et al (2014) Depression and the risk of coronary heart disease: a meta-analysis of prospective cohort studies. BMC Psychiatry 14:7

Gaulton KJ, Ferreira T, Lee Y et al (2015) Genetic fine mapping and genomic annotation defines causal mechanisms at type 2 diabetes susceptibility loci. Nat Genet 47:1415–1425

Glaus J, Vandeleur CL, Lasserre AM et al (2015) Aspirin and statin use and the subsequent development of depression in men and women: results from a longitudinal population-based study. J Affect Disord 182:126–131

Golden SH, Lazo M, Carnethon M et al (2008) Examining a bidirectional association between depressive symptoms and diabetes. JAMA 299:2751–2759

Goswami DB, May WL, Stockmeier CA et al (2010) Transcriptional expression of serotonergic regulators in laser-captured microdissected dorsal raphe neurons of subjects with major depressive disorder: sex-specific differences. J Neurochem 112:397–409

Haefner S, Baghai TC, Schule C et al (2008) Impact of gene-gender effects of adrenergic polymorphisms on hypothalamic-pituitary-adrenal axis activity in depressed patients. Neuropsychobiology 58:154–162

Hara K, Fujita H, Johnson TA et al (2014) Genome-wide association study identifies three novel loci for type 2 diabetes. Hum Mol Genet 23:239–246

Herbert J, Ban M, Brown GW et al (2012) Interaction between the BDNF gene Val/66/Met polymorphism and morning cortisol levels as a predictor of depression in adult women. Br J Psychiatry 201:313–319

Hong W, Fan J, Yuan C et al (2014) Significantly decreased mRNA levels of BDNF and MEK1 genes in treatment-resistant depression. Neuroreport 25:753–755

Hu Y, Xing H, Dong X et al (2015) Pioglitazone is an effective treatment for patients with post-stroke depression combined with type 2 diabetes mellitus. Exp Ther Med 10:1109–1114

Huffman JC, Celano CM, Beach SR et al (2013) Depression and cardiac disease: epidemiology, mechanisms, and diagnosis. Cardiovasc Psychiatry Neurol 2013:1–14

Hung YY, Kang HY, Huang KW et al (2014) Association between toll-like receptors expression and major depressive disorder. Psychiatry Res 220:283–286

Hwang JY, Sim X, Wu Y et al (2015) Genome-wide association meta-analysis identifies novel variants associated with fasting plasma glucose in East Asians. Diabetes 64:291–298

Iwahashi K, Nishizawa D, Narita S et al (2014) Haplotype analysis of GSK-3β gene polymorphisms in bipolar disorder lithium responders and nonresponders. Clin Neuropharmacol 37:108–110

Jeanneteau FD, Lambert WM, Ismaili N et al (2012) BDNF and glucocorticoids regulate corticotrophin-releasing hormone (CRH) homeostasis in the hypothalamus. Proc Natl Acad Sci U S A 109:1305–1310

Kato M, Fukuda T, Wakeno M et al (2009) Effect of 5-HT1A gene polymorphisms on antidepressant response in major depressive disorder. Am J Med Genet B Neuropsychiatr Genet 150B:115–123

Kato M, Serretti A, Nonen S et al (2015) Genetic variants in combination with early partial improvement as a clinical utility predictor of treatment outcome in major depressive disorder: the result of two pooled RCTs. Transl Psychiatry 5:e513

Kelly CB, Mcdonnell AP, Johnston TG et al (2004) The MTHFR C677T polymorphism is associated with depressive episodes in patients from Northern Ireland. J Psychopharmacol (Oxford, England) 18:567–571

Kemp DE, Gao K, Chan PK et al (2010) Medical comorbidity in bipolar disorder: relationship between illnesses of the endocrine/metabolic system and treatment outcome. Bipolar Disord 12:404–413

Kim HK, Kim SJ, Lee YJ et al (2011a) Influence of the interaction between the serotonin 1A receptor C-1019G polymorphism and negative life stressors on the development of depression. Neuropsychobiology 64:1–8

Kim YJ, Go MJ, Hu C et al (2011b) Large-scale genome-wide association studies in east Asians identify new genetic loci influencing metabolic traits. Nat Genet 43:990–995

Kishi T, Yoshimura R, Fukuo Y et al (2013) The serotonin 1A receptor gene confer susceptibility to mood disorders: results from an extended meta-analysis of patients with major depression and bipolar disorder. Eur Arch Psychiatry Clin Neurosci 263:105–118

Klenke S, Siffert W (2011) SNPs in genes encoding G proteins in pharmacogenetics. Pharmacogenomics 12:633–654

Kloiber S, Ripke S, Kohli MA et al (2013) Resistance to antidepressant treatment is associated with polymorphisms in the leptin gene, decreased leptin mRNA expression, and decreased leptin serum levels. Eur Neuropsychopharmacol 23:653–662

Knoblauch H, Busjahn A, Munter S et al (1997) Heritability analysis of lipids and three gene loci in twins link the macrophage scavenger receptor to HDL cholesterol concentrations. Arterioscler Thromb Vasc Biol 17:2054–2060

Knol MJ, Twisk JWR, Beekman ATF et al (2006) Depression as a risk factor for the onset of type 2 diabetes mellitus. A meta-analysis. Diabetologia 49:837–845

Ko A, Cantor RM, Weissglas-Volkov D et al (2014) Amerindian-specific regions under positive selection harbour new lipid variants in Latinos. Nat Commun 5:3983

Kohler O, Benros ME, Nordentoft M et al (2014) Effect of anti-inflammatory treatment on depression, depressive symptoms, and adverse effects: a systematic review and meta-analysis of randomized clinical trials. JAMA Psychiatry 71:1381–1391

Kooner JS, Chambers JC, Aguilar-Salinas CA et al (2008) Genome-wide scan identifies variation in MLXIPL associated with plasma triglycerides. Nat Genet 40:149–151

Kopczak A, Stalla GK, Uhr M et al (2015) IGF-I in major depression and antidepressant treatment response. Eur Neuropsychopharmacol J Eur Coll Neuropsychopharmacol 25:864–872

Kupper NHM, Willemsen G, Van Den Berg M et al (2004) Heritability of ambulatory heart rate variability. Circulation 110:2792–2796

Lavebratt C, Sjöholm LK, Soronen P et al (2010) CRY2 is associated with depression. PLoS One 5:e9407

Lemonde S, Du L, Bakish D et al (2004) Association of the C(-1019)G 5-HT1A functional promoter polymorphism with antidepressant response. Int J Neuropsychopharm Off Sci J Coll Int Neuropsychopharm 7:501–506

Levy D, Ehret GB, Rice K et al (2009) Genome-wide association study of blood pressure and hypertension. Nat Genet 41:677–687

Lewis SJ, Lawlor DA, Davey Smith G et al (2006) The thermolabile variant of MTHFR is associated with depression in the British Women's Heart and Health Study and a meta-analysis. Mol Psychiatry 11:352–360

Li Z, Li Y, Chen L et al (2015) Prevalence of depression in patients with hypertension: a systematic review and meta-analysis. Medicine 94:e1317

Liu XH, Xu YF, Cui DH et al (2010) Association of cyclic adenosine monophosphate response element-binding protein gene and major depressive disorder. Chin J Med Gen 27:263–266

Liu JJ, Buisman-Pijlman F, Hutchinson MR (2014) Toll-like receptor 4: innate immune regulator of neuroimmune and neuroendocrine interactions in stress and major depressive disorder. Front Neurosci 8:309

Locke AE, Kahali B, Berndt SI et al (2015) Genetic studies of body mass index yield new insights for obesity biology. Nature 518:197–206

Lohoff FW (2010) Overview of the genetics of major depressive disorder. Curr Psychiatry Rep 12:539–546

Lok A, Bockting CLH, Koeter MWJ et al (2013) Interaction between the MTHFR C677T polymorphism and traumatic childhood events predicts depression. Transl Psychiatry 3:e288

López-Figueroa AL, Norton CS, López-Figueroa MO et al (2004) Serotonin 5-HT1A, 5-HT1B, and 5-HT2A receptor mRNA expression in subjects with major depression, bipolar disorder, and schizophrenia. Biol Psychiatry 55:225–233

Lopez-Leon S, Aulchenko YS, Tiemeier H et al (2010) Shared genetic factors in the co-occurrence of symptoms of depression and cardiovascular risk factors. J Affect Disord 122:247–252

Lu X, Wang L, Lin X et al (2015) Genome-wide association study in Chinese identifies novel loci for blood pressure and hypertension. Hum Mol Genet 24:865–874

Mahajan A, Go MJ, Zhang W et al (2014) Genome-wide trans-ancestry meta-analysis provides insight into the genetic architecture of type 2 diabetes susceptibility. Nat Genet 46:234–244

Maher BS, Hughes HB, Zubenko WN et al (2010) Genetic linkage of region containing the CREB1 gene to depressive disorders in families with recurrent, early-onset, major depression: a re-analysis and confirmation of sex-specific effect. Am J Med Genet B Neuropsychiatr Genet 153:10–16

Manning AK, Hivert M-F, Scott RA et al (2012) A genome-wide approach accounting for body mass index identifies genetic variants influencing fasting glycemic traits and insulin resistance. Nat Genet 44:659–669

Marenberg ME, Risch N, Berkman LF et al (1994) Genetic susceptibility to death from coronary heart disease in a study of twins. N Engl J Med 330:1041–1046

Mezuk B, Eaton WW, Albrecht S et al (2008) Depression and type 2 diabetes over the lifespan: a meta-analysis. Diabetes Care 31:2383–2390

Mitjans M, Arias B, Jiménez E et al (2015) Exploring genetic variability at PI, GSK3, HPA, and glutamatergic pathways in lithium response: association with IMPA2, INPP1, and GSK3B genes. J Clin Psychopharmacol 35:600–604

Mitschelen M, Yan H, Farley JA et al (2011) Long-term deficiency of circulating and hippocampal insulin-like growth factor I induces depressive behavior in adult mice: a potential model of geriatric depression. Neuroscience 185:50–60

Moses-Kolko EL, Wisner KL, Price JC et al (2008) Serotonin 1A receptor reductions in postpartum depression: a positron emission tomography study. Fertil Steril 89:685–692

Murphy GM Jr, Sarginson JE, Ryan HS et al (2013) BDNF and CREB1 genetic variants interact to affect antidepressant treatment outcomes in geriatric depression. Pharmacogenet Genomics 23:301–313

Murray CJL, Barber RM, Foreman KJ et al (2015) Global, regional, and national disability-adjusted life years (DALYs) for 306 diseases and injuries and healthy life expectancy (HALE) for 188 countries, 1990–2013: quantifying the epidemiological transition. Lancet 386: 2145–2191

Newton-Cheh C, Johnson T, Gateva V et al (2009) Genome-wide association study identifies eight loci associated with blood pressure. Nat Genet 41:666–676

Ng MCY, Shriner D, Chen BH et al (2014) Meta-analysis of genome-wide association studies in African Americans provides insights into the genetic architecture of type 2 diabetes. PLoS Genet 10:e1004517

Nikpay M, Goel A, Won H-H et al (2015) A comprehensive 1,000 Genomes-based genome-wide association meta-analysis of coronary artery disease. Nat Genet 47:1121–1130

Nouwen A, Winkley K, Twisk J et al (2010) Type 2 diabetes mellitus as a risk factor for the onset of depression: a systematic review and meta-analysis. Diabetologia 53:2480–2486

Otsuki K, Uchida S, Wakabayashi Y et al (2010) Aberrant REST-mediated transcriptional regulation in major depressive disorder. J Psychiatr Res 44:378–384

Pandey GN, Dwivedi Y, Rizavi HS et al (2010) Brain-derived neurotrophic factor gene and protein expression in pediatric and adult depressed subjects. Prog Neuro-Psychopharmacol Biol Psychiatry 34:645–651

Pandey GN, Rizavi HS, Ren X et al (2014) Toll-like receptors in the depressed and suicide brain. J Psychiatr Res 53:62–68

Parsaik AK, Singh B, Murad MH et al (2014) Statins use and risk of depression: a systematic review and meta-analysis. J Affect Disord 160:62–67

Pasco JA, Jacka FN, Williams LJ et al (2010) Clinical implications of the cytokine hypothesis of depression: the association between use of statins and aspirin and the risk of major depression. Psychother Psychosom 79:323–325

Perroud N, Aitchison KJ, Uher R et al (2009) Genetic predictors of increase in suicidal ideation during antidepressant treatment in the GENDEP project. Neuropsychopharm Off Publ Am Coll Neuropsychopharmacol 34:2517–2528

Peter D, Finn JP, Klisak I et al (1993) Chromosomal localization of the human vesicular amine transporter genes. Genomics 18:720–723

Plante GE (2005) Depression and cardiovascular disease: a reciprocal relationship. Metab Clin Exp 54:45–48

Poulsen P, Ohm Kyvik K, Vaag A et al (1999) Heritability of type II (non-insulin-dependent) diabetes mellitus and abnormal glucose tolerance - a population-based twin study. Diabetologia 42:139–145

Pruitt K, Brown G, Tatusova T et al. (2012) The reference sequence (RefSeq) database. In: National Center for Biotechnology Information (US), Nucleic Acids Research 40. http://www.ncbi.nlm.nih.gov/pmc/articles/PMC3245008/

Raote I, Bhattacharya A, Panicker MM (2007) Serotonin 2A (5-HT2A) Receptor function: ligand-dependent mechanisms and pathways. In: Serotonin receptors in neurobiology. CRC Press, Boca Raton, pp 1–17

Rivera M, Cohen-Woods S, Kapur K et al (2011) Depressive disorder moderates the effect of the FTO gene on body mass index. Mol Psychiatry 17:604–611
Rosmond R, Björntorp P (2000) The hypothalamic-pituitary-adrenal axis activity as a predictor of cardiovascular disease, type 2 diabetes and stroke. J Intern Med 247:188–197
Rudisch B, Nemeroff CB (2003) Epidemiology of comorbid coronary artery disease and depression. Biol Psychiatry 54:227–240
Rugulies R (2002) Depression as a predictor for coronary heart disease: a review and meta-analysis. Am J Prev Med 23:51–61
Samaan Z, Anand SS, Anand S et al (2013) The protective effect of the obesity-associated rs9939609 a variant in fat mass- and obesity-associated gene on depression. Mol Psychiatry 18:1281–1286
Samaan Z, Lee YK, Gerstein HC et al (2015) Obesity genes and risk of major depressive disorder in a multiethnic population: a cross-sectional study. J Clin Psychiatry 76:e1611–e1618
Sarchiapone M, Carli V, Roy A et al (2008) Association of polymorphism (Val66Met) of brain-derived neurotrophic factor with suicide attempts in depressed patients. Neuropsychobiology 57:139–145
Saus E, Soria V, Escaramís G et al (2010) A haplotype of glycogen synthase kinase 3β is associated with early onset of unipolar major depression. Genes Brain Behav 9:799–807
Scherrer JF, Xian H, Bucholz KK et al (2003) A twin study of depression symptoms, hypertension, and heart disease in middle-aged men. Psychosom Med 65:548–557
Schmidt HD, Shelton RC, Duman RS (2011) Functional biomarkers of depression: diagnosis, treatment, and pathophysiology. Neuropsychopharmacology 36:2375–2394
Schumann G, Binder EB, Holte A et al (2014) Stratified medicine for mental disorders. Eur Neuropsychopharmacol 24:5–50
Scott RA, Lagou V, Welch RP et al (2012) Large-scale association analyses identify new loci influencing glycemic traits and provide insight into the underlying biological pathways. Nat Genet 44:991–1005
Serretti A, Chiesa A, Calati R et al (2011) A preliminary investigation of the influence of CREB1 gene on treatment resistance in major depression. J Affect Disord 128:56–63
Shyn SI, Shi J, Kraft JB et al (2011) Novel loci for major depression identified by genome-wide association study of sequenced treatment alternatives to relieve depression and meta-analysis of three studies. Mol Psychiatry 16:202–215
Sivakumaran S, Agakov F, Theodoratou E et al (2011) Abundant pleiotropy in human complex diseases and traits. Am J Hum Genet 89:607–618
Smoller JW (2013) Identification of risk loci with shared effects on five major psychiatric disorders: a genome-wide analysis. Lancet 381:1371–1379
Soranzo N, Sanna S, Wheeler E et al (2010) Common variants at 10 genomic loci influence hemoglobin A1C levels via glycemic and nonglycemic pathways. Diabetes 59:3229–3239
Soria V, Martínez-Amorós E, Escaramís G et al (2010) Differential association of circadian genes with mood disorders: CRY1 and NPAS2 are associated with unipolar major depression and CLOCK and VIP with bipolar disorder. Neuropsychopharmacol Off Publ Am Coll Neuropsychopharmacol 35:1279–1289
Speliotes EK, Willer CJ, Berndt SI et al (2010) Association analyses of 249,796 individuals reveal 18 new loci associated with body mass index. Nat Genet 42:937–948
Stearns FW (2010) One hundred years of pleiotropy: a retrospective. Genetics 186:767–773
Su S, Lampert R, Lee F et al (2010) Common genes contribute to depressive symptoms and heart rate variability: the twins heart study. Twin Res Hum Genet Off J Int Soc Twin Stud 13:1–9
Sullivan PF, Neale MC, Kendler KS (2000) Genetic epidemiology of major depression: review and meta-analysis. Am J Psychiatr 157:1552–1562
Suzuki Y, Sawamura K, Someya T (2004) The effects of a 5-hydroxytryptamine 1A receptor gene polymorphism on the clinical response to fluvoxamine in depressed patients. Pharmacogenomics J 4:283–286
Szczepanska-Sadowska E, Cudnoch-Jedrzejewska A, Ufnal M et al (2010) Brain and cardiovascular diseases: common neurogenic background of cardiovascular, metabolic and inflammatory diseases. J Physiol Pharmacol 61:509–521

Van Rijn MJE, Schut AFC, Aulchenko YS et al (2007) Heritability of blood pressure traits and the genetic contribution to blood pressure variance explained by four blood-pressure-related genes. J Hypertens 25:565–570

Voight BF, Scott LJ, Steinthorsdottir V et al (2010) Twelve type 2 diabetes susceptibility loci identified through large-scale association analysis. Nat Genet 42:579–589

Wain LV, Verwoert GC, O'reilly PF et al (2011) Genome-wide association study identifies six new loci influencing pulse pressure and mean arterial pressure. Nat Genet 43:1005–1011

Wakeno M, Kato M, Okugawa G et al (2008) The alpha 2A-adrenergic receptor gene polymorphism modifies antidepressant responses to milnacipran. J Clin Psychopharmacol 28:518–524

Welter D, Macarthur J, Morales J et al (2014) The NHGRI GWAS Catalog, a curated resource of SNP-trait associations. Nucleic Acids Res 42:D1001–D1006

Wen W, Zheng W, Okada Y et al (2014) Meta-analysis of genome-wide association studies in East Asian-ancestry populations identifies four new loci for body mass index. Hum Mol Genet 23:5492–5504

Whiteford HA, Degenhardt L, Rehm J et al (2013) Global burden of disease attributable to mental and substance use disorders: findings from the Global Burden of Disease Study 2010. Lancet 382:1575–1586

Willer CJ, Sanna S, Jackson AU et al (2008) Newly identified loci that influence lipid concentrations and risk of coronary artery disease. Nat Genet 40:161–169

Willer CJ, Schmidt EM, Sengupta S et al (2013) Discovery and refinement of loci associated with lipid levels. Nat Genet 45:1274–1283

Williams LJ, Pasco JA, Mohebbi M et al (2016) Statin and aspirin use and the risk of mood disorders among men. Int J Neuropsychopharmacol 1–4. http://www.ncbi.nlm.nih.gov/pubmed/?term=26839250

Willyard C (2014) Heritability: the family roots of obesity. Nature 508:S58–S60

Woo YS, Seo HJ, Mcintyre RS et al (2016) Obesity and its potential effects on antidepressant treatment outcomes in patients with depressive disorders: a literature review. Int J Mol Sci 17. http://www.mdpi.com/1422-0067/17/1/80

Wray NR, Lee SH, Mehta D et al (2014) Research review: polygenic methods and their application to psychiatric traits. J Child Psychol Psychiatry 55:1068–1087

Wu Y-L, Ding X-X, Sun Y-H et al (2013) Association between MTHFR C677T polymorphism and depression: an updated meta-analysis of 26 studies. Prog Neuropsychopharmacol Biol Psychiatry 46:78–85

Yang C, Xu Y, Sun N et al (2010) The combined effects of the BDNF and GSK3B genes modulate the relationship between negative life events and major depressive disorder. Brain Res 1355:1–6

Yen Y-C, Rebok GW, Gallo JJ et al (2007) ApoE4 allele is associated with late-life depression: a population-based study. Am J Geriatr Psychiatry Off J Am Assoc Geriatr Psychiatry 15:858–868

Zelinski EL, Deibel SH, Mcdonald RJ (2014) The trouble with circadian clock dysfunction: multiple deleterious effects on the brain and body. Neurosci Biobehav Rev 40:80–101

Zhang K, Yang C, Xu Y et al (2010) Genetic association of the interaction between the BDNF and GSK3B genes and major depressive disorder in a Chinese population. J Neural Transm (Vienna: 1996) 117:393–401

Zheng J-S, Arnett DK, Lee Y-C et al (2013) Genome-wide contribution of genotype by environment interaction to variation of diabetes-related traits. PLoS One 8:e77442

Zill P, Baghai TC, Engel R et al (2003) Beta-1-adrenergic receptor gene in major depression: influence on antidepressant treatment response. American journal of medical genetics. Part B. Neuropsychiatr Genet Off Publ Int Soc Psychiatr Genet 120B:85–89

Zou Y-F, Wang Y, Liu P et al (2010) Association of BDNF Val66Met polymorphism with both baseline HRQOL scores and improvement in HRQOL scores in Chinese major depressive patients treated with fluoxetine. Hum Psychopharmacol 25:145–152

Zubenko GS, Hughes HB, Stiffler JS et al (2003) Sequence variations in CREB1 cosegregate with depressive disorders in women. Mol Psychiatry 8:611–618

Emotional Word Processing in Cardiovascular Disease, Depression, and Depression Subtypes

16

Henning Teismann, Britta Radenz, Johanna Kissler, and Klaus Berger

Contents

Abstract

In the recent past, evaluation and processing of emotional content have received much attention in clinical psychology and (cognitive) neuroscience. For instance, using experimental designs and stimuli such as emotional pictures or words, it has been consistently shown that patients with depression are characterized by intensified evaluation and elaboration of particularly unpleasant, high-arousing information. However, although population-based research has uncovered the close, bidirectional link between depression and cardiopathy, emotional content

H. Teismann (✉) • B. Radenz • K. Berger
Institute of Epidemiology and Social Medicine, University of Münster,
Albert-Schweitzer-Campus 1, Building D3, Münster 48149, Germany
e-mail: h.teismann@uni-muenster.de

J. Kissler
Department of Psychology, University of Bielefeld, Bielefeld 33501, Germany

Center of Excellence Cognitive Interaction Technology (CITEC),
University of Bielefeld, Bielefeld 33619, Germany

B.T. Baune, P.J. Tully (eds.), *Cardiovascular Diseases and Depression*,
DOI 10.1007/978-3-319-32480-7_16

evaluation and processing investigations did not yet focus on cardiovascular disease (CVD) or coronary heart disease. Moreover, measures of emotional content evaluation or processing have not yet been included into large, observational psychocardiologic investigations.

In this chapter, we present analyses of *valence* (i.e., unpleasant to neutral to pleasant) and *arousal* (i.e., calm to exciting) ratings of words, which were part of the baseline core examination program of the BiDirect Study, a large prospective observational study designed to investigate the relationship between depression and (subclinical) arteriosclerosis. The BiDirect Study integrates three cohorts of adults between 35 and 65 years (depression patients vs. CVD patients vs. control subjects); here, the data of 2,165 BiDirect subjects were included.

The valence and arousal rating analysis showed that (i) patients with depression rated in particular the high-arousing unpleasant words to be more unpleasant and more arousing compared to CVD patients or control subjects. Moreover, there were indications:

1. For (ii) reduced valence ratings and increased arousal ratings in women compared to men (particularly for high-arousing unpleasant words)
2. For (iii) increased valence ratings in the oldest compared to younger participants
3. For (iv) the amplified processing of positive information in older CVD patients
4. For (v) the amplified processing of positive and neutral information in female CVD patients
5. For (vi) an association between health state that was assessed as good and reduced arousal by unpleasant material in patients with a severe disease (i.e., depression or CVD)

Even after taking several limitations into account, the present findings basically confirm robust results from previous experimental investigations (e.g., showing an equivalent of the well-established processing bias for negative information in depression patients). Furthermore, there are first hints for novel results, which may indicate that our efforts of moving beyond laboratory affective science toward *emotional epidemiology* may uncover effects that were otherwise not very likely to be detected. A future challenge will be to thoroughly explore the potential of emotional content evaluation and processing data with regard to quality of life or disease risk prediction in the context of psychocardiology.

16.1 Introduction

What emotions are and which brain structures are involved in their development and processing are questions that have been asked since long. In the recent past, the field of affective science has quickly grown (DeSteno et al. 2013), and more and more scientists from different disciplines such as psychology, (cognitive) neuroscience, electrophysiology, or neuroimaging joined in, leading to considerable knowledge gain regarding the nature, structure, functions, experience, and regulation of emotions (Barrett et al. 2007).

Certain emotion theories have postulated the existence of a set of discrete, basic emotions (i.e., sadness (help seeking), fear (avoiding), anger (fighting), disgust (rejecting), enjoyment (playing), and surprise (orienting) (Levenson 2011)). Other models emphasized the dimensional structure of emotions (Rubin and Talarico 2009). Dimensional models of emotions are nowadays an accepted concept (Citron 2012), and research has shown that humans are able to reliably distinguish the *valence* (i.e., pleasant vs. unpleasant) and the *arousal* (i.e., calming vs. exciting) associated with core affective states (Lang et al. 1997). In the tradition of Osgood et al. (1975) and Lang (1979), it has become common practice to routinely measure these two key affective dimensions of subjective experience and to use them as a common metric to evaluate the emotional content of stimuli. The evaluation is often conducted using numerical rating scales, which allow the quick assessment of a large number of stimuli. The typical finding is that highly arousing stimuli (e.g., the words *torture* or *love*) are rated as being either highly pleasant or highly unpleasant, while low-arousing stimuli (e.g., *building* or *normal*) usually receive rather neutral valence ratings, resulting in a U-shaped valence by arousal plot (Kissler et al. 2006).

Regarding stimulus material that is suitable for experimental investigations of emotions, it has been argued that words (which are completely symbolic and whose meaning and emotional significance are acquired by learning) may be rather heterogeneous and thus less potent emotional stimuli as compared to pictorial or facial stimuli (Lifshitz 1966; Vanderploeg et al. 1987). The latter evoke responses that are at least partly based on biological preparedness (Ohman and Mineka 2001). More specifically, it is reasonable to assume that visually presented words are less arousing than corresponding, potentially complex and colored pictures or even photographs. Hence, emotion research has mainly focused on the processing of nonlinguistic stimuli (Kissler et al. 2007). However, a considerable number of electrophysiological studies (Kissler et al. 2007) demonstrated amplified cortical responses during the processing of words with an emotional load, and studies directly comparing the effects of words versus pictorial material showed similar arousal effects for both stimulus classes at late (Hinojosa et al. 2009) and even early (Schacht and Sommer 2009) processing stages. Responses evoked by words may not be as pronounced as responses recorded during the processing of emotional pictures or faces, but they are reliably observable (Kissler et al. 2006). Thus, words have been demonstrated to constitute an eligible means to investigate emotional processing.

Emotions matter for health, and effects of emotion on health and well-being can be both direct and indirect (Levenson 2011). In the shorter terms, emotion experience is directly associated with adaptive physiological alterations, e.g., regarding cardiac functioning, blood pressure, immune response, or HPA axis. In the longer term, depending on the nature, frequency, and time course of the emotional state, initially adaptive physiologic responses can lead to maladaptive outcomes if not adequately regulated. Effects of emotion on health can also manifest indirectly, e.g., via shaping thoughts, decisions, and behaviors (DeSteno et al. 2013).

Both negative and positive emotions matter for health. Negative emotions (e.g., anxiety or depression) are associated with subjective experience of negative valence ("unhappiness") and may influence the development of infectious disease (Cohen et al. 1993), declines in lung function (Kubzansky et al. 2006), diabetes (Mezuk et al. 2008), arthritis (Karakus and Patton 2011), and cancer (Kroenke et al. 2005). The strongest evidence available showed that negative emotions influenced the development of cardiovascular disease (CVD) (Roest et al. 2010). On the other hand, positive emotions (e.g., enjoyment) are associated with subjective experience of positive valence ("happiness") and likely have a protective effect on health (Cohen and Pressman 2006). Again, the strongest available evidence showed an association with CVD, with studies generally indicating that positive affect reduced the risk of developing CVD (Boehm and Kubzansky 2012).

Many recent cognitive and affective science studies recruited samples of patients with affective disorders such as anxiety or depression to investigate the *evaluation or processing of emotional content*. Among other results, these studies yielded conclusive evidence demonstrating that depression is characterized by the intensified elaboration of negatively toned information, by difficulties in withdrawing attention from negative material ("rumination" (Zetsche et al. 2012)), and by deficits in cognitive control during the processing of negative information (Joormann and D'Avanzato 2010; Gotlib and Joormann 2010). Depression-related specifics in emotional content evaluation and processing become manifest particularly in the form of (explicit) memory bias (Gotlib and Joormann 2010; Sumner 2012). For instance, during verbal memory tasks, patients with depression typically remember more negative than positive words, while the opposite holds true for nondepressed individuals (Denny and Hunt 1992; Matt et al. 1992; Dalgleish and Watts 1990; Blaney 1986). Furthermore, depressed but not anxious patients exhibited an enhanced recognition of negative compared to positive facial expressions (Gilboa-Schechtman et al. 2002).

There is a large and ever-growing body of psychocardiologic studies yielding evidence for the relationship between emotional distress (i.e., anxiety, depression) and heart disease. For instance, depression following myocardial infarction was a significant predictor of mortality (Frasure-Smith et al. 1993; Lesperance et al. 1996; Schleifer et al. 1989), and patients with heart disease reported an overall poorer quality of life (Stewart et al. 1989; Sirois and Burg 2003). Interestingly however, according to our literature research there seem to be merely very few studies (Constans et al. 1999; Ginting et al. 2013) that were specifically designed to investigate evaluation or processing of emotional content in CVD patients. Using an emotional Stroop paradigm (Williams et al. 1996), one study (Ginting et al. 2013) demonstrated that coronary heart disease (CHD) patients exhibited a specific attentional bias toward CHD-related threatening words.

Noteworthy, emotion processing or affective science has not yet received much attention in the field of population-based research. Furthermore, to our knowledge observational studies or even epidemiologic cohort studies with larger sample sizes investigating emotional content evaluation or processing in depression or CVD are scarce if at all existing. The available studies investigating emotional content evaluation or processing were usually small, aimed at homogeneous disease phenotypes, and adopted experimental designs under highly controlled laboratory conditions.

For this chapter, we initially explored data regarding the evaluation of emotionally charged written words. The data were collected as part of the baseline assessment of the BiDirect Study (Teismann et al. 2014), a cohort study designed to investigate the bidirectional relationship between depression and (subclinical) arteriosclerosis. The BiDirect Study includes three large cohorts: (i) patients with depression, (ii) patients with CVD, and (iii) community-dwelling control subjects. Here, in addition to contrasting the cohorts, patients with two different subtypes of depression (melancholic vs. atypical depression) were compared with regard to affective word evaluation. The results are discussed including (i) options to adequately model the data and (ii) the potential that considering the evaluation and processing of emotional content may have for the prediction of disease risk or quality of life in the context of psychocardiology.

16.2 Emotional Word Processing in the BiDirect Study

16.2.1 Background

Psychocardiologic research has shown that depression and CVD are related, and ample evidence indicated that the link is bidirectional (Hare et al. 2013). For instance, depression appears to be a risk for CVD onset (Davidson et al. 2005) and a predictor of poorer CVD outcome (Baune et al. 2012). In turn, many CVD patients develop subsequent depression (Carney and Freedland 2003), and patients with CVD plus depression have an increased risk for further cardiovascular events compared to CVD patients without depression (Baune et al. 2012).

Studies addressing the bidirectional depression-CVD association mainly focused on potentially shared biological mechanisms, which may underlie a partly joint causal relationship. However, in addition to biological processes, there could also be other pathways that might lead from one disease to the other. For instance, certain lifestyle behaviors typically characterizing patients with depression (e.g., smoking, physical inactivity, poor diet) may increase the risk to experience future cardiovascular events. The other way around, certain cognitions may typically characterize CVD patients (e.g., prevailing thoughts regarding burdens such as heart symptoms, losses such as quality of life or independence, or threats such as further cardiac events), leading to an increased risk to develop subsequent depression (Teismann et al. 2014). Another possibility, which so far has received little attention, is that certain styles regarding the evaluation or processing of emotional content may be relevant in this context.

16.2.2 Rationale and Design of the BiDirect Study

The BiDirect Study (Teismann et al. 2014; Wersching and Berger 2012) is a prospective epidemiologic study, which was designed to investigate the bidirectional relationship between depression and (subclinical) arteriosclerosis. The BiDirect Study integrates three cohorts of adults who were aged 35–65 years at the time point of recruitment: (i) patients with depression, (ii) patients with CVD due to arteriosclerosis, and (iii) community-dwelling control subjects randomly drawn from the registry of the city of Münster, North Rhine-Westphalia, Germany. In total, 2,165 BiDirect participants (989 patients with depression, 340 patients with CVD, and 836 control subjects) were included in the present analyses.

16.2.3 Methods

16.2.3.1 Evaluation of Emotional Word Content

Besides markers of depressive symptoms, (subclinical) arteriosclerosis, cognitive functioning, or lifestyle, which are rather commonly used in epidemiologic investigations of issues relevant to psychocardiology, the BiDirect Study core examination program included measures of the evaluation of emotional content. Specifically, subjective ratings of 12 written German nouns were inquired from the participants. A nine-point rating scale (1 = "very unpleasant" … 5 = "neutral" … 9 = "very pleasant") quantified the perceived *valence* for each presented word. Another nine-point rating scale was used to assess the perceived *arousal* (1 = "not arousing" … 9 = "very arousing") for each individual noun.

The nouns used here are a subset of the *buzzwords* that were introduced by Kissler et al. (2007). These nouns had been pre-categorized into high-arousing pleasant words, low-arousing neutral words, or high-arousing unpleasant words. Each of these three categories was represented by four nouns (Fig. 16.1). Before using the nouns in the BiDirect Study, we conducted a pretest in a convenience sample of 52 participants (64 %, females; 48 %, <40 years; 44 %, between 40 and 60 years; 8 %, >60 years) in order to evaluate whether the valence and arousal categorizations could be reproduced in a sample of older subjects that was more representative of the BiDirect Study participants. The results of the pretest indicated that the valence and arousal scores were sufficiently similar to those reported by Kissler et al. (2007). Noteworthy, the 12 nouns were comparable regarding concreteness, word length (in letters), and word frequency (per million), the latter based on counts for written German according to the CELEX database (Baayen et al. 1995).

16.2.3.2 Determination of Depression Subtype

During BiDirect-Baseline, symptom-based determination of depression subtypes was conducted using selected modules of the MINI International Neuropsychiatric Interview (German version 5.0.0) (Ackenheil and Stotz-Ingenlath 1999), selected

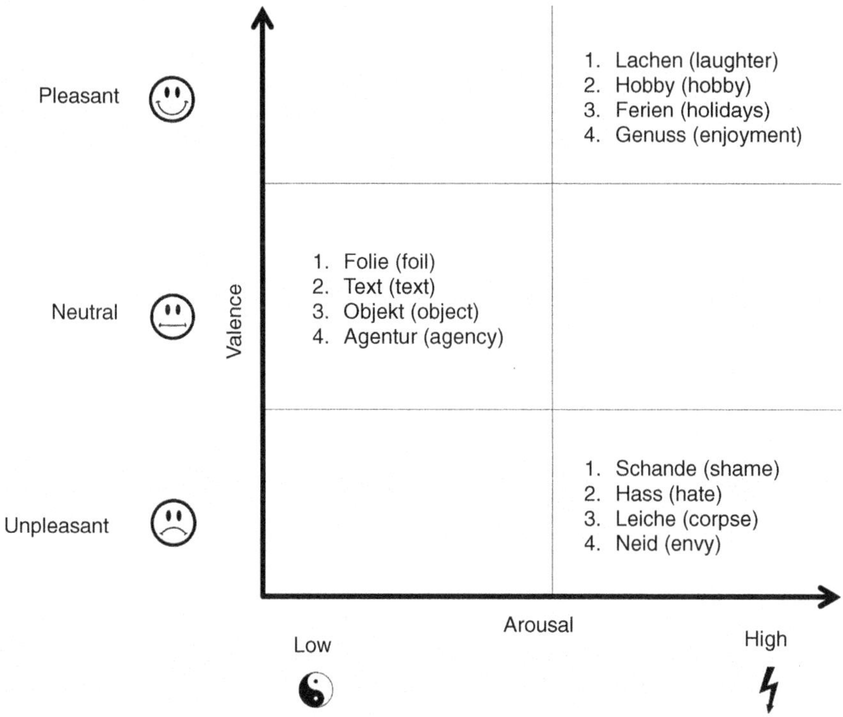

Fig. 16.1 Mapping of the 12 nouns to arousal-valence space. In each case four nouns represented the categories (i) high-arousing unpleasant, (ii) low-arousing neutral, and (iii) high-arousing pleasant

Inventory of Depressive Symptomatology (Rush et al. 1986) items, and the 17 items version of the Hamilton Depression Rating Scale (HAM-D) (Hamilton 1960). In short, for the purpose of the BiDirect Study, patients who met either all ("certain" subtypes) or all but one ("probable" subtypes) DSM-IV diagnostic criteria for depression with either atypical or melancholic features were assigned the particular diagnoses. Patients who did not meet these criteria were classified as undifferentiated; patients who met the criteria for atypical and melancholic depression at the same time were classified as mixed (Teismann et al. 2014). From the patients included in the present analyses, 82 had atypical depression, and 576 had melancholic depression.

16.2.3.3 Assessment of Perceived Health State

Perceived health state was quantified using the "thermometer" (a visual analogue scale ranging from 0="worst imaginable health state" to 100="best imaginable health state") from the EQ-5D-3L (Rabin and De Charro 2001), a questionnaire which measures perceived health-related quality of life. For analysis, perceived health state ratings were categorized into quartiles.

16.2.3.4 Analysis Strategy

For the purpose of this chapter, we analyzed both the valence and arousal ratings given for the pleasant, neutral, and unpleasant words. First, we compared the mean valence and arousal ratings between sexes, age categories, cohorts, and depression subtypes. Second, we stratified the mean valence and arousal ratings (i) by cohort and sex and (ii) by cohort and age. And third, we associated the mean valence and arousal ratings per cohort with a measure of perceived health state, the "thermometer" from the EQ-5D-3L questionnaire (Rabin and De Charro 2001) (thereby adjusting for effects of both sex and age). Noteworthy, due to low number ($N = 82$), we refrained from further stratifying patients with atypical depression due to age and sex; in lieu thereof, we contrasted the patients with melancholic depression ($N = 576$) with the whole cohort of (non-differentiated) depression patients ($N = 989$).

16.2.4 Results

16.2.4.1 Comparison of Mean Valence and Arousal Ratings Between Sexes and Between Age Categories

Table 16.1 shows mean valence and arousal ratings for the three different word categories (unpleasant vs. neutral vs. pleasant) split by sex (male vs. female) or age category (35–44 years vs. 45–54 years vs. 55–65 years), respectively. Regarding sex, across word categories women rated the words to be less pleasant compared to men. This tendency was most pronounced in case of words which had been pre-categorized as unpleasant. Women rated the words also to be more arousing compared to men. This tendency was also most pronounced in case of words which had been pre-categorized as unpleasant. Regarding age, across word categories the oldest participants rated the words to be more pleasant compared to younger participants. This effect was most pronounced in case of words which had been pre-categorized as neutral. Moreover, the youngest patients rated the words to be less arousing compared to older patients. This effect was also most pronounced in case of words which had been pre-categorized as neutral.

16.2.4.2 Comparison of Mean Valence and Arousal Ratings Between Cohorts and Between Depression Subtypes

Table 16.2 shows mean valence and arousal ratings for the three different word categories (unpleasant vs. neutral vs. pleasant) split by cohort (depression vs. CVD vs. control) or depression subtype (atypical vs. melancholic depression), respectively. Regarding cohort, across word categories patients with depression rated the words to be less pleasant compared to CVD patients and control subjects. This tendency was most pronounced in case of words which had been pre-categorized as unpleasant. Moreover, across word categories patients with depression rated the words to be more arousing compared to CVD patients and control subjects. This tendency was also most pronounced in case of words which had been pre-categorized as unpleasant. Interestingly, there was one noticeable deviation from the overall pattern: CVD patients rated words which had been pre-categorized as

Table 16.1 Mean valence and arousal ratings (± SD) for the three different word categories split by sex or age, respectively

		Sex			Age			
		Male (N=1,104)	Female (N=1,061)	Total	35–44 years (N=484)	45–54 years (N=838)	55–65 years (N=843)	Total
Valence	Unpleasant words	2.75 (1.57)	2.47 (1.58)	2.61 (1.58)	2.52 (1.42)	2.60 (1.56)	2.67 (1.69)	2.61 (1.58)
	Neutral words	5.23 (0.84)	5.17 (0.84)	5.20 (0.84)	5.14 (0.82)	5.13 (0.79)	5.30 (0.90)	5.20 (0.84)
	Pleasant words	7.59 (1.59)	7.73 (1.55)	7.66 (1.57)	7.65 (1.46)	7.65 (1.57)	7.67 (1.65)	7.66 (1.57)
	Total	5.19 (0.61)	5.12 (0.59)		5.10 (0.57)	5.13 (0.57)	5.21 (0.65)	
Arousal	Unpleasant words	5.30 (2.32)	5.81 (2.47)	5.55 (2.41)	5.43 (2.40)	5.64 (2.38)	5.53 (2.43)	5.55 (2.41)
	Neutral words	3.12 (1.64)	3.01 (1.69)	3.07 (1.66)	2.84 (1.69)	2.98 (1.67)	3.29 (1.62)	3.07 (1.66)
	Pleasant words	5.84 (2.17)	5.62 (2.36)	5.73 (2.27)	5.70 (2.28)	5.81 (2.23)	5.67 (2.30)	5.73 (2.27)
	Total	4.75 (1.36)	4.82 (1.51)		4.66 (1.52)	4.81 (1.37)	4.83 (1.45)	

Table 16.2 Mean valence and arousal ratings (± SD) for the three different word categories split by cohort or depression subtype, respectively

		Cohort				Depression subtype		
		Depression (N=989)	CVD (N=340)	Control (N=836)	Total	Atypical depression (N=82)	Melancholic depression (N=576)	Total
Valence	Unpleasant words	2.40 (1.51)	2.78 (1.55)	2.79 (1.64)	2.61 (1.58)	2.38 (1.35)	2.40 (1.54)	2.40 (1.52)
	Neutral words	5.09 (0.82)	5.25 (0.82)	5.31 (0.86)	5.20 (0.84)	5.09 (0.81)	5.13 (0.81)	5.12 (0.81)
	Pleasant words	7.58 (1.50)	7.73 (1.55)	7.72 (1.66)	7.66 (1.57)	7.60 (1.16)	7.55 (1.58)	7.56 (1.53)
	Total	5.02 (0.60)	5.25 (0.55)	5.27 (0.60)		5.02 (0.48)	5.02 (0.62)	
Arousal	Unpleasant words	5.92 (2.43)	5.16 (2.37)	5.27 (2.34)	5.55 (2.41)	5.30 (2.62)	6.06 (2.38)	5.96 (2.42)
	Neutral words	3.12 (1.70)	3.06 (1.60)	3.01 (1.65)	3.07 (1.66)	2.98 (1.61)	3.14 (1.64)	3.12 (1.64)
	Pleasant words	5.67 (2.28)	6.04 (2.16)	5.68 (2.29)	5.73 (2.27)	5.81 (2.31)	5.67 (2.29)	5.69 (2.29)
	Total	4.90 (1.42)	4.76 (1.36)	4.66 (1.47)		4.69 (1.52)	4.96 (1.41)	

pleasant to be distinctly more arousing compared to patients with depression and control subjects. Regarding depression subtype, across word categories there was no difference in valence ratings between patients with atypical compared to patients with melancholic depression. However, patients with melancholic depression rated the words to be more arousing compared to patients with atypical depression. This tendency was most pronounced in case of words which had been pre-categorized as unpleasant.

16.2.4.3 Stratification of Mean Valence and Arousal Ratings by Sex and Cohort

Figure 16.2 displays mean valence and arousal ratings for the three different word categories (unpleasant vs. neutral vs. pleasant) stratified by sex (male vs. female) and cohort (non-differentiated depression vs. melancholic depression vs. CVD vs. control). There were striking effects of sex: unlike male CVD patients, female CVD patients gave increased arousal ratings for neutral and pleasant words relative to depression patients and control subjects.

16.2.4.4 Stratification of Mean Valence and Arousal Ratings by Age Category and Cohort

Figure 16.3 displays mean valence and arousal ratings for the three different word categories (unpleasant vs. neutral vs. pleasant) stratified by age category (35–44 vs. 45–54 vs. 55–65 years) and cohort (non-differentiated depression vs. melancholic depression vs. CVD vs. control). Basically, striking effects of age were not visible. Effects of age appeared rather in the arousal compared to the valence dimension. Interestingly, the increased arousal ratings of CVD patients for pleasant words relative to depression patients and control subjects were not visible in the youngest age stratum. And moreover, the youngest CVD patients tended to give lower arousal ratings for unpleasant and neutral words than older CVD patients.

16.2.4.5 Associations Between Mean Valence and Arousal Ratings and Perceived Health State

The exploration of the associations between the mean valence ratings, the mean arousal ratings, and the perceived health state (Fig. 16.4) uncovered interesting effects. Across cohorts, (i) deviations were rather found for emotionally charged compared to neutral words; (ii) deviations were more likely to be found for those subjects who perceived their health status as being comparably good as compared to subjects who perceived it as comparably bad; and (iii) deviations tended to represent relatively reduced arousal and relatively increased pleasantness. In case of the patient cohorts, effects were visible for both the unpleasant and the pleasant words; in the control subjects, effects appeared for the pleasant words only. Effects were most pronounced and most restricted to the arousal dimension in case of the CVD patients. In case of melancholic depression, effects seem to represent a slightly more pronounced pattern of the effects observed for the whole cohort of (non-differentiated) depression patients.

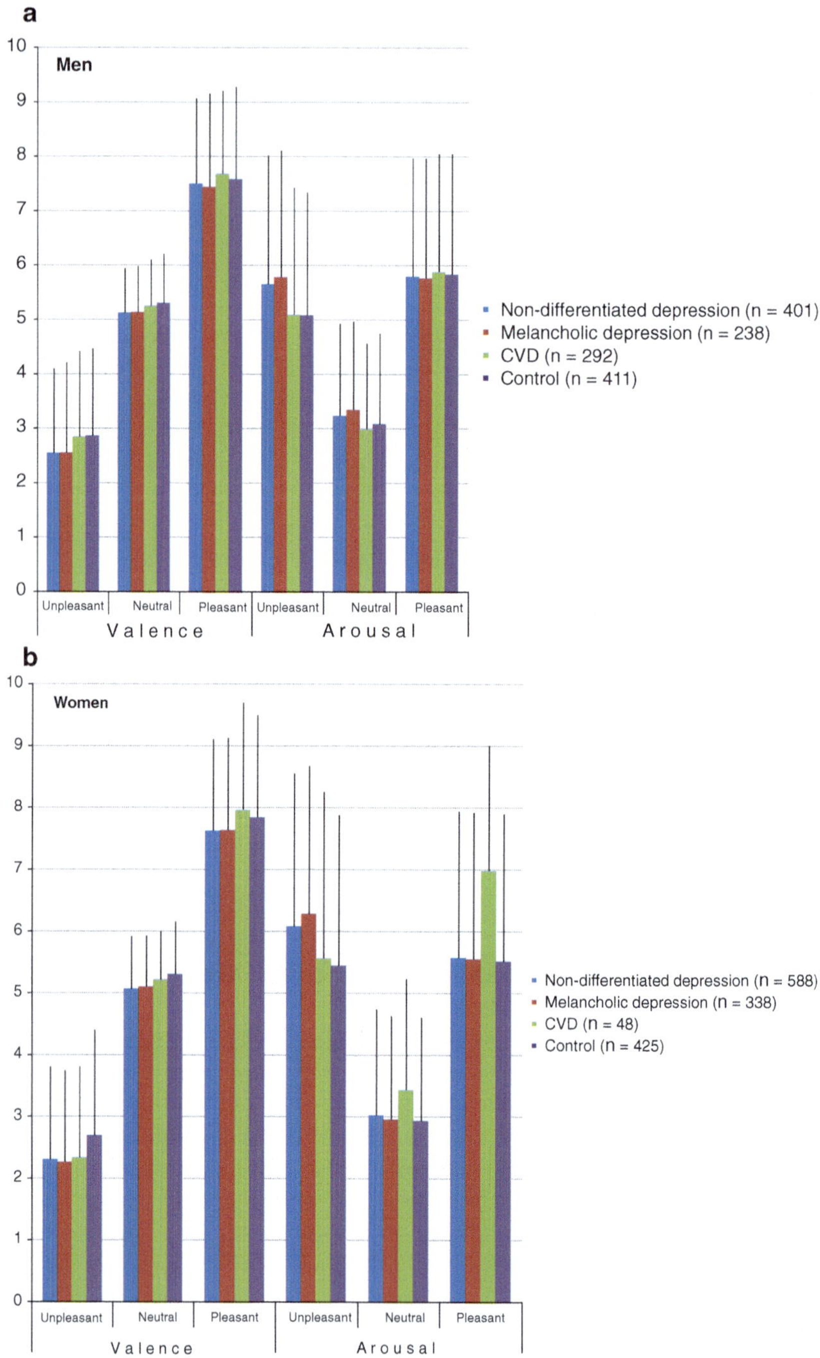

Fig. 16.2 (**a**, **b**) Mean valence and arousal ratings stratified by sex, emotion dimension, word category, and cohort. Patients with melancholic depression constitute a subgroup of the whole cohort of depression patients (= "non-differentiated depression"). *Error bars* denote standard deviations

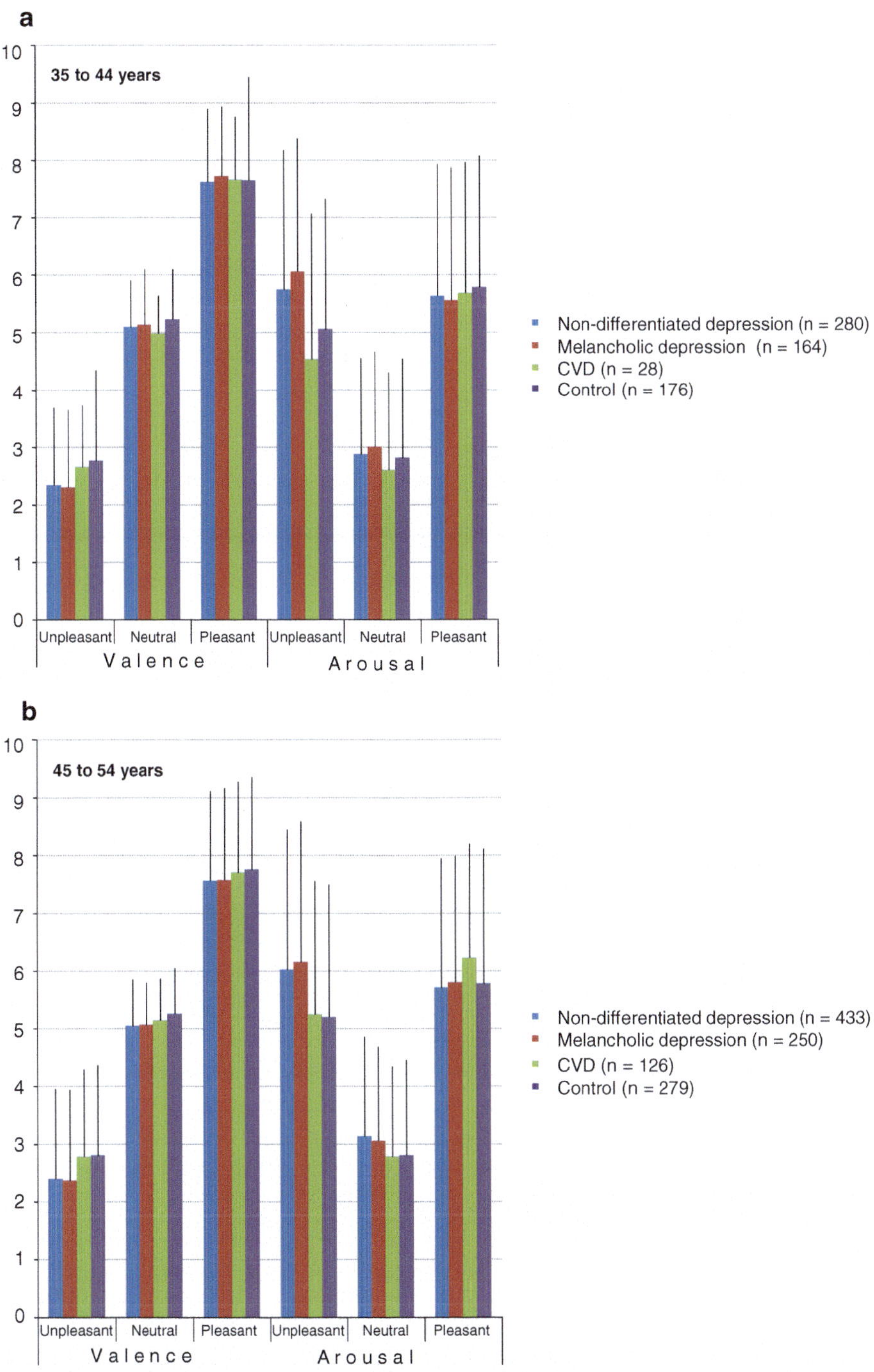

Fig. 16.3 (**a**–**c**) Mean valence and arousal ratings stratified by age category, emotion dimension, word category, and cohort. Patients with melancholic depression constitute a subgroup of the whole cohort of depression patients (= "non-differentiated depression"). *Error bars* denote standard deviations

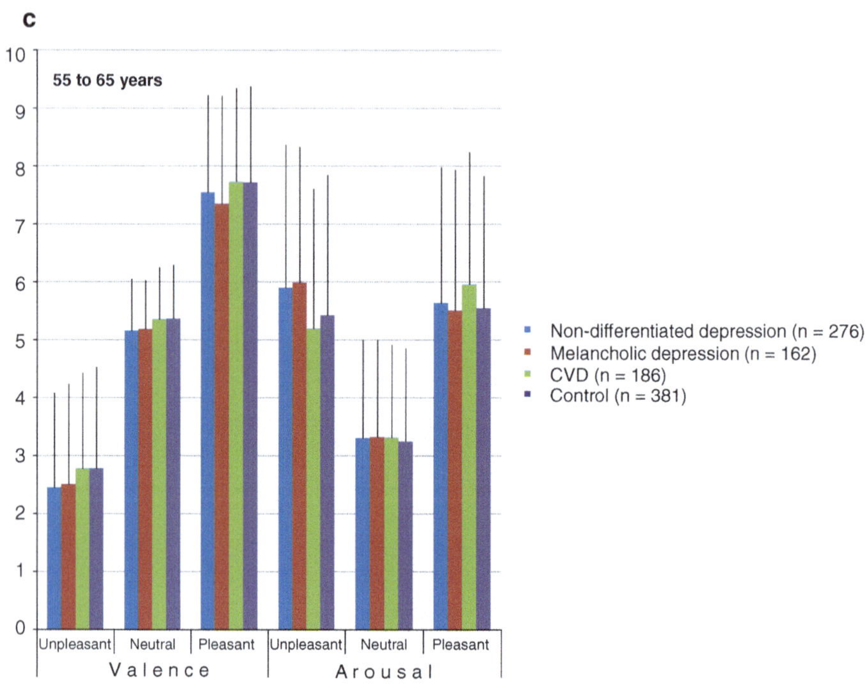

Fig. 16.3 (continued)

16.2.5 Discussion

The main result of our initial data analysis conducted for the purpose of this chapter generally fits to a robust finding from previous experimental investigations: patients with depression rated the words (in particular words pre-categorized as high-arousing unpleasant) to be distinctly less pleasant and more arousing compared to CVD patients or control subjects. We interpret this finding as an equivalent of the well-established processing bias for negative information in depression patients (for review, see Gotlib and Joormann (2010)), which typically manifests clinically in the form of "ruminations" (Zetsche et al. 2012) and which typically reveals itself as recall or recognition bias during laboratory experiments (Gotlib and Joormann 2010; Sumner 2012; Denny and Hunt 1992; Matt et al. 1992; Dalgleish and Watts 1990; Blaney 1986; Gilboa-Schechtman et al. 2002).

Additionally, we found indications for reduced valence ratings (i.e., "less pleasant") and increased arousal ratings in women compared to men, again particularly for high-arousing unpleasant words. Also this finding fits to robust results from previous investigations, as sex differences in emotional processing have been consistently reported (Gohier et al. 2013). For instance, a recent study found that women rated particularly high-arousing, unpleasant pictures to be more unpleasant and more arousing compared to men (Gomez et al. 2013). Moreover, being confronted with aversive content (e.g., fearful or sickened faces), healthy women tended to show more intense (Schienle et al. 2005; Rohrmann et al. 2009) or more sensitive (Gohier et al. 2013) behavioral responses, greater ERP amplitudes (Lithari et al. 2010), or superior performance (Burton et al. 2005; Collignon et al. 2010). Here, we demonstrated that such effects are also detectable using unpleasant *word* stimuli. This is noteworthy, since experience has shown that patient samples tend to perceive unpleasant pictorial or facial stimuli to be quite distressing. It has been hypothesized that sex differences in emotional processing may contribute to the increased susceptibility of women for emotional disorders (Gohier et al. 2013). Population-based studies have consistently shown that major depression is about two times as common in women compared to men (e.g., Kuehner (2003)).

Notably, the number of studies dealing with age-related differences in affective experience remains to be comparably limited. So far, the focus has been on emotional valence rather than arousal, and the majority of studies dealt with negative rather than positive affect (Kessler and Staudinger 2009). Available data converge to indicate that young adults scored highest in negative affect and that negative affect decreased from younger ages to middle age, thereby stabilizing also into older ages (Kessler and Staudinger 2009). Interestingly, our initial analysis yielded indications for increased valence ratings (i.e., "more pleasant") in the oldest (i.e., 55–65 years) compared to younger participants (35–54 years). This result fits to the results of previous investigations. Noteworthy, our analyses showed that the effects of age on valence ratings were evident particularly in case of the low-arousing words. This finding resembles the results of a recent study by Kensinger (2008), which found an age effect during the recall of non-arousing, but not during the recall of arousing words: young adults remembered non-arousing negative words better than non-arousing positive ones; the opposite held true for older adults, which demonstrated a "positivity effect." Eventually, we also found reduced arousal ratings in the youngest (35–44 years) compared to older participants (45–65 years), again most pronounced in case of low-arousing words.

Moreover, further results of our initial data analysis indicated that our efforts of moving beyond laboratory affective science toward "emotional epidemiology" may uncover effects that were otherwise not very likely to be detected. Examples are (i) the indications for the amplified processing of positive information in older CVD patients (Fig. 16.3), (ii) the amplified processing of positive and neutral information in female CVD patients (Fig. 16.2), or (iii) the association between health state that was assessed as good and reduced arousal by unpleasant material in patients with a severe disease (i.e., depression or CVD) (Fig. 16.4). At first sight, obvious explanations for these findings did not suggest themselves. However, it is conceivable that the theory behind the so-called *age-related positivity effect* (Reed and Carstensen 2012) may be extended to include also life-threatening disease. If the positivity effect at older ages arose because life was perceived to be finite, a similar process may be initiated by the experience of a sudden health threat, the prototype of which is myocardial infarction, which is usually accompanied by fierce pain and agony. Nevertheless, despite being alluring this line of thought apparently remains speculative.

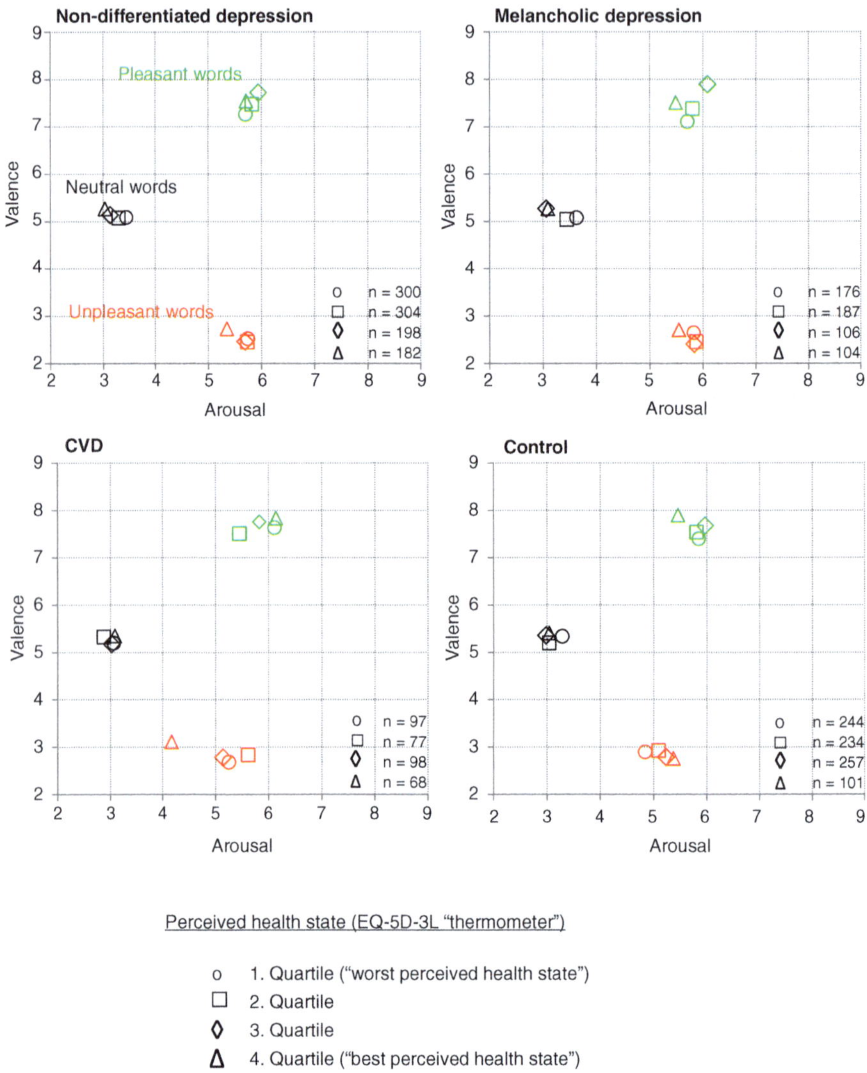

Fig. 16.4 Associations between mean valence ratings, mean arousal ratings, and perceived health state for four cohorts of participants. Patients with melancholic depression constitute a subgroup of the whole cohort of depression patients (= "non-differentiated depression"). *Colors* represent word categories; symbols denote perceived health state categories (EQ-5D-3L "thermometer," quartilized). Mean values were adjusted for sex (assuming male) and age (evaluated at the cohort age mean)

From our point of view, the present results are noteworthy for several reasons. First of all, the evaluation and processing of emotional content have so far almost exclusively been studied under highly standardized laboratory conditions, including among other things (i) recruitment of rather small, homogeneous, and easy-to-manage participant samples, (ii) allocation of enough time and personnel resources for careful subject instruction and the gathering of a sufficient amount of data points, and (iii) the use of proper experimental designs to completely control the influence of potential confounds (e.g., by randomization). Therefore, it is motivating to state that such data can be obtained with sufficient data quality also in the context of an observational, epidemiologic cohort study, which is typically characterized by obstacles such as, e.g., (i) the need to recruit and manage large, heterogeneous samples of participants, (ii) restricted time and personnel resources for instruction and measurement, and (iii) the necessity to consider and therefore adequately measure many potentially confounding variables.

Nonetheless, it has to be emphasized that the findings reported here are preliminary. First, our results remain to be descriptive at this stage of analysis. Second, it should be noted that some of the effects that *popped out* in our initial data analysis are based on a comparably low number of subjects. Third, the mean valence and arousal ratings were indeed stratified by age and sex, and the valence and arousal – perceived health state associations were indeed adjusted for effects of age and sex, but it is obvious that several other variables might act as effect moderators or mediators. Besides usual suspects such as age, sex, or education level, for instance, certain comorbidities (e.g., hyperthyreosis) or heavy smoking, both of which lead to bodily sensations such as accelerated pulse or tachycardia, may be associated with higher arousal ratings. The other way around, certain medications that attenuate, for example, central nervous system activity (e.g., antipsychotics) or heavy exercising (which may lead to a relatively low resting pulse), may be associated with lower arousal ratings. And these or other variables (e.g., severity of depressive/anxiety symptoms, childhood trauma, sleep quality, etc.) may be related to valence ratings in a similar vein.

Thus, one challenge will be to adequately model the valence and arousal ratings. Once the modeling is complete, it will be of great interest for us to thoroughly explore the potential of our emotional content evaluation data with regard to important psychocardiologic issues. For example, it will be worthwhile to investigate whether our emotional content evaluation data would hold additional value, for instance, in (i) predicting the quality of life of depression or CVD patients or in (ii) predicting the risk for depression patients to suffer myocardial infarction or the risk for CVD patients to develop depression.

Unfortunately, due to the low number of patients with atypical depression, we were not able to scrutinize the potential association between emotional content evaluation and depression subtypes. There are hints for a comparatively reduced overall sensitivity to the arousal dimension in patients with atypical compared to patients with melancholic depression (Table 16.2); however, at the current stage of analysis (and considering the large difference in number of cases), we prefer to refrain from interpreting any depression subtype-related effects. Nonetheless, we would like to emphasize that atypical and melancholic subtypes of depression reflect distinct, "antithetic" entities (Gold and Chrousos 2013) and that the systematic comparison of atypical and melancholic subtypes is essential to consider and further establish their differential pathophysiology (Gold 2014).

16.2.6 Limitations

The here briefly described evaluation of emotional content in the context of the BiDirect Study is characterized by certain limitations. First, the nouns that were used in the BiDirect Study were insofar nonspecific as they did not closely relate to topics known to dominate the cognitions of depression patients or CVD patients. Depression patients typically ruminate about experienced or anticipated *loss*, while CVD patients may be preoccupied rather with *threat*-related thoughts. It is reasonable to assume that larger differences between depression and CVD patients (and possibly between patients with atypical versus melancholic depression) would have emerged in case of more on-topic stimuli. On the other hand, cohort or subtype differences in the evaluation of off-topic emotional stimuli would be very interesting; we have found here first hints for such effects, and it may be possible to better carve them out by means of adequate data modeling. Moreover, we used only relatively few words (i.e., four) per category. It is conceivable that the utilization of a larger number of stimuli would have led to more precise intraindividual mean valence and arousal estimates, which in turn may have facilitated the assessment of effect size or significance. On the other hand, we have the advantage of having recruited a large amount of subjects, leading to more precise interindividual estimations.

Furthermore, the fact that the nouns had been used in a learning and memory task prior to being rated with regard to valence and arousal may have reduced differences in their evaluation. On the other hand, it is equally possible that differences were amplified. In any case, the fact that the emotional words were used in different tasks in parallel opens the possibility to consider the results of one task during the analysis of another, and it also opens up the possibility for conjoint analyses.

The task that we used here was explicit and not performance based. It is conceivable that the results of an implicit, performance-based task such as the emotional Stroop paradigm (for review, see Williams et al. (1996)) would be less likely to be biased by, e.g., voluntarily controlled responding, response tendencies, or deficient task comprehension. Thus, such a task may be better suited to detect potentially subtle emotional content processing differences between cohorts and depression subtypes. On the other hand, it appears at least not very likely that participants would have voluntarily manipulated their ratings or that the current task was too difficult to comprehend for a significant number of participants.

Conclusion

The present chapter describes the initial analyses of emotional content evaluation data collected in the context of a large, observational psychocardiologic study. From our point of view, this project holds innovative potential, because it establishes ties between affective science and psychocardiology. Moreover, the initial results appear promising, since existing knowledge is corroborated, and as novel and interesting starting points emerge.

References

Ackenheil M, Stotz-Ingenlath G (1999) MINI mini international neuropsychiatric interview, German version 5.0.0 DSM IV. Psychiatrische Universitätsklinik München, München

Baayen R, Piepenbrock R, Gulikers L (1995) CELEX2 LDC96L14. Web Download. Linguistic Data Consortium, Philadelphia

Barrett LF, Mesquita B, Ochsner KN, Gross JJ (2007) The experience of emotion. Annu Rev Psychol 58:373–403

Baune BT, Stuart M, Gilmour A, Wersching H, Arolt V, Berger K (2012) Moderators of the rela tionship between depression and cardiovascular disorders: a systematic review. Gen Hosp Psychiatry 34:478–492

Blaney PH (1986) Affect and memory: a review. Psychol Bull 99:229–246

Boehm JK, Kubzansky LD (2012) The heart's content: the association between positive psychological well-being and cardiovascular health. Psychol Bull 138:655–691

Burton LA, Rabin L, Wyatt G, Frohlich J, Bernstein Vardy S, Dimitri D (2005) Priming effects for affective vs. neutral faces. Brain Cogn 59:322–329

Carney RM, Freedland KE (2003) Depression, mortality, and medical morbidity in patients with coronary heart disease. Biol Psychiatry 54:241–247

Citron FMM (2012) Neural correlates of written emotion word processing: a review of recent electrophysiological and hemodynamic neuroimaging studies. Brain Lang 122:211–226

Cohen S, Pressman SD (2006) Positive affect and health. Curr Dir Psychol Sci 15:122–125

Cohen S, Tyrrell DA, Smith AP (1993) Negative life events, perceived stress, negative affect, and susceptibility to the common cold. J Pers Soc Psychol 64:131–140

Collignon O, Girard S, Gosselin F, Saint-Amour D, Lepore F, Lassonde M (2010) Women process multisensory emotion expressions more efficiently than men. Neuropsychologia 48:220–225

Constans JI, Mathews A, Brantley PJ, James T (1999) Attentional reactions to an mi. J Psychosom Res 46:415–423

Dalgleish T, Watts FN (1990) Biases of attention and memory in disorders of anxiety and depression. Clin Psychol Rev 10:589–604

Davidson KW, Rieckmann N, Rapp MA (2005) Definitions and distinctions among depressive syndromes and symptoms: implications for a better understanding of the depression-cardiovascular disease association. Psychosom Med 67(Suppl 1):S6–S9

Denny EB, Hunt RR (1992) Affective valence and memory in depression: dissociation of recall and fragment completion. J Abnorm Psychol 101:575–580

DeSteno D, Gross JJ, Kubzansky L (2013) Affective science and health: the importance of emotion and emotion regulation. Health Psychol 32:474–486

Frasure-Smith N, Lespérance F, Talajic M (1993) Depression following myocardial infarction. Impact on 6-month survival. JAMA 270:1819–1825

Gilboa-Schechtman E, Erhard-Weiss D, Jeczemien P (2002) Interpersonal deficits meet cognitive biases: memory for facial expressions in depressed and anxious men and women. Psychiatry Res 113:279–293

Ginting H, Näring G, Becker ES (2013) Attentional bias and anxiety in individuals with coronary heart disease. Psychol Health 28:1306–1322

Gohier B, Senior C, Brittain PJ, Lounes N, El-Hage W, Law V, Phillips ML, Surguladze SA (2013) Gender differences in the sensitivity to negative stimuli: cross-modal affective priming study. Eur Psychiatry 28:74–80

Gold PW (2015) The organization of the stress system and its dysregulation in depressive illness. Mol Psychiatry 20(1):32–47. doi: 10.1038/mp.2014.163. Epub 2014 Dec 9

Gold PW, Chrousos GP (2013) Melancholic and atypical subtypes of depression represent distinct pathophysiological entities: CRH, neural circuits, and the diathesis for anxiety and depression. Mol Psychiatry 18:632–634

Gomez P, von Gunten A, Danuser B (2013) Content-specific gender differences in emotion ratings from early to late adulthood. Scand J Psychol 54:451–458

Gotlib IH, Joormann J (2010) Cognition and depression: current status and future directions. Annu Rev Clin Psychol 6:285–312

Hamilton M (1960) A rating scale for depression. J Neurol Neurosurg Psychiatry 23:56–62

Hare DL, Toukhsati SR, Johansson P, Jaarsma T (2013) Depression and cardiovascular disease: a clinical review. Eur Heart J. doi:10.1093/eurheartj/eht462

Hinojosa JA, Carretié L, Valcárcel MA, Méndez-Bértolo C, Pozo MA (2009) Electrophysiological differences in the processing of affective information in words and pictures. Cogn Affect Behav Neurosci 9:173–189

Joormann J, D'Avanzato C (2010) Emotion regulation in depression: examining the role of cognitive processes. Cogn Emot 24:913–939

Karakus MC, Patton LC (2011) Depression and the onset of chronic illness in older adults: a 12-year prospective study. J Behav Health Serv Res 38:373–382

Kensinger EA (2008) Age differences in memory for arousing and nonarousing emotional words. J Gerontol B Psychol Sci Soc Sci 63:P13–P18

Kessler E-M, Staudinger UM (2009) Affective experience in adulthood and old age: the role of affective arousal and perceived affect regulation. Psychol Aging 24:349–362

Kissler J, Assadollahi R, Herbert C (2006) Emotional and semantic networks in visual word processing: insights from ERP studies. Prog Brain Res 156:147–183

Kissler J, Herbert C, Peyk P, Junghofer M (2007) Buzzwords: early cortical responses to emotional words during reading. Psychol Sci 18:475–480

Kroenke CH, Bennett GG, Fuchs C, Giovannucci E, Kawachi I, Schernhammer E, Holmes MD, Kubzansky LD (2005) Depressive symptoms and prospective incidence of colorectal cancer in women. Am J Epidemiol 162:839–848

Kubzansky LD, Sparrow D, Jackson B, Cohen S, Weiss ST, Wright RJ (2006) Angry breathing: a prospective study of hostility and lung function in the normative aging study. Thorax 61:863–868

Kuehner C (2003) Gender differences in unipolar depression: an update of epidemiological findings and possible explanations. Acta Psychiatr Scand 108:163–174

Lang PJ (1979) Presidential address, 1978. A bio-informational theory of emotional imagery. Psychophysiology 16:495–512

Lang PJ, Bradley MM, Cuthbert BN (1997) Motivated attention: affect, activation, and action. In: Lang PJ, Simons RF, Balaban MT (eds) Attention and orienting: sensory and motivational processes. NJ. Erlbaum, Hillsdale, pp 97–135

Lesperance F, Frasure-Smith N, Talajic M (1996) Major depression before and after myocardial infarction: its nature and consequences. Psychosom Med 58:99–110

Levenson RW (2011) Basic emotion questions. Emot Rev 3:379–386

Lifshitz K (1966) The averaged evoked cortical response to complex visual stimuli. Psychophysiology 3:55–68

Lithari C, Frantzidis CA, Papadelis C, Vivas AB, Klados MA, Kourtidou-Papadeli C, Pappas C, Ioannides AA, Bamidis PD (2010) Are females more responsive to emotional stimuli? A neurophysiological study across arousal and valence dimensions. Brain Topogr 23:27–40

Matt GE, Vázquez C, Campbell WK (1992) Mood-congruent recall of affectively toned stimuli: a meta-analytic review. Clin Psychol Rev 12:227–255

Mezuk B, Eaton WW, Albrecht S, Golden SH (2008) Depression and type 2 diabetes over the lifespan: a meta-analysis. Diabetes Care 31:2383–2390

Ohman A, Mineka S (2001) Fears, phobias, and preparedness: toward an evolved module of fear and fear learning. Psychol Rev 108:483–522

Osgood CE, Miron MS, May WH (1975) Cross-cultural universals of affective meaning. University of Illinois Press, Urbana

Rabin R, De Charro F (2001) EQ-5D: a measure of health status from the EuroQol Group. Ann Med 33:337–343

Reed AE, Carstensen LL (2012) The theory behind the age-related positivity effect. Front Psychol 3:339

Roest AM, Martens EJ, de Jonge P, Denollet J (2010) Anxiety and risk of incident coronary heart disease. A meta-analysis. J Am Coll Cardiol 56:38–46
Rohrmann S, Hopp H, Schienle A, Hodapp V (2009) Emotion regulation, disgust sensitivity, and psychophysiological responses to a disgust-inducing film. Anxiety Stress Coping 22:215–236
Rubin DC, Talarico JM (2009) A comparison of dimensional models of emotion: evidence from emotions, prototypical events, autobiographical memories, and words. Memory 17:802–808
Rush A, Giles D, Schlesser M (1986) The inventory for depressive symptomatology (IDS): preliminary findings. Psychiatry Res 18:65–87
Schacht A, Sommer W (2009) Emotions in word and face processing: early and late cortical responses. Brain Cogn 69:538–550
Schienle A, Schäfer A, Stark R, Walter B, Vaitl D (2005) Gender differences in the processing of disgust- and fear-inducing pictures: an fMRI study. Neuroreport 16:277–280
Schleifer SJ, Macari-Hinson MM, Coyle DA, Slater WR, Kahn M, Gorlin R, Zucker HD (1989) The nature and course of depression following myocardial infarction. Arch Intern Med 149:1785–1789
Sirois BC, Burg MM (2003) Negative emotion and coronary heart disease: a review. Behav Modif 27:83–102
Stewart A, Greenfield S, Hays R, Rogers W, Berry S, McGlynn E, Ware J (1989) Functional status and well-being of patients with chronic conditions. JAMA 7:907–913
Sumner JA (2012) The mechanisms underlying overgeneral autobiographical memory: an evaluative review of evidence for the CaR-FA-X model. Clin Psychol Rev 32:34–48
Teismann H, Wersching H, Nagel M, Arolt V, Heindel W, Baune BT, Wellmann J, Hense H-W, Berger K (2014) Establishing the bidirectional relationship between depression and subclinical arteriosclerosis – rationale, design, and characteristics of the BiDirect study. BMC Psychiatry 14:174
Vanderploeg RD, Brown WS, Marsh JT (1987) Judgments of emotion in words and faces: ERP correlates. Int J Psychophysiol 5:193–205
Wersching H, Berger K (2012) New cohorts. The BiDirect study. Bundesgesundheitsbl Gesundheitsforsch Gesundheitsschutz 55:822–823
Williams JMG, Mathews A, MacLeod C (1996) The emotional stroop task and psychopathology. Psychol Bull 120:3–24
Zetsche U, D'Avanzato C, Joormann J (2012) Depression and rumination: relation to components of inhibition. Cogn Emot 26:758–767

Nutrition and Depression: Current Evidence on the Association of Dietary Patterns with Depression and Its Subtypes

17

Corinna Rahe and Klaus Berger

Contents

C. Rahe (✉) • K. Berger
Institute of Epidemiology and Social Medicine, University of Münster, Albert-Schweitzer-Campus 1, Building D3, 48149 Münster, Germany
e-mail: corinna.rahe@uni-muenster.de

B.T. Baune, P.J. Tully (eds.), *Cardiovascular Diseases and Depression*, DOI 10.1007/978-3-319-32480-7_17

Abstract
Modifiable lifestyle factors, in particular nutrition, may be promising prevention and intervention targets not only for physical but also for mental health. The diet-depression relationship is very complex and even may be of bidirectional nature. Growing evidence suggests a potential role of nutrition in the development, course, and treatment of depression, whereas present depressive symptoms may also predict the development of an unhealthy lifestyle including poor diet quality. While previous research mainly investigated the effects of individual nutrients or foods on depression, the recent research focus shifted toward the investigation of the overall diet, because dietary patterns may better reflect the complexity of the habitual diet in daily life. In this chapter, we aim to summarize the current evidence on the diet-depression relationship, with major focus on overall diet rather than single nutrients. Furthermore, we briefly discuss potential underlying mechanisms and point out the interplay of nutrition and depression with the development of somatic comorbidities, in particular cardiovascular disease. A shortcoming of previous research on the diet-depression relationship is that most studies commonly treated depression as a homogeneous disease entity, although it actually is a very heterogeneous illness. In this context, we further want to highlight the role of distinct subtypes of depression in regard to the diet-depression relationship and reflect important implications for public health, clinical practice, and future research.

Abbreviations

CI	Confidence interval
CRP	C-reactive protein
CVD	Cardiovascular disease
DNA	Deoxyribonucleic acid
DSM-IV	*Diagnostic and Statistical Manual of Mental Disorders, Fourth Edition*
HPA axis	Hypothalamic-pituitary-adrenal axis
HR	Hazard ratio
IL-6	Interleukin-6
MeDi	Mediterranean diet
OR	Odds ratio
RCT	Randomized controlled trial
ROS	Reactive oxygen species
RR	Relative risk
SSRI	Selective serotonin reuptake inhibitor
TNF-α	Tumor necrosis factor alpha

17.1 Introduction

Mental health problems in general and depressive disorders in particular are an increasing public health challenge all over the world. Unipolar depressive disorders (in the following abbreviated as depression) strongly contribute to the global disease burden (Ferrari et al. 2013) and seriously affect both the individual and the society (Lepine and Briley 2011). Approaches to reduce the health problem of depression have mainly focused on treatment rather than on prevention (Jacka et al. 2012). However, its high prevalence, limitations in treatment response, as well as its relation to the development of other poor health conditions (e.g., cardiovascular diseases (CVD), diabetes, or suicidal behavior) highlight the importance of preventive approaches (Popa and Ladea 2012). Hence, research on potential risk factors and the development of effective prevention strategies against depression are urgently needed.

Modifiable lifestyle factors may be such risk factors that can be considered as possible intervention targets (van Gool et al. 2007; Sarris et al. 2015). Whereas lifestyle factors are established risk factors for common somatic diseases such as CVD or cancer, the investigation of the link between lifestyle and mental health is a rather new research area (Sanchez-Villegas and Martínez-González 2013). Especially nutrition may be related not only to physical but also to mental health (Sarris et al. 2015). As a consequence, a novel discipline named "nutritional psychiatry research" is rapidly developing, which aims to comprehensively investigate the relationship between nutrition and mental illnesses such as depression (Logan and Jacka 2014).

In this chapter, we aim to summarize the current evidence on the diet-depression relationship, with major focus on overall diet rather than single nutrients. Furthermore, we briefly discuss potential underlying mechanisms and point out the interplay of nutrition and depression with the development of somatic comorbidities, in particular CVD. A shortcoming of previous research on the diet-depression relationship is that most studies commonly treated depression as a homogeneous disease entity, although it actually is a very heterogeneous illness. In this context, we further want to highlight the role of distinct subtypes of depression in regard to the diet-depression relationship and reflect important implications for public health, clinical practice, and future research.

17.2 The Diet-Depression Relationship: Overview of the Current Evidence

The relationship between diet and depression is complex. Nutrition may be related to the development, course, and treatment of depression. Moreover, the diet-depression relationship is likely to be of bidirectional nature: On the one side, diet may be a risk factor for the onset and course of depression, and, on the other side, depression itself may lead to changes in lifestyle including poor dietary habits (Lopresti et al. 2013; Jacka et al. 2015).

Prior research on the diet-depression relationship primarily focused on the effects of individual nutrients or foods on depression. In recent years, there has been a shift toward a more comprehensive approach that investigates the association of depression and overall diet considered as dietary patterns or diet quality. This approach aims to assess the habitual diet as one overall exposure by analyzing how nutrients or foods are consumed in combination (Hu 2002; Kant 2004). There are different approaches to assess the overall diet (Hu 2002; Ocké 2013). A priori approaches are based on the calculation of diet scores or indices and usually assess the diet quality and/or the adherence to predefined nutritional recommendations (e.g., Mediterranean Diet Score, Healthy Eating Index, Diet Quality Index). A posteriori approaches use statistical techniques (e.g., factor analysis, principal component analysis, or cluster analysis) without a priori hypotheses to derive empirically based dietary patterns which are unique to the specific study population. A third approach (e.g., reduced rank regression) combines a priori and a posteriori methods by using response variables, such as specific biomarkers, which are known intermediate factors for the outcome of interest (Hoffmann et al. 2004).

Overall, the approach of dietary pattern analysis consolidates several methodological advantages (Hu 2002): Dietary patterns consider that people eat meals which include a variety of different nutrients and may better reflect the complexity of the habitual diet. Given that nutrients are likely to interact with each other and potentially have synergetic effects, the overall diet may have a larger impact on health than single dietary factors.

Individual nutrients most frequently examined in relation to depression are omega-3 fatty acids and vitamins, in particular B vitamins and folate; foods commonly investigated are fruit, vegetables, and fish (for detailed information, please see, e.g., Murakami and Sasaki 2010; Sanhueza et al. 2013). The following literature overview mainly focuses on summarizing the current evidence on the relationship between depression and overall diet instead of individual nutrients.

17.2.1 Diet in the Prevention of Depression

In the last few years, various studies reported that the habitual diet may predict the onset of depression or depressive symptoms (Sánchez-Villegas et al. 2009; Jacka et al. 2010; Le Port et al. 2012; Akbaraly et al. 2013). First systematic reviews and meta-analyses have been published recently, which summarize the available literature on the association between dietary patterns and depression in adults (Psaltopoulou et al. 2013; Quirk et al. 2013; Lai et al. 2014; Rahe et al. 2014). Overall, these reviews concluded that healthy or prudent dietary patterns (with high intakes of fruit, vegetables, fish, and whole grains and low intakes of processed foods) as well as the Mediterranean diet (MeDi) may have protective effects against depression, whereas Western dietary patterns (with high intakes of processed foods, meat, meat products, refined grains, and high-sugar/high-fat foods) may increase the depression risk. Pooled results of two meta-analyses showed similar results: One meta-analysis reported a significant association of the MeDi with a reduced depression risk (RR = 0.68; 95 % CI, 0.54–0.86) (Psaltopoulou et al. 2013). Another meta-analysis showed a significant association between healthy dietary patterns and lower odds of depression (OR = 0.84; 95 % CI, 0.76–0.92), but closely missed to detect a significant positive association of Western dietary patterns with higher odds of depression (OR = 1.17; 95 % CI, 0.97–1.68) (Lai et al. 2014).

The abovementioned reviews and meta-analyses included most of all cross-sectional studies. However, studies with cross-sectional design cannot determine the temporal sequence of the diet-depression relationship. Several new prospective studies have been published recently which are not included in reviews so far. In line with previous results, some of these prospective studies also reported associations between Western dietary patterns and an increased depression risk (Jacka et al. 2014a) as well as prudent dietary patterns and a decreased depression risk (Jacka et al. 2014a; Ruusunen et al. 2014). However, other new high-quality prospective studies did not support a clear association of dietary patterns with depression (Chan et al. 2014; Chocano-Bedoya et al. 2013). For example, a study of Chocano-Bedoya and colleagues, who examined a large sample of more than 50,000 participants from the longitudinal Nurses' Health Study, did not find associations between a prudent or a Western dietary pattern and depression (Chocano-Bedoya et al. 2013). All in all, current studies on the diet-depression relationship are very heterogeneous and strongly differ in their methodology, i.e., in terms of psychiatric assessment, dietary assessment, statistical analyses, or adjustment for possible confounding variables.

The majority of the existent evidence is built on observational studies, which include the possibility of (residual) confounding and/or chance findings. Although observational studies have supported a relationship between diet and depression, research in the form of intervention studies is scarce up to now. A recent systematic review aimed to summarize the yet available evidence on randomized controlled trials (RCT) investigating the effects of dietary interventions (with whole-diet approaches) on depression and anxiety (Opie et al. 2014). Depression outcomes in the included studies were assessed by several different depression scales, mostly in study samples of individuals with present physical but not psychological diseases (e.g., diabetes, obesity, or cancer). The authors concluded that there is some promising evidence from RCTs that dietary interventions may improve depression outcomes. However, evidence was not consistent, with about half of the included studies observing significant improvements in favor of the treatment groups.

For example, the PREDIMED (Prevención con Dieta Mediterránea) trial is an intervention study on the role of the MeDi in the prevention of CVD (Sánchez-Villegas et al. 2013). In this context, additional analyses regarding the role of the MeDi on depression risk were performed. Participants at high risk for cardiovascular events were randomly assigned to one of the following intervention groups: (A) MeDi with supplementation of virgin olive oil, (B) MeDi with supplementation of nuts, or (C) low-fat diet (= control group). No significant association between the MeDi and incident depression was found for the overall study sample (A: HR = 0.91; 95 % CI, 0.67–1.24; B: HR = 0.78; 95 % CI, 0.55–1.10), but the authors reported a significant inverse association for intervention group B (MeDi plus nuts) within one sensitivity analysis that was restricted to participants with type 2 diabetes (B: HR = 0.59; 95 % CI, 0.36–0.98) (Sánchez-Villegas et al. 2013). Additional intervention studies are urgently needed to further enlighten the diet-depression relationship.

Given the fact that depressive disorders often develop early in the life span, even in childhood (Kim-Cohen et al. 2003; Merikangas et al. 2010), the investigation of the relationship between diet and mental health in children and adolescents is highly relevant. One systematic review summarized the existing evidence on the relationship between dietary patterns and mental health in children and adolescents, focusing on internalizing disorders including low mood, depression, and anxiety (O'Neil et al. 2014b). The authors concluded that the available evidence suggests a consistent association between unhealthy dietary patterns and poorer mental health as well as an inverse association between healthy diets and better mental health in children; the second association was less consistent than the first one (O'Neil et al. 2014b). These results highlight the potential of dietary interventions targeting mental health early in the life span.

A very new area of research focuses on even earlier life stages, namely, the perinatal period, when the brain is rapidly developing (O'Neil et al. 2014a). According to the Barker hypothesis, the fetus adapts to the intrauterine environment; if the unborn child is exposed to an unfavorable environment in utero (e.g., by undernutrition), this "fetal programming" might predispose the child to chronic diseases in later life (Barker 1997, 2002). There are established links between fetal programming and later somatic diseases such as CVD, highlighting the importance of maternal diet during pregnancy for health and disease in offspring (Barker 1997, 2002; Capra et al. 2013). By contrast, only few studies applied this hypothesis to mental health so far. Two recent studies reported that maternal diet during pregnancy may influence the risk for mental and behavioral problems in children, suggesting a potential role of the maternal diet for externalizing (e.g., aggression, attention deficit) but not for internalizing (e.g., depression, anxiety) problems in childhood (Jacka et al. 2013; Steenweg-de Graaff et al. 2014). Evidence is still limited, but these findings may highlight the impact of maternal diet during pregnancy on fetal development and later mental health. The improvement of dietary intake during pregnancy may have the potential to be an additional strategy in the primary prevention of mental disorders (O'Neil et al. 2014a).

17.2.2 Depression and Its Impact on Diet

Although a growing body of literature highlights an important role of nutrition in the development of depression, there is also evidence for the reverse direction, i.e., depression leading to poor dietary habits. It has been reported that depressive symptoms or depressive disorders are associated with unhealthy lifestyle behaviors, such as smoking, risky alcohol consumption, reduced physical activity, and poorer dietary habits (Bonnet et al. 2005; Kilian et al. 2006).

In terms of dietary intake, studies showed that individuals with depressive symptoms are more likely to make unfavorable food choices than non-depressed individuals. For example, the presence of depressive symptoms was associated with a lower consumption of fruit and vegetables (Konttinen et al. 2010) and a higher consumption of sweet and non-sweet energy-dense foods (i.e., sweets, chocolate, salty snacks, and fast food) (Konttinen et al. 2010; Crawford et al. 2011).

Evidence on the association of depression and overall diet (as the outcome of interest) is conflicting and mostly limited to cross-sectional studies so far (Quirk et al. 2013). Whereas some studies failed to detect an association between depression and overall diet quality (Whitaker et al. 2014), others did find significant associations linking (Pagoto et al. 2009; Appelhans et al. 2012; Yu et al. 2014). For example, Appelhans and colleagues reported that greater depression severity was significantly associated with poorer diet quality in obese women with major depression (Appelhans et al. 2012). Moreover, they reported that the observed association was mainly driven by higher intakes of sugar, saturated fats, and sodium (Appelhans et al. 2012). Similarly to the results of adult samples, there is also some evidence on a relationship between mental health problems and poor diet in children and adolescents: In their systematic review, O'Neil and colleagues reported that two (out of three) identified studies observed a significant inverse association between worse mental health and poorer dietary habits in children (O'Neil et al. 2014b).

17.2.3 Diet in the Treatment of Depression

The impact of nutrition in the treatment of depression is still unclear but remains an interesting field of research, since depression has been linked to poor nutritional status (Sarris et al. 2009). Clinical management of depression generally involves pharmacotherapy and psychotherapy as first-line treatments, while it often neglects the potential role of lifestyle factors in this context (Berk et al. 2013a; Sarris et al. 2014). A large part of depressed patients do not sufficiently respond to first-line treatment approaches such as antidepressant medication (Rush 2007; Lee et al. 2012). Thus, a consideration of additional treatment strategies is desirable, and modifiable lifestyle factors such as physical activity or diet may be interesting intervention targets. The call for the consideration of diet and specific nutrients in the treatment of depression is rising (Rucklidge et al. 2015).

However, evidence regarding the impact of dietary interventions (in terms of whole-diet approaches) on the improvement of mental health outcomes is still limited (Opie et al. 2014). As already mentioned in Sect. 17.2.1, a recent systematic review examined the effect of whole-diet interventions on depression as well as anxiety and concluded that there may be some evidence from RCTs that dietary interventions improve depression outcomes (Opie et al. 2014). However, the majority of the included studies investigated the effects of diet on depressive outcomes in samples of non-depressed subjects. Only one included study specifically examined the effects of healthy lifestyle recommendations (including diet, physical activity, sunlight exposure, and sleep) on participants with a depressive disorder, reporting reduced depressive symptoms and a higher rate of remitters after six month in the active group (García-Toro et al. 2012). Unfortunately, the single effect of the included dietary intervention was not distinguished. Further studies examining the impact of whole-diet interventions on patients with clinically diagnosed depression are needed, preferably in the form of high-quality RCTs. Some promising studies are currently performed (e.g., O'Neil et al. 2013).

The potential therapeutic effect of specific nutrients was examined more extensively in the past. In particular, studies on the effects of polyunsaturated fatty acids (e.g., omega-3 fatty acids) have received much attention (Appleton et al. 2010; Bloch and Hannestad 2012; Politi et al. 2013). Further nutrients examined in this context (either as monotherapies or as adjuvant therapies) were folate, B vitamins, magnesium, zinc, or specific amino acids, for instance (Sarris et al. 2009). However, most of this research yielded limited or conflicting results. Moreover, it should be considered that these treatment approaches are built on the supplementation of specific nutrients and not on the habitual dietary intake. Given the complex nature of nutrition with possible nutrient interactions, it is conceivable that especially broad-spectrum micronutrient treatments, which provide a multitude of essential nutrients rather than single ones, may be promising as adjunct therapies in the treatment of depression. However, to date there is only scarce evidence on the effectiveness of such multi-nutrient approaches in clinical samples of patients with depressive disorders (Rucklidge and Kaplan 2013).

17.3 Mechanisms Linking Nutrition and Depression

Depression has a multifactorial origin (Lopresti et al. 2013), involving genetic, psychological, physiological, environmental, and social factors. As summarized in the above-outlined literature overview, current evidence emphasizes a potential role of nutrition as one important environmental lifestyle factor in the development and progression of depression. Since there is a substantial body of evidence on an association between nutrition and depression, we have to better understand the biological pathways, which specifically explain how nutrition can influence mental health and vice versa. Although the actual underlying mechanisms are still not sufficiently understood, it is plausible that diet may influence mental health and mood, since a variety of nutrients (in particular, amino acids, fatty acids, vitamins, and minerals (Sarris et al. 2015)) are essential substances for brain structure, function, and activity. Therefore, several biological mechanisms linking diet and depression have been proposed in the past, including pathways related to neurotransmitter regulation, inflammatory processes, oxidative stress, gut microbiome, mitochondrial disturbances, neuroprogression, or stress-response system regulation, for instance. In the following sections, the most promising biological pathways (i.e., neurotransmitters, inflammation, oxidative stress, and gut microbiome) will be summarized and discussed briefly (see Fig. 17.1). For further and more detailed information on potential pathways, please see recent reviews (e.g., Lopresti et al. 2013; Kaplan et al. 2015).

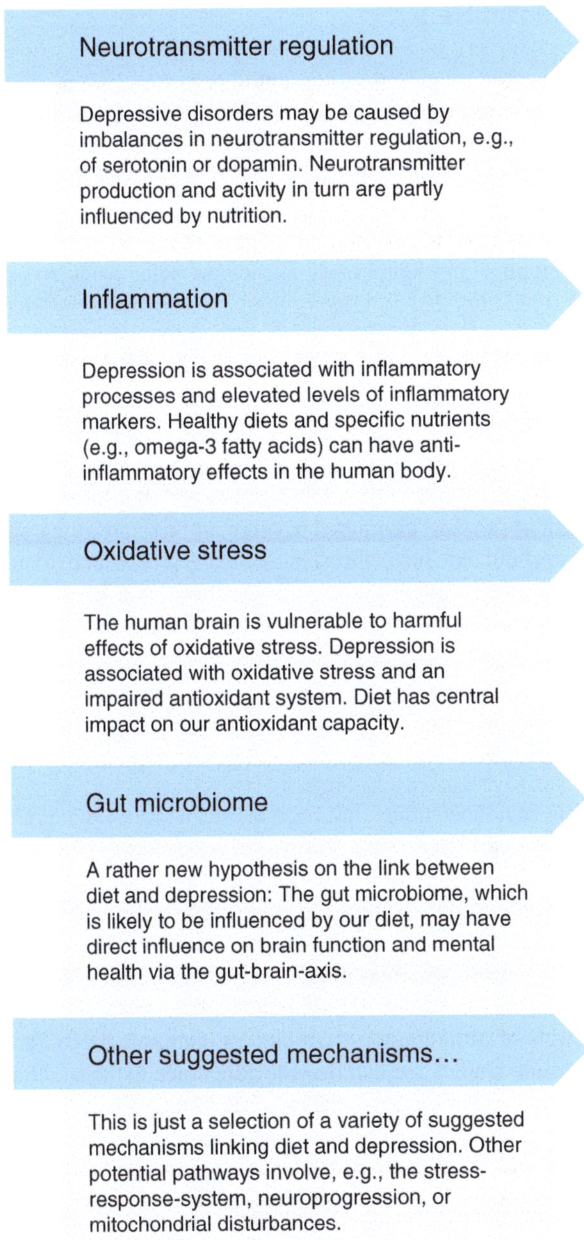

Fig. 17.1 An overview of suggested mechanisms linking diet and depression

17.3.1 Neurotransmitters

One of the oldest hypotheses in terms of potential pathways linking diet and depression implies that depressive disorders were caused by imbalances in neurotransmitter regulation, especially for serotonin or dopamine (Lopresti et al. 2013). After it had been observed that depression is associated with low levels of serotonin, the serotonin hypothesis was postulated, which is one of the most extensively studied pathways related to depression and resulted in the development of specific treatment strategies by developing antidepressants known as selective serotonin reuptake inhibitors (SSRI) (Fakhoury 2015). Dietary intake, particularly the intake of carbohydrates and specific amino acids, can have important impact on the production and activity of neurotransmitters such as serotonin (Lopresti et al. 2013). It has been proposed that carbohydrate-rich diets are associated with reduced depressive symptoms, maybe by promoting the brain levels of the amino acid tryptophan, resulting in an increased serotonin synthesis, as tryptophan is a precursor of serotonin (Wurtman and Wurtman 1995; Benton and Donohoe 1999). Since protein-rich diets are relatively low in tryptophan compared to other amino acids, the consumption of high-protein diets would not have the same effect (Benton and Donohoe 1999). However, the practical relevance of these observations is unclear, since levels of potentially interesting nutrients in the habitual diet are relatively low (Benton and Donohoe 1999).

17.3.2 Inflammation

Another hypothesis on how diet may influence mental health and depression focuses on inflammatory processes (Berk et al. 2013b). Several studies showed that depression is associated with inflammation and elevated levels of inflammatory markers such as C-reactive protein (CRP) or interleukin-6 (IL-6) (Haapakoski et al. 2015). Inflammation in turn can be influenced by the habitual diet. There is evidence that the intake of specific nutrients such as fiber, omega-3 fatty acids, magnesium, carotenoids, or flavonoids may have anti-inflammatory effects and, thus, are associated with decreased levels of inflammatory biomarkers (Galland 2010). A recent meta-analysis of intervention studies yielded that the adherence to the MeDi is associated with a reduction of the inflammatory markers CRP and IL-6 (Schwingshackl and Hoffmann 2014). Similarly, a recent systematic review on dietary patterns and inflammation concluded that current evidence supports an inverse association between fruit and vegetable-based patterns with inflammation, while Western diets, in particular meat-based diets, were positively associated with inflammation (Barbaresko et al. 2013).

One recent study of Lucas and colleagues examined the association between an "inflammatory dietary pattern" and depression in women from the Nurses' Health Study (n=43,685) (Lucas et al. 2014). This inflammatory dietary pattern (derived by reduced rank regression) was characterized by high intakes of red meat, refined grains, soft drinks, and margarine as well as low intakes of green and yellow vegetables, olive oil, coffee, and wine, and was associated with the inflammatory biomarkers CRP, IL-6, and tumor necrosis factor alpha (TNF-α). Overall, the inflammatory dietary pattern showed a significant association with an increased risk for the development of depression, suggesting that inflammation may underlie the diet-depression relationship.

17.3.3 Oxidative Stress

Next to inflammation, oxidative stress is considered a key component of depression (Maes et al. 2011a). Inflammation often goes along with the induction of oxidative stress associated with the generation of highly reactive free radicals, so-called reactive oxygen species (ROS). These ROS have several physiological roles, and under normal conditions the human metabolism has several defense mechanisms (i.e., antioxidant systems) to keep them balanced. Oxidative stress occurs if impaired defense pathways lead to imbalances in favor of increased ROS levels, which in turn cause damages in lipids, proteins, or DNA (Maes et al. 2011a). The brain and its nerve cells seem to be especially vulnerable to the harmful effects of oxidative stress.

Depression has been shown to be associated with lowered levels of antioxidants (e.g., vitamin E) and reduced activity of antioxidant enzymes (e.g., glutathione peroxidase) (Maes et al. 2000, 2011a, 2011b; Cumurcu et al. 2009; Prohan et al. 2014). As a consequence of the impaired antioxidant system, depression seems to be associated with an impaired protection against ROS and, thus, increased oxidative stress. As our diet can deliver a variety of antioxidants, it plays a crucial role and has important influence on the antioxidant capacity and oxidative stress level in the human organism (Lopresti et al. 2013). In particular, the MeDi (with its high proportion of fruit and vegetables as well as olive oil as the main source of fat) has been shown to be associated with an increased antioxidant intake as well as decreased oxidative stress levels (Fito et al. 2007; Dai et al. 2008; Esposito et al. 2011).

17.3.4 Gut Microbiome

A rather new suggestion how diet affects mood and mental health focuses on the gut microbiome (Dash et al. 2015). The human intestine is colonized by around 100 trillion bacteria building the gut microbiome (Foster and McVey Neufeld 2013), which has major influence on diverse important functions of the human organism, i.e., by developing the immune system or by maintaining the intestinal barrier function (Dash et al. 2015; Kaplan et al. 2015). Changes in the gut microbiome are supposed to be associated with the increasing incidence of inflammatory diseases (Maslowski and Mackay 2011), including CVD, diabetes, or arthritis. For example, dysbiosis of the gut microbiota can induce immune responses and inflammatory processes in the human organism, e.g., by harming the intestinal barrier function (Kaplan et al. 2015). Recently, research on the gut-brain axis has reached much attention, confirming the importance of the gut microbiome for brain function and mental health via endocrine, immune, or neural pathways (Cryan and Dinan 2012; Foster and McVey Neufeld 2013).

Throughout the life course, the human gut microbiome is influenced by different factors such as age, genetics, stress, hygiene, or medication (Maslowski and Mackay 2011). Moreover and possibly most important, the habitual diet is supposed to have considerable influence on the composition of the gut microbiome (Moschen et al. 2012). This discovery offers new opportunities for the prevention and treatment of depression, because it indicates that the gut microbiome can be manipulated by diet and the intake of special dietary components such as fermented foods, prebiotics, or probiotics (Maslowski and Mackay 2011; Moschen et al. 2012; Selhub et al. 2014; Dash et al. 2015; Kaplan et al. 2015). Furthermore, research has highlighted that in particular long-term dietary patterns rather than short-term intake might influence the microbiota composition (Moschen et al. 2012). Supportive evidence comes from one study reporting significant differences in fecal microbiota between European children (consuming a Western diet) and children from rural Africa (consuming a traditional plant-based diet rich in fruit, vegetables, and dietary fiber); higher microbiota diversity and less pathogenic bacteria were reported for the African children (De Filippo et al. 2010). However, although first evidence advocates that the relationship between diet and depression may be partly mediated by the gut microbiome, further research on how diet is influencing microbiota composition toward a "healthy gut" is needed.

17.3.5 Impact of Depressive Symptoms on Dietary Intake

The above-outlined mechanisms explain how diet may influence the development or progression of depression. However, there is also some evidence on how depression or depressive symptoms may lead to unfavorable food habits. In this context, suggested mechanisms may involve physiological, psychological, as well as sensory pathways (Gibson 2006).

An interesting factor may be the phenomenon of emotional eating, which means to preferably consume energy-dense comfort foods rich in fat and sugar (e.g., sweets, salty snacks, or fast food) in response to negative emotions or distress. It has been confirmed in several studies that depressive symptoms are associated with patterns of emotional eating and as a consequence with unhealthy food choices (Ouwens et al. 2009; Konttinen et al. 2010).

Moreover, it has been proposed that the excessive consumption of carbohydrate-rich foods (called carbohydrate craving) may be a form of self-medication (Moller 1992; Wurtman and Wurtman 1995). These observations may be especially related to the subtype of atypical depression (Moller 1992). The consumption of snack foods such as chocolate, pastries, or chips, which are particularly rich in carbohydrates (but also in fat), may have antidepressant-like effects by increasing serotonin levels in the brain (please see also Sect. 17.3.1) (Wurtman and Wurtman 1995).

However, the hypothesis of antidepressant-like serotonergic effects of chocolate or other carbohydrate-rich foods has been discussed controversially, because several arguments indicate flaws in this theoretical hypothesis (Parker et al. 2006).

As one important underlying physiological explanation, the hypothalamic-pituitary-adrenal (HPA) axis has been proposed to play an important role as a link between depression, stress, appetite, and eating behavior (Whitaker et al. 2014). Depression is associated with an increased activity of the HPA axis, indicated by higher cortisol levels in depressed subjects compared to healthy controls (Knorr et al. 2010; Stetler and Miller 2011). Cortisol in turn has influence on our food choices, as there is evidence that cortisol stimulates our appetite regulation and predicts an overall increased food intake, particularly of palatable and energy-dense foods (George et al. 2010). However, underlying biological pathways that link depressive symptoms and dietary intake have not been sufficiently understood. Further, there is evidence that specific subtypes of depression may have different underlying pathophysiological processes and, thus, may be related to specific biological parameters such as the HPA axis differently (Stetler and Miller 2011; Lamers et al. 2013).

17.4 Rethinking the Diet-Depression Relationship: The Role of Distinct Subtypes of Depression

In the context of the diet-depression relationship, the role of distinct subtypes of depression is an important but unsolved research issue. Prior studies commonly treated depression as a homogeneous disease entity. Currently, this view has been increasingly criticized, since depression actually is a very heterogeneous illness, e.g., in terms of symptom profiles, clinical picture, treatment response, or underlying pathophysiology (Baumeister and Parker 2012). Distinct subtypes of depression even differ in relation to nutritional aspects, e.g., in relation to appetite, craving, or weight management. Thus, the consideration of distinct symptom profiles and subtypes of depression seems to be promising.

A variety of depression subtyping models has been described in the literature, such as symptom-based (e.g., melancholic and atypical depression), aetiologically-based (e.g., early trauma depression, perinatal depression), or time-of-onset-based approaches (e.g., early vs. late onset depression, seasonal affective disorder) (Baumeister and Parker 2012). Data-driven techniques on specific symptom dimensions have proposed further subtypes but did not provide conclusive evidence of their existence (van Loo et al. 2012).

An established subtype classification is based on the *Diagnostic and Statistical Manual of Mental Disorders, Fourth Edition* (DSM-IV) (American Psychiatric Association 2000), which differentiates subtypes in terms of symptom profiles, e.g., into major depression with melancholic features or atypical features. An overview of the distinct symptom profiles of melancholic and atypical depression according

Table 17.1 Melancholic and atypical depression according to DSM-IV (American Psychiatric Association 2000)

Criteria	Melancholic depression	Atypical depression
A criteria	Loss of pleasure in (almost) all activities (and/or)	Mood reactivity
	Lack of reactivity to usually pleasurable stimuli	
B criteria	*Accompanied by at least three of the following symptoms:*	*Accompanied by at least two of the following symptoms:*
	Distinct quality of depressed mood	Significant weight gain or increased appetite
	Depression worse in the morning	Hypersomnia
	Early morning awakening	Leaden paralysis
	Marked psychomotor retardation or agitation	Interpersonal rejection sensitivity
	Significant anorexia or weight loss	
	Excessive or inappropriate guilt	

to DSM-IV is shown in Table 17.1. As one can see, both subtypes differ in symptoms related to dietary aspects: Melancholic depression is characterized by decreased appetite and weight loss, whereas atypical depression is characterized by increased appetite and weight gain. Although the contrasting symptom profiles suggest that diet and depression could be associated differently in distinct depression subtypes, prior research did hardly address this issue when examining the diet-depression relationship.

In the past, literature highlighted that especially the atypical subtype is related to emotional eating, craving, and increased consumption of comfort foods (Moller 1992; Parker and Crawford 2007). In particular, symptoms such as irritability and rejection sensitivity, a symptom criterion for the atypical depression subtype according to DSM-IV, have been shown to be predictors of craving for comfort foods such as chocolate (Parker and Crawford 2007).

One recent study examined associations between overall diet and depression while considering distinct depression subtypes (Rahe et al. 2015). In this study, no differences in diet quality were found between non-depressed control subjects and patients with depression if depression was considered as homogeneous disease condition. Interestingly, differences were found after considering different subtypes of depression (melancholic, atypical, mixed, and undifferentiated depression). Patients with atypical depression reported significantly poorer diet quality than patients with melancholic depression. In line with the results mentioned above, these differences were mainly explained by higher intakes of comfort foods such as chocolate and cake in patients with atypical depression. Furthermore, overall diet quality of patients with melancholic depression was significantly better than of the other depression subtypes as well as of the non-depressed controls, suggesting that these patients may consume less low-quality comfort foods, possibly due to their decreased appetite, which in turn may have positive influence on their overall diet quality.

Another special case of depressive disorders that has been examined in relation to overall diet is perinatal depression (also known as maternal depression), covering both antenatal depression during pregnancy and postnatal depression in the first weeks or months postpartum (Baumeister and Parker 2012). During the perinatal period, women are at greater risk of experiencing mental health problems, which can negatively affect both the women's and their children's health (Leung and Kaplan 2009). Except for the special onset period, no subtype-specific symptoms of perinatal depression have been defined.

In the past, it has been proposed that nutrient deficiencies during pregnancy, a phase while nutritional requirements are actually increased in order to ensure maternal metabolic needs as well as adequate child growth, may be related to greater risk of maternal depression (Leung and Kaplan 2009). Such nutrient deficiencies are known to be relatively common in individuals consuming Western-type diets that are low in vitamins and minerals (Leung and Kaplan 2009). A recent systematic review evaluated the association between overall diet quality during pregnancy and maternal depression during the perinatal period (Baskin et al. 2015). There is still little evidence from only a small number of studies. On the basis of the available literature, the authors reported that there is limited evidence for a positive association between poor diet and antenatal depression as well as for an inverse association between healthy diets and antenatal depression; further, there is conflicting evidence for an association between healthy diets and postnatal depression (Baskin et al. 2015).

17.5 Interplay of Nutrition, Depression, and Cardiovascular Disease

As outlined in the previous sections, nutrition and depression are linked within a complex relationship. This relationship appears to be even more complex, if we additionally consider its interplay with the development and progression of somatic diseases, in particular CVD.

Research has shown that individuals with depression are at greater risk of an increased overall mortality (Cuijpers et al. 2013) as well as of several chronic diseases such as obesity, type 2 diabetes or CVD (Penninx et al. 2013). Depression and these somatic diseases are highly comorbid and may share biological pathways. Moreover, these relationships are also supposed to be of bidirectional nature. A considerable body of evidence has pointed out that, on the one hand, patients with CVD have an increased risk to develop a depressive episode and, on the other hand, patients with depression have an increased risk to experience cardiovascular events later on (Hare et al. 2014). Currently, this is an extensively investigated research topic: For example, the ongoing prospective BiDirect Study was exclusively

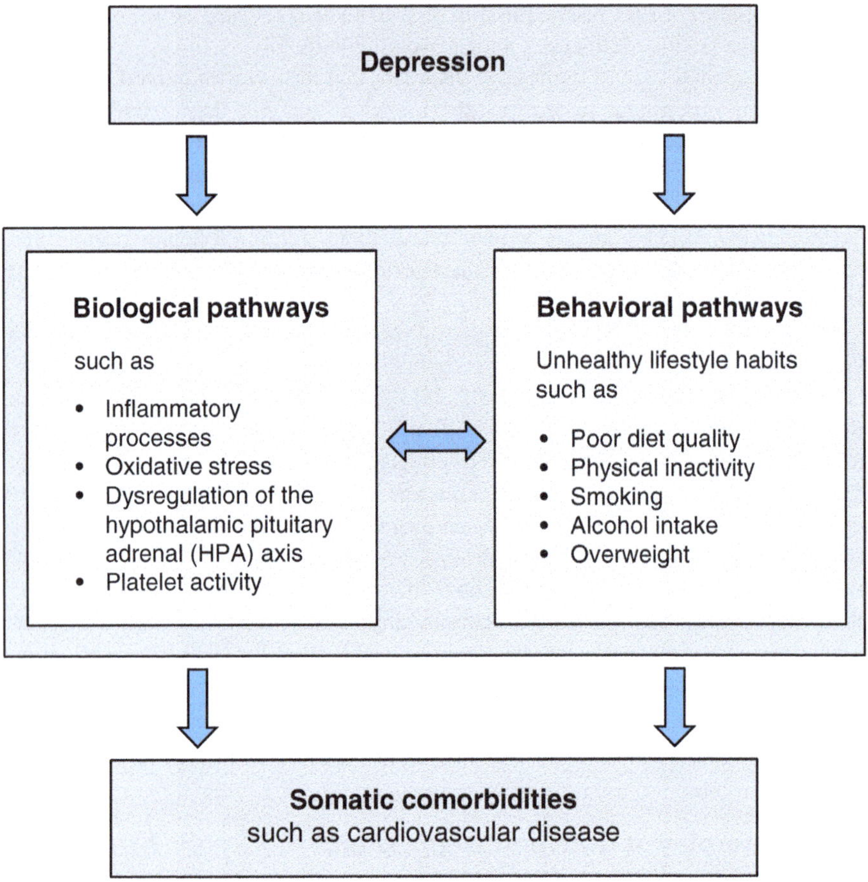

Fig. 17.2 Pathways linking depression and somatic comorbidities (adapted from Lett et al. 2004; Kuehl et al. 2012)

designed to establish the bidirectional relationship between depression and (subclinical) arteriosclerosis (Teismann et al. 2014).

The underlying pathways remain unclear, but it has been suggested that there are biological as well as behavioral pathways linking depression and CVD (see Fig. 17.2) (Lett et al. 2004; Kuehl et al. 2012). As pointed out in Sect. 17.2.2, patients with depression may develop an overall unhealthy lifestyle with risk factor profiles that include obesity, poor diet, physical inactivity, and smoking (Bonnet et al. 2005; Kilian et al. 2006). Since the abovementioned lifestyle factors are established CVD risk factors, this condition may explain (at least to some degree) the increased risk of CVD in individuals with depression (Whooley et al. 2008; Ye et al. 2013; Rutledge et al. 2014). In terms of nutrition, especially low intakes of dietary fiber, omega-3 fatty acids, and fruit and vegetables have been highlighted as potential meditating factors in the relationship between depression and CVD (Rutledge et al. 2014; Frasure-Smith et al. 2004).

Since distinct subtypes of depression may vary in terms to their lifestyle habits and anthropometric characteristics, certain subtypes may be at greater risk of developing somatic comorbidities. In this context, it has been highlighted that in particular individuals with atypical depression show unfavorable CVD risk profiles, e.g., in terms of poorer anthropometric measures such as higher BMI, fat mass, and waist circumference (Lasserre et al. 2014), possibly due to physical inactivity (Glaus et al. 2013) and/or increased appetite and calorie intake. Likewise, in several studies, atypical depression was associated with a higher prevalence of the metabolic syndrome, an additional important CVD risk factor (Lamers et al. 2010, 2013; Glaus et al. 2013). Overall, these findings suggested that in particular patients with atypical rather than melancholic depression have unfavorable CVD risk profiles and, therefore, should get special attention, since this subtype of depression may be a strong predictor of later CVD. However, the prevention of subsequent CVD events in patients with depression is supposed to be challenging, since patients with depression show a poor compliance and are less likely to follow recommendations regarding healthy lifestyle modifications (Ziegelstein et al. 2000).

17.6 Implications for Public Health, Clinical Practice, and Future Research

Although there is emerging evidence on a relationship between nutrition and depression, there are several unsolved research questions and shortcomings of previous studies, which should be addressed in future studies. In the following, we want to highlight important implications for public health, clinical practice, and future research.

17.6.1 Public Health

Because of its high prevalence and its significant contribution to the global disease burden, the consideration of depression as a "public health priority" (Ferrari et al. 2013) is of major importance. Prior efforts to tackle the health problem of depression have primarily focused on treatment rather than on prevention. A shift toward a focus on multidisciplinary preventive approaches on the population level seems desirable and necessary (Logan and Jacka 2014). Lifestyle factors in general and diet in particular should be considered as promising intervention targets, since they are generally modifiable and, thus, may offer great potential for prevention.

In the last decades, Western societies have undergone behavioral changes toward physical inactivity in daily life and unhealthy dietary habits with a high consumption of processed foods rich in saturated fats, added sugar, and sodium (Popkin et al. 2012; Sarris et al. 2015; Logan and Jacka 2014). Globalization of the food system and changes in regard to food production, transportation, and marketing were contributors to this "nutrition transition" and advanced the development of a food environment that ensures a wide availability of relatively inexpensive, palatable, energy-dense, but nutrient-poor foods, whereas traditional diets with a high consumption of fruit, vegetables, legumes, and whole-grain products more and more disappear (Popkin et al. 2012; Logan and Jacka 2014; Jacka et al. 2014b). Key public health targets should include policy actions toward improving food and lifestyle environments, including greater funding for programs which target on promoting the implementation of healthier dietary habits back toward traditional dietary patterns as well as on reducing existing barriers which hinder people from engaging a healthier lifestyle (van Gool et al. 2007; Jacka et al. 2012, 2014b; Sarris et al. 2015).

Given that there is emerging evidence on a crucial relationship between diet and depression, it is argued to build a shared framework for physical and mental health by implementing the common mental disorders (i.e., depression and anxiety) into the league of the highly prevalent common non-communicable diseases (Jacka et al. 2012; O'Neil et al. 2015). Although the existing evidence on the diet-depression relationship is not entirely consistent and mechanisms are not completely understood, emerging studies conclude that it is "feasible and timely" to develop prevention strategies involving dietary changes on population level (Jacka et al. 2012). Lessons can be learned from already existing approaches related to other chronic diseases (Hayward et al. 2014).

Since nutrition is related to both mental and physical health, the incorporation of nutrition in evidence-based prevention strategies against depression would overlap with already existing strategies regarding other non-communicable diseases such as CVD, where lifestyle factors are already well-established key contributors. Nevertheless, it has to be considered that depression has a multifactorial origin and that diet can only be one single factor in a comprehensive prevention strategy. However, given its high prevalence and its serious consequences, even small effects can be important in the prevention of depression on a population level.

17.6.2 Clinical Practice

Although the call for preventive approaches is rising, the clinical management of patients with depressive disorders is also highly relevant. The clinical management of depression should more strongly incorporate the monitoring of lifestyle behaviors in patients with depression and give guidance to implement an overall healthy lifestyle including a healthy diet. Given the fact that unfavorable lifestyle habits are established risk factors for the development of common chronic diseases, continuous monitoring of lifestyle and diet behavior should be a common part in the clinical management of patients with depression. Moreover, clinical practice should also consider the relevance of distinct depression subtypes, since subtypes may be related to lifestyle habits differently and, therefore, may have different risk profiles for developing comorbidities.

Such "lifestyle medicine" approaches should be included in treatment guidelines next to the common first-line treatments. Up to now, the clinical management of depression has largely been focused on pharmacological treatment and psychotherapy, but rarely includes the consideration of lifestyle factors including diet (Berk et al. 2013a). Given that antidepressant medications have a limited efficacy and can be accompanied by side effects, alternative treatment strategies for mental health problems should be considered (Rucklidge and Kaplan 2013). Based on the current literature, it is demanded to implement nutritional medicine into psychiatric standard practice (Sarris et al. 2015).

17.6.3 Research

Although evidence on the diet-depression relationship arises continuously, there are still unsolved research questions as well as methodological shortcomings, which should be properly addressed in future research. Firstly, it is relevant to conduct methodologically sound studies in the form of RCTs and prospective observational studies, which should include large sample sizes, proper assessment methods (for both dietary and psychiatric assessment), and thorough control for potential confounding factors (if applicable). Moreover, these studies should consider the actual direction of the diet-depression relationship. Since it is argued that the link between diet and depression may be bidirectional (i.e., poor diet may predict depression and/or depression may predict poor diet), research must address the issue of reverse causality (Jacka et al. 2015).

Furthermore, it seems important that studies apply appropriate methods for depression classification. Prior studies on the diet-depression relationship mainly used depression scales in order to assess depressive symptoms as a marker of major depression. Only few studies applied more appropriate methods such as the clinical interview, which is known to be the gold standard method in depression diagnostic (Joiner et al. 2005; Stuart et al. 2014).

In this context, future research should also consider the differentiation of distinct depression subtypes (Penninx et al. 2013). Up to this point, research findings on the diet-depression relationship are not entirely consistent. The variability of existing results could be partly explained by the heterogeneity of depression (Penninx et al. 2013), since distinct depression subtypes may be related to diet differently. To take into account subtypes of depression in research may help to prevent blurred results and, thus, may improve the understanding of the diet-depression relationship.

Conclusions

There is emerging evidence of a complex relationship between nutrition and depression, suggesting that diet plays a crucial role in the development and progression of depressive disorders. In turn, depression itself is supposed to be a predictor of developing an unhealthy lifestyle and unfavorable cardiovascular risk factor profiles including poor diet. Hence, nutrition may be one mediating factor in the observed link between depression and CVD.

Prior research on the diet-depression relationship has commonly treated depression as a homogeneous disease entity, although there is evidence that distinct subtypes of depression vary in terms of their lifestyle habits and anthropometric characteristics. In particular, atypical depression is highlighted to be characterized by more unfavorable cardiovascular risk profiles, including obesity, poorer diet, and physical inactivity, and may be at greater risk of developing somatic comorbidities such as CVD. As a consequence, the consideration of distinct depression subtypes may be helpful in order to better understand the link between nutrition, depression, and CVD as well as its underlying mechanisms.

Further research is needed to enlighten the diet-depression relationship. However, research is just the first step and only builds the basis for further important approaches regarding treatment and prevention of depression. There is an urgent need to push forward both translational medicine approaches and policy actions in the field of nutritional psychiatry. Thus, it seems important that research results are disseminated to important stakeholders such as clinicians, politicians, and the wider public, in order to ensure that important research findings can be implemented in clinical practice as well as in public health interventions.

References

Akbaraly TN, Sabia S, Shipley MJ, Batty GD, Kivimaki M (2013) Adherence to healthy dietary guidelines and future depressive symptoms: evidence for sex differentials in the Whitehall II study. Am J Clin Nutr 97(2):419–427

American Psychiatric Association (2000) Diagnostic and statistical manual of mental disorders: DSM-IV-TR, 4th edn, Text revision. American Psychiatric Association, Washington, DC

Appelhans BM, Whited MC, Schneider KL, Ma Y, Oleski JL, Merriam PA, Waring ME, Olendzki BC, Mann DM, Ockene IS, Pagoto SL (2012) Depression severity, diet quality, and physical activity in women with obesity and depression. J Acad Nutr Diet 112(5):693–698

Appleton KM, Rogers PJ, Ness AR (2010) Updated systematic review and meta-analysis of the effects of n-3 long-chain polyunsaturated fatty acids on depressed mood. Am J Clin Nutr 91(3):757–770

Barbaresko J, Koch M, Schulze MB, Nöthlings U (2013) Dietary pattern analysis and biomarkers of low-grade inflammation: a systematic literature review. Nutr Rev 71(8):511–527

Barker D (1997) Maternal nutrition, fetal nutrition, and disease in later life. Nutrition 13(9):807–813

Barker D (2002) Fetal programming of coronary heart disease. Trends Endocrinol Metab 13(9):364–368

Baskin R, Hill B, Jacka FN, O'Neil A, Skouteris H (2015) The association between diet quality and mental health during the perinatal period. A systematic review. Appetite 91:41–47

Baumeister H, Parker G (2012) Meta-review of depressive subtyping models. J Affect Disord 139(2):126–140

Benton D, Donohoe RT (1999) The effects of nutrients on mood. Public Health Nutr 2(3A):403–409

Berk M, Sarris J, Coulson CE, Jacka FN (2013a) Lifestyle management of unipolar depression. Acta Psychiatr Scand 127(Suppl 443):38–54

Berk M, Williams LJ, Jacka FN, O'Neil A, Pasco JA, Moylan S, Allen NB, Stuart AL, Hayley AC, Byrne ML, Maes M (2013b) So depression is an inflammatory disease, but where does the inflammation come from? BMC Med 11:200

Bloch MH, Hannestad J (2012) Omega-3 fatty acids for the treatment of depression: systematic review and meta-analysis. Mol Psychiatry 17(12):1272–1282

Bonnet F, Irving K, Terra J, Nony P, Berthezène F, Moulin P (2005) Anxiety and depression are associated with unhealthy lifestyle in patients at risk of cardiovascular disease. Atherosclerosis 178(2):339–344

Capra L, Tezza G, Mazzei F, Boner AL (2013) The origins of health and disease: the influence of maternal diseases and lifestyle during gestation. Ital J Pediatr 39:7
Chan R, Chan D, Woo J (2014) A prospective cohort study to examine the association between dietary patterns and depressive symptoms in older Chinese people in Hong Kong. PLoS One 9(8):e105760
Chocano-Bedoya PO, O'Reilly EJ, Lucas M, Mirzaei F, Okereke OI, Fung TT, Hu FB, Ascherio A (2013) Prospective study on long-term dietary patterns and incident depression in middle-aged and older women. Am J Clin Nutr 98(3):813–820
Crawford GB, Khedkar A, Flaws JA, Sorkin JD, Gallicchio L (2011) Depressive symptoms and self-reported fast-food intake in midlife women. Prev Med 52(3–4):254–257
Cryan JF, Dinan TG (2012) Mind-altering microorganisms: the impact of the gut microbiota on brain and behaviour. Nat Rev Neurosci 13(10):701–712
Cuijpers P, Vogelzangs N, Twisk J, Kleiboer A, Li J, Penninx BW (2013) Differential mortality rates in major and subthreshold depression: meta-analysis of studies that measured both. Br J Psychiatry 202(1):22–27
Cumurcu BE, Ozyurt H, Etikan I, Demir S, Karlidag R (2009) Total antioxidant capacity and total oxidant status in patients with major depression: impact of antidepressant treatment. Psychiatry Clin Neurosci 63(5):639–645
Dai J, Jones DP, Goldberg J, Ziegler TR, Bostick RM, Wilson PW, Manatunga AK, Shallenberger L, Jones L, Vaccarino V (2008) Association between adherence to the Mediterranean diet and oxidative stress. Am J Clin Nutr 88(5):1364–1370
Dash S, Clarke G, Berk M, Jacka FN (2015) The gut microbiome and diet in psychiatry: focus on depression. Curr Opin Psychiatry 28(1):1–6
De Filippo C, Cavalieri D, Di Paola M, Ramazzotti M, Poullet JB, Massart S, Collini S, Pieraccini G, Lionetti P (2010) Impact of diet in shaping gut microbiota revealed by a comparative study in children from Europe and rural Africa. Proc Natl Acad Sci U S A 107(33):14691–14696
Esposito K, Di Palo C, Maiorino MI, Petrizzo M, Bellastella G, Siniscalchi I, Giugliano D (2011) Long-term effect of mediterranean-style diet and calorie restriction on biomarkers of longevity and oxidative stress in overweight men. Cardiol Res Pract 2011:293916
Fakhoury M (2015) Revisiting the serotonin hypothesis: implications for major depressive disorders. Mol Neurobiol doi:10.1007/s12035-015-9152-z
Ferrari AJ, Charlson FJ, Norman RE, Patten SB, Freedman G, Murray CJL, Vos T, Whiteford HA (2013) Burden of depressive disorders by country, sex, age, and year: findings from the global burden of disease study 2010. PLoS Med 10(11):e1001547
Fito M, de La Torre R, Covas M (2007) Olive oil and oxidative stress. Mol Nutr Food Res 51(10):1215–1224
Foster JA, McVey Neufeld K (2013) Gut-brain axis: how the microbiome influences anxiety and depression. Trends Neurosci 36(5):305–312
Frasure-Smith N, Lespérance F, Julien P (2004) Major depression is associated with lower omega-3 fatty acid levels in patients with recent acute coronary syndromes. Biol Psychiatry 55(9):891–896
Galland L (2010) Diet and inflammation. Nutr Clin Pract 25(6):634–640
García-Toro M, Ibarra O, Gili M, Serrano MJ, Oliván B, Vicens E, Roca M (2012) Four hygienic-dietary recommendations as add-on treatment in depression: a randomized-controlled trial. J Affect Disord 140(2):200–203
George SA, Khan S, Briggs H, Abelson JL (2010) CRH-stimulated cortisol release and food intake in healthy, non-obese adults. Psychoneuroendocrinology 35(4):607–612
Gibson EL (2006) Emotional influences on food choice: sensory, physiological and psychological pathways. Physiol Behav 89(1):53–61
Glaus J, Vandeleur C, Gholam-Rezaee M, Castelao E, Perrin M, Rothen S, Bovet P, Marques-Vidal P, von Känel R, Merikangas K, Mooser V, Waterworth DM, Waeber G, Vollenweider P, Preisig M (2013) Atypical depression and alcohol misuse are related to the cardiovascular risk in the general population. Acta Psychiatr Scand 128(4):282–293
Haapakoski R, Mathieu J, Ebmeier KP, Alenius H, Kivimaki M (2015) Cumulative meta-analysis of interleukins 6 and 1beta, tumour necrosis factor alpha and C-reactive protein in patients with major depressive disorder. Brain Behav Immun 49:206–215

Hare DL, Toukhsati SR, Johansson P, Jaarsma T (2014) Depression and cardiovascular disease: a clinical review. Eur Heart J 35(21):1365–1372

Hayward J, Jacka FN, Waters E, Allender S (2014) Lessons from obesity prevention for the prevention of mental disorders: the primordial prevention approach. BMC Psychiatry 14:254

Hoffmann K, Schulze MB, Schienkiewitz A, Nothlings U, Boeing H (2004) Application of a new statistical method to derive dietary patterns in nutritional epidemiology. Am J Epidemiol 159(10):935–944

Hu FB (2002) Dietary pattern analysis: a new direction in nutritional epidemiology. Curr Opin Lipidol 13(1):3–9

Jacka FN, Pasco JA, Mykletun A, Williams LJ, Hodge AM, O'Reilly SL, Nicholson GC, Kotowicz MA, Berk M (2010) Association of Western and traditional diets with depression and anxiety in women. Am J Psychiatry 167(3):305–311

Jacka FN, Mykletun A, Berk M (2012) Moving towards a population health approach to the primary prevention of common mental disorders. BMC Med 10:149

Jacka FN, Ystrom E, Brantsaeter AL, Karevold E, Roth C, Haugen M, Meltzer HM, Schjolberg S, Berk M (2013) Maternal and early postnatal nutrition and mental health of offspring by age 5 years: a prospective cohort study. J Am Acad Child Adolesc Psychiatry 52(10):1038–1047

Jacka FN, Cherbuin N, Anstey KJ, Butterworth P (2014a) Dietary patterns and depressive symptoms over time: examining the relationships with socioeconomic position, health behaviours and cardiovascular risk. PLoS One 9(1):e87657

Jacka FN, Sacks G, Berk M, Allender S (2014b) Food policies for physical and mental health. BMC Psychiatry 14:132

Jacka FN, Cherbuin N, Anstey KJ, Butterworth P (2015) Does reverse causality explain the relationship between diet and depression? J Affect Disord 175:248–250

Joiner TE, Walker RL, Pettit JW, Perez M, Cukrowicz KC (2005) Evidence-based assessment of depression in adults. Psychol Assess 17(3):267–277

Kant AK (2004) Dietary patterns and health outcomes. J Am Diet Assoc 104(4):615–635

Kaplan BJ, Rucklidge JJ, Romijn A, McLeod K (2015) The emerging field of nutritional mental health: inflammation, the microbiome, oxidative stress, and mitochondrial function. Clin Psychol Sci 3(6):964–980

Kilian R, Becker T, Kruger K, Schmid S, Frasch K (2006) Health behavior in psychiatric in-patients compared with a German general population sample. Acta Psychiatr Scand 114(4):242–248

Kim-Cohen J, Caspi A, Moffitt TE, Harrington H, Milne BJ, Poulton R (2003) Prior juvenile diagnoses in adults with mental disorder: developmental follow-back of a prospective-longitudinal cohort. Arch Gen Psychiatry 60(7):709–717

Knorr U, Vinberg M, Kessing LV, Wetterslev J (2010) Salivary cortisol in depressed patients versus control persons: a systematic review and meta-analysis. Psychoneuroendocrinology 35(9):1275–1286

Konttinen H, Männistö S, Sarlio-Lähteenkorva S, Silventoinen K, Haukkala A (2010) Emotional eating, depressive symptoms and self-reported food consumption. A population-based study. Appetite 54(3):473–479

Kuehl LK, Penninx BWJH, Otte C (2012) Depression: risk factor for cardiovascular disease. Nervenarzt 83(11):1379–1384

Lai JS, Hiles S, Bisquera A, Hure AJ, McEvoy M, Attia J (2014) A systematic review and meta-analysis of dietary patterns and depression in community-dwelling adults. Am J Clin Nutr 99(1):181–197

Lamers F, de Jonge P, Nolen WA, Smit JH, Zitman FG, Beekman ATF, Penninx BWJH (2010) Identifying depressive subtypes in a large cohort study: results from the Netherlands Study of Depression and Anxiety (NESDA). J Clin Psychiatry 71(12):1582–1589

Lamers F, Vogelzangs N, Merikangas KR, de Jonge P, Beekman ATF, Penninx BWJH (2013) Evidence for a differential role of HPA-axis function, inflammation and metabolic syndrome in melancholic versus atypical depression. Mol Psychiatry 18(6):692–699

Lasserre AM, Glaus J, Vandeleur CL, Marques-Vidal P, Vaucher J, Bastardot F, Waeber G, Vollenweider P, Preisig M (2014) Depression with atypical features and increase in obesity,

body mass index, waist circumference, and fat mass: a prospective, population-based study. JAMA Psychiatry 71(8):880–888
Le Port A, Gueguen A, Kesse-Guyot E, Melchior M, Lemogne C, Nabi H, Goldberg M, Zins M, Czernichow S (2012) Association between dietary patterns and depressive symptoms over time: a 10-year follow-up study of the GAZEL cohort. PLoS One 7(12):e51593
Lee T, Nkouibert Assam P, Gersing KR, Chan E, Burchett BM, Sim K, Feng L, Krishnan KR, Rush AJ (2012) The effectiveness of antidepressant monotherapy in a naturalistic outpatient setting. Prim Care Companion CNS Disord 14(5): doi: 10.4088/PCC.12m01364
Lepine J, Briley M (2011) The increasing burden of depression. Neuropsychiatr Dis Treat 7(Suppl 1):3–7
Lett HS, Blumenthal JA, Babyak MA, Sherwood A, Strauman T, Robins C, Newman MF (2004) Depression as a risk factor for coronary artery disease: evidence, mechanisms, and treatment. Psychosom Med 66(3):305–315
Leung BM, Kaplan BJ (2009) Perinatal depression: prevalence, risks, and the nutrition link – a review of the literature. J Am Diet Assoc 109(9):1566–1575
Logan AC, Jacka FN (2014) Nutritional psychiatry research: an emerging discipline and its intersection with global urbanization, environmental challenges and the evolutionary mismatch. J Physiol Anthropol 33:22
Lopresti AL, Hood SD, Drummond PD (2013) A review of lifestyle factors that contribute to important pathways associated with major depression: diet, sleep and exercise. J Affect Disord 148(1):12–27
Lucas M, Chocano-Bedoya P, Schulze MB, Mirzaei F, O'Reilly ÉJ, Okereke OI, Hu FB, Willett WC, Ascherio A (2014) Inflammatory dietary pattern and risk of depression among women. Brain Behav Immun 36:46–53
Maes M, de Vos N, Pioli R, Demedts P, Wauters A, Neels H, Christophe A (2000) Lower serum vitamin E concentrations in major depression. Another marker of lowered antioxidant defenses in that illness. J Affect Disord 58(3):241–246
Maes M, Galecki P, Chang YS, Berk M (2011a) A review on the oxidative and nitrosative stress (O&NS) pathways in major depression and their possible contribution to the (neuro)degenerative processes in that illness. Prog Neuropsychopharmacol Biol Psychiatry 35(3):676–692
Maes M, Mihaylova I, Kubera M, Uytterhoeven M, Vrydags N, Bosmans E (2011b) Lower whole blood glutathione peroxidase (GPX) activity in depression, but not in myalgic encephalomyelitis/chronic fatigue syndrome: another pathway that may be associated with coronary artery disease and neuroprogression in depression. Neuro Endocrinol Lett 32(2):133–140
Maslowski KM, Mackay CR (2011) Diet, gut microbiota and immune responses. Nat Immunol 12(1):5–9
Merikangas KR, He J, Burstein M, Swanson SA, Avenevoli S, Cui L, Benjet C, Georgiades K, Swendsen J (2010) Lifetime prevalence of mental disorders in U.S. adolescents: results from the National Comorbidity Survey Replication-Adolescent Supplement (NCS-A). J Am Acad Child Adolesc Psychiatry 49(10):980–989
Moller SE (1992) Serotonin, carbohydrates, and atypical depression. Pharmacol Toxicol 71(Suppl 1):61–71
Moschen AR, Wieser V, Tilg H (2012) Dietary factors: major regulators of the gut's microbiota. Gut Liver 6(4):411–416
Murakami K, Sasaki S (2010) Dietary intake and depressive symptoms: a systematic review of observational studies. Mol Nutr Food Res 54(4):471–488
O'Neil A, Berk M, Itsiopoulos C, Castle D, Opie R, Pizzinga J, Brazionis L, Hodge A, Mihalopoulos C, Chatterton ML, Dean OM, Jacka FN (2013) A randomised, controlled trial of a dietary intervention for adults with major depression (the "SMILES" trial): study protocol. BMC Psychiatry 13:114
O'Neil A, Itsiopoulos C, Skouteris H, Opie RS, McPhie S, Hill B, Jacka FN (2014a) Preventing mental health problems in offspring by targeting dietary intake of pregnant women. BMC Med 12:208
O'Neil A, Quirk SE, Housden S, Brennan SL, Williams LJ, Pasco JA, Berk M, Jacka FN (2014b) Relationship between diet and mental health in children and adolescents: a systematic review. Am J Public Health 104(10):e31–e42

O'Neil A, Jacka FN, Quirk SE, Cocker F, Taylor C, Oldenburg B, Berk M (2015) A shared framework for the common mental disorders and non-communicable disease: key considerations for disease prevention and control. BMC Psychiatry 15:15

Ocké MC (2013) Evaluation of methodologies for assessing the overall diet: dietary quality scores and dietary pattern analysis. Proc Nutr Soc 72(2):191–199

Opie RS, O'Neil A, Itsiopoulos C, Jacka FN (2014) The impact of whole-of-diet interventions on depression and anxiety: a systematic review of randomised controlled trials. Public Health Nutr 18(11):2074–2093

Ouwens MA, van Strien T, van Leeuwe JFJ (2009) Possible pathways between depression, emotional and external eating. A structural equation model. Appetite 53(2):245–248

Pagoto SL, Ma Y, Bodenlos JS, Olendzki B, Rosal MC, Tellez T, Merriam P, Ockene IS (2009) Association of depressive symptoms and lifestyle behaviors among Latinos at risk of type 2 diabetes. J Am Diet Assoc 109(7):1246–1250

Parker G, Crawford J (2007) Chocolate craving when depressed: a personality marker. Br J Psychiatry 191:351–352

Parker G, Parker I, Brotchie H (2006) Mood state effects of chocolate. J Affect Disord 92(2–3):149–159

Penninx BW, Milaneschi Y, Lamers F, Vogelzangs N (2013) Understanding the somatic consequences of depression: biological mechanisms and the role of depression symptom profile. BMC Med 11:129

Politi P, Rocchetti M, Emanuele E, Rondanelli M, Barale F (2013) Randomized placebo-controlled trials of omega-3 polyunsaturated fatty acids in psychiatric disorders: a review of the current literature. Curr Drug Discov Technol 10(3):245–253

Popa TA, Ladea M (2012) Nutrition and depression at the forefront of progress. J Med Life 5(4):414–419

Popkin BM, Adair LS, Ng SW (2012) Global nutrition transition and the pandemic of obesity in developing countries. Nutr Rev 70(1):3–21

Prohan M, Amani R, Nematpour S, Jomehzadeh N, Haghighizadeh MH (2014) Total antioxidant capacity of diet and serum, dietary antioxidant vitamins intake, and serum hs-CRP levels in relation to depression scales in university male students. Redox Rep 19(3):133–139

Psaltopoulou T, Sergentanis TN, Panagiotakos DB, Sergentanis IN, Kosti R, Scarmeas N (2013) Mediterranean diet, stroke, cognitive impairment, and depression: a meta-analysis. Ann Neurol 74(4):580–591

Quirk SE, Williams LJ, O'Neil A, Pasco JA, Jacka FN, Housden S, Berk M, Brennan SL (2013) The association between diet quality, dietary patterns and depression in adults: a systematic review. BMC Psychiatry 13:175

Rahe C, Unrath M, Berger K (2014) Dietary patterns and the risk of depression in adults: a systematic review of observational studies. Eur J Nutr 53(4):997–1013

Rahe C, Baune BT, Unrath M, Arolt V, Wellmann J, Wersching H, Berger K (2015) Associations between depression subtypes, depression severity and diet quality: cross-sectional findings from the BiDirect Study. BMC Psychiatry 15:38

Rucklidge JJ, Kaplan BJ (2013) Broad-spectrum micronutrient formulas for the treatment of psychiatric symptoms: a systematic review. Expert Rev Neurother 13(1):49–73

Rucklidge JJ, Kaplan BJ, Mulder RT (2015) What if nutrients could treat mental illness? Aust N Z J Psychiatry 49(5):407–408

Rush AJ (2007) Limitations in efficacy of antidepressant monotherapy. J Clin Psychiatry 68(Suppl 10):8–10

Rutledge T, Kenkre TS, Thompson DV, Bittner VA, Whittaker K, Eastwood J, Eteiba W, Cornell CE, Krantz DS, Pepine CJ, Johnson BD, Handberg EM, Bairey Merz CN (2014) Depression, dietary habits, and cardiovascular events among women with suspected myocardial ischemia. Am J Med 127(9):840–847

Ruusunen A, Lehto SM, Mursu J, Tolmunen T, Tuomainen T, Kauhanen J, Voutilainen S (2014) Dietary patterns are associated with the prevalence of elevated depressive symptoms and the risk of getting a hospital discharge diagnosis of depression in middle-aged or older Finnish men. J Affect Disord 159:1–6

Sanchez-Villegas A, Martínez-González MA (2013) Diet, a new target to prevent depression? BMC Med 11:3

Sánchez-Villegas A, Delgado-Rodríguez M, Alonso A, Schlatter J, Lahortiga F, Serra Majem L, Martínez-González MA (2009) Association of the Mediterranean dietary pattern with the incidence of depression: the Seguimiento Universidad de Navarra/University of Navarra follow-up (SUN) cohort. Arch Gen Psychiatry 66(10):1090–1098

Sánchez-Villegas A, Martínez-González MA, Estruch R, Salas-Salvadó J, Corella D, Covas MI, Arós F, Romaguera D, Gómez-Gracia E, Lapetra J, Pintó X, Martínez JA, Lamuela-Raventós RM, Ros E, Gea A, Wärnberg J, Serra-Majem L (2013) Mediterranean dietary pattern and depression: the PREDIMED randomized trial. BMC Med 11:208

Sanhueza C, Ryan L, Foxcroft DR (2013) Diet and the risk of unipolar depression in adults: systematic review of cohort studies. J Hum Nutr Diet 26(1):56–70

Sarris J, Schoendorfer N, Kavanagh DJ (2009) Major depressive disorder and nutritional medicine: a review of monotherapies and adjuvant treatments. Nutr Rev 67(3):125–131

Sarris J, O'Neil A, Coulson CE, Schweitzer I, Berk M (2014) Lifestyle medicine for depression. BMC Psychiatry 14:107

Sarris J, Logan AC, Akbaraly TN, Amminger GP, Balanzá-Martínez V, Freeman MP, Hibbeln J, Matsuoka Y, Mischoulon D, Mizoue T, Nanri A, Nishi D, Ramsey D, Rucklidge JJ, Sanchez-Villegas A, Scholey A, Su K, Jacka FN, on behalf of The International Society for Nutritional Psychiatry Research (2015) Nutritional medicine as mainstream in psychiatry. Lancet Psychiatry 2(3):271–274

Schwingshackl L, Hoffmann G (2014) Mediterranean dietary pattern, inflammation and endothelial function: a systematic review and meta-analysis of intervention trials. Nutr Metab Cardiovasc Dis 24(9):929–939

Selhub EM, Logan AC, Bested AC (2014) Fermented foods, microbiota, and mental health: ancient practice meets nutritional psychiatry. J Physiol Anthropol 33:2

Steenweg-de Graaff J, Tiemeier H, Steegers-Theunissen RPM, Hofman A, Jaddoe VWV, Verhulst FC, Roza SJ (2014) Maternal dietary patterns during pregnancy and child internalising and externalising problems. The Generation R Study. Clin Nutr 33(1):115–121

Stetler C, Miller GE (2011) Depression and hypothalamic-pituitary-adrenal activation: a quantitative summary of four decades of research. Psychosom Med 73(2):114–126

Stuart AL, Pasco JA, Jacka FN, Brennan SL, Berk M, Williams LJ (2014) Comparison of self-report and structured clinical interview in the identification of depression. Compr Psychiatry 55(4):866–869

Teismann H, Wersching H, Nagel M, Arolt V, Heindel W, Baune BT, Wellmann J, Hense H, Berger K (2014) Establishing the bidirectional relationship between depression and subclinical arteriosclerosis - rationale, design, and characteristics of the BiDirect Study. BMC Psychiatry 14:174

van Gool CH, Kempen GI, Bosma H, van Boxtel MP, Jolles J, van Eijk JT (2007) Associations between lifestyle and depressed mood: longitudinal results from the Maastricht Aging Study. Am J Public Health 97(5):887–894

van Loo HM, de Jonge P, Romeijn J, Kessler RC, Schoevers RA (2012) Data-driven subtypes of major depressive disorder: a systematic review. BMC Med 10:156

Whitaker KM, Sharpe PA, Wilcox S, Hutto BE (2014) Depressive symptoms are associated with dietary intake but not physical activity among overweight and obese women from disadvantaged neighborhoods. Nutr Res 34(4):294–301

Whooley MA, de Jonge P, Vittinghoff E, Otte C, Moos R, Carney RM, Ali S, Dowray S, Na B, Feldman MD, Schiller NB, Browner WS (2008) Depressive symptoms, health behaviors, and risk of cardiovascular events in patients with coronary heart disease. JAMA 300(20):2379–2388

Wurtman RJ, Wurtman JJ (1995) Brain serotonin, carbohydrate-craving, obesity and depression. Obes Res 3(Suppl 4):477S–480S

Ye S, Muntner P, Shimbo D, Judd SE, Richman J, Davidson KW, Safford MM (2013) Behavioral mechanisms, elevated depressive symptoms, and the risk for myocardial infarction or death in individuals with coronary heart disease: the REGARDS (Reason for Geographic and Racial Differences in Stroke) study. J Am Coll Cardiol 61(6):622–630

Yu ZM, Parker L, Dummer TJB (2014) Depressive symptoms, diet quality, physical activity, and body composition among populations in Nova Scotia, Canada: report from the Atlantic Partnership for Tomorrow's Health. Prev Med 61:106–113

Ziegelstein RC, Fauerbach JA, Stevens SS, Romanelli J, Richter DP, Bush DE (2000) Patients with depression are less likely to follow recommendations to reduce cardiac risk during recovery from a myocardial infarction. Arch Intern Med 160(12):1818

Cardiometabolic Risk and Monitoring in Psychiatric Disorders

18

Katherine Samaras

Contents

Abstract

Severe psychiatric disorders are associated with a mortality gap of 20–30 years, attributable to premature cardiac disease and diabetes mellitus. Both are substantially related to obesity and its metabolic complications, which occur following the initiation of psychotropic medications, particularly antipsychotics.

The risk of incident heart disease in people with severe mental illness is 1.6–2.2 times higher, with higher risk in men. The excess risk is related to higher rates of traditional and modifiable cardiovascular risk factors, including higher rates of smoking, diabetes, hyperlipidaemia, hypertension and obesity, with

K. Samaras, MBBS, PhD, FRACP
Department of Endocrinology, St Vincent's Hospital,
390 Victoria Street, Darlinghurst, NSW 2010 Sydney, Australia

Diabetes and Obesity Program, Garvan Institute of Medical Research,
384 Victoria Street, Darlinghurst, NSW, Sydney, Australia
e-mail: k.samaras@garvan.org.au

B.T. Baune, P.J. Tully (eds.), *Cardiovascular Diseases and Depression*,
DOI 10.1007/978-3-319-32480-7_18

poorer diet and greater sedentariness. This chapter reviews the major studies of cardiac disease in people with severe mental illness and discusses their strengths and limitations.

Diabetes risk is also increased in severe mental illness, related to greater rates of obesity, sedentariness and poor diet. Exposure to antidepressant medications and antipsychotic medications appears to increase diabetes risk 1.4- to 1.6-fold overall, though there is evidence that some medications have a much stronger association with incident diabetes. The major studies pertaining to diabetes risk in people with severe mental illness are discussed.

Strategies for detection of weight gain and metabolic decline are discussed and screening algorithms presented. Early detection of change in traditional and modifiable cardiometabolic risk factors is essential for early intervention, for the preservation of physical health in people with severe mental illness. Lifestyle intervention at psychotropic medication initiation prevents weight gain and cardiometabolic decline. This will translate to abbreviation of the premature cardiovascular mortality in people with severe mental illness, as has already occurred in the general population.

18.1 Introduction

Severe psychiatric disorders, such depression, schizophrenia and bipolar disease, are associated with a substantive burden of premature cardiometabolic diseases, including atherothrombotic cardiac disease, diabetes mellitus, hypertension, hyperlipidaemia and obesity. These contribute to an excess of premature mortality that has been estimated at 20–30 years (Colton and Manderscheid 2006; Thornicroft 2011; Hennekens 2007; Brown et al. 2010; Saha et al. 2007; Brown 1997). The majority of these deaths are attributable to cardiovascular disease (Colton and Manderscheid 2006). Of great concern, this mortality gap has widened over the last decade (Saha et al. 2007; Lawrence et al. 2013), despite medical advances in cardiovascular management and public health programmes that have benefited the majority of the general community.

Public health programmes have, for over two to three decades, focused attention on different aspects of physical health. These include strategies for smoking prevention, smoking cessation, dietary improvement, cholesterol reduction, increased physical activity, lipid and diabetes screening and obesity prevention and intervention. The attention of primary care and general practitioners has focused on cardiometabolic risk factor assessment and management, with early intervention for the prevention of cardiovascular disease and diabetes. Medical advances in the medical and interventional treatment of cardiovascular disease have also reduced morbidity and mortality in the general population. Advances in the understanding of diabetes development have led to practices of early intervention in prediabetes and earlier detection and treatment of diabetes. These standard practices have not been as seamlessly shared with people with severe mental illness.

The premature mortality and mortality gap from cardiovascular death in people with severe mental illness has been termed a "scandal" and considered by learned advocates to "contravene international conventions for the 'right to health'" (Thornicroft 2011). Widespread disparities have been reported in health service access, service delivery and management in people with severe mental illness, shown to contribute substantially to poorer physical health and health outcomes. Multiple unmet health needs exist for people with severe mental illness, not only for intervention, but also for prevention.

International efforts are addressing the factors that promote premature cardiometabolic disease in people with SMI. These include mandates for regular physical health care, cardiometabolic screening and intervention and prevention programmes. Increasingly, the model of unified physical and mental health care of the individual with severe mental illness is promoted, developing synergies and collaborations across multiple disciplines and allied health specialists.

Cardiometabolic screening, early intervention and prevention are steps towards redressing the excess burden of cardiometabolic disease in severe mental illness. This chapter will provide the reader with a detailed understanding of the cardiometabolic risk present in people with severe mental illness. It will examine:

Section 18.2: Cardiometabolic diseases and obesity in severe mental illness.
- 1.1. Cardiovascular risk factors in mental illness
- 1.2. The trajectory of cardiovascular risk factors following antipsychotic medication initiation
- 1.3. Diabetes mellitus in severe mental illness
  - 1.3.1 Depression and diabetes mellitus
  - 1.3.2 Antidepressant medications and diabetes risk
  - 1.3.3 Psychotic illness and diabetes mellitus
- 1.4. Weight gain, obesity and antipsychotic medications

Section 18.3: Screening and early intervention strategies. Algorithms that promote early identification of people with increased cardiometabolic risk. Screening tools operationalised internationally will be presented.

18.2 Cardiometabolic Diseases and Obesity in Severe Mental Illness

In people with the severe mental illnesses of depression, schizophrenia and bipolar disease, an excess of cardiovascular disease mortality has been shown repeatedly and consistently by a number of epidemiological studies (Colton and Manderscheid 2006; Saha et al. 2007; Brown 1997; Surtees et al. 2008; Osby et al. 2000; Osborn et al. 2007; Angst et al. 2002; Brown et al. 2000; Capasso et al. 2008; Casey et al. 2004; Laursen et al. 2009; Lawrence et al. 2003). A large meta-analysis found the standardised mortality rate for cardiovascular disease of 1.79 in people with schizophrenia using data from 37 studies with approximately 23,000 deaths (Saha et al. 2007). An analysis of mortality in bipolar disease found similar results with a standardised coronary mortality rate of 1.61 after 34–38 years of follow-up (Angst et al. 2002). Data on people with depression are consistent, with sexual dimorphism evident: the standardised coronary mortality rate was 1.7 in women and 2.21 in men (Angst et al. 2002). A further study reported that myocardial infarction rates were 4.5-fold higher in men with depression (Pratt et al. 1996).

18.2.1 Cardiovascular Risk Factors in Mental Illness

Raised cardiovascular risk in people with depression and severe mental illness are, at least in part, driven by factors associated with their mental illness, including sedentariness (McDevitt et al. 2006; Lindamer et al. 2008; Faulkner and Cohn 2006; Brown et al. 1999; Daumit et al. 2005), high rates of smoking (Brown et al. 1999; de Leon and Diaz 2005; Compton et al. 2006 ; Goff et al. 2005) and poor diet (Brown et al. 1999; Casagrande et al. 2011). An additional factor is the effect of medications in promoting weight gain, with its consequent effects on a deteriorated cardiometabolic profile.

The lifestyle factors promoting a greater risk cardiometabolic risk are important to understand. A number are listed in Table 18.1.

The lifestyle behaviours manifested by people with severe mental illness include sedentariness and lower physical activity, which define risk for a great number of chronic diseases as well as physical health outcomes. For example, less than 30 % of adults with schizophrenia take part in regular physical activity compared to 62 % of those without schizophrenia (Lindamer et al. 2008). Further, less than 25 % of adults receiving antipsychotic medications meet the recommended 150 min of moderate intensity exercise per week (Faulkner and Cohn 2006). Extrinsic factors promoting sedentariness are similar to those shared with the rest of the community, such as lack of access to areas for exercise, perceptions of environmental danger and low physical activity literacy; however, some factors that are intrinsic to the mental illness may contribute, such as paranoia and social phobias, or its treatment (such as the sedating effects of some medications).

18.2.2 The Trajectory of Cardiovascular Risk Factors Following Antipsychotic Medication Initiation

Lifestyle factors aside, the published literature demonstrates rapid onset of metabolic disturbances induced within as short a period as 12 weeks after initiation of antipsychotic medications on blood lipids (Perez-Iglesias et al. 2007). Detrimental effects are seen on insulin resistance within the first year of treatment (Perez-Iglesias et al. 2009). Increases in insulin resistance are predicted by the gain in adiposity following initiation of antipsychotic medications (Haupt et al. 2007; Newcomer et al. 2009). Antipsychotics have also been shown to induce fasting and postprandial hyperinsulinaemia within 12 days and prior to any weight gain (Teff et al. 2013). Importantly, the latter study was conducted in volunteers without psychiatric disease, indicating that adverse metabolic effects are independent of mental illness.

Table 18.1 Contributors to cardiometabolic risk in people with severe mental illness

Factor	Mechanisms
Antipsychotic and antidepressant medications	• Increased appetite and lower satiety
	• Weight gain and induction of overweight/obesity
	• Hypertriglyceridemia
	• Hyperinsulinaemia
	• Hyperglycaemia
	• Sympathetic activation (antidepressants)
	• Sedation (antidepressants and antipsychotics)
Sedentary lifestyle	
Extrinsic to mental health:	Social exclusion and isolation
	• Lack of access to areas for physical activity
	• Perception of lack of safety
	• Low literacy on physical activity
Intrinsic to mental health and its treatment:	• Sedating effects of medication
	• Impaired and reduced motivation
	• Symptoms of psychosis (delusions and hallucinations limiting activity)
Poor nutrition	• Lower healthy eating literacy
	• Lower food preparation literacy
	• Restricted access to fresh food
	• Restricted access to cooking facilities
	• Impaired and reduced motivation (illness or medication)
	• Financial restraint/poverty
Smoking continuance	• Disparities in offering of smoking cessation
Disparities in health care access: primary care	• Financial restraint/poverty
	• Challenging waiting room environments
	• Challenges in engagement, bidirectional
	• Challenges in treatment: late presentation
	• Treatment discrimination (see below)
Disparities in health care access: specialist care	• Poverty/financial restraint
	• Difficulties in negotiating hospital systems
	• Challenging waiting room environments
	• Challenges in engagement, bidirectional
	• Challenges in treatment: late presentation
	• Treatment discrimination (see below)
Disparities in health care access: prevention and early intervention	• Poor engagement
	• Late presentation: lost opportunities
	• Few specific programs
	• Treatment discrimination (see below)
Disparities in receiving benchmark health services (Treatment discrimination)	• Entrenched clinician attitudes of hopelessness
	• Non-prescription when indicated
	• Fewer treatment-to-target medication changes

Higher rates of metabolic syndrome are also observed in a multitude of studies and reports (Correll et al. 2006, 2008; De Hert et al. 2006, 2008, 2009; Vancampfort et al. 2013; Patel et al. 2009; Fleischhacker et al. 2013; Meyer et al. 2008; Newcomer et al. 2004; Newcomer 2005, 2007). A large meta-analysis reported the rates of cardiometabolic abnormalities in people with medication-naïve first-episode psychosis and multi-episode psychosis, compared with rates in the general population (Vancampfort et al. 2013). Data from over 185,000 unique individuals with schizophrenia were analyzed, with general population control data from nearly 4,000,000 people. Rates of hypertension were similar in both first- and multi-episode psychosis (36 % and 41 %, respectively) and higher than that observed in the general population, with a calculated odds ratio of 1.36. Rates of hypertriglyceridaemia in multi-episode psychosis were substantially higher than that in first-episode psychosis (39 % compared to 11 %). The odds ratio for hypertriglyceridaemia in multi-episode psychosis was 2.73 compared to the general population. Rates of abnormally low HDL-cholesterol in first- and multi-episode psychosis were 16 % and 42 %, respectively. The odds ratio for abnormally low HDL-cholesterol in multi-episode psychosis was 2.35 compared to the general population (Vancampfort et al. 2013). These analyses represent a synthesis of data from 136 studies and support the findings from a plethora of studies indicating a deteriorated profile of modifiable cardiovascular risk factors.

In addition to the evidence for a more prevalent and early deterioration of traditional cardiovascular risk factors, there is also evidence that medication type influences cardiovascular end points in people with severe mental illness. Second-generation antipsychotic medications appear to load a greater risk on incident hypertension, hyperlipidaemia, heart disease and stroke, compared to antidepressant medications (Correll et al. 2015). In an analysis of health outcomes derived from a health-care claims database, data from over 284,000 people aged 18–65 years were examined. Over 31,000 had exposure to second-generation antipsychotic medications, and over 253,000 had exposure to antidepressant medications. Following adjustment for multiple important covariates, including sex, age and mental illness, the hazard ratios for people exposed to antipsychotics compared to antidepressants were 1.16 for hypertension, 117 for coronary artery disease, 1.34 for hypertensive heart disease and 1.46 for stroke (Correll et al. 2015). These data suggest that medication type adds a further factor to the determinants of cardiovascular and metabolic risk in people with severe mental illness.

The documented high rates of cardiometabolic risk factors in people with severe mental illness together with the evidence of premature death from cardiovascular disease have cemented international efforts for cardiovascular risk factor screening and intervention in people with severe mental illness. This will be discussed in detail in Sect. 18.3 of this chapter.

18.2.3 Diabetes Mellitus in Severe Mental Illness

Diabetes mellitus (diabetes) is a common condition of elevated glucose level development when the pancreas is unable to secrete sufficient insulin to meet needs. Insulin need is determined by an individual's insulin resistance and dietary intake. Insufficient insulin secretion can be absolute (ketosis-prone or type 1 diabetes) or relative (non-ketotic or type 2). Table 18.2 shows the international diagnostic cut-offs for a diagnosis of diabetes.

Type 1 diabetes mellitus is frequently due to autoimmune destruction of the insulin-secreting beta cells in the pancreas, but can also be due to pancreatic damage (recurrent pancreatitis, cystic fibrosis, trauma or surgery). The onset of type 1 diabetes mellitus is often in childhood or youth, but even the autoimmune form can occur in late adulthood (latent autoimmune diabetes of adulthood). Type 2 diabetes mellitus most frequently occurs in adulthood, has a strong genetic background and its time of onset is accelerated by lifestyle factors such as obesity and sedentariness. In the context of the global epidemic of obesity, type 2 diabetes mellitus is occurring in younger and younger people, even in childhood. Type 2 diabetes is often preceded by a 5–10-year prodrome of "prediabetes", which can be detected as impaired fasting glucose or impaired glucose tolerance (Table 18.2). If prediabetes is detected, a number of efficacious strategies can be undertaken to prevent progression to overt diabetes mellitus. Proven interventions that substantially reduce diabetes risk in people with prediabetes include modest weight reduction through caloric restriction and increased physical activity, with additional benefit demonstrated with concomitant treatment with the medication metformin (Knowler et al. 2002).

Diabetes carries an increased risk of macrovascular and microvascular complications. Both macrovascular and microvascular complications are often present at the time of type 2 diabetes diagnosis, indicating that the lipid, glycaemic and inflammatory disturbances present during the prodrome of diabetes adversely affect large and small calibre vascular health. The microvascular complications of hyperglycaemia include retinopathy, nephropathy and neuropathy. Further, high glucose levels

Table 18.2 International criteria for diagnosis of diabetes mellitus and other glucose disorders

	Fasting glucose[a]	2 h glucose[b]	Random glucose	HbA1c
Normal	WHO: <6.0 mmol/L ADA: <5.6 mmol/L			
Diabetes mellitus	>7.0 mmol/L >126 mg/dL	>11.1 mmol/L >200 mg/dL	>11.1 mmol/L >200 mg/dL with symptoms[c]	>6.5 %
Impaired fasting glucose	WHO: 6.0–6.9 mmol/L ADA: 5.6–6.9 mmol/L 100–125 mg/dL			
Impaired glucose tolerance		7.8–11.0 mmol/L 140–200 mg/dL		

[a]Fasting is defined as no caloric intake for at least 8 h
[b]Following a 75 g anhydrous glucose load dissolved in water
[c]Symptoms can includepolyuria, polydipsia or unexplained weight loss
HbA1c glycated haemoglobin
ADA American Diabetes Association
WHO World Health Organisation

impair cognition and mental functioning and cause fatigue. Diabetes is also associated with rates of depression, in a bidirectional relationship that is under intense investigation discussed below.

Diabetes is a challenging condition that requires daily attention. Diabetes care focuses on education for self-care and monitoring, careful eating to manage glucose levels and address obesity, medications for glucose control and cardiovascular risk reduction and complications screening. In this regard, people suffering from mental illness are those most vulnerable to poor outcomes from diabetes including complications, as capacity for self-care and health-seeking behaviours may be impaired, limited or constrained.

18.2.3.1 Diabetes and Depression

Depression frequently accompanies diabetes and vice versa. For example, studies of people attending a diabetes outpatient service have reported that about one third meet criteria for a subthreshold or a major depressive disorder (Fisher et al. 2008; Ali et al. 2006; Nouwen et al. 2010; Pouwer et al. 2010). Further, people with depression more frequently also have diabetes (Holt et al. 2009). This bidirectional relationship that has been observed between diabetes and depression has been under intense examination to determine whether one promotes the other or whether there are shared underlying mechanisms.

A number of risk factors are shared between diabetes and depression, including smoking, higher caloric intake and sedentariness (Strine et al. 2008). Depression is also characterised by a number of physiological disturbances which promote insulin resistance and diabetes risk. These include altered stress hormone physiology, including overactivation of the sympathetic system, the adrenal medulla and the hypothalamic-pituitary-adrenal axis, in addition to increased circulating pro-inflammatory cytokines (Golden 2007).

Synchronous diabetes and depression augur for worse outcomes. An increased mortality risk has been reported in people with both diabetes and depression (Katon et al. 2005). A number of factors appear to contribute to the observed increase in mortality risk; these include suboptimal diabetes management and self-care (Ciechanowski et al. 2000) in addition to greater financial health-care burden (Egede et al. 2002) contributing to worse sociodemographic determinants of health.

18.2.3.2 Antidepressant Medications and Diabetes Risk

In addition to the shared risk factors between depression and diabetes, antidepressant medications are implicated in diabetes risk. Medications currently used to treat depression fall into three pharmacological categories: tricyclic antidepressants, serotonin-selective reuptake inhibitors and noradrenaline-selective reuptake inhibitors (Table 18.3). The data suggest that all pharmacological classes of antidepressant medications are associated with weight gain and insulin resistance (Serretti and Mandelli 2010), which increase diabetes risk. The literature contains a large number of cross-sectional studies, case-controlled studies, prospective observational studies and subgroup comparisons of randomised intervention studies that support an association between antidepressant medications and diabetes (Andersohn et al. 2009;

Table 18.3 Medications used to management severe mental illness that can impact weight and cardiometabolic risk

Antipsychotics		Antidepressants		Mood stabilisers
First generation	Second generation	Tricyclics	SSRI/NSRI	
Haloperidol	Aripiprazole	Amitriptyline	Citalopram	*Anticonvulsants*
Chloropromazine	Clozapine	Amoxapine	Escitalopram	Sodium valproate
Perphenazine	Risperidone	Doxepin	Fluoxetine	Topiramate
Fluphenazine	Quetiapine	Imipramine	Paroxetine	Valproic acid
Thioridazine	Olanzapine	Nortriptyline	Sertaline	Lamotrigine
	Clozapine	Trimipramine	Venlafaxine	
	Amisulpride			*Others*
	Ziprasidone			Lithium carbonate

SSRI serotonin-selective re-uptake inhibitors
NSRI noradrenaline-selective re-uptake inhibitors

Barnard et al. 2013; Kivimaki et al. 2010; Pan et al. 2012; Pyykkonen et al. 2012; Raeder et al. 2006; Rubin et al. 2008, 2010). However, these studies do not establish causation (Barnard et al. 2013). Further, the majority of randomised controlled trials of antidepressants have actively excluded people with diabetes.

Cross-sectional studies showed an association between antidepressant use and elevated 2-h glucose levels, higher blood lipid levels, blood pressure and waist circumference (Pyykkonen et al. 2012) and a 40 % higher rate of diabetes in people receiving antidepressant medications (Raeder et al. 2006).

Considering the data in case-controlled studies, a number of studies have consistently shown that people receiving antidepressant medications have a doubling of diabetes risk. The UK General Practice Research Database has provided extremely useful data, showing that diabetes risk was increased by about 80 % in the 165,000 people treated with antidepressants, compared to healthy controls (Andersohn et al. 2009). An important aspect of this large study was that diabetes ascertainment was not by universal screening, but by recorded diabetes diagnosis, abnormal HbA1c or antidiabetic medication prescription. As is a common ascertainment limitation in many observational studies, universal fasting glucose or HbA1c levels were not evaluated. An interesting finding of this study was that diabetes risk was similar between the pharmacological classes or selective serotonin reuptake inhibitors and tricyclic antidepressants, and further, the risk of diabetes appeared to be mitigated by shorter duration of antidepressant exposure.

A further enlightening study in people with depression sought to determine what factors were associated with diabetes development, with careful matching of confounders including age, sex, sociodemographic and occupational status (Kivimaki et al. 2010). The study found that antidepressant use was associated with twofold increased risk of incident diabetes in those with milder forms of depression and a threefold diabetes risk increase in those with severe depression. In contrast, in people with depression who did not receive antidepressant therapy, the risk of incident diabetes was only increased by 20 % (Kivimaki et al. 2010).

The largest prospective observational study to date is represented by pooled data from the Nurses' Health Study I, Nurses' Health Study II and the Health Professionals Study, with follow-up of in excess of 1.6 million person-years (Pan et al. 2012). It was found that the incident diabetes risk was almost tripled in women receiving antidepressant medications but that risk estimates were reduced after adjusting for traditional diabetes risk factors of BMI, lipids and hypertension (Pan et al. 2012).

Diabetes prevention interventions have also provided interesting data that add to the concerns that antidepressant medication increase diabetes risk. The Diabetes Prevention Program was a large-scale intervention that randomised people with prediabetes to either intensive lifestyle intervention (dietary change, increased physical activity and modest weight loss) with and without metformin, standard lifestyle intervention with and without metformin or metformin alone. The Program showed that intensive lifestyle intervention reduced the risk of progression of prediabetes to overt diabetes by approximately 50 % (Knowler et al. 2002). The addition of metformin to intensive lifestyle intervention augmented diabetes prevention (Knowler et al. 2002). The wealth of data collected in the Diabetes Prevention Program has since been interrogated to examine whether antidepressant therapy affected incident diabetes rates within the randomisation framework (Rubin et al. 2008). Only participants with mild depression were included in the Program. Those taking antidepressant medications and randomised to lifestyle intervention alone (either intensive or standard) had incident diabetes rates that were two- to fourfold higher than participants in the same intervention group who were not receiving antidepressants. However, participants taking antidepressant medications who were randomised to any metformin-containing intervention arm had similar incident diabetes risk to those not taking antidepressants (Rubin et al. 2008). These data support that metformin blunts the diabetes risk increase that has been observed with antidepressants medications. Further, these data suggest the diabetes risk associated with antidepressants is not blunted by lifestyle measures alone.

Ten-year follow-up data are also available from the Diabetes Prevention Program, with 82 % of the original cohort re-examined. Analyses showed that continuous antidepressant medication use was associated with a more than doubling of incident diabetes risk in participants on lifestyle intervention alone, with diabetes risk reduced by metformin (Rubin et al. 2010). These very interesting data cannot be extrapolated to people with severe depression, since they were actively excluded from the Diabetes Prevention Trial.

18.2.3.3 Psychotic Illness and Diabetes Mellitus

A number of studies have documented people receiving antipsychotic medications have a two- to fivefold higher risk of incident diabetes (Gianfrancesco et al. 2003; Kessing et al. 2010; Lambert et al. 2006; Nielsen et al. 2010; Ramaswamy et al. 2006; Smith et al. 2008; Yood et al. 2009; Bobo et al. 2013). In examining the published literature, it is important to recall that the standard risk factors for diabetes include obesity, family history, sedentariness and an energy dense diet. Thus, any risk estimate of diabetes in severe mental illness treated with antipsychotic medications needs to be considered for covariates included in the analyses. The literature on antipsychotic medications and weight gain is reviewed below.

Diabetes diagnosis relies on testing fasting glucose levels, glucose levels following an oral glucose load or, more recently, testing of glycated haemoglobin (HbA1c). The diagnostic cut-offs used internationally are summarised in Table 18.2. A challenge in interpreting the published literature that describes diabetes risk in severe mental illness is ascertainment. For example, most studies have not screened all participants, relying on self-report or reported use of antidiabetic medications. This may miss people with undiagnosed diabetes. Further, most studies testing glucose levels have not performed glucose tolerance tests. The use of glycated haemoglobin has only recently been promulgated and has the advantage of not relying on fasting. A further challenge is the adequacy of the control group, which may in itself have a higher diabetes risk.

In examining the literature, generational differences are evident between antipsychotic medications, with second-generation antipsychotic medications consistently showing higher risk for diabetes. For example, the risk of diabetes with second-generation medications was 1.3, compared to first-generation medications (Smith et al. 2008). Studies have also identified specific antipsychotic medications as promoting greater diabetes risk. For example, clozapine has been found to be associated with the highest risk for diabetes, with relative risk of diabetes of 1.45 (compared to the general population) (Kessing et al. 2010). Olanzapine and risperidone also increase diabetes risk (1.29- and 1.23-fold, respectively) (Kessing et al. 2010). By contrast, aripiprazole, amisulpride and quetiapine use was associated with diabetes risk that was similar to normal population (Kessing et al. 2010).

Systematic review of 22 RCTs of different APM against placebo suggest no particular agent promoted diabetes incidence; however, most trials were of short duration. In contrast, post-marketing data from the Federal Drugs Administration has demonstrated diabetes-related adverse outcome reporting ratios that are substantially higher for olanzapine (ORR, 9.6), risperidone (ORR, 3.8), quetiapine (ORR, 3.5), clozapine (ORR, 3.1), ziprasidone (ORR, 2.4), aripiprazole (ORR, 2.4) and haloperidol (ORR, 2.0) (Baker et al. 2009). Post-marketing reporting biases are acknowledged, however, along with confounding by preferentially prescribing "low-risk" agents to people considered at "high-risk" of diabetes.

In this regard, studies of glucose levels following antipsychotic initiation in first-episode psychosis are helpful in overcoming the challenges of prescribing biases and past medication exposures. A large study of 7,139 people with first-episode psychosis from the Danish Psychiatric Central Research Registry reported greater rates of diabetes with olanzapine and clozapine, following a mean of 6.6 years (Nielsen et al. 2010). Diabetes ascertainment was by attendance to a diabetes clinic or initiation of antidiabetic medication. Controls were registry participants without diabetes. The risk of incident diabetes within the first year of exposure was 1.41 for olanzapine and 1.6 for first-generation antipsychotic medications (periciazine, perphenazine, prochlorperazine and zuclopenthixol), compared to registry participants not taking these medications (Nielsen et al. 2010). The risk of diabetes within 3 months of antipsychotic medication initiation was 1.44 for olanzapine and 1.67 for clozapine (Nielsen et al. 2010).

Further, the literature supports greater risk of diabetes in younger antipsychotic medication recipients. For example, the risk of diabetes in youth <24 years of age treated with antipsychotic medication is increased 8.9-fold, compared to children and youth not receiving these medications (Hammerman et al. 2008). A second study of children and youth receiving antipsychotic medications for a range of disorders reported a threefold higher diabetes incidence, compared to age-matched controls receiving other psychotropic medications (mostly antidepressant medications) (Bobo et al. 2013). The study included large numbers of children and youth treated with antipsychotic medications for nonpsychotic illnesses, including behavioural disorders. This study also found that the onset of diabetes was rapid, within 12 months of antipsychotic medication initiation (Bobo et al. 2013). Importantly, as antidepressant medications also associated with increased diabetes risk, estimates of the risk of diabetes were likely to be underestimated (Samaras et al. 2014). Further, ascertainment relied on insurance records of antidiabetic medications. Routine glucose screening was not undertaken and symptomatic presentation prompted diabetes diagnosis. It is relevant to consider that symptomatic presentation of diabetes occurs when the renal glucose threshold is surpassed, producing polyuria and thirst. In children and youth, the renal threshold is crossed at glucose levels exceeding 17–18 mmol/L. Without universal glucose screening, the real incidence of diabetes was likely to have been underestimated due to undiagnosed cases (Samaras et al. 2014).

In summary, the risk of diabetes is increased in people with depression, severe mental illness and recipients of antidepressant and antipsychotic medications. The elevated risk of premature-onset diabetes in people with depression and severe mental illness requires regular glucose screening. Glucose screening in all recipients of psychotropic and antipsychotic medication is now part of international initiatives to improve physical health in people with severe mental illness (De Hert et al. 2011a, 2012; Curtis et al. 2012; Pringsheim et al. 2011b).

18.2.4 Weight Gain and Antipsychotic Medications

A body of epidemiological evidence shows that people with severe mental illness have higher risk of obesity, with the risk of obesity (body mass index >30 kg/m^2) estimated at 2.8–3.5 higher than the general population for schizophrenia (De Hert et al. 2011b) and 1.2–1.5 times higher in bipolar disorder (Maina et al. 2008).

All antipsychotic medications can cause weight gain. Whilst first- and second-generation antipsychotic medications differ for their potential to induce severe motor complications, both classes appear to be for capacity to produce weight gain and metabolic risk. Rates of obesity in youth receiving antipsychotics are alarming, with overweight and obese rates 55 % in males and 42 % in females in a first-episode psychosis youth cohort after a median of 8 months of antipsychotic medication (Curtis et al. 2011b). Body mass index was directly related to the length of medication exposure (Curtis et al. 2011b).

Longitudinal controlled studies that report metabolic outcomes in treatment-naïve patients with first-episode psychosis following antipsychotic initiation show that substantial weight gain occurs in the majority of patients rapidly. Table 18.4 shows the weight gain by antipsychotic medication and observation duration in a number of prospective observational studies, with the majority of studies performed in antipsychotic-naïve patients. All studies consistently showed weight gain over the observation period, which varied from 11 to 104 weeks (Table 18.4). For example, a study of 272 antipsychotic-naïve youth showed significant weight gain over approximately 11 weeks for all four antipsychotic medications studied: aripiprazole, olanzapine, quetiapine and risperidone (Correll et al. 2009). Weight gain ranged from 4.4 kg (3.7–5.2) on aripiprazole to 8.5 kg (7.4–9.7) on olanzapine, significantly higher than the 0.2-kg weight gained in the control group (Correll et al. 2009).

Significant and rapid weight gain was reported in a further study of 400 treatment-naïve participants in the 12 weeks after antipsychotic medication initiation: of 3.9 kg with risperidone, 3.6 kg with quetiapine and 7.1 kg with olanzapine (Patel et al. 2009). Another large study of treatment-naïve people with first-episode psychosis reported high rates of clinically adverse weight gain (>7 %) from baseline weight by 12 months: in 86 % of olanzapine recipients, 65 % of quetiapine recipients, 53 % of haloperidol recipients and 37 % of all ziprasidone recipients (Kahn et al. 2008).

A systematic critical appraisal of the published literature of studies in people with first-episode psychosis and chronic psychotic disorders showed that the rapidity and degree of weight gain was inversely related with disease chronicity, evaluating weight observations made in randomised controlled trials (Alvarez-Jimenez et al. 2008). The weight gain occurring within 12–24 months following medication initiation in first-episode psychosis ranged 10.2–15.4 kg with olanzapine, 6.6–8.9 with risperidone and 4.0–9.7 kg with haloperidol (Alvarez-Jimenez et al. 2008). In contrast, the weight gain observed with the same medications over 12–18 months was substantially less in patients chronically treated with these medications: 2.0–6.2 kg with olanzapine, 0.4–3.9 kg with risperidone and −0.7 to 0.4 kg with haloperidol (Alvarez-Jimenez et al. 2008). In considering these data, it is important to note that chronic patients started their weight trajectory at a higher weight than treatment-naïve patients. The same study showed that clinically significant weight gain was found in up to 60 % of treatment-naïve individuals in the first 10–16 weeks of treatment, increasing to 60–100 % after 1–2 years of antipsychotic medication exposure (Alvarez-Jimenez et al. 2008).

The European First-Episode Schizophrenia Trial (EUFEST) randomised young people with first-episode psychosis to amisulpride, haloperidol, olanzapine, quetiapine or ziprasidone (Fleischhacker et al. 2013). A large proportion of participants (67 %) had prior but only short-term antipsychotic medication exposure. At 52 weeks, the average weight gains observed in increasing order were: ziprasidone 2.5 kg, haloperidol 6.4 kg, quetiapine 7.1 kg, amisulpride 7.7 kg and olanzapine 11.2 kg (Fleischhacker et al. 2013). Of concern, rapid weight gain is also observed in treatment-naïve paediatric populations (Correll et al. 2009; Sikich et al. 2008). Greater metabolic disturbances including weight gain and hyperglycaemia are observed with clozapine and olanzapine (Gohlke et al. 2012; Rummel-Kluge et al. 2010).

The effects of obesity on seeding future diseases is well known, particularly where its onset is in relative youth – for dyslipidaemia, dysglycaemia and hypertension (Weiss et al. 2004). Early onset obesity predicts adult coronary artery disease. The early and adverse effects of these medications on weight, obesity, lipids and

Table 18.4 Prospective observational studies of weight gain following initiation of antipsychotic medications in treatment-naïve patients with severe mental illness

Medication	Authors	Year	Number	Age (years)	Observation length (weeks)	Weight gain (kg)	
						Medication	Control
Amisulpride							
	Fleischhacker et al.[a]	2013	55/498	26	26	6.5	-
	Fleischhacker et al. [a]	2013	48/498	26	52	7.7	-
Aripiprazole							
	Correll et al.	2009	41/272	14	11	4.4	0.2
Haloperidol							
	Kahn	2008					
	Fleischhacker et al. [a]	2013	34/498	26	26	5.0	-
	Fleischhacker et al. [a]	2013	22/498	26	52	6.4	-
Olanzapine							
	Correll et al.	2009	45/272	14	11	8.5	0.2
	Patel et al.	2009	400		12	7.1	-
	Patel et al.	2009	400		52	11.0	-
	Fleischhacker et al. [a]	2013	69/498	26	26	9.6	-
	Fleischhacker et al. [a]	2013	59/498	26	52	11.2	-

Quetiapine							
	Correll et al.	2009	36/272	14	11	6.1	0.2
	Patel et al.	2009	400		12	3.6	-
	Patel et al.	2009	400		52	5.5	-
	Fleischhacker et al. [a]	2013	45/498	26	26	6.6	-
	Fleischhacker et al. [a]	2013	40/498	26	52	7.1	-
Risperidone							
	Correll et al.	2009	135/272	14	11	5.3	0.2
	Patel et al.	2009	400		12	3.9	-
	Patel et al.	2009	400		52	6.4	-
Ziprasidone							
	Fleischhacker et al. [a]	2013	35/498	26	26	1.9	
	Fleischhacker et al. [a]	2013	31/498	26	52	2.5	

[a] partially medication-naïve: 67 % had past antipsychotic exposure

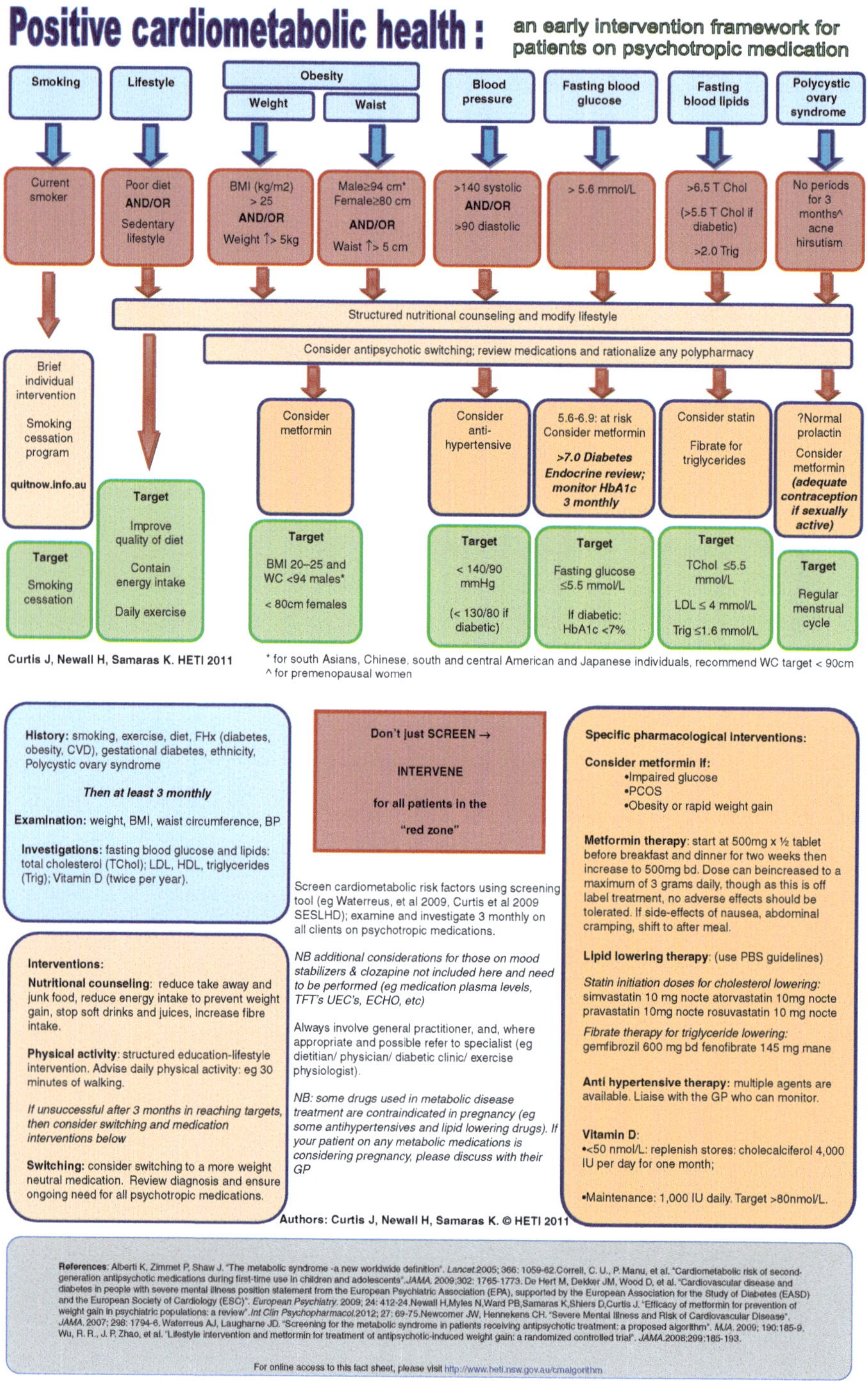

Fig. 18.1 Positive cardiometabolic health. An early intervention framework. "Don't Just Screen, Intervene"

insulin metabolism are major contributors to the seeding of diseases such as cardiovascular disease, diabetes and possibly future cancer.

18.3 Screening for Cardiometabolic Disease in People with Severe Mental Illness

The high prevalence of modifiable cardiometabolic risk factors in people with severe mental illness is driven by weight gain, but also to lack of screening and under-treatment. The key to reducing cardiometabolic complications in people with mental illness relies on the prevention or attenuation of weight gain and, most importantly, screening and intervention. Numerous authors and national bodies have recommended screening for early identification of modifiable cardiometabolic risk in people with severe mental illness (De Hert et al. 2009, 2011a, b; Curtis et al. 2012; Pringsheim et al. 2011a, b; Crawford et al. 2014; American Diabetes Association, American Psychiatric Association, American Association of Clinical Endocrinologists, North American Association for the Study of Obesity 2004).

A review of the published literature demonstrates considerable variation in the rates of cardiometabolic screening in people with severe mental illness (Mitchell et al. 2012; Baller et al. 2015). One study examined cardiometabolic screening rates that were substantially and consistently below the standard of the American Diabetes Association/American Psychiatric Association/American Association of Clinical Endocrinologists/North American Association for the Study of Obesity (Baller et al. 2015). The recommendations of this consensus group are summarised in Table 18.5 (American Diabetes Association, American Psychiatric Association, American Association of Clinical Endocrinologists, North American Association for the Study of Obesity 2004). For example, rates of any glucose screening ranged 18–28 % (Morrato et al. 2008, 2009; Moeller et al. 2011; Barnett et al. 2010) and lipids 6–39 % (Morrato et al. 2008; Moeller et al. 2011; Barnett et al. 2010). Health setting appears to influence screening rates. For example, high screening rates are evident from the (United States of America) Veterans Health System (Kilbourne et al. 2011). In contrast, extremely low rates of metabolic screening have been documented in resource poor settings, where rates for complete screening across weight, blood pressure, glucose and lipids were only 0.6 % (Saloojee et al. 2014). Screening rates in people with severe mental illness have also been found to be substantially lower to that in other high cardiovascular risk patients. In a large national audit that compared risk factor screening in over 422,000 people with severe mental illness and nearly 2.5 million people with diabetes, screening rates for obesity, hypertension, blood glucose and lipids were 75 % in severe mental illness and 97 % in diabetes (Mitchell and Hardy 2013). In considering these screening rates, it is important to consider that provision of screening in these conditions is incentivized by payment in the United Kingdom's primary health-care system.

The introduction of cardiometabolic risk screening guidelines appears to have influenced screening rates for some factors. For example, the rate of glucose screening increased by 15 % following the introduction of guidelines; however, there were insufficient data on other risk factors (Mitchell et al. 2012).

18.3.1 Cardiometabolic Screening Tools and Clinical Algorithms

A number of clinical algorithms, essentially workplace tools, are available to guide clinicians and mental health-care workers in cardiometabolic screening in people with severe mental illness (Curtis et al. 2011a, 2012, 2014; Pringsheim et al. 2011b; American Diabetes Association, American Psychiatric Association, American Association of Clinical Endocrinologists, North American Association for the Study of Obesity 2004; National Institute for Health and Clinical Excellence n.d.). These are summarised in Table 18.5 and serve as trigger points not only for standardised screening in people with severe mental illness but also for intervention with defined treatment targets for optimising cardiovascular and diabetes outcomes (Curtis et al. 2012; National Institute for Health and Clinical Excellence n.d.). Examples are seen in the Australian tool "Don't just Screen, Intervene" (Curtis et al. 2011a) (Fig. 18.1) and its UK (National Institute for Health and Clinical Excellence n.d.) and adolescent adaptations (Curtis et al. 2014). These practical resources can be downloaded from the internet (National Institute for Health and Clinical Excellence n.d.; Curtis et al. 2011a, 2014). These clinical algorithms contain prompts on screening method and its frequency and thresholds for intervention and suggest appropriate interventions and evidence-based treatment targets. The adolescent algorithm contains links to national and international databases for age-specific thresholds for weight, body mass index, blood pressure and blood parameters (Curtis et al. 2014).

18.3.2 Successful Interventions for Obesity and Cardiometabolic Risk

Weight loss interventions applied to the setting of severe mental illness have been shown to be efficacious, just as in the general population. For example, a tailored behavioural intervention with weight management counselling and group exercise for 18 months significantly reduced weight in obese people with schizophrenia or bipolar disorder (Daumit et al. 2013). Weight loss was initially slower than that observed in such interventions in the general population, but continued steadily over the study duration with less plateau than observed in general. Further, the weight loss achieved was similar to that observed in the general population. A second study compared the effects of a weight loss intervention in obese people with psychotic illness against people without psychiatric disease, with greater weight loss success in those with psychotic illness (Zhang et al. 2012). Other weight loss interventions in patients with severe mental illness have been limited to less than 6-month duration

Table 18.5 Recommendations for cardiometabolic screening in people with severe mental illness from the published literature

Authors	Year	Weight and/or waist	Glucose	Lipids	Blood pressure	Other
ADA/APA/AACE/ NAASO[a][91]	2004	At APM initiation Then at 1,2,3 months Then every 3 months	At APM initiation Then at 3 months after any new APM	At APM initiation Then at 3 months Then every 5 years	At APM initiation Then at 3 months Then annually	
New South Wales Health (Australia) Curtis et al[103]	2012	At APM initiation Then every 3 months	At APM initiation Then every 3 months	At APM initiation Then every 3 months	At APM initiation Then every 3 months	Smoking abstinence: every 3 months Diet: every 3 months Sedentariness: every 3 months Polycystic ovary syndrome
National Institute for Health and Clinical Excellence (UK) [102]	2014	At APM initiation 1–2 weekly in first 8 weeks of a new APM Then every 3 months	At APM initiation Then every 3 months	At APM initiation Then every 3 months	At APM initiation Then every 3 months	Prompts for considering APM change with defined metabolic decline or rapid weight gain
The Canadian Alliance for Monitoring Effectiveness and Safety of Antipsychotics in Children[92]	2011	At APM initiation Then at 1,2,3,6,9,12 months	At APM initiation Then at 1,3,6,12 months	At APM initiation Then at 1,3,6,12 months	At APM initiation Then at 1,2,3,6,9,12 months	Child-specific
New South Wales Health (Australia) Curtis et al[104]	2014	At APM initiation 1–2 weekly in first 8 weeks of a new APM Then every 3 months	At APM initiation Then at 1,3,6,12 months	At APM initiation Then at 1,3,6,12 months	At APM initiation Then at 1,3,6,12 months	Adolescent-specific Smoking abstinence: every 3 months Diet: every 3 months Sedentariness: every 3 months Polycystic ovary syndrome

[a]American Diabetes Association/American Psychiatric Association/American Association of Clinical Endocrinologists/North American Association for the Study of Obesity

APM antipsychotic medication

(Zhang et al. 2012; Cabassa et al. 2010; Daumit et al. 2011; Faulkner et al. 2007; McKibbin et al. 2006; Verhaeghe et al. 2011; Wu et al. 2008b; Curtis et al. 2015).

Importantly, a recent study showed that the weight gain that occurs at antipsychotic medication initiation in first-episode psychosis can be prevented by a structured and individualised lifestyle intervention (Curtis et al. 2015). Rises in cardiometabolic risk factors were prevented (Curtis et al. 2015). In concert with the studies above, it is clear that lifestyle interventions can improve or prevent obesity in people with severe mental illness.

Further, lifestyle interventions with metformin have demonstrated both weight and cardiometabolic benefits. A randomised controlled trial of metformin at antipsychotic medication initiation showed a 4 kg lesser weight gain in the metformin-treated arm, compared to placebo (Wu et al. 2008b). Metformin plus lifestyle intervention appear to have additive benefits. In a randomised controlled trial of participants with schizophrenia receiving long-term antipsychotic medications, placebo was associated with 2.4–3.8-kg weight gain over 12 weeks, participants randomised to metformin lost 2.5–3.9 kg, and participants randomised to metformin plus lifestyle lost 3.4–5.7 kg (Wu et al. 2008a). A systematic review of the studies of metformin in psychiatric cohorts to manage obesity ad cardiometabolic risk found strong evidence of benefit (Newall et al. 2012).

Thus, it appears that lifestyle intervention should be implemented in all individuals receiving antipsychotic therapy as a standard of care. This is mandated in several of the clinical algorithms for cardiometabolic screening (National Institute for Health and Clinical Excellence n.d.; Curtis et al. 2011a, 2014). Lifestyle intervention at the time of psychotropic medication initiation appears imperative in preventing cardiometabolic risk in this high-risk group.

Conclusion

People with severe mental illnesses such as depression and diabetes have shortened life expectancy through premature cardiovascular disease and diabetes. There are a number of screening and intervention opportunities which will improve access to appropriate treatment of modifiable cardiovascular and diabetes risk factors.

Appropriate cardiometabolic screening and intervention will start addressing the conditions that result in premature loss of life in this population and redress the inequalities in physical health care, morbidity and mortality that exist. A number of thematically similar cardiometabolic screening algorithms are in use internationally and can be used to guide appropriate screening and intervention to maintain or improve modifiable cardiometabolic risk factors in people with severe mental illness.

Engagement of the diverse and specialised skill sets in the different professions that serve people with severe mental illness, with collaboration between and within specialities, education of the wider workforce, enthusiasm and commitment can improve the physical health and outcomes of people with severe mental illness – an obligation as a matter of health equity and social justice.

Disclosures No conflicts of interest to declare.

References

Ali S, Stone MA, Peters JL, Davies MJ, Khunti K (2006) The prevalence of co-morbid depression in adults with type 2 diabetes: a systematic review and meta-analysis. Diabet Med 23(11):1165–1173

Alvarez-Jimenez M, Gonzalez-Blanch C, Crespo-Facorro B, Hetrick S, Rodriguez-Sanchez JM, Perez-Iglesias R et al (2008) Antipsychotic-induced weight gain in chronic and first-episode psychotic disorders: a systematic critical reappraisal. CNS Drugs 22(7):547–562

American Diabetes Association, American Psychiatric Association, American Association of Clinical Endocrinologists, North American Association for the Study of Obesity (2004) Consensus development conference on antipsychotic drugs and obesity and diabetes. Diabetes Care 27(2):596–601

Andersohn F, Schade R, Suissa S, Garbe E (2009) Long-term use of antidepressants for depressive disorders and the risk of diabetes mellitus. Am J Psychiatry 166(5):591–598

Angst F, Stassen HH, Clayton PJ, Angst J (2002) Mortality of patients with mood disorders: follow-up over 34–38 years. J Affect Disord 68(2–3):167–181

Baker RA, Pikalov A, Tran QV, Kremenets T, Arani RB, Doraiswamy PM (2009) Atypical antipsychotic drugs and diabetes mellitus in the US Food and Drug Administration Adverse Event database: a systematic Bayesian signal detection analysis. Psychopharmacol Bull 42(1):11–31

Baller JB, McGinty EE, Azrin ST, Juliano-Bult D, Daumit GL (2015) Screening for cardiovascular risk factors in adults with serious mental illness: a review of the evidence. BMC Psychiatry 15:55, Pubmed Central PMCID: 4376086

Barnard K, Peveler RC, Holt RI (2013) Antidepressant medication as a risk factor for type 2 diabetes and impaired glucose regulation: systematic review. Diabetes Care 36(10):3337–3345, Pubmed Central PMCID: 3781547

Barnett M, VonMuenster S, Wehring H, Popish S, McDonald K, Walker VM et al (2010) Assessment of monitoring for glucose and lipid dysregulation in adult Medi-Cal patients newly started on antipsychotics. Ann Clin Psychiatry 22(1):9–18

Bobo WV, Cooper WO, Stein CM, Olfson M, Graham D, Daugherty J et al (2013) Antipsychotics and the risk of type 2 diabetes mellitus in children and youth. JAMA Psychiatry 70(10): 1067–1075

Brown S (1997) Excess mortality of schizophrenia. A meta-analysis. Br J Psychiatry 171:502–508

Brown S, Birtwistle J, Roe L, Thompson C (1999) The unhealthy lifestyle of people with schizophrenia. Psychol Med 29(3):697–701

Brown S, Inskip H, Barraclough B (2000) Causes of the excess mortality of schizophrenia. Br J Psychiatry 177:212–217

Brown S, Kim M, Mitchell C, Inskip H (2010) Twenty-five year mortality of a community cohort with schizophrenia. Br J Psychiatry 196(2):116–121

Cabassa LJ, Ezell JM, Lewis-Fernandez R (2010) Lifestyle interventions for adults with serious mental illness: a systematic literature review. Psychiatr Serv 61(8):774–782, Pubmed Central PMCID: 3632414

Capasso RM, Lineberry TW, Bostwick JM, Decker PA, St Sauver J (2008) Mortality in schizophrenia and schizoaffective disorder: an Olmsted County, Minnesota cohort: 1950–2005. Schizophr Res 98(1–3):287–294

Casagrande SS, Anderson CA, Dalcin A, Appel LJ, Jerome GJ, Dickerson FB et al (2011) Dietary intake of adults with serious mental illness. Psychiatr Rehabil J 35(2):137–140

Casey DE, Haupt DW, Newcomer JW, Henderson DC, Sernyak MJ, Davidson M et al (2004) Antipsychotic-induced weight gain and metabolic abnormalities: implications for increased mortality in patients with schizophrenia. J Clin Psychiatry 65(Suppl 7):4–18, quiz 9–20

Ciechanowski PS, Katon WJ, Russo JE (2000) Depression and diabetes: impact of depressive symptoms on adherence, function, and costs. Arch Intern Med 160(21):3278–3285

Colton CW, Manderscheid RW (2006) Congruencies in increased mortality rates, years of potential life lost, and causes of death among public mental health clients in eight states. Prev Chronic Dis 3(2):A42, Pubmed Central PMCID: 1563985

Compton MT, Daumit GL, Druss BG (2006) Cigarette smoking and overweight/obesity among individuals with serious mental illnesses: a preventive perspective. Harv Rev Psychiatry 14(4):212–222

Correll CU, Frederickson AM, Kane JM, Manu P (2006) Metabolic syndrome and the risk of coronary heart disease in 367 patients treated with second-generation antipsychotic drugs. J Clin Psychiatry 67(4):575–583

Correll CU, Frederickson AM, Kane JM, Manu P (2008) Equally increased risk for metabolic syndrome in patients with bipolar disorder and schizophrenia treated with second-generation antipsychotics. Bipolar Disord 10(7):788–797

Correll CU, Manu P, Olshanskiy V, Napolitano B, Kane JM, Malhotra AK (2009) Cardiometabolic risk of second-generation antipsychotic medications during first-time use in children and adolescents. JAMA 302(16):1765–1773, Pubmed Central PMCID: 3055794

Correll CU, Joffe BI, Rosen LM, Sullivan TB, Joffe RT (2015) Cardiovascular and cerebrovascular risk factors and events associated with second-generation antipsychotic compared to antidepressant use in a non-elderly adult sample: results from a claims-based inception cohort study. World Psychiatry 14(1):56–63, Pubmed Central PMCID: 4329898

Crawford MJ, Jayakumar S, Lemmey SJ, Zalewska K, Patel MX, Cooper SJ et al (2014) Assessment and treatment of physical health problems among people with schizophrenia: national cross-sectional study. Br J Psychiatry 205(6):473–477

Curtis J, Newall H, Samaras K. New South Wales Health (NSW Government) (2011) Positive Cardiometabolic Health; an early intervention framework for patients on psychotropic medication. www.heti.nsw.gov.au/resources-library/positive-cardio-metabolic-algorithm-2011/

Curtis J, Henry C, Watkins A, Newall H, Samaras K, Ward PB (2011b) Metabolic abnormalities in an early psychosis service: a retrospective, naturalistic cross-sectional study. Early Interv Psychiatry 5(2):108–114

Curtis J, Newall HD, Samaras K (2012) The heart of the matter: cardiometabolic care in youth with psychosis. Early Interv Psychiatry 6(3):347–353

Curtis J, Newall H, Samaras K. New South Wales Health (NSW Government) (2014) Adolescent version: positive cardiometabolic health. www.heti.nsw.gov.au/adolescentcmalgorithm

Curtis J, Watkins A, Rosenbaum S, Teasdale S, Kalucy M, Samaras K et al (2016) Evaluating an individualized lifestyle and life skills intervention to prevent antipsychotic-induced weight gain in first-episode psychosis. Early Interv Psychiatry 10:267–276

Daumit GL, Goldberg RW, Anthony C, Dickerson F, Brown CH, Kreyenbuhl J et al (2005) Physical activity patterns in adults with severe mental illness. J Nerv Ment Dis 193(10):641–646

Daumit GL, Dalcin AT, Jerome GJ, Young DR, Charleston J, Crum RM et al (2011) A behavioral weight-loss intervention for persons with serious mental illness in psychiatric rehabilitation centers. Int J Obes (Lond) 35(8):1114–1123, Pubmed Central PMCID: 3409245

Daumit GL, Dickerson FB, Wang NY, Dalcin A, Jerome GJ, Anderson CA et al (2013) A behavioral weight-loss intervention in persons with serious mental illness. N Engl J Med 368(17):1594–1602, Pubmed Central PMCID: 3743095

De Hert M, van Winkel R, Van Eyck D, Hanssens L, Wampers M, Scheen A et al (2006) Prevalence of diabetes, metabolic syndrome and metabolic abnormalities in schizophrenia over the course of the illness: a cross-sectional study. Clin Pract Epidemiol Ment Health 2:14, Pubmed Central PMCID: 1533826

De Hert M, Schreurs V, Sweers K, Van Eyck D, Hanssens L, Sinko S et al (2008) Typical and atypical antipsychotics differentially affect long-term incidence rates of the metabolic syndrome in first-episode patients with schizophrenia: a retrospective chart review. Schizophr Res 101(1–3):295–303

De Hert M, Dekker JM, Wood D, Kahl KG, Holt RI, Moller HJ (2009) Cardiovascular disease and diabetes in people with severe mental illness position statement from the European Psychiatric Association (EPA), supported by the European Association for the Study of Diabetes (EASD) and the European Society of Cardiology (ESC). Eur Psychiatry 24(6):412–424

De Hert M, Vancampfort D, Correll CU, Mercken V, Peuskens J, Sweers K et al (2011a) Guidelines for screening and monitoring of cardiometabolic risk in schizophrenia: systematic evaluation. Br J Psychiatry 199(2):99–105

De Hert M, Correll CU, Bobes J, Cetkovich-Bakmas M, Cohen D, Asai I et al (2011b) Physical illness in patients with severe mental disorders. I. Prevalence, impact of medications and disparities in health care. World Psychiatry 10(1):52–77, Pubmed Central PMCID: 3048500

De Hert M, Detraux J, van Winkel R, Yu W, Correll CU (2012) Metabolic and cardiovascular adverse effects associated with antipsychotic drugs. Nat Rev Endocrinol 8(2):114–126

de Leon J, Diaz FJ (2005) A meta-analysis of worldwide studies demonstrates an association between schizophrenia and tobacco smoking behaviors. Schizophr Res 76(2–3):135–157

Egede LE, Zheng D, Simpson K (2002) Comorbid depression is associated with increased health care use and expenditures in individuals with diabetes. Diabetes Care 25(3):464–470

Faulkner G, Cohn TA (2006) Pharmacologic and nonpharmacologic strategies for weight gain and metabolic disturbance in patients treated with antipsychotic medications. Can J Psychiatry 51(8):502–511

Faulkner G, Cohn T, Remington G (2007) Interventions to reduce weight gain in schizophrenia. Schizophr Bull 33(3):654–656, Pubmed Central PMCID: 2526141

Fisher L, Skaff MM, Mullan JT, Arean P, Glasgow R, Masharani U (2008) A longitudinal study of affective and anxiety disorders, depressive affect and diabetes distress in adults with Type 2 diabetes. Diabet Med 25(9):1096–1101, Pubmed Central PMCID: 2635496

Fleischhacker WW, Siu CO, Boden R, Pappadopulos E, Karayal ON, Kahn RS et al (2013) Metabolic risk factors in first-episode schizophrenia: baseline prevalence and course analysed from the European First-Episode Schizophrenia Trial. Int J Neuropsychopharmacol 16(5):987–995

Gianfrancesco F, Grogg A, Mahmoud R, Wang RH, Meletiche D (2003) Differential effects of antipsychotic agents on the risk of development of type 2 diabetes mellitus in patients with mood disorders. Clin Ther 25(4):1150–1171

Goff DC, Sullivan LM, McEvoy JP, Meyer JM, Nasrallah HA, Daumit GL et al (2005) A comparison of ten-year cardiac risk estimates in schizophrenia patients from the CATIE study and matched controls. Schizophr Res 80(1):45–53

Gohlke JM, Dhurandhar EJ, Correll CU, Morrato EH, Newcomer JW, Remington G et al (2012) Recent advances in understanding and mitigating adipogenic and metabolic effects of antipsychotic drugs. Front Psychiatry 3:62, Pubmed Central PMCID: 3385013

Golden SH (2007) A review of the evidence for a neuroendocrine link between stress, depression and diabetes mellitus. Curr Diabetes Rev 3(4):252–259

Hammerman A, Dreiher J, Klang SH, Munitz H, Cohen AD, Goldfracht M (2008) Antipsychotics and diabetes: an age-related association. Ann Pharmacother 42(9):1316–1322

Haupt DW, Fahnestock PA, Flavin KA, Schweiger JA, Stevens A, Hessler MJ et al (2007) Adiposity and insulin sensitivity derived from intravenous glucose tolerance tests in antipsychotic-treated patients. Neuropsychopharmacology 32(12):2561–2569

Hennekens CH (2007) Increasing global burden of cardiovascular disease in general populations and patients with schizophrenia. J Clin Psychiatryy 68(Suppl 4):4–7

Holt RI, Phillips DI, Jameson KA, Cooper C, Dennison EM, Peveler RC et al (2009) The relationship between depression and diabetes mellitus: findings from the Hertfordshire Cohort Study. Diabet Med 26(6):641–648

Kahn RS, Fleischhacker WW, Boter H, Davidson M, Vergouwe Y, Keet IP et al (2008) Effectiveness of antipsychotic drugs in first-episode schizophrenia and schizophreniform disorder: an open randomised clinical trial. Lancet 371(9618):1085–1097

Katon WJ, Rutter C, Simon G, Lin EH, Ludman E, Ciechanowski P et al (2005) The association of comorbid depression with mortality in patients with type 2 diabetes. Diabetes Care 28(11):2668–2672

Kessing LV, Thomsen AF, Mogensen UB, Andersen PK (2010) Treatment with antipsychotics and the risk of diabetes in clinical practice. Br J Psychiatry 197(4):266–271

Kilbourne AM, Lai Z, Bowersox N, Pirraglia P, Bauer MS (2011) Does colocated care improve access to cardiometabolic screening for patients with serious mental illness? Gen Hosp Psychiatry 33(6):634–636, Pubmed Central PMCID: 3208760

Kivimaki M, Hamer M, Batty GD, Geddes JR, Tabak AG, Pentti J et al (2010) Antidepressant medication use, weight gain, and risk of type 2 diabetes: a population-based study. Diabetes Care 33(12):2611–2616, Pubmed Central PMCID: 2992199

Knowler WC, Barrett-Connor E, Fowler SE, Hamman RF, Lachin JM, Walker EA et al (2002) Reduction in the incidence of type 2 diabetes with lifestyle intervention or metformin. N Engl J Med 346(6):393–403, Pubmed Central PMCID: 1370926

Lambert BL, Cunningham FE, Miller DR, Dalack GW, Hur K (2006) Diabetes risk associated with use of olanzapine, quetiapine, and risperidone in veterans health administration patients with schizophrenia. Am J Epidemiol 164(7):672–681

Laursen TM, Munk-Olsen T, Agerbo E, Gasse C, Mortensen PB (2009) Somatic hospital contacts, invasive cardiac procedures, and mortality from heart disease in patients with severe mental disorder. Arch Gen Psychiatry 66(7):713–720

Lawrence DM, Holman CD, Jablensky AV, Hobbs MS (2003) Death rate from ischaemic heart disease in Western Australian psychiatric patients 1980–1998. Br J Psychiatry 182:31–36

Lawrence D, Hancock KJ, Kisely S (2013) The gap in life expectancy from preventable physical illness in psychiatric patients in Western Australia: retrospective analysis of population based registers. Br Med J 346:f2539, Pubmed Central PMCID: 3660620

Lindamer LA, McKibbin C, Norman GJ, Jordan L, Harrison K, Abeyesinhe S et al (2008) Assessment of physical activity in middle-aged and older adults with schizophrenia. Schizophr Res 104(1–3):294–301, Pubmed Central PMCID: 2560984

Maina G, Salvi V, Vitalucci A, D'Ambrosio V, Bogetto F (2008) Prevalence and correlates of overweight in drug-naive patients with bipolar disorder. J Affect Disord 110(1–2):149–155

McDevitt J, Snyder M, Miller A, Wilbur J (2006) Perceptions of barriers and benefits to physical activity among outpatients in psychiatric rehabilitation. J Nurs Scholarsh 38(1):50–55

McKibbin CL, Patterson TL, Norman G, Patrick K, Jin H, Roesch S et al (2006) A lifestyle intervention for older schizophrenia patients with diabetes mellitus: a randomized controlled trial. Schizophr Res 86(1–3):36–44

Meyer JM, Davis VG, Goff DC, McEvoy JP, Nasrallah HA, Davis SM et al (2008) Change in metabolic syndrome parameters with antipsychotic treatment in the CATIE Schizophrenia Trial: prospective data from phase 1. Schizophr Res 101(1–3):273–286, Pubmed Central PMCID: 3673564

Mitchell AJ, Hardy SA (2013) Screening for metabolic risk among patients with severe mental illness and diabetes: a national comparison. Psychiatr Serv 64(10):1060–1063

Mitchell AJ, Delaffon V, Vancampfort D, Correll CU, De Hert M (2012) Guideline concordant monitoring of metabolic risk in people treated with antipsychotic medication: systematic review and meta-analysis of screening practices. Psychol Med 42(1):125–147

Moeller KE, Rigler SK, Mayorga A, Nazir N, Shireman TI (2011) Quality of monitoring for metabolic effects associated with second generation antipsychotics in patients with schizophrenia on public insurance. Schizophr Res 126(1–3):117–123

Morrato EH, Newcomer JW, Allen RR, Valuck RJ (2008) Prevalence of baseline serum glucose and lipid testing in users of second-generation antipsychotic drugs: a retrospective, population-based study of Medicaid claims data. J Clin Psychiatry 69(2):316–322

Morrato EH, Newcomer JW, Kamat S, Baser O, Harnett J, Cuffel B (2009) Metabolic screening after the American Diabetes Association's consensus statement on antipsychotic drugs and diabetes. Diabetes Care 32(6):1037–1042, Pubmed Central PMCID: 2681020

National Institute for Health and Clinical Excellence (UK) (n.d.) An intervention framework for patients with psychosis on antipsychotic medication in "CG178 Psychosis and schizophrenia in adults: full guideline". http://guidance.nice.org.uk/CG178/InterventionFramework/pdf/English

Newall H, Myles N, Ward PB, Samaras K, Shiers D, Curtis J (2012) Efficacy of metformin for prevention of weight gain in psychiatric populations: a review. Int Clin Psychopharmacol 27(2):69–75

Newcomer JW (2005) Second-generation (atypical) antipsychotics and metabolic effects: a comprehensive literature review. CNS Drugs 19(Suppl 1):1–93

Newcomer JW (2007) Antipsychotic medications: metabolic and cardiovascular risk. J Clin Psychiatry 68(Suppl 4):8–13

Newcomer JW, Nasrallah HA, Loebel AD (2004) The Atypical Antipsychotic Therapy and Metabolic Issues National Survey: practice patterns and knowledge of psychiatrists. J Clin Psychopharmacol 24(5 Suppl 1):S1–S6

Newcomer JW, Ratner RE, Eriksson JW, Emsley R, Meulien D, Miller F et al (2009) A 24-week, multicenter, open-label, randomized study to compare changes in glucose metabolism in patients with schizophrenia receiving treatment with olanzapine, quetiapine, or risperidone. J Clin Psychiatry 70(4):487–499, Pubmed Central PMCID: 3703648

Nielsen J, Skadhede S, Correll CU (2010) Antipsychotics associated with the development of type 2 diabetes in antipsychotic-naive schizophrenia patients. Neuropsychopharmacology 35(9):1997–2004, Pubmed Central PMCID: 3055629

Nouwen A, Winkley K, Twisk J, Lloyd CE, Peyrot M, Ismail K et al (2010) Type 2 diabetes mellitus as a risk factor for the onset of depression: a systematic review and meta-analysis. Diabetologia 53(12):2480–2486, Pubmed Central PMCID: 2974923

Osborn DP, Levy G, Nazareth I, Petersen I, Islam A, King MB (2007) Relative risk of cardiovascular and cancer mortality in people with severe mental illness from the United Kingdom's General Practice Research Database. Arch Gen Psychiatry 64(2):242–249

Osby U, Correia N, Brandt L, Ekbom A, Sparen P (2000) Mortality and causes of death in schizophrenia in Stockholm county, Sweden. Schizophr Res 45(1–2):21–28

Pan A, Sun Q, Okereke OI, Rexrode KM, Rubin RR, Lucas M et al (2012) Use of antidepressant medication and risk of type 2 diabetes: results from three cohorts of US adults. Diabetologia 55(1):63–72, Pubmed Central PMCID: 3229672

Patel JK, Buckley PF, Woolson S, Hamer RM, McEvoy JP, Perkins DO et al (2009) Metabolic profiles of second-generation antipsychotics in early psychosis: findings from the CAFE study. Schizophr Res 111(1–3):9–16

Perez-Iglesias R, Crespo-Facorro B, Amado JA, Garcia-Unzueta MT, Ramirez-Bonilla ML, Gonzalez-Blanch C et al (2007) A 12-week randomized clinical trial to evaluate metabolic changes in drug-naive, first-episode psychosis patients treated with haloperidol, olanzapine, or risperidone. J Clin Psychiatry 68(11):1733–1740

Perez-Iglesias R, Mata I, Pelayo-Teran JM, Amado JA, Garcia-Unzueta MT, Berja A et al (2009) Glucose and lipid disturbances after 1 year of antipsychotic treatment in a drug-naive population. Schizophr Res 107(2–3):115–121

Pouwer F, Geelhoed-Duijvestijn PH, Tack CJ, Bazelmans E, Beekman AJ, Heine RJ et al (2010) Prevalence of comorbid depression is high in out-patients with Type 1 or Type 2 diabetes mellitus. Results from three out-patient clinics in the Netherlands. Diabet Med 27(2): 217–224

Pratt LA, Ford DE, Crum RM, Armenian HK, Gallo JJ, Eaton WW (1996) Depression, psychotropic medication, and risk of myocardial infarction. Prospective data from the Baltimore ECA follow-up. Circulation 94(12):3123–3129

Pringsheim T, Panagiotopoulos C, Davidson J, Ho J, group Cg (2011a) Evidence-based recommendations for monitoring safety of second generation antipsychotics in children and youth. J Can Acad Child Adolesc Psychiatry 20(3):218–233, Pubmed Central PMCID: 3143700

Pringsheim T, Panagiotopoulos C, Davidson J, Ho J, Canadian Alliance for Monitoring Effectiveness, Safety of Antipsychotics in Children guideline group (2011b) Evidence-based recommendations for monitoring safety of second-generation antipsychotics in children and youth. Paediatr Child Health 16(9):581–589, Pubmed Central PMCID: 3223902

Pyykkonen AJ, Raikkonen K, Tuomi T, Eriksson JG, Groop L, Isomaa B (2012) Association between depressive symptoms and metabolic syndrome is not explained by antidepressant medication: results from the PPP-Botnia Study. Ann Med 44(3):279–288

Raeder MB, Bjelland I, Emil Vollset S, Steen VM (2006) Obesity, dyslipidemia, and diabetes with selective serotonin reuptake inhibitors: the Hordaland Health Study. J Clin Psychiatry 67(12):1974–1982

Ramaswamy K, Masand PS, Nasrallah HA (2006) Do certain atypical antipsychotics increase the risk of diabetes? A critical review of 17 pharmacoepidemiologic studies. Ann Clin Psychiatry 18(3):183–194

Rubin RR, Ma Y, Marrero DG, Peyrot M, Barrett-Connor EL, Kahn SE et al (2008) Elevated depression symptoms, antidepressant medicine use, and risk of developing diabetes during the diabetes prevention program. Diabetes Care 31(3):420–426, Pubmed Central PMCID: 2373986

Rubin RR, Ma Y, Peyrot M, Marrero DG, Price DW, Barrett-Connor E et al (2010) Antidepressant medicine use and risk of developing diabetes during the diabetes prevention program and diabetes prevention program outcomes study. Diabetes Care 33(12):2549–2551, Pubmed Central PMCID: 2992187

Rummel-Kluge C, Komossa K, Schwarz S, Hunger H, Schmid F, Lobos CA et al (2010) Head-to-head comparisons of metabolic side effects of second generation antipsychotics in the treatment of schizophrenia: a systematic review and meta-analysis. Schizophr Res 123(2–3):225–233, Pubmed Central PMCID: 2957510

Saha S, Chant D, McGrath J (2007) A systematic review of mortality in schizophrenia: is the differential mortality gap worsening over time? Arch Gen Psychiatry 64(10):1123–1131

Saloojee S, Burns JK, Motala AA (2014) Very low rates of screening for metabolic syndrome among patients with severe mental illness in Durban, South Africa. BMC Psychiatry 14:228, Pubmed Central PMCID: 4149236

Samaras K, Correll CU, Mitchell AJ, De Hert M, HeAL Collaborators Healthy Active Lives for People With Severe Mental Illness (2014) Diabetes risk potentially underestimated in youth and children receiving antipsychotics. JAMA Psychiatry 71(2):209–210

Serretti A, Mandelli L (2010) Antidepressants and body weight: a comprehensive review and meta-analysis. J Clin Psychiatry 71(10):1259–1272

Sikich L, Frazier JA, McClellan J, Findling RL, Vitiello B, Ritz L et al (2008) Double-blind comparison of first- and second-generation antipsychotics in early-onset schizophrenia and schizo-affective disorder: findings from the treatment of early-onset schizophrenia spectrum disorders (TEOSS) study. Am J Psychiatry 165(11):1420–1431

Smith M, Hopkins D, Peveler RC, Holt RI, Woodward M, Ismail K (2008) First- vs. second-generation antipsychotics and risk for diabetes in schizophrenia: systematic review and meta-analysis. Br J Psychiatry 192(6):406–411

Strine TW, Mokdad AH, Dube SR, Balluz LS, Gonzalez O, Berry JT et al (2008) The association of depression and anxiety with obesity and unhealthy behaviors among community-dwelling US adults. Gen Hosp Psychiatry 30(2):127–137

Surtees PG, Wainwright NW, Luben RN, Wareham NJ, Bingham SA, Khaw KT (2008) Depression and ischemic heart disease mortality: evidence from the EPIC-Norfolk United Kingdom prospective cohort study. Am J Psychiatry 165(4):515–523

Teff KL, Rickels MR, Grudziak J, Fuller C, Nguyen HL, Rickels K (2013) Antipsychotic-induced insulin resistance and postprandial hormonal dysregulation independent of weight gain or psychiatric disease. Diabetes 62(9):3232–3240, Pubmed Central PMCID: 3749337

Thornicroft G (2011) Physical health disparities and mental illness: the scandal of premature mortality. Br J Psychiatry 199(6):441–442

Vancampfort D, Wampers M, Mitchell AJ, Correll CU, De Herdt A, Probst M et al (2013) A meta-analysis of cardio-metabolic abnormalities in drug naive, first-episode and multi-episode patients with schizophrenia versus general population controls. World Psychiatry 12(3):240–250, Pubmed Central PMCID: 3799255

Verhaeghe N, De Maeseneer J, Maes L, Van Heeringen C, Annemans L (2011) Effectiveness and cost-effectiveness of lifestyle interventions on physical activity and eating habits in persons with severe mental disorders: a systematic review. Int J Behav Nutr Phys Act 8:28, Pubmed Central PMCID: 3094265

Weiss R, Dziura J, Burgert TS, Tamborlane WV, Taksali SE, Yeckel CW et al (2004) Obesity and the metabolic syndrome in children and adolescents. N Engl J Med 350(23):2362–2374

Wu RR, Zhao JP, Jin H, Shao P, Fang MS, Guo XF et al (2008a) Lifestyle intervention and metformin for treatment of antipsychotic-induced weight gain: a randomized controlled trial. JAMA 299(2):185–193

Wu RR, Zhao JP, Guo XF, He YQ, Fang MS, Guo WB et al (2008b) Metformin addition attenuates olanzapine-induced weight gain in drug-naive first-episode schizophrenia patients: a double-blind, placebo-controlled study. Am J Psychiatry 165(3):352–358

Yood MU, DeLorenze G, Quesenberry CP Jr, Oliveria SA, Tsai AL, Willey VJ et al (2009) The incidence of diabetes in atypical antipsychotic users differs according to agent – results from a multisite epidemiologic study. Pharmacoepidemiol Drug Saf 18(9):791–799

Zhang JP, Weiss JJ, McCardle M, Klopchin H, Rosendahl E, Maayan L et al (2012) Effectiveness of a cognitive behavioral weight management intervention in obese patients with psychotic disorders compared to patients with nonpsychotic disorders or no psychiatric disorders: results from a 12-month, real-world study. J Clin Psychopharmacol 32(4):458–464, Pubmed Central PMCID: 3389573

Monitoring for Metabolic Dysfunction and Cardiovascular Disease in Bipolar Disorder: A Shared Illness Process Approach

19

Tim Outhred, Claire McAulay, Danielle Gessler, and Gin S. Malhi

Contents

Abstract

The alarming rates of physical health comorbidity in bipolar disorder, primarily metabolic and cardiovascular illness, place a heavy burden on patient quality of life and healthcare. Despite clear advice and the widespread availability for monitoring and intervention, clinicians continue to overlook the physical health of

T. Outhred • C. McAulay • D. Gessler • G.S. Malhi (✉)
Academic Department of Psychiatry, Kolling Institute, Northern Sydney Local Health District, St Leonards, NSW 2065, Australia

Sydney Medical School Northern, The University of Sydney, Sydney, NSW 2006, Australia

CADE Clinic, Royal North Shore Hospital, Northern Sydney Local Health District, CADE Clinic Level 3, Main Hospital Building, St Leonards, NSW 2065, Australia
e-mail: gin.malhi@sydney.edu.au

B.T. Baune, P.J. Tully (eds.), *Cardiovascular Diseases and Depression*,
DOI 10.1007/978-3-319-32480-7_19

patients with psychiatric disorders and psychological problems. Therefore, the associations between these chronic mental illnesses and the role of physical health monitoring and intervention strategies warrant evaluation.

The aim of this chapter is to review metabolic and cardiovascular disease monitoring practices in bipolar disorder. In doing so, the links between bipolar disorder, metabolic function, and cardiovascular disease and potential shared illness processes are examined. On the basis of this, clinical and research recommendations are outlined. With greater understanding of the shared illness processes for bipolar disorder and metabolic and cardiovascular dysfunction, improvements in the monitoring and treatment of patients with bipolar disorder may be developed. By considering a shared illness process approach, bipolar disorder-specific solutions for more informative monitoring and targeted healthcare options may be implemented into routine psychiatric practice. This will facilitate better lifelong management of the psychological and physical health of patients with bipolar disorder.

19.1 Introduction

Bipolar disorder is a debilitating psychiatric illness characterised by sustained and often extreme mood swings described as episodes of mania and depression. There has been an increasing awareness that bipolar disorder also causes considerable physical harm, with patients developing metabolic syndrome and cardiovascular disease at alarming rates. These medical comorbidities are associated with progressive disease course and premature mortality in patients with bipolar disorder. Due to these concerns, clinical practice guidelines (e.g. NICE 2006, 2015) suggest that patients with bipolar disorder be monitored not only for illness progression and treatment efficacy but also across an array of metabolic and cardiovascular parameters such as blood pressure, body morphology, and lipid profile and blood glucose concentration (see Table 19.1). Research over the last decade has increased understanding of the compounding factors that contribute to the metabolic dysfunction and cardiovascular disease in bipolar disorder, ranging from treatment side effects

Table 19.1 A typical physical health monitoring regimen of clinical practice guidelines depicts the frequency at which key parameters are assessed

Parameters	Initial assessment	Treatment commencement (every 1–3 months)	Annually
Body morphology Lifestyle factors Fasting blood glucose Blood lipid profile Liver, renal, and thyroid function	◆	◆	◆

to socioeconomic factors (e.g. McElroy et al. 2002; NICE 2006, 2015). Additionally, the findings of endocrine dysregulation, the impact of stress on the autonomic nervous system, and sedentary behaviour and overeating are showing increasing overlap between bipolar disorder and metabolic and cardiovascular illness processes (Bengesser et al. 2015; Choi et al. 2013; Fagiolini et al. 2008; Mansur et al. 2015; Taylor and MacQueen 2006; Wildes et al. 2008). These findings suggest that there are common mechanisms that may precipitate or at least perpetuate metabolic dysfunction in bipolar disorder. Despite the availability of metabolic and cardiovascular disease monitoring and an array of interventions, primary care clinicians continue to observe their patients with bipolar disorder decline in physical health. This may be due to the paucity of effective long-term management strategies available to clinicians designed for this population, along with the absence of novel pharmacological treatments. Therefore, the associations between these patient illnesses, along with clinical management strategies, deserve evaluation.

Considering the various challenges in treating a comorbid population with distinctly treatment-resistant illnesses (Fagiolini et al. 2005; Lakka et al. 2002; Murray et al. 2010), successful management strategies for metabolic health must be implemented early in the disease course in order to curb further disability and mortality and perhaps partially ameliorate illness progression (Malik et al. 2004; Wong et al. 2003). Though understanding of the associations between metabolic function, cardiovascular disease, and bipolar disorder is increasing, fundamental changes to monitoring strategy—aside from frequency of and parameters for testing (as depicted in Table 19.1)—are yet to be realised. Incorporating metabolic and cardiovascular disease monitoring and intervention as a standard practice in the management of bipolar is clearly a clinically beneficial goal; however, the underlying approach deserves evaluation in light of an emerging picture of shared illness processes (see Fig. 19.1 for an overview). While practices for monitoring and slowing the advancement of each illness are evaluated, an approach that takes shared illness processes into account may afford novel and effective strategies that further curb comorbidity and illness progression. Hence, the aim of this chapter is to review metabolic and cardiovascular disease monitoring in bipolar disorder and how this could be better deployed. In doing so, the chapter will aim to illustrate the associations between bipolar disorder, metabolic function, and cardiovascular disease; the endocrine and autonomic nervous system dysregulation as potential shared illness processes; the factors that contribute to comorbidities; and how clinical management can both exacerbate and curb comorbid disease progression.

19.2 Epidemiology and Monitoring of Metabolic Dysfunction and Cardiovascular Disease in Bipolar Disorder

Metabolic and cardiovascular health measures are assessed routinely in primary care with blood pressure, body morphology, blood glucose and lipid profile, and lifestyle behaviours monitored regularly to provide indications of physical health status in the general population. Bipolar disorder significantly compromises general

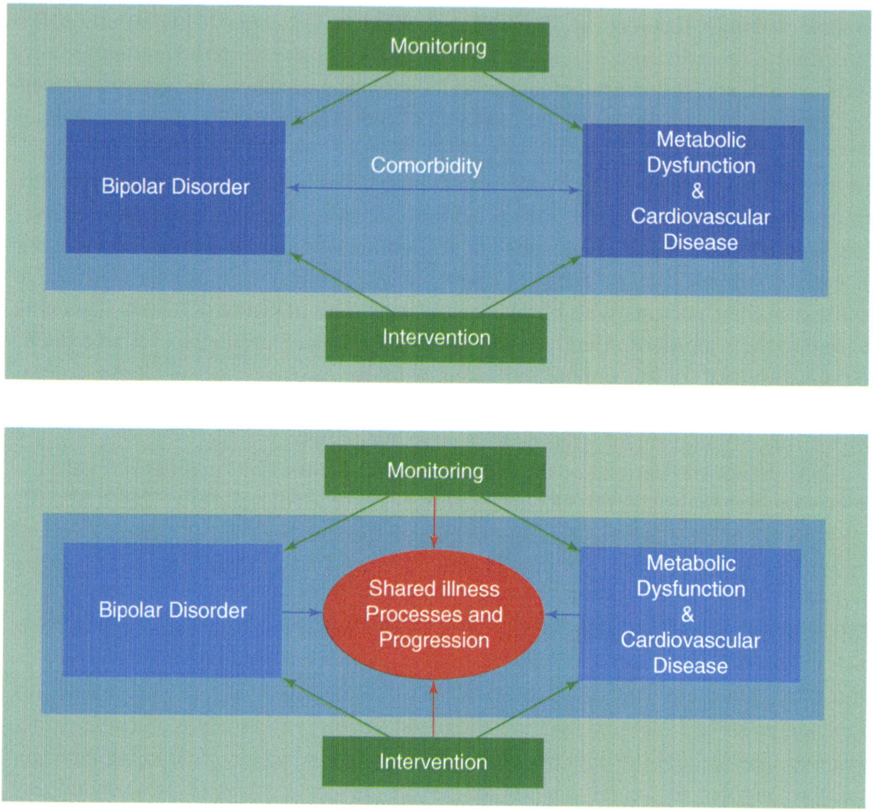

Fig. 19.1 An overview of a shared illness process approach to the understanding and management of bipolar disorder and physical health comorbidities – primarily metabolic dysfunction and cardiovascular disease. Panel (**a**) routine clinical approach**.** Patient illnesses (in *blue*; 1) bipolar disorder and (2) metabolic dysfunction and cardiovascular disease (*blue*) have high rates of comorbidity. In noting this comorbidity, management (*green*) concerns frequency and parameters for monitoring and interventions targeting each illness, typically across different domains of care (e.g. primary and secondary care). Panel (**b**) a shared illness processes approach. Shared illness processes may explain, at least in part, the comorbidity of (1) bipolar disorder and (2) metabolic dysfunction and cardiovascular disease (*blue*) and may underpin progression on both fronts (*red*). With greater understanding of these shared illness processes, they could be directly targeted with management (*red arrows*)—monitoring and intervening at times when the illnesses are exacerbating or compounding each other (e.g. diet and lifestyle behaviour changes during bipolar disorder illness episodes). The aim of this would then be to curb simultaneous progression of both illnesses early in its illness course, perhaps an approach lending itself to a more coordinated or integrated care (e.g. specialist bipolar disorder services)

functioning, but behavioural engagement with physical healthcare interventions is challenging for both patients and clinicians alike (Berk et al. 2004; Byrne et al. 2006; Fagiolini et al. 2005; Murray et al. 2010). Hence, despite efforts from both parties, patients with bipolar disorder deteriorate in terms of their physical health even while maintaining psychological wellbeing. The treatment of bipolar disorder with atypical antipsychotics is thought to often lead to metabolic syndrome and cardiovascular disease (Cardenas et al. 2008; Correll et al. 2006, 2008; Fagiolini et al. 2008; Keck and McElroy 2003; Lee et al. 2010; Nemeroff 2003; Yumru et al. 2007), which are significant causes of premature death in this population (Fagiolini et al. 2008; Weiner et al. 2011). Notably, metabolic syndrome and cardiovascular disease appear to have overlapping courses and shared risk factors, with serious or fatal cardiovascular events typically following a history of metabolic dysfunction and hypertension (Malik et al. 2004; Wong et al. 2003). Metabolic syndrome is variably defined as a cluster of symptoms—with some adjustment for age and gender. Across classifications (Alberti and Zimmet 1998; Expert Panel on Detection, Evaluation, and Treatment of High Blood Cholesterol in Adults 2001; Reaven 1988), the core features of metabolic syndrome are hypertension, obesity, hyperglycaemia, and dyslipidaemia. Along with hypertension and hypertensive heart disease, common cardiovascular disease presentations in bipolar disorder are fatal cardiac events (e.g. myocardial infarction), stroke, and heart failure (Fiedorowicz et al. 2009; Goldstein et al. 2009; Vancampfort et al. 2013). Bipolar disorder can be considered to carry additional, perhaps multiplicative illness and healthcare burden. However, epidemiological findings suggest that in the wider population, much of metabolic syndrome and cardiovascular disease is preventable or can at least be effectively managed, through implementation of lifestyle strategies and treatment and monitoring in those at high risk (Malik et al. 2004; Wong et al. 2003). However, epidemiological findings of the relationship between bipolar disorder and declining physical health paint a disturbing picture.

19.2.1 Epidemiological Findings

Rates of metabolic dysfunction and the development of metabolic syndrome and cardiovascular disease in bipolar disorder are well documented (Fiedorowicz et al. 2008; McIntyre et al. 2010; Vancampfort et al. 2013). The estimated prevalence of metabolic dysfunction in bipolar disorder ranges from 22 to 49 % (Cardenas et al. 2008; Correll et al. 2008; Garcia-Portilla et al. 2008; Grover et al. 2012; John et al. 2009). The rate of full metabolic syndrome is estimated to be twofold of that in the general population (McIntyre et al. 2010), with increased rates in older patients (Lee et al. 2010; Vancampfort et al. 2013), and is associated with poorer illness course (McElroy et al. 2015) and increased reports of suicide attempt (Fagiolini et al. 2005).

Similarly there is an increased prevalence of cardiovascular disease among patients with bipolar disorder (Fiedorowicz et al. 2009; Goldstein et al. 2009), who are at five times greater risk of developing the illness (Vancampfort et al. 2013). Indeed, health risks associated with metabolic syndrome predict poorer cardiovascular outcomes (Birkenaes et al. 2007; Garcia-Portilla et al. 2009; Weiner et al. 2011) and effectively double the risk (Correll et al. 2006). Increased cardiovascular disease risk has been more commonly detected in older patients with bipolar disorder, where younger samples have not shown early risk factors (Murray et al. 2012), suggesting that the course of the disease over time perhaps increases cardiovascular risk, possibly via arterial stiffness (Sodhi et al. 2012). In having examined multiplicative risk for bipolar disorder illness course and metabolic dysfunction and cardiovascular disease, predictive factors are discussed below.

19.2.2 Iatrogenic Factors Associated with Metabolic Dysfunction and Cardiovascular Disease in Bipolar Disorder

Causes for the increased prevalence of both metabolic syndrome and cardiovascular disease appear to be multifactorial, and various studies have sought to identify the iatrogenic (e.g. Correll et al. 2006, 2008; Fagiolini et al. 2008; Yumru et al. 2007) and non-iatrogenic causes (e.g. Fiedorowicz et al. 2008; McIntyre et al. 2010; Murray et al. 2009, 2012). In order to explain the poorer health outcomes seen in bipolar disorder, the role of pharmacotherapy treatment has been the focus of recent research, which has looked at the obesogenic (weight gain inducing) properties of psychoactive medication as well as the differential outcomes of atypical antipsychotics (e.g. clozapine, olanzapine), mood stabilisers (e.g. lithium, sodium valproate), and drug polytherapy (e.g. Cardenas et al. 2008). Common adverse effects of frequently prescribed treatments on metabolic and cardiovascular parameters are shown in Table 19.2.

While the obesogenic properties of psychotropic medication are well reported (e.g. Keck and McElroy 2003; Nemeroff 2003), inconsistent attributions of pharmacotherapy treatment to weight gain have raised doubt as to the extent to which

Table 19.2 Some of the frequently prescribed medications for bipolar disorder along with common adverse effects on metabolic and cardiovascular parameters

		Parameter			
Class	Medications	Body morphology	Blood pressure	Fasting blood glucose	Blood lipid profile
Mood stabilisers	Lithium	◆			
Anticonvulsants	Carbamazepine	◆			
	Lamotrigine				
	Valproate				
Atypical antipsychotics	Aripiprazole				
	Clozapine				
	Lurasidone[a]				
	Olanzapine	◆	◆	◆	◆
	Quetiapine				
	Risperidone				
	Ziprasidone				

Based on search on MIMS Online and reported frequencies of adverse effects >5 %

[a]From manufacturer's product information

weight gain is wholly iatrogenic and what proportion is attributable to the aetiology of the illness (Birkenaes et al. 2007; Correll et al. 2008). Many studies have pointed to the weight gain-inducing properties of psychoactive medication, in particular in terms of metabolic and cardiovascular outcomes (Cardenas et al. 2008; Correll et al. 2006, 2008; Fagiolini et al. 2008; Lee et al. 2010; Yumru et al. 2007); however, there appear to be differential findings depending on the antipsychotic administered and whether this occurred in the context of polypharmacy. Atypical antipsychotics, known for inducing weight gain, have been the focus of metabolic syndrome research in bipolar disorder, with consistent findings of metabolic disturbance in those prescribed with these medications for a long term (Cardenas et al. 2008; Fagiolini et al. 2008; Keck and McElroy 2003). Second-generation antipsychotic use has been associated with weight gain and a higher cardiovascular risk burden, as well as an increased risk of metabolic syndrome prevalence, such that 67 % of second-generation antipsychotic users met criteria for metabolic syndrome, as compared to 42 % of nonusers (Fiedorowicz et al. 2008). Olanzapine and clozapine were more likely to lead to metabolic syndrome relative to carbamazepine, which was associated with a lower prevalence (Cardenas et al. 2008). The seemingly modest effects of carbamazepine have been attributed to specific pharmacokinetic properties, which are able to reduce the likelihood of adverse lipid or glucose disturbances (Cardenas et al. 2008).

Differential effects of psychoactive pharmacotherapy with metabolic syndrome and cardiovascular illness in bipolar disorder have been investigated in the context of polypharmacy. In some instances, metabolic syndrome prevalence was found to be significantly less with polypharmacy, for example, when antipsychotics were taken in combination with mood stabilisers, as compared to antipsychotics taken alone (Kemp et al. 2010; Yumru et al. 2007). In others, medication polypharmacy has appeared to be associated with greater risk (e.g. Correll et al. 2008). However, some aversive or preventative effects may be due to the agents—with other effects, it may be that having an additional agent offers the ability to lower the doses of the active (mood stabilising) but aversive (e.g. obesogenic) agent. Therefore, when examining polypharmacy, relative or typical changes to dosing should be taken into account.

Further, when metabolic syndrome prevalence has been assessed between patients with schizophrenia and bipolar disorder, weight gain could not be explained by psychotropic medication alone (Birkenaes et al. 2007; Correll et al. 2008). Despite the divergent drug treatment received in a study conducted by Birkenaes and colleagues (2007), in particular where bipolar disorder treatment had no known metabolic disturbances and schizophrenia patients received atypical antipsychotics known to induce weight gain, there was no difference in prevalence of metabolic or cardiovascular risk factors. This incongruence was also demonstrated with findings of equal prevalence of metabolic syndrome in bipolar disorder and schizophrenia patients, in spite of patients with bipolar disorder being significantly more likely than patients with schizophrenia to receive mood stabilisers and less likely to receive antipsychotics or antipsychotic polypharmacy (Correll et al. 2008). This is important as these findings suggest that iatrogenic factors cannot wholly explain the association between bipolar disorder and metabolic dysfunction and cardiovascular disease (Taylor and MacQueen 2006); instead, illness processes that underpin bipolar disorder may in part perpetuate metabolic dysfunction and cardiovascular disease. In order to test this hypothesis, researchers have called for treatment and illness-naïve studies in order to ascertain the extent of this association. In a treatment-naïve study, obesity was significantly more prevalent in drug-naïve patients with bipolar disorder than in another drug-naïve psychiatric patient group (OCD), and the number of depressive episodes was associated with greater prevalence of obesity (Maina et al. 2008). The authors suggested that the prevalence of obesity in bipolar patients might be more influenced by the illness itself, or at least mediating behavioural diet and lifestyle factors, than by pharmacological treatment. Taken together, these findings appear to indicate common illness processes in bipolar disorder and comorbid metabolic dysfunction and associated cardiovascular disease, where pharmacotherapy treatment cannot wholly account for these comorbidities. While it has been suggested that there is a common diathesis, relating potentially to the hypothalamic–pituitary–adrenal axis (HPA) dysfunction and cortical regulation abnormalities in this illness (as discussed in Sect. 19.3), the degree of this shared pathophysiology is unclear in the absence of treatment and illness-naïve research paradigms. In clinical practice, however, monitoring and interventions targeted at metabolic dysfunction and cardiovascular disease in bipolar disorder may help to prevent the development of these debilitating and fatal comorbidities and curb comorbid disease progression.

19.2.3 Current State of Metabolic Monitoring in Bipolar Disorder

Given the high risk of metabolic dysfunction and cardiovascular disease in bipolar disorder, it has been established in clinical practice guidelines (e.g. NICE 2006, 2015) that clinicians should routinely perform physical assessment. Clinical practice guidelines typically institute a frequency- and parameter-based approach to monitoring (as depicted in Table 19.1). An initial assessment should include height and weight, thyroid, liver and renal function tests, blood pressure, full blood count, plasma glucose levels, lipid profile, and smoking status and alcohol use. Cardiology, neurology, and radiology referrals are also considered. Clinical practice guidelines (e.g. NICE 2006) recommend patients to have an annual review of weight, blood pressure, lipid levels, plasma glucose levels, and smoking status and alcohol use. When initiating and monitoring treatments, clinicians should conduct assessments every 1–3 months for metabolic and cardiovascular changes and ensure ECGs are performed for at-risk patients (e.g. NICE 2006). Though these measures are widely instated and easily performed (assuming patient compliance), making decisions based on results poses a particular challenge. Currently, clinicians attempt to manage, largely modifying lifestyle factors and instituting treatment and monitoring, much like they would in the wider population. This is reasonable as metabolic syndrome and cardiovascular disease is preventable or at least can be effectively managed in this manner. However, given the particularly high risk that bipolar disorder confers, as well as its inherent high comorbidity and worsening health outcomes overtime, perhaps this nonspecific approach is insufficient. It appears that clinicians are at odds with the nature of the disorder, the potential impact of treatment, and the underlying illness processes of both the disorder and physical health comorbidities. Therefore, we must better interrogate underlying illness processes in order to proceed, with perhaps a more specific solution.

19.3 Potential Mechanisms and Shared Illness Processes in Bipolar Disorder and Metabolic and Cardiovascular Health

It is thought that good physical and psychological health is essentially founded on the optimal basal activity and responsiveness of an HPA axis and autonomic-mediated stress system (Chrousos 2009). Given that bipolar disorder is one of both recurrent acute (episodic) and chronic stress, it is unsurprising that deterioration across these integrated components occurs. Bipolar disorder has been characterised as having a progressive clinical course in that presentations tend to worsen over time. It has been argued that each acute episode further degrades the course of bipolar, with associated impacts on functioning. This progressive course is thought to be paralleled by deteriorating neurobiological pathways of glucocorticoid elevation, oxidative stress, nitrosative stress, and inflammation, which are associated with diminished function of neurotransmission and neurotrophic pathways that underpin behaviour (Berk et al. 2011). As bipolar disorder is characterised by and known to lead to degradation of forebrain regulatory control (Berk et al. 2011; Outhred et al. 2014), the progressive nature of deterioration of the basal activity and responsiveness of the stress system are manifest. In terms of cardiovascular and metabolic function, there are well-characterised inflammatory, oxidative and nitrosative, and endocrine changes that progressively disrupt these functions, underpinned by acute and chronic HPA axis and autonomic stress responses. In cross-sectional studies, physical health parameters have shown to deteriorate with worsening bipolar presentation (e.g. Fagiolini et al. 2003, 2005).

In order to understand the associations between bipolar disorder, metabolic dysfunction, and cardiovascular disease, researchers are attempting to interrogate shared illness processes (Chrousos 2009). In the context of bipolar disorder, the HPA axis and the autonomic nervous system are thought to play roles in the precipitation, perpetuation, and progression of clinical presentation and endocrine, metabolic, and cardiovascular function. The HPA axis cascade and autonomic nervous system are integrated, and the functioning of both is interrelated (Ahrens et al. 1995; Kallner et al. 2000). Together, they underpin a shared illness process of psychiatric and physical health: the stress response. The stress response is an integration of behavioural and physiological response within a system of central and peripheral HPA axis and autonomic nervous system components (Chrousos 2009; Mayer and Fanselow 2003). These neural and endocrine components are interconnected, the products of which are the central executive; emotion and sleep-wake systems; the growth, reproductive, and thyroid hormone axes; and the gastrointestinal, cardiovascular, respiratory, metabolic, and immune systems (Chrousos 2009). The HPA axis is a hormone-based cascade of positive and negative feedback interactions between three endocrine glands: the hypothalamus and the pituitary and adrenal glands. The HPA cascade is activated by stress responses and plays a major role in the longer-term impacts of chronic stress, leading to deterioration in metabolic and cardiovascular function, as well as psychological health. In terms of the autonomic nervous system, stress manifests in physiological changes through neural integration of stressors and signals to and from the periphery at the brainstem, with control mechanisms based in the forebrain (for a review, see Kemp and Quintana 2013). Parasympathetic signals to the heart, for instance, allow optimal basal activity and reactivity and adaptation to stress (see Kemp and Quintana 2013). Chronic stress is thought to be associated with dysfunction of the autonomic nervous system, through disturbed central and peripheral nervous system integration pathways, and ongoing damage to the cardiovasculature, through multiple HPA axis-mediated pathways including oxidative and nitrosative stress and inflammation (see Kemp and Quintana 2013). Indeed, a number of findings in patients with bipolar disorder and metabolic and cardiovascular dysfunction point to shared illness processes (Mansur et al. 2015), in terms of oxidative and nitrosative markers (e.g. Bengesser et al. 2015), inflammatory markers (e.g. Choi et al. 2013), and glucocorticoid pathways (see Mansur et al. 2015; Taylor and MacQueen 2006). Glucocorticoid pathways appear to be particularly explanatory given that chronically elevated levels, as a result of acute and chronic stress, disrupt insulin, leptin, lipoprotein lipase, and autonomic nervous system function, which each interact and contribute to metabolic and cardiovascular dysfunction and disease (Mansur et al. 2015; Taylor and MacQueen 2006).

It is becoming apparent that the stress responses that occur in bipolar disorder lead to further deterioration of the illness and at the same time impact metabolic and cardiovascular health. Deterioration of the stress system is, at least in part, a shared illness process of bipolar disorder and metabolic and cardiovascular diseases, and together they show a progressive course due to the diminishing ability for the stress system to respond and adapt. Confounding this notion is that the interventions and monitoring practices that are being delivered to treat bipolar disorder may, at least in some respects, exacerbate or ameliorate deterioration of components of the stress system, and this should be taken into account. Given that physical health deterioration is associated with worsening bipolar disorder presentation (Fagiolini et al. 2003, 2005), shared illness processes should be further investigated in longitudinal research, with the aim to identify potential interventions. This is critical given the absence of novel pharmacological options. With greater consideration of shared illness processes for bipolar disorder and metabolic and cardiovascular dysfunction (see Fig. 19.1), the manner in which bipolar disorder patients are treated and monitored may be improved.

19.4 Towards Monitoring and Intervention Approaches for Shared Illness Processes

Despite the frequency at which monitoring and opportunities to intervene occur in clinical practice, adverse metabolic and cardiovascular health in patients with bipolar disorder appears to worsen. Current frameworks and guidelines for monitoring take a frequency-based approach, with consideration of the optimal frequency at which patients should be monitored across an array of parameters (see Fig. 19.1). This approach is widely recommended as regimens can be easily embedded and adopted in practice, and these also apply in the general population. However, this approach may not be capturing the key times at which the bipolar illness is severely compounding morbidity. Given that shared illness processes of bipolar disorder and metabolic and cardiovascular health are becoming more apparent, acute episodes may lead to increased deterioration in health over the long term—not just the duration of the illness. Hence, morbidity may be more apparent when acute bipolar episodes coincide with changes to the activation and responsiveness of the stress system as well as concurrent changes to lifestyle behaviour. Therefore, monitoring patients' lifestyle behaviour and metabolic and cardiovascular parameters during times of acute illness and relative health, not just at regular time intervals, is likely to be informative (see Fig. 19.1). In doing so, clinicians and patients may have a better insight into the specific behaviour changes and their impact on metabolic and cardiovascular health and thus better target intervention. In terms of monitoring the effect of medications and interventions, with changes to psychotropic medication and improvement in mood stability, behavioural factors will also differ. Hence, it may be more informative to examine changes in lifestyle factors and metabolic and cardiovascular parameters together with medication efficacy and side effect assessments than to simply infer changes at fixed time points within a frequency-based monitoring regime. In doing so, clinicians and patients may have greater insight into how metabolic and cardiovascular parameters change with intervention, medication, and bipolar disorder illness and lifestyle factors. Though further research is needed, this approach may be considered given that patients who remain well in the longer term report continuous management of lifestyle factors and stressors, in and between episodes (Murray et al. 2010; Russell and Browne 2005). As an episode arises, self-management of diet and physical activity may become severely impaired in many patients, likely affecting metabolic and cardiovascular parameters. This is when patients who remain well report seeking assistance from clinicians and significant others (Murray et al. 2010; Russell and Browne 2005). Taken together, it appears that current frequency-based metabolic and cardiovascular parameter monitoring practices are effective to an extent, but may be improved and better deployed when considering the potential for concurrent shared illness processes (see Fig. 19.1). This should be further investigated as with more informative monitoring, treatment, and lifestyle interventions, and other typical management strategies may be better targeted.

In the wider population, metabolic health is increasingly being treated by multidisciplinary teams who attempt to monitor and address the various factors and sequelae associated with this disease, including those within biological, environmental, behavioural, and psychological domains. Cognitive and behavioural approaches have received increasing attention, with results demonstrating that small but significant changes are achievable. Monitoring is key to this approach, with both clinicians and patients facilitating the process. Treatments that target motivation, while incorporating basic nutritional and activity monitoring and goals, and a weight-maintenance phase are recommended for bipolar disorder (e.g. NICE 2006, 2015). The efficacy of these treatments in depressed populations is promoted; however, most research studies specifically exclude those with current mood disruption, major psychiatric illnesses, or antipsychotic use, which typically encompasses bipolar disorder. This practice, while maintaining greater homogeneity within research samples, unfortunately excludes those who are perhaps most needing intervention and has prevented understanding about lifestyle-mediated metabolic disruption and cardiovascular illness in bipolar disorder. Recently, research has expanded to assess the impact of lifestyle interventions for patients with 'severe mental illness', which includes schizophrenia and bipolar disorder (Cabassa et al. 2010; Kelly et al. 2014). Arguably, given that weight gain typically increases over time, treatments that stop weight gain can make a valuable contribution to patient health (Yilmaz et al. 2011). Despite a lack of more specific investigation, it appears that cognitive- and behavioural-based approaches may be well suited to identifying, monitoring, and modifying the illness-related lifestyle behaviours observed in bipolar disorder presentations. Given promise to improve overall health and perhaps indirectly improve bipolar disorder illness processes, these possibilities should be further investigated.

The monitoring and treatment of metabolic disruption in bipolar disorder may be further complicated by its high comorbidity with eating disorders (e.g. 14.3 %; McElroy et al. 2011). Binge eating-type disorders and behaviours are particularly common in bipolar disorder (McElroy et al. 2011) and a key contributing factor to obesity (McElroy et al. 2002). Eating disorders are also associated with increased cardiovascular risk, low levels of treatment seeking, and high suicidality, together compounding the existing burden of bipolar disorder. While bingeing does not always present as a clinically significant eating disorder in bipolar disorder, subthreshold bingeing is still relevant to weight gain and should be regularly assessed by clinicians (Castrogiovanni et al. 2009; Wildes et al. 2008). Eating disorder and behaviour may be associated with added guilt and shame, making detection challenging without targeted assessment and monitoring, and certain antipsychotics have been found to increase the risk of bingeing (Theisen et al. 2003). Hence, eating behaviour disturbances may serve as a hidden obstacle to any treatment aligned to improve metabolic and cardiovascular outcomes in bipolar disorder.

19.5 Recommendations

19.5.1 Research Recommendations

Not surprisingly, the management of metabolic and cardiovascular health in bipolar disorder is more difficult than in the general population, perhaps due to the compounding effects of shared illness processes. Therefore, further research on shared illness processes needs to be conducted; in particular, metabolic and cardiovascular parameters should be examined both during acute episodes and periods of relative health, and compared over time against key, interacting moderators (e.g. illness onset, introduction of treatment, diet and lifestyle changes, mood stability, bingeing). This may afford greater insight into the manner in which these factors change over the course of illness and in response to treatment. Investigations along these lines are likely to facilitate the development of predictive models alongside the development of more granular and informative monitoring. Such research is necessary to determine the added benefits of monitoring for a shared illness process, over the simple frequency-based approach currently recommended in clinical practice guidelines. Translating this into clinical practice, in addition to metabolic and cardiovascular measures, monitoring may involve concurrent charting of mood, treatment, diet and lifestyle changes, and other relevant moderators (e.g. bingeing). Given the technological advancements in smart-wearable technologies and their affordable widespread availability, these devices can now be used to monitor mood, lifestyle behaviours, and metabolic and cardiovascular health in real-world settings over long periods of time.

In order to determine the role of shared illness processes, further research monitoring the impacts of treatments to manage both bipolar disorder illness and metabolic and cardiovascular health is also needed. In terms of biological treatments, promising findings include the administration of statins, given that they may improve mental health as well as decrease physical health sequelae for patients with major depressive disorder (Redlich et al. 2014; Stafford and Berk 2011). The reverse may also occur, with findings that patients with cardiovascular disease may have decreased mental health sequelae with statin administration (Redlich et al. 2014). With further research along these lines, shared illness processes may be better understood, facilitating improvement of clinical management strategies.

19.5.2 Clinical Recommendations

Given the significant overlap between mental ill-health and physical disease, a shared illness process approach for understanding the causes of bipolar disorder and its associated metabolic and cardiovascular dysfunction is likely to be the most beneficial in clinical settings (see Fig. 19.1). Thus, it is important to determine monitoring and management strategies that target this shared illness process. Recommendations from clinical practice guidelines advise clinicians to monitor general health (as depicted in Table 19.1) and consider dietetic and exercise interventions. However, the challenge for clinicians is how to apply these to patients with bipolar disorder, whose changing mental state may have a great bearing on lifestyle- and health-related behaviour. The notion that patients who are adequately treated as regards their bipolar disorder are better able to maintain their physical health is likely to be true, but only to a point. The long-term physical health of patients with bipolar disorder is also dependent upon how patients maintain their physical health when they become psychologically unwell (depression or mania), and how the medications that they are prescribed impact their illness course and health outcomes on both fronts. When monitoring the effects of bipolar disorder illness and treatments, physicians may consider monitoring metabolic and cardiovascular status in both acute episodes and during periods of relative health against potential moderators (e.g. treatment, diet and lifestyle changes, mood stability, bingeing). Therefore, monitoring and management strategies may be adapted to take into consideration this shared illness processes in order to better inform management strategies. In terms of biological treatment, statins, for example, may be considered alongside mood stabilisers such as lithium, given the potential for both to improve mental health and decrease physical health sequelae in the long term. In terms of psycho-educational and psychological treatment, equipping patients to face inevitable stressors when they become psychologically unwell, and have changes to lifestyle routine, will ensure maintenance of better overall health, given that this is what patients who remain well are reporting (Murray et al. 2010; Russell and Browne 2005). Given that metabolic and cardiovascular dysfunction in bipolar disorder appears to be greater than that of other mood disorders, a shared illness approach to monitoring and management of bipolar disorder is likely to be of significant benefit.

The recent shift towards community care for patients with bipolar disorder, compiled with decreasing specialist long-term care—for example, in the form of lithium clinics—has cut cost in the short term but will be more costly in the long term. For instance, naturalistic studies suggest that patients who regularly engage with lithium clinics have reduced morbidity and mortality from all causes (e.g. Ahrens et al. 1995; Kallner et al. 2000). The likely reason for this is better engagement with population-specific psycho-educational and dietetic interventions along with frequent systematic monitoring, which together increase the efficacy of treatment and ensure maintenance of good physical health. Alongside monitoring lithium and psychological symptoms, lithium clinics were traditionally also preventing deterioration in physical health, and so perhaps it is time such clinics are resurrected and positioned so as to function in combination with community care, to target the management of shared illness processes in bipolar disorder.

Bipolar disorder-specific clinics such as lithium clinics may be well equipped to monitor and manage long-term physical health in this population, by integrating metabolic and cardiovascular parameters with bipolar disorder illness- and treatment-related changes. For example, food frequency charts for the home (involving the family unit), for monitoring and illustrating size of meal portions and proportions of food types on plates (e.g. protein to carbohydrates to vegetables), are a simple example of cost-effective advice and intervention that can be delivered, alongside necessary psycho-education. The latter specifically aims to enhance insight into the manner in which mood state and changes to medication impact desired meal portions, and emphasising and ensuring consistent comparison with a pictorial chart promote regulation of meal portion. Simple and easily deployed psychological, psycho-educational, and dietetic interventions designed for bipolar disorder such as this are needed, and perhaps specialist bipolar disorder clinics are best positioned to monitor and deliver them. In doing so, bipolar disorder illness may have less of an impact on metabolic and cardiovascular health.

Conclusions

Bipolar disorder is associated with noticeable physical health morbidity and mortality, involving primarily metabolic dysfunction and cardiovascular disease. Pharmacological treatment may be a double-edged sword, where the aim to maintain psychological health may be at the cost of physical health. Despite this, clinicians still face a losing battle, whereby psychological health wavers when physical health deteriorates. Increasingly, there appear to be shared illness processes between bipolar disorder and metabolic and cardiovascular health, where each condition has an iteratively deleterious and compounding effect. In the near term, the amelioration and prevention of metabolic dysfunction and cardiovascular disease in bipolar disorder pose a great clinical challenge, especially in the context of current management. However, improved monitoring, decision-making, and targeted psychological and dietetic intervention will likely better curb physical health morbidity and mortality. This should be a focus of clinical research, given that findings thus far have been promising and also that there is little in the way of novel pharmacological options. Further research on effective monitoring and intervention for metabolic and cardiovascular health is required, and management targeted at shared illness processes may be more effective in the longer term. To this end, bipolar disorder-specific clinics (such as lithium clinics) are well positioned to become part of the solution to deliver better monitoring and improved healthcare options for patients with bipolar disorder. In doing so, both psychological and physical health of patients with bipolar disorder can be managed more effectively with better eventual outcomes in both domains.

References

Ahrens B, Grof P, Moller HJ, Müller-Oerlinghausen B, Wolf T (1995) Extended survival of patients on long-term lithium treatment. Can J Psychiatr 40(5):241–246

Alberti KG, Zimmet PZ (1998) Definition, diagnosis and classification of diabetes mellitus and its complications. Part 1: diagnosis and classification of diabetes mellitus provisional report of a WHO consultation. Diabet Med 15(7):539–553, http://doi.org/10.1002/(SICI)1096-9136(199807)15:7<539::AID-DIA668>3.0.CO;2-S

Bengesser SA, Lackner N, Birner A, Fellendorf FT, Platzer M, Mitteregger A et al (2015) Peripheral markers of oxidative stress and antioxidative defense in euthymia of bipolar disorder—gender and obesity effects. J Affect Disord 172:367–374

Berk M, Berk L, Castle D (2004) A collaborative approach to the treatment alliance in bipolar disorder. Bipolar Disord 6(6):504–518, http://doi.org/10.1111/j.1399-5618.2004.00154.x

Berk M, Kapczinski F, Andreazza AC, Dean OM, Giorlando F, Maes M et al (2011) Pathways underlying neuroprogression in bipolar disorder: focus on inflammation, oxidative stress and neurotrophic factors. Neurosci Biobehav Rev 35(3):804–817, http://doi.org/10.1016/j.neubiorev.2010.10.001

Birkenaes AB, Opjordsmoen S, Brunborg C, Engh JA, Jonsdottir H, Ringen PA et al (2007) The level of cardiovascular risk factors in bipolar disorder equals that of schizophrenia: a comparative study. J Clin Psychiatry 68(6):917–923

Byrne N, Regan C, Livingston G (2006) Adherence to treatment in mood disorders. Curr Opin Psychiatry 19(1):44

Cabassa LJ, Ezell JM, Lewis-Fernández R (2010) Lifestyle interventions for adults with serious mental illness: a systematic literature review. Psychiatr Serv 61(8):774–782

Cardenas J, Frye MA, Marusak SL, Levander EM, Chirichigno JW, Lewis S et al (2008) Modal subcomponents of metabolic syndrome in patients with bipolar disorder. J Affect Disord 106(1–2):91–97, http://doi.org/10.1016/j.jad.2007.05.030

Castrogiovanni S, Soreca I, Troiani D, Mauri M (2009) Binge eating, weight gain and psychosocial adjustment in patients with bipolar disorder. Psychiatry Res 169(1):88–90, http://doi.org/10.1016/j.psychres.2008.06.016

Choi J, Joseph L, Pilote L (2013) Obesity and C-reactive protein in various populations: a systematic review and meta-analysis. Obes Rev 14(3):232–244, http://doi.org/10.1111/obr.12003

Chrousos GP (2009) Stress and disorders of the stress system. Nat Rev Endocrinol 5(7):374–381, http://doi.org/10.1038/nrendo.2009.106

Correll CU, Frederickson AM, Kane JM, Manu P (2006) Metabolic syndrome and the risk of coronary heart disease in 367 patients treated with second-generation antipsychotic drugs. J Clin Psychiatry 67(4):575–583

Correll CU, Frederickson AM, Kane JM, Manu P (2008) Equally increased risk for metabolic syndrome in patients with bipolar disorder and schizophrenia treated with second-generation antipsychotics. Bipolar Disord 10(7):788–797, http://doi.org/10.1111/j.1399-5618.2008.00625.x

Expert Panel on Detection, Evaluation, and Treatment of High Blood Cholesterol in Adults (2001) Executive summary of the third report of the National Cholesterol Education Program (NCEP) expert panel on detection, evaluation, and treatment of high blood cholesterol in adults (adult treatment panel III). JAMA 285(19):2486–2497

Fagiolini A, Kupfer DJ, Houck PR, Novick DM, Frank E (2003) Obesity as a correlate of outcome in patients with bipolar I disorder. Am J Psychiatr 160(1):112–117

Fagiolini A, Frank E, Scott JA, Turkin S, Kupfer DJ (2005) Metabolic syndrome in bipolar disorder: findings from the Bipolar Disorder Center for Pennsylvanians. Bipolar Disord 7(5):424–430, http://doi.org/10.1111/j.1399-5618.2005.00234.x

Fagiolini A, Chengappa KNR, Soreca I, Chang J (2008) Bipolar disorder and the metabolic syndrome. CNS Drugs 22(8):655–669, http://doi.org/10.2165/00023210-200822080-00004

Fiedorowicz JG, Palagummi NM, Forman-Hoffman VL, Miller DD, Haynes WG (2008) Elevated prevalence of obesity, metabolic syndrome, and cardiovascular risk factors in bipolar disorder. Ann Clin Psychiatry 20(3):131–137, http://doi.org/10.1080/10401230802177722

Fiedorowicz JG, Solomon DA, Endicott J, Leon AC, Li C, Rice JP, Coryell WH (2009) Manic/hypomanic symptom burden and cardiovascular mortality in bipolar disorder. Psychosom Med 71(6):598–606, http://doi.org/10.1097/PSY.0b013e3181acee26

Garcia-Portilla MP, Sáiz PA, Benabarre A, Sierra P, Perez J, Rodriguez A et al (2008) The prevalence of metabolic syndrome in patients with bipolar disorder. J Affect Disord 106(1–2):197–201, http://doi.org/10.1016/j.jad.2007.06.002

Garcia-Portilla MP, Sáiz PA, Bascaran MT, Martínez AS, Benabarre A, Sierra P et al (2009) Cardiovascular risk in patients with bipolar disorder. J Affect Disord 115(3):302–308, http://doi.org/10.1016/j.jad.2008.09.008

Goldstein BI, Fagiolini A, Houck P, Kupfer DJ (2009) Cardiovascular disease and hypertension among adults with bipolar I disorder in the United States. Bipolar Disord 11(6):657–662, http://doi.org/10.1111/j.1399-5618.2009.00735.x

Grover S, Aggarwal M, Chakrabarti S, Dutt A, Avasthi A, Kulhara P et al (2012) Prevalence of metabolic syndrome in bipolar disorder: an exploratory study from North India. Prog Neuro-Psychopharmacol Biol Psychiatry 36(1):141–146, http://doi.org/10.1016/j.pnpbp.2011.10.013

John AP, Koloth R, Dragovic M, Lim SCB (2009) Prevalence of metabolic syndrome among Australians with severe mental illness. Med J Aust 190(4):176–179

Kallner G, Lindelius R, Petterson U, Stockman O, Tham A (2000) Mortality in 497 patients with affective disorders attending a lithium clinic or after having left it. Pharmacopsychiatry 33(1):8–13, http://doi.org/10.1055/s-2000-7965

Keck PE, McElroy SL (2003) Bipolar disorder, obesity, and pharmacotherapy-associated weight gain. J Clin Psychiatry 64(12):1426–1435

Kelly EL, Fenwick KM, Barr N, Cohen H, Brekke JS (2014) A systematic review of self-management health care models for individuals with serious mental illnesses. Psychiatr Serv 65(11):1300–1310, http://doi.org/10.1176/appi.ps.201300502

Kemp AH, Quintana DS (2013) The relationship between mental and physical health: insights from the study of heart rate variability. Int J Psychophysiol 89(3):288–296, http://doi.org/10.1016/j.ijpsycho.2013.06.018

Kemp DE, Eudicone JM, McQuade RD, Chambers JS, Baker RA (2010) Metabolic syndrome and its potential effect on treatment response to aripiprazole a post hoc analysis of the stabilization phase of a long-term, double-blind study in patients with bipolar disorder (CN138-010). J Clin Psychopharmacol 30(5):631–634, http://doi.org/10.1097/JCP.0b013e3181f0569f

Lakka H, Laaksonen DE, Lakka TA, Niskanen LK, Kumpusalo E, Tuomilehto J, Salonen JT (2002) The metabolic syndrome and total and cardiovascular disease mortality in middle-aged men. JAMA 288(21):2709–2716

Lee NY, Kim SH, Cho B, Lee YJ, Chang JS, Kang UG et al (2010) Patients taking medications for bipolar disorder are more prone to metabolic syndrome than Korea's general population. Prog Neuro-Psychopharmacol Biol Psychiatry 34(7):1243–1249, http://doi.org/10.1016/j.pnpbp.2010.06.029

Maina G, Salvi V, Vitalucci A, D'Ambrosio V, Bogetto F (2008) Prevalence and correlates of overweight in drug-naïve patients with bipolar disorder. J Affect Disord 110(1–2):149–155, http://doi.org/10.1016/j.jad.2007.12.233

Malik S, Wong ND, Franklin SS, Kamath TV, L'Italien GJ, Pio JR, Williams GR (2004) Impact of the metabolic syndrome on mortality from coronary heart disease, cardiovascular disease, and all causes in united states adults. Circulation 110(10):1245–1250, http://doi.org/10.1161/01.CIR.0000140677.20606.0E

Mansur RB, Brietzke E, McIntyre RS (2015) Is there a "metabolic-mood syndrome?" A review of the relationship between obesity and mood disorders. Neurosci Biobehav Rev 52:89–104, http://doi.org/10.1016/j.neubiorev.2014.12.017

Mayer EA, Fanselow MS (2003) Dissecting the components of the central response to stress. Nat Neurosci 6(10):1011–1012, http://doi.org/10.1038/nn1003-1011

McElroy SL, Frye MA, Suppes T, Dhavale D, Keck PEJ, Leverich GS et al (2002) Correlates of overweight and obesity in 644 patients with bipolar disorder. J Clin Psychiatry 63(3):207–213

McElroy SL, Frye MA, Hellemann G, Altshuler L, Leverich GS, Suppes T et al (2011) Prevalence and correlates of eating disorders in 875 patients with bipolar disorder. J Affect Disord 128(3):191–198, http://doi.org/10.1016/j.jad.2010.06.037

McElroy SL, Kemp DE, Friedman ES, Reilly-Harrington NA, Sylvia LG, Calabrese JR et al (2015) Obesity, but not metabolic syndrome, negatively affects outcome in bipolar disorder. Acta Psychiatr Scand 133(2):144–153, http://doi.org/10.1111/acps.12460

McIntyre RS, Danilewitz M, Liauw SS, Kemp DE, Nguyen HTT, Kahn LS et al (2010) Bipolar disorder and metabolic syndrome: an international perspective. J Affect Disord 126(3):366–387

Murray DP, Weiner M, Prabhakar M, Fiedorowicz JG (2009) Mania and mortality: why the excess cardiovascular risk in bipolar disorder? Curr Psychiatr Rep 11(6):475–480

Murray G, Suto M, Hole R, Hale S, Amari E, Michalak EE (2010) Self-management strategies used by "high functioning" individuals with bipolar disorder: from research to clinical practice. Clin Psychol Psychother 18(2):95–109, http://doi.org/10.1002/cpp.710

Murray DP, Metz NS, Haynes WG, Fiedorowicz JG (2012) Vascular function is not impaired early in the course of bipolar disorder. J Psychosom Res 72(3):195–198, http://doi.org/10.1016/j.jpsychores.2011.12.006

Nemeroff CB (2003) Safety of available agents used to treat bipolar disorder: focus on weight gain. J Clin Psychiatry 64(5):532–539

NICE (2006) Bipolar disorder: the management of bipolar disorder in adults, children and adolescents, in primary and secondary care: clinical guideline 38. National Institute of Health and Care Excellence, London

NICE (2015) Bipolar disorder: the assessment and management of bipolar disorder in adults, children and young people in primary and secondary care. NICE clinical guideline 185. National Institute of Health and Care Excellence, London

Outhred T, Kemp AH, Malhi GS (2014) Physiological correlates of bipolar spectrum disorders and their treatment. In: Kumari V, Boutros N, Bob P (eds) Current topics in behavioral neurosciences. Springer, Berlin, pp 1–56, http://doi.org/10.1007/7854_2014_297

Reaven GM (1988) Role of insulin resistance in human disease. Diabetes 37(12):1595–1607

Redlich C, Berk M, Williams LJ, Sundquist J, Sundquist K, Li X (2014) Statin use and risk of depression: a Swedish national cohort study. BMC Psychiatr 14:348, http://doi.org/10.1186/s12888-014-0348-y

Russell SJ, Browne JL (2005) Staying well with bipolar disorder. Aust N Z J Psychiatry 39(3):187–193, http://doi.org/10.1111/j.1440-1614.2005.01542.x

Sodhi SK, Linder J, Chenard CA, Miller DD, Haynes WG, Fiedorowicz JG (2012) Evidence for accelerated vascular aging in bipolar disorder. J Psychosom Res 73(3):175–179, http://doi.org/10.1016/j.jpsychores.2012.06.004

Stafford L, Berk M (2011) The use of statins after a cardiac intervention is associated with reduced risk of subsequent depression: proof of concept for the inflammatory and oxidative hypotheses of depression? J Clin Psychiatry 72(9):1229–1235, http://doi.org/10.4088/JCP.09m05825blu

Taylor V, MacQueen G (2006) Associations between bipolar disorder and metabolic syndrome: a review. J Clin Psychiatry 67(7):1034–1041

Theisen FM, Linden A, König IR, Martin M, Remschmidt H, Hebebrand J (2003) Spectrum of binge eating symptomatology in patients treated with clozapine and olanzapine. J Neural Transm 110(1):111–121, http://doi.org/10.1007/s00702-002-0792-6

Vancampfort D, Vansteelandt K, Correll CU, Mitchell AJ, De Herdt A, Sienaert P et al (2013) Metabolic syndrome and metabolic abnormalities in bipolar disorder: a meta-analysis of prevalence rates and moderators. Am J Psychiatr 170(3):265–274, http://doi.org/10.1176/appi.ajp.2012.12050620

Weiner M, Warren L, Fiedorowicz JG (2011) Cardiovascular morbidity and mortality in bipolar disorder. Ann Clin Psychiatry 23(1):40–47

Wildes JE, Marcus MD, Fagiolini A (2008) Prevalence and correlates of eating disorder co-morbidity in patients with bipolar disorder. Psychiatry Res 161(1):51–58, http://doi.org/10.1016/j.psychres.2007.09.003

Wong ND, Pio JR, Franklin SS, L'Italien GJ, Kamath TV, Williams GR (2003) Preventing coronary events by optimal control of blood pressure and lipids in patients with the metabolic syndrome. Am J Cardiol 91(12):1421–1426

Yilmaz J, Povey L, Dalgliesh J (2011) Adopting a psychological approach to obesity. Nurs Stand 25(21):42–46, http://doi.org/10.7748/ns2011.01.25.21.42.c8289

Yumru M, Savas HA, Kurt E, Kaya MC, Selek S, Savas E et al (2007) Atypical antipsychotics related metabolic syndrome in bipolar patients. J Affect Disord 98(3):247–252, http://doi.org/10.1016/j.jad.2006.08.009

Assessment and Psychological Interventions for Depression Comorbid with Cardiovascular Disease

20

Evelyn Smith and Ian Kneebone

Contents

Abstract

Depression is common in those with cardiovascular disease and is independently associated with increased cardiovascular morbidity and mortality. On this account identifying and treating depression are of utmost importance in this group. In this chapter we consider tools to screen for depression in cardiac patients and review the evidence of the effectiveness of psychological interventions for depression in those with cardiovascular disease, including stroke.

E. Smith (✉)
Clinical and Health Psychology Research Initiative,
School of Social Sciences and Psychology, Western Sydney University,
Richmond, NSW, Australia
e-mail: evelyn.smith@unsw.edu.au

I. Kneebone
Discipline of Clinical Psychology, Graduate School of Health,
University of Technology Sydney, Ultimo, NSW, Australia

B.T. Baune, P.J. Tully (eds.), *Cardiovascular Diseases and Depression*,
DOI 10.1007/978-3-319-32480-7_20

There are numerous cardiovascular disease (CVD) risk factors that can be modified or managed, including high blood pressure, high cholesterol, smoking, obesity, physical inactivity, diabetes, unhealthy diets and harmful use of alcohol (World Heart Federation 2015). Research has found that 90 % of CVD is preventable by modifying these risk factors (Mendis et al. 2011; McGill et al. 2008).

Many people need help with changing behaviours that increase the risk of CVD, including stopping smoking, increasing physical activity and eating healthily. There is also a psychological component to many of these risk factors. For example, some individuals use smoking, alcohol and food to cope with their *emotions* (Holahan et al. 2003; Konttinen et al. 2010), and some people hold *beliefs* that interfere with their health (Carpenter 2010; Dennis and Goldberg 1996; Horne and Weinman 1999). Individuals may also need support to manage other health problems (e.g. diabetes, high blood pressure) and mental illnesses (e.g. anxiety, depression and personality disorders). Mental illness can also exacerbate the negative behaviours that impact on these risk factors. For example, depression may interfere with engaging in physical activity and may impact on diet (Jacka and Berk 2013).

Depression after CVD is a predictor of a 1-year cardiac mortality (Kop et al. 2010), and one study found that even mild symptoms of depression can predict mortality, morbidity and poorer clinical outcomes in those with myocardial infarction (Lespérance et al. 2007). Evidence suggests that around 15–20 % of cardiac patients experience clinical depression (Tully and Baker 2012) and around 31 % of stroke patients experience significant symptoms (Hackett and Pickles 2014). Depression is a major predictor of poor adherence in patients with CVD, be it to drug therapy or lifestyle changes (Kronish et al. 2006). Depression after stroke appears to influence morbidity and mortality (Morris et al. 1993) and affects functional outcome (Herrmann et al. 1998). Consequently, treating depression in the context of CVD is important. There are many benefits associated with treating depression, including improved quality of life, improved adherence to other therapies and, potentially, improved CVD outcomes (Gulliksson et al. 2011). Psychological treatment has been found to be better at treating depression effectively in the long term compared to antidepressants (Spielmans et al. 2011).

Psychologists can provide psychological care and support to individuals with CVD and comorbid depression, and the evidence for the effectiveness is summarised below. Studies on CVD usually include myocardial infarction, a revascularisation procedure [coronary artery bypass grafting or percutaneous transluminal coronary angioplasty], or having been diagnosed with coronary heart disease. There is also an emerging evidence base to support the effectiveness of psychological interventions for depression after stroke. Below we review how to screen for depression in cardiac and stroke patients and how depression can be managed in these samples.

20.1 Screening for Depression in Cardiac and Stroke Patients

The consensus statement from the National Heart Foundation of Australia (NHFA) reported the need for routine screening for depression in all patients with cardiovascular disease. Screening should occur at first presentation,

2–3 months after the event and then on a yearly basis (Colquhoun et al. 2013). Similarly, the National Stroke Foundation's (2010) Clinical Guidelines for Stroke Management have recommended screening for depression with a validated instrument, though no time frames are specified. However, after screening it is imperative that patients be properly referred and treated and that there should be pathways to do this appropriately (Colquhoun et al. 2013). Some medical professionals have said that the screen-and-treat models of depression are insufficient without a proper follow-up and referral pathways. It is advised that medical practitioners refer a patient with symptoms of depression to a local psychologist; however, there is no clear research of when to refer them.

There are many free screening tools for depression in CVD patients available, for example:

- *Patient Health Questionnaire-9 and Patient Health Questionnaire-2* (PHQ-9; Kroenke et al. 2001, PHQ-2; Kroenke et al. 2003): The PHQ-9 is a self-administered tool for assessing depression. The PHQ-2 uses only the first two items of PHQ-9 and it is commonly used for screening. It inquires about the degree to which an individual has experienced depressed mood and anhedonia over the past 2 weeks (Gilbody et al. 2007). PHQ-9 scores >10 had a sensitivity of 88 % and a specificity of 88 % for major depression, and it has been shown to be a reliable and valid tool (Kroenke et al. 2001).
- *Cardiac Depression Scale* (CDS; Hare and Davis 1996): The CDS is a 26-item inventory to assess depressive symptoms in cardiac patients. Respondents answer questions, in an interview, and indicate the appropriate number on a Likert scale that expresses the strength of their response to an item. There are seven positively worded items (e.g. 'My concentration is as good as it ever was'), which are reverse coded for aggregation and statistical analysis. A cut-off score of 95 has 97 % sensitivity and 85 % specificity for major depression (Hare and Davis 1996). Unfortunately, no other evidence regarding the CDS to detect major depression in CVD currently exists.
- *Geriatric Depression Scale – short form* (GDS-sf; Yesavage and Sheikh 1986): The GDS-sf, a short form of the GDS, is a 15-item inventory used to screen for mild to moderate depression symptoms. The reliability and validity of the GDS-sf have been demonstrated among the elderly (Marc et al. 2008), individuals with dementia (Lesher and Berryhill 1994) and chronic heart failure outpatients (Haworth et al. 2007). A score of more than five suggests that a clinical assessment should be undertaken.
- *Depression Anxiety Stress Scale* (DASS-42; Lovibond and Lovibond 1995; Kutlubaev and Hackett 2014): DASS-42 is a 42-item self-report instrument designed to measure the three related negative emotional states of depression, anxiety and tension/stress. There is also a short version with 21 items that has been found to be reliable and valid (Antony et al. 1998; Gloster et al. 2008). The DASS is the most commonly used screening measure in Australian hospitals.

With respect to stroke, a number of self-report instruments have received empirical support in screening for depression, including the PHQ-9 to detect major depression and the GDS-sf to identify milder symptoms (Burton and Tyson 2015). Due to the diversity of the findings in the literature, however, clear recommendations for cut-offs on these cannot currently be made. Despite this, as a guide, a cut-off of >9 on PHQ-9 has been suggested (Williams et al. 2005) and on the GDS-sf a cut-off slightly lower than for CVD, of >4 (Lee and Park 2008). The lack of clear guidance on cut-offs on depression screening instruments in stroke (Burton and Tyson 2015) is less of an issue than it may seem as cut-offs can be set dependent on the purpose of screening and the resources available. For instance, lower cut-offs can be used where a higher number of false positives can be tolerated in order that true positives are not overlooked. A number of other instruments can be used to screen for depression after stroke:

- *Hospital Anxiety and Depression Scale – Depression subscale (HADS-D;* Zigmond and Snaith 1983): The HADS was developed specifically to assess mood symptoms in people with physical illness. It consists of 14 items with two subscales: anxiety (seven items) and depression (seven items). Patient's scores range 0–3 with reference to each item and their experience in the last 7 days. The depression subscale has a range of 0–21. As noted above a literature review failed to give clear guidance on the cut-offs for depression in stroke populations; however >8 is commonly used (Kneebone et al. 2010). One attraction of the HADS is that it also includes an anxiety measure; however it has been criticised as it can require initial and recurrent costs (Burton and Tyson 2015).

The fact that many with stroke have cognitive and communication problems means that some patients are not accessible to screening for depression via self-report measures. On this account observational measures and simplified measures using visual stimuli have been developed to screen for depression.

- *Stroke Aphasic Depression Questionnaire Hospital, 10-item version* (SADQ-H10; Lincoln et al. 2000) and the *Stroke Aphasic Depression Questionnaire, 10-item version* (SADQ-10; Sutcliffe and Lincoln 1998). The SADQs are observer rating scales to identify depression in people with communication disorder after stroke. The former is designed for the use in inpatient settings and utilises staff observations; the latter is designed for community use, to be completed by carers or someone who knows the patient well. The H10 utilises more specific categories with respect to screen items, e.g. '2–4 times a week', whereas the 10, less specific ones such as 'sometimes' and 'rarely'. Research has supported the reliability of these different categories (Lincoln et al. 2012).
- *Depression Intensity Scale Circles* (DISCs; Turner-Stokes et al. 2005): The DISCs consists of six circles of equivalent size displayed vertically. Each circle has an increasing proportion of grey shading, from no shading at the bottom of

the display to completely shading at the top. The degree of shading indicates the level of depression. A further version of the DISCs incorporates a sad and smiley face as anchor points. A cut-off of >1 for significant depression is recommended for use with this instrument.

It should be noted screening instruments in themselves do not diagnose depression. Patients who receive a positive screening will need further evaluation and will need to be referred for a formal clinical assessment by a psychologist or psychiatrist.

A relatively recent development in stroke is the determining of screening protocols to detect mood disorder after stroke (Kneebone et al. 2012; Lincoln et al. 2012). These consist of specific information on what instrument to use with which patient based on presentation factors such as age, cognitive and communication deficits. Figure 20.1 displays one such protocol developed for screening in an acute setting (Galvin et al. 2014). Based on whether a severe cognitive or communication disorder is present, self-report measures or observational measures are utilised. The protocol also incorporates a procedure to screen for the presence of suicidal ideas. The protocol also includes how to interpret results and the actions required based on these. Along with relatively brief training, such protocols support those not trained or not practising in mental health (who make up the majority of stroke clinicians) to feel confident in conducting screens and thus support compliance with guidelines (Kneebone et al. 2013).

20.2 Psychological Interventions for Depression in Those with CVD

There are many different types of psychological interventions that have been used in CVD patients and individuals at risk of CVD. A recent Cochrane systematic review and meta-analysis (Whalley et al. 2014) found that psychological intervention did result in moderate improvements in depression in those with CVD. There were also significantly fewer deaths attributed to cardiac causes among treated patients. However, it found no strong evidence that psychological intervention reduced all-cause mortality or nonfatal infarction in patients with CVD.

This review also found that certain styles of psychological treatment for comorbid depression and CVD are not always beneficial. For example, including other family members in treatment, allowing the clients to lead the discussion or providing support were negatively associated with depression outcomes (Whalley et al. 2014). However, not all psychological interventions are equally effective. A systematic review and meta-analysis found that among high-quality trials, only cognitive behavioural therapy was effective, but only a small effect was found (Dickens et al. 2013). We will look closely at cognitive behavioural therapy, a widely accepted evidence-based treatment option. There are other interventions that have been investigated, including problem solving, skills training and relaxation, all showing small effect sizes when including both low- and high-quality studies (Dickens et al. 2013).

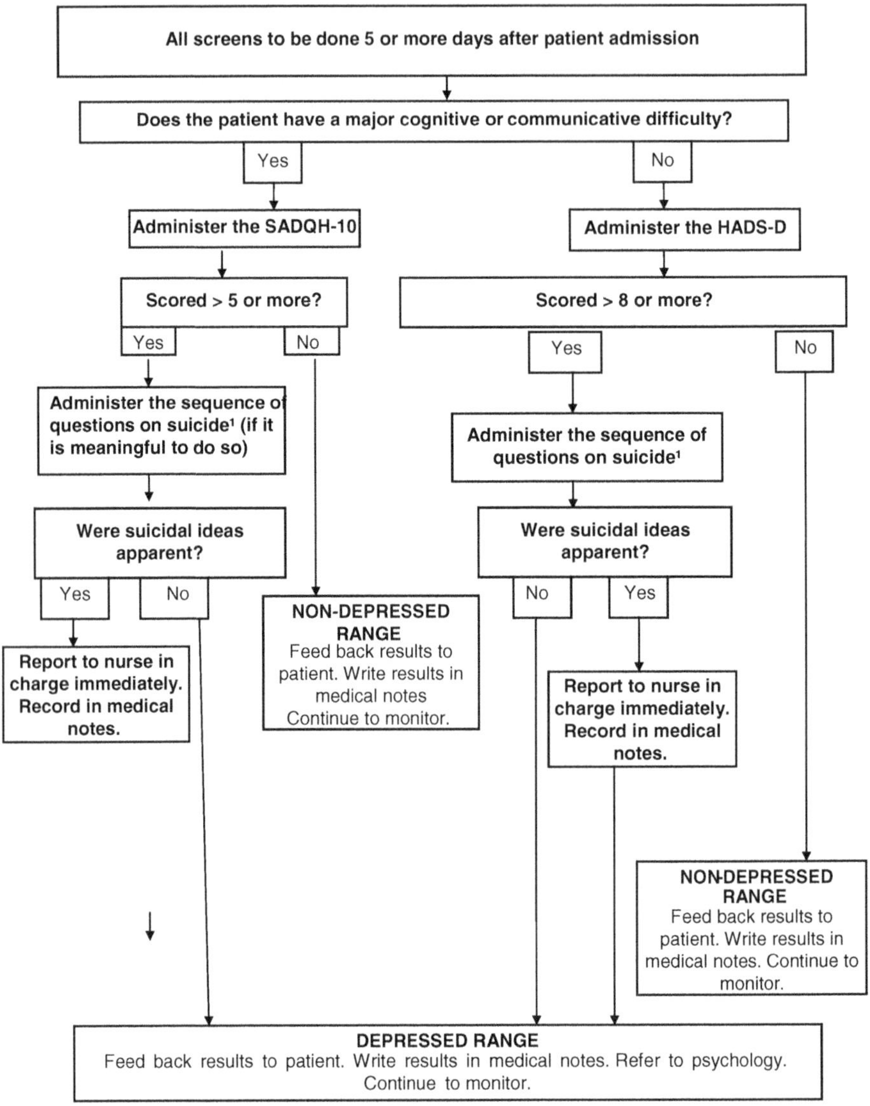

Fig. 20.1 Flow chart for post-stroke depression screening derived from Galvin et al. (2014). *HADS-D* hospital anxiety and depression scale – depression subscale, *SADQ-H10* stroke aphasic depression questionnaire hospital, 10-item version

For those individuals with CVD and depression who are not ready for change, motivational interviewing (Miller and Rollnick 2009) can be delivered before cognitive behavioural therapy.

20.2.1 Cognitive Behavioural Therapy (CBT)

Cognitive behavioural therapy (CBT) is a short-term, individualised, collaborative intervention designed at modifying unhelpful thoughts, behaviours and emotions that maintain a condition. There is strong evidence that CBT is effective at treating depression (Cuijpers et al. 2013). Cardiac patients usually have beliefs, emotions and behaviours that maintain their depression. CBT can also focus on changing health-related behaviours, including alcohol consumption, eating, physical activity, smoking and problem-solving ability.

Cognitive behavioural therapy has been used to treat depression in older patients with elevated CVD risk (Strachowski et al. 2008). Fifty seven percent of participants were in remission after 16 sessions of individual CBT ($n=23$), compared to only 4 % of the waitlist control ($n=25$) (Strachowski et al. 2008). In the Enhancing Recovery in Coronary Heart Disease (ENRICHD) patients trial, individuals with myocardial infarction treated with CBT had fewer depressive symptoms than those receiving usual care at 6 months posttreatment. However, differences in depression did not translate to differences in CVD outcomes (Berkman et al. 2003).

Another study compared traditional care to traditional care plus a CBT program, with 20 2-h sessions during 1 year, in persons with recurrent CVD (Gulliksson et al. 2011). The study included 362 individuals aged 75 years or younger. During a mean 94 months of follow-up, the intervention group had a 41 % lower rate of fatal and nonfatal first recurrent CVD events, 45 % fewer recurrent acute myocardial infarctions and a 28 % lower all-cause mortality (not statistically significant) than the control group after adjustment for confounding variables.

Cognitive behaviour therapy (CBT) is efficacious in the acute treatment of depression and provides a viable alternative to antidepressant medication. More importantly, CBT has an enduring effect that protects against subsequent relapse following the end of active treatment, something that cannot be said for medications (Driessen and Hollon 2010). However, some people may not be ready or be ambivalent towards change; in this case motivational interviewing can be used before implementing CBT.

20.2.2 Motivational Interviewing

Motivational interviewing is a person-centred approach that facilitates intrinsic motivation and aims at changing people's perceptions of their behaviour (Miller and Rollnick 2009). The first stage involves discussing the discrepancy of the patients' beliefs to the patients' behaviour. This is done in an empathic way and direct confrontation is avoided as it may induce resistance. Instead, the individual is encouraged to reflect on their situation and talk about ways they want to change. Motivational interviewing enhances self-efficacy, autonomy and competency by setting goals, providing feedback, eliciting change talk and exploring possibilities (Miller and Rollnick 2009).

A systematic review and meta-analysis showed that motivational interviewing had a significant and clinically relevant effect in three out of four studies, for both physiological and psychological diseases (Rubak et al. 2005). Motivational interviewing has been applied to patients with CVD in order to modify their ill-health lifestyle to decrease the risk of CVD occurrence (for a review see Thompson et al. 2011). For example, one study found that motivational interviewing in cardiac rehabilitation patients was effective at reducing depression symptoms; however, surprisingly they were found to have an increase in anxiety level when compared to controls (Chair et al. 2012). Motivational interviewing was also effective at changing other CVD risk factors, including physical activity and cholesterol (Hardcastle et al. 2013), smoking (Bredie et al. 2011; Groeneveld et al. 2011), body weight (Groeneveld et al. 2010) and snack intake (Groeneveld et al. 2011), but long-term follow-ups are needed.

Motivational interviewing has also been integrated into cognitive behavioural therapy and applied to individuals with depression (Westra 2004; Arkowitz and Westra 2004). Whether integrating these treatments in the context of CVD and comorbid depression would be beneficial remains to be examined.

20.3 Psychological Interventions for Stroke

20.3.1 Prevention of Depression After Stroke

Attention to depression in stroke has taken two main approaches, prevention and treatment. Preventative approaches take a variety of forms including the provision of support groups, befriending, art therapy, music therapy and attending to the overall experience of patients of what is important to them in their rehabilitation (Kneebone, in press). Specific psychological therapies have some support here including motivational interviewing and problem solving. The intention of motivational interviewing in this instance is not to change health-related behaviours but to support the management of adversity. It involves a therapist countering ambivalence alongside developing optimism and confidence to overcome challenges (Miller and Rollnick 2012; Watkins and French 2009). Motivational interviewing after stroke has been demonstrated to prevent depression and reduce morbidity in a randomised controlled trial (Watkins et al. 2007).

Problem solving is a systematic way of tackling issues that are amenable to change. Problem solving is a structured approach which generally involves a number of stages: problem definition, identifying solutions via brainstorming, solution evaluation, response selection, developing a plan and then acting upon it (Montgomery and Evans 1984). Along with motivational interviewing, problem solving is considered to have an evidence base for the prevention of depression after stroke (Hackett et al. 2008).

New developments in the prevention of depression after stroke are under evaluation, for example, the aphasia action success knowledge (ASK) intervention case series study, designed to prevent depression in people with aphasia and their carers after stroke. It is delivered by speech pathologists, and includes the development of a stroke narrative, attention to enjoyable activities and accessing social support after stroke (Grohn et al. 2013; Simmons-Mackie 2013). The strategy is currently being subject to RCT evaluation (Worrall et al. 2016).

20.3.2 Treatment of Depression After Stroke

Until recently there was no real evidence base for psychological intervention for depression after stroke. Despite promising case series support for its efficacy (Lincoln et al. 1997; Rasquin et al. 2009), the only randomised controlled trial of cognitive behaviour therapy to date failed to indicate a treatment response (Lincoln and Flannaghan 2003). In contrast, one behavioural component often used in CBT, behavioural activation, has found to be useful in isolation, when tested via randomised controlled trial in those with stroke with significant aphasia (Thomas et al. 2013). Why CBT has been less successful has been debated in the literature. However, the consensus does seem to be that while CBT is one of the most proven of therapies in the non-stroke population (Butler et al. 2006; Gloaguen et al. 1998), it requires substantial modification if it is to be successful with people who have had a stroke (Broomfield et al. 2011; Kneebone 2016). Such modified treatment is yet to be evaluated.

A holistic approach to both prevention and treatment of distress after stroke has been proposed. This is based on the stepped care model developed for mental health in the UK (Davison 2000; National Health Service 2014), which proposes that each person with stroke receives psychosocial care in accordance with the nature and severity of symptoms (Gillham and Clark 2011). An elaboration on this latter model is presented in Fig. 20.2. Level 1 directs services to all persons with stroke and is aimed at general support and prevention, level 2 those with clinically significant symptoms of anxiety or depression and level 3 those with more severe symptoms or conditions that require specialist care. Level 4 addresses the needs of a small but significant group of stroke survivors, those presenting with serious challenging behaviours. The elaboration provides indications for how to determine the appropriate level for a particular presentation (Kneebone, in press).

20.4 Clinical Implications

Health practitioners working with CVD patients who choose to follow NHFA guidelines and screen for depression in cardiac patients should only do this when there are appropriate referral pathways in place. Psychological treatment, such as cognitive behavioural therapy, does reduce depressive symptoms in individuals with CVD and can improve an individual's quality of life. Research on depression in psychological interventions to manage and prevent depression in stroke requires further research but shows promise.

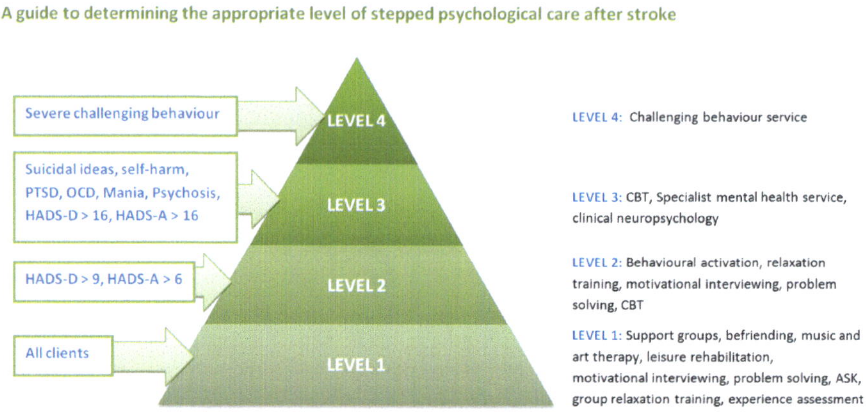

Fig. 20.2 A revised model for stepped psychological care after stroke. Kneebone (in press). Stepped psychological care after stroke. *Disabil Rehabil* (Reproduced with permission. Note: *ASK* action success knowledge programme for people with aphasia, *HADS* hospital anxiety and depression scale, *HADS-D* hospital anxiety and depression scale – depression subscale, *HADS-A* hospital anxiety and depression scale – anxiety subscale, *CBT* cognitive behaviour therapy, *PTSD* post-traumatic stress disorder, *OCD* obsessive-compulsive disorder)

References

Antony MM, Bieling PJ, Cox BJ, Enns MW, Swinson RP (1998) Psychometric properties of the 42-item and 21-item versions of the depression anxiety stress scales in clinical groups and a community sample. Psychol Assess 10:176–181

Arkowitz H, Westra HA (2004) Integrating motivational interviewing and cognitive behavioral therapy in the treatment of depression and anxiety. J Cogn Psychother 18:337–350

Berkman LF, Blumenthal J, Burg M, Carney RM, Catellier D, Cowan MJ, Czajkowski SM, Debusk R, Hosking J, Jaffee A, Kaufmann PG, Mitchell P, Norman J, Powell LH, Raczynski JM, Schneiderman N (2003) Effects of treating depression and low perceived social support on clinical events after myocardial infarction: the Enhancing Recovery in Coronary Heart Disease Patients (ENRICHD) randomized trial. JAMA: J Am Med Assoc 289:3106–3116

Bredie SJH, Fouwels AJ, Wollersheim H, Schippers GM (2011) Effectiveness of nurse based motivational interviewing for smoking cessation in high risk cardiovascular outpatients: a randomized trial. Eur J Cardiovasc Nurs 10:174–179

Broomfield NM, Laidlaw K, Hickabottom E, Murray MF, Pendrey R, Whittick JE, Gillespie DC (2011) Post stroke depression: the case for augmented, individually tailored cognitive behavioural therapy. Clin Psychol Psychother 18:202–217

Burton LJ, Tyson S (2015) Screening for mood disorders after stroke: a systematic review of psychometric properties and clinical utility. Psychol Med 45:29–49

Butler AC, Chapman JE, Forman EM, Beck AT (2006) The empirical status of cognitive-behavioral therapy: a review of meta-analyses. Clin Psychol Rev 26:17–31

Carpenter CJ (2010) A meta-analysis of the effectiveness of health belief model variables in predicting behavior. Health Commun 25:661–669

Chair SY, Chan SW-C, Thompson DR, Leung K-P, Ng SK-C, Choi KC (2012) Short-term effect of motivational interviewing on clinical and psychological outcomes and health-related quality of life in cardiac rehabilitation patients with poor motivation in Hong Kong: a randomized controlled trial. Eur J Prev Cardiol 19:1383–1392

Colquhoun DM, Bunker SJ, Clarke DM, Glozier N, Hare DL, Hickie IB, Tatoulis J, Thompson DR, Tofler GH, Wilson A, Branagan MG (2013) Screening, referral and treatment for depression in patients with coronary heart disease. Med J Aust 198:483–484
Cuijpers P, Berking M, Andersson G, Quigley L, Kleiboer A, Dobson KS (2013) A meta-analysis of cognitive-behavioural therapy for adult depression, alone and in comparison with other treatments. Can J Psychiatry/La Revue canadienne de psychiatrie 58:376–385
Davison GC (2000) Stepped care: doing more with less? J Consult Clin Psychol 68:580
Dennis KE, Goldberg AP (1996) Weight control self-efficacy types and transitions affect weight-loss outcomes in obese women. Addict Behav 21:103–116
Dickens C, Cherrington A, Adeyemi I, Roughley K, Bower P, Garrett C, Bundy C, Coventry P (2013) Characteristics of psychological interventions that improve depression in people with coronary heart disease: a systematic review and meta-regression. Psychosom Med 75(2):211–221. doi:10.1097/PSY.0b013e31827ac009.Epub2013Jan16
Driessen E, Hollon SD (2010) Cognitive behavioral therapy for mood disorders: efficacy, moderators and mediators. Psychiatr Clin North Am 33:537–555
Galvin R, Marsden D, Hambridge J, Quinn R, Bareham N, Wood D, Jordan L, Boyle K, Kneebone I, Cadilhac D (2014) The protocol for an implementation project: Identification of Altered Mood After Stroke (IAMAS). Int J Stroke 9:14
Gilbody S, Richards D, Brealey S, Hewitt C (2007) Screening for depression in medical settings with the Patient Health Questionnaire (PHQ): a diagnostic meta-analysis. J Gen Intern Med 22:1596–1602
Gillham S, Clark L (2011) Psychological care after stroke: improving stroke services for people with cognitive and mood disorders. NHS Improvement–Stroke, Leicester
Gloaguen V, Cottraux J, Cucherat M, Blackburn I-M (1998) A meta-analysis of the effects of cognitive therapy in depressed patients. J Affect Disord 49:59–72
Gloster AT, Rhoades HM, Novy D, Klotsche J, Senior A, Kunik M, Wilson N, Stanley MA (2008) Psychometric properties of the depression anxiety and stress scale-21 in older primary care patients. J Affect Disord 110:248–259
Groeneveld I, Proper K, Van der Beek A, Van Mechelen W (2010) Sustained body weight reduction by an individual-based lifestyle intervention for workers in the construction industry at risk for cardiovascular disease: results of a randomized controlled trial. Prev Med 51:240–246
Groeneveld I, Proper K, van der Beek A, Hildebrandt V, van Mechelen W (2011) Short and long term effects of a lifestyle intervention for construction workers at risk for cardiovascular disease: a randomized controlled trial. BMC Public Health 11:836
Grohn B, Brown K, Finch E, Worrall L, Simmons-mackie N (2013) Aphasia ASK (Access, Success, Knowledge) program: an intervention program designed to help meet the needs of people with aphasia early during rehabilitation. Speech Pathol Aust Conf, Broadbeach, Queensland, Australia.
Gulliksson M, Burell G, Vessby B, Lundin L, Toss H, Svärdsudd K (2011) Randomized controlled trial of cognitive behavioral therapy vs standard treatment to prevent recurrent cardiovascular events in patients with coronary heart disease: secondary prevention in uppsala primary health care project (suprim). Arch Intern Med 171:134–140
Hackett ML, Pickles K (2014) Part I: frequency of depression after stroke: an updated systematic review and meta-analysis of observational studies. Int J Stroke 9:1017–1025
Hackett ML, Anderson CS, House A, Halteh C (2008) Interventions for preventing depression after stroke. Cochrane Libr
Hardcastle SJ, Taylor AH, Bailey MP, Harley RA, Hagger MS (2013) Effectiveness of a motivational interviewing intervention on weight loss, physical activity and cardiovascular disease risk factors: a randomised controlled trial with a 12-month post-intervention follow-up. Int J Behav Nutr Phys Act 10:1–16
Hare DL, Davis CR (1996) Cardiac depression scale: validation of a new depression scale for cardiac patients. J Psychosom Res 40:379–386

Haworth J, Moniz-Cook E, Clark A, Wang M, Cleland J (2007) An evaluation of two self report screening measures for mood in an out-patient chronic heart failure population. Int J Geriatr Psychiatry 22:1147–1153
Herrmann N, Black SE, Lawrence J, Szekely C, Szalai JP (1998) The Sunnybrook stroke study: a prospective study of depressive symptoms and functional outcome. Stroke 29:618–624
Holahan CJ, Moos RH, Holahan CK, Cronkite RC, Randall PK (2003) Drinking to cope and alcohol use and abuse in unipolar depression: a 10-year model. J Abnorm Psychol 112:159–165
Horne R, Weinman J (1999) Patients' beliefs about prescribed medicines and their role in adherence to treatment in chronic physical illness. J Psychosom Res 47:555–567
Jacka FN, Berk M (2013) Depression, diet and exercise. Med J Aust 199:S21–S23
Kneebone II (2016) A framework to support cognitive behavior therapy for emotional disorder after stroke. Cogn Behav Pract 23:99–109
Kneebone I. Stepped psychological care after stroke. Disabil Rehabil (in press)
Kneebone I, Baker J, O'Malley H (2010) Screening for depression after stroke: developing protocols for the occupational therapist. Br J Occup Ther 73:71–76
Kneebone II, Neffgen LM, Pettyfer SL (2012) Screening for depression and anxiety after stroke: developing protocols for use in the community. Disabil Rehabil 34:1114–1120
Kneebone I, Stone N, Robertson S, Walker-Samuel N (2013) Screening for depression after stroke: occupational therapists' performance to protocols. Occup Ther Mental Health 29:106–113
Konttinen H, Männistö S, Sarlio-Lähteenkorva S, Silventoinen K, Haukkala A (2010) Emotional eating, depressive symptoms and self-reported food consumption. A population-based study. Appetite 54:473–479
Kop WJ, Stein PK, Tracy RP, Barzilay JI, Schulz R, Gottdiener JS (2010) Autonomic nervous system dysfunction and inflammation contribute to the increased cardiovascular mortality risk associated with depression. Psychosom Med 72:626
Kroenke K, Spitzer RL, Williams JBW (2001) The PHQ-9: validity of a brief depression severity measure. J Gen Intern Med 16:606–613
Kroenke K, Spitzer RL, Williams JBW (2003) The patient health questionnaire-2: validity of a two-item depression screener. Med Care 41:1284–1292
Kronish IM, Rieckmann N, Halm EA, Shimbo D, Vorchheimer D, Haas DC, Davidson KW (2006) Persistent depression affects adherence to secondary prevention behaviors after acute coronary syndromes. J Gen Intern Med 21:1178–1183
Kutlubaev MA, Hackett ML (2014) Part II: predictors of depression after stroke and impact of depression on stroke outcome: an updated systematic review of observational studies. Int J Stroke 9:1026–1036
Lee Y, Park K (2008) Does physical activity moderate the association between depressive symptoms and disability in older adults? Int J Geriatr Psychiatry 23:249–256
Lesher EL, Berryhill JS (1994) Validation of the geriatric depression scale-short form among inpatients. J Clin Psychol 50:256–260
Lespérance F, Frasure-Smith N, Koszycki D, Laliberté M-A, VAN Zyl LT, Baker B, Swenson JR, Ghatavi K, Abramson BL, Dorian P (2007) Effects of citalopram and interpersonal psychotherapy on depression in patients with coronary artery disease: the Canadian Cardiac Randomized Evaluation of Antidepressant and Psychotherapy Efficacy (CREATE) trial. JAMA 297:367–379
Lincoln N, Flannaghan T (2003) Cognitive behavioral psychotherapy for depression following stroke A randomized controlled trial. Stroke 34:111–115
Lincoln N, Flannaghan T, Sutcliffe L, Rother L (1997) Evaluation of cognitive behavioural treatment for depression after stroke: a pilot study. Clin Rehabil 11:114–122
Lincoln N, Sutcliffe L, Unsworth G (2000) Validation of the Stroke Aphasic Depression Questionnaire (SADQ) for use with patients in hospital. Clin Neuropsychol Assess 1:88–96
Lincoln NB, Kneebone II, Macniven JA, Morris RC (2012) Psychological management of stroke. Wiley-Blackwell, Chichester, UK
Lovibond PF, Lovibond SH (1995) The structure of negative emotional states: comparison of the Depression Anxiety Stress Scales (DASS) with the Beck depression and anxiety inventories. Behav Res Ther 33:335–343

Marc LG, Raue PJ, Bruce ML (2008) Screening performance of the 15-item geriatric depression scale in a diverse elderly home care population. Am J Geriatr Psychiatry 16:914–921
Mcgill HC, Mcmahan CA, Gidding SS (2008) Preventing heart disease in the 21st century: implications of the Pathobiological Determinants of Atherosclerosis in Youth (PDAY) study. Circulation 117:1216–1227
Mendis S, Puska P, Norrving B (2011) Global atlas on cardiovascular disease prevention and control. Geneva, World Health Organization
Miller WR, Rollnick S (2009) Ten things that motivational interviewing is not. Behav Cogn Psychother 37:129–140
Miller WR, Rollnick S (2012) Motivational interviewing: helping people change. Guilford press, New York
Montgomery B, Evans L (1984) You and stress: a guide to successful living. Nelson, Melbourne, Australia
Morris PL, Robinson RG, Andrzejewski P, Samuels J, Price TR (1993) Association of depression with 10-year poststroke mortality. Am J Psychiatry 150:124–129
National Health Service (2014) Improving access to psychological therapies [Online]. National Health Service. Available: http://www.iapt.nhs.uk/iapt/. Accessed 27 Apr 2015
National Stroke Foundation (2010) Clinical guidelines for stroke management [Online]. Available: http://strokefoundation.com.au/site/media/clinical_guidelines_stroke_managment_2010_interactive.pdf. Accessed 27 Nov 2014
Rasquin S, van de Sande P, Praamstra A, van Heugten C (2009) Cognitive-behavioural intervention for depression after stroke: five single case studies on effects and feasibility. Neuropsychol Rehabil 19:208–222
Rubak S, Sandbæk A, Lauritzen T, Christensen B (2005) Motivational interviewing: a systematic review and meta-analysis. Br J Gen Pract 55:305–312
Simmons-Mackie N (2013) A systems approach to training potential communication partners of people with aphasia. SIG 12 Perspect Augmentative Altern Commun 22:21–29
Spielmans GI, Berman MI, Usitalo AN (2011) Psychotherapy versus second-generation antidepressants in the treatment of depression: a meta-analysis. J Nerv Ment Dis 199:142–149
Strachowski D, Khaylis A, Conrad A, Neri E, Spiegel D, Taylor CB (2008) The effects of cognitive behavior therapy on depression in older patients with cardiovascular risk. Depress Anxiety 25:E1–E10
Sutcliffe L, Lincoln N (1998) The assessment of depression in aphasic stroke patients: the development of the stroke aphasic depression questionnaire. Clin Rehabil 12:506–513
Thomas SA, Walker MF, Macniven JA, Haworth H, Lincoln NB (2013) Communication and Low Mood (CALM): a randomized controlled trial of behavioural therapy for stroke patients with aphasia. Clin Rehabil 27:398–408
Thompson DR, Chair SY, Chan SW, Astin F, Davidson PM, Ski CF (2011) Motivational interviewing: a useful approach to improving cardiovascular health? J Clin Nurs 20:1236–1244
Tully PJ, Baker RA (2012) Depression, anxiety, and cardiac morbidity outcomes after coronary artery bypass surgery: a contemporary and practical review. J Geriatr Cardiol 9(2): 197–208
Turner-Stokes L, Kalmus M, Hirani D, Clegg F (2005) The Depression Intensity Scale Circles (DISCs): a first evaluation of a simple assessment tool for depression in the context of brain injury. J Neurol Neurosurg Psychiatry 76:1273–1278
Watkins CL, French B (2009) Psychological intervention poststroke ready for action? Stroke 40:2951–2952
Watkins CL, Auton MF, Deans CF, Dickinson HA, Jack CI, Lightbody CE, Sutton CJ, van den Broek MD, Leathley MJ (2007) Motivational interviewing early after acute stroke a randomized, controlled trial. Stroke 38:1004–1009
Westra H (2004) Managing resistance in cognitive behavioural therapy: the application of motivational interviewing in mixed anxiety and depression. Cogn Behav Ther 33:161–175
Whalley B, Thompson DR, Taylor RS (2014) Psychological interventions for coronary heart disease: cochrane systematic review and meta-analysis. Int J Behav Med 21:109–121

Williams LS, Brizendine EJ, Plue L, Bakas T, Tu W, Hendrie H, Kroenke K (2005) Performance of the PHQ-9 as a screening tool for depression after stroke. Stroke 36:635–638
World Heart Federation (2015) Cardiovascular disease risk factors [Online]. World Heart Federation. Available: http://www.world-heart-federation.org/cardiovascular-health/cardiovascular-disease-risk-factors/. Accessed 27 Apr 2015
Worrall L, Ryan B, Hudson K, Kneebone II, Simmons-Mackie N, Khan A, Hoffman T, Power E, Togher L, Rose M (2016) Reducing the psychosocial impact of aphasia on mood and quality of life in people with aphasia and the impact of caregiving in family members through the aphasia action success knowledge (Aphasia ASK) program: study protocol for a randomized controlled trial. Trials
Yesavage JA, Sheikh JI (1986) Geriatric Depression Scale (GDS). Clin Gerontol 5:165–173
Zigmond AS, Snaith RP (1983) The hospital anxiety and depression scale. Acta Psychiatr Scand 67:361–370

Moving Beyond Mood: Is it Time to Recommend Cognitive Training for Depression in Older Adults?

21

Sharon L. Naismith and Loren Mowszowski

Contents

S.L. Naismith (✉) • L. Mowszowski
Healthy Brain Ageing Program, School of Psychology, Charles Perkins Centre and Brain and Mind Research Centre, University of Sydney, Sydney, NSW, Australia
e-mail: sharon.naismith@sydney.edu.au

B.T. Baune, P.J. Tully (eds.), *Cardiovascular Diseases and Depression*,
DOI 10.1007/978-3-319-32480-7_21

Abstract
Major depression is often associated with neuropsychological deficits, most commonly in the areas of executive functioning (e.g. set-shifting, problem-solving, decision-making), information processing speed, new learning and memory. These cognitive deficits may be even more pronounced in older adults with depression and particularly in those with cardiovascular risk factors, where cognitive impairment is linked with multiple pathophysiologies including white matter lesions and alterations in key grey matter brain structures. In this group, underlying neurodegenerative pathology is also an important consideration. Of concern, cognitive deficits are predictive of treatment responsiveness and may persist despite depressive symptom resolution. However, most traditional treatments for depression (i.e. antidepressants and psychological therapies) do not focus on cognition. By contrast, cognitive training is a novel non-pharmacological therapy that may be used to directly target cognition and psychosocial functioning, by promoting neural plasticity. In this chapter, we review the evidence for cognitive training in depression with additional reference to work in healthy samples and those with neuropsychiatric and neurodegenerative disease. Studies using both computer-based and strategy-based training approaches are discussed. To date, there is a lack of well-controlled studies utilising cognitive training for people with depression. Nonetheless, 13 studies employing computer-based cognitive training programs reveal promising results, particularly for improving memory and mood. Further randomised controlled trials in those with depression are now required, to examine the potential magnitude of cognitive improvement and to determine which individual, clinical and treatment-related factors may influence treatment efficacy.

The hallmark symptoms of major depression (MD) are widely recognised to include persistent low mood and anhedonia (i.e. loss of pleasure or enjoyment of usual daily activities or hobbies). In addition to these core symptoms, persons with depression typically present with 'second-tier' symptoms such as feelings of guilt, worthlessness or suicidal ideation, amotivation, fatigue, appetite changes, weight loss or weight gain, altered sleep and circadian rhythms, sexual dysfunction and generalised pain (American Psychiatric Association 2013). Importantly, many patients also describe difficulties with aspects of cognition, including reduced concentration, feeling slowed down, having poor memory or with alterations in higher-level thinking skills such as poor decision-making and problem-solving (American Psychiatric Association 2013). Cognitive deficits in MD are a significant clinical issue, with data showing they are associated with disability (Naismith et al. 2007), psychosocial functioning (Bosworth et al. 2002) and poor functional outcomes (Baldwin et al. 2004; Baune et al. 2010).

Using formal neuropsychological tests, cognitive difficulties in MD are often characterised as resembling a 'fronto-subcortical' profile, with deficits in executive functioning, processing speed and memory being most pronounced (Naismith et al.

2003; Veiel 1997). Indeed, around one fifth of patients exhibit 'impairments' (i.e. >2 standard deviation (SD) decline relative to premorbid levels of general cognitive functioning) on at least two cognitive domains (Veiel 1997).

Executive dysfunction in older people with depression encompasses a wide array of functions including deficits in planning, organisation, sequencing, response inhibition, problem-solving and set-shifting (Herrmann et al. 2007; Naismith et al. 2003; Pisljar et al. 2008; Salloway et al. 1996). In particular, meta-analytic studies have shown that around 15 % of patients with depression perform in the 'impaired' ranges on tests of set-shifting and response inhibition (Veiel 1997). In older people with severe depressive disorders, deficits in the 'impaired' (<2 SD relative to normative samples) range are a prominent finding (Naismith et al. 2003). In the older person, executive deficits may be particularly severe in those with later ages of onset (Naismith et al. 2003; Salloway et al. 1996), and are of particular concern since they tend to be associated with a suboptimal prognosis, treatment resistance and lower remission rates (Baldwin et al. 2004; Sheline et al. 2010; Sneed et al. 2007). Additionally, such features have been linked to poor psychosocial functioning and difficulties in instrumental activities of daily living (Kiosses et al. 2000, 2001; Lockwood et al. 2000; Mackin and Arean 2009).

Slowed processing speed is a common feature of depression, particularly in later life. It has been linked to markers of cerebrovascular disease (Hickie et al. 2001) and is a key feature of 'vascular depression' (see below). Slowed processing speed may also be associated with poor treatment response (Hickie et al. 1995; Sheline et al. 2010; Simpson et al. 1997; Story et al. 2008), thus affirming the utility of considering cognitive function when determining treatment responsiveness. Processing speed is a prominent feature in severe depressive episodes and particularly melancholic and psychotic subtypes (Jeste et al. 1996; Naismith et al. 2003). However, this domain of cognitive functioning may at least partially improve with symptom resolution (McDermott and Ebmeier 2009).

Whilst older patients with depression typically complain of poor memory, which is in turn linked with disability (Naismith et al. 2007), formal neuropsychological testing reveals average deficits in the order of around 0.5 standard deviation units below normal (Naismith et al. 2006; Veiel 1997). However, the literature pertaining to the pattern of memory deficits in older people with depression is somewhat heterogeneous. This may relate to multiple pathophysiologies underpinning memory difficulties including the effects of cardiovascular disease (CVD), the early neurodegenerative changes and the chronic effects of depressive illness on the hippocampus (Naismith et al. 2012; Schmaal et al. 2015). Memory performance is associated with neurochemical markers of neuronal integrity (Jayaweera et al. 2015b) as well as volumetric changes in the hippocampus (Hickie et al. 2005a, b; Jayaweera et al. 2015a). In fact, over short-term follow-up periods, hippocampal volume has been linked to persistent memory change (O'Brien et al. 2004) as well as progression to dementia (Steffens et al. 2011). The mechanism by which depression itself may cause memory decline is unclear but could at least partially reflect downregulation of the hypothalamic-pituitary-adrenal axis, as well as the associated neurotoxic effects of glucocorticoids and reduced expression of brain-derived neurotrophic factor (BDNF) (Duman et al. 2006; Dwivedi 2013; Molendijk et al. 2014). Since antidepressants may promote hippocampal neurogenesis and plasticity (Pilar-Cuéllar et al. 2013) and appear to be associated with restored levels of BDNF (Castrén and Rantamäki 2010), their use may even be neuroprotective against changes in hippocampal volume and memory (Duman et al. 2006; Elcombe et al. 2014a, b; Sheline et al. 2012; Tanti and Belzung 2013). However, more prospective data is required in this area; certainly at a community level, emerging epidemiological data does not support the notion that antidepressant use is associated with slower rates of cognitive decline (Saczynski et al. 2015), though notably these relationships may differ markedly in clinical samples.

When evaluating memory in older people, the literature suggests that key phenotypic features are linked with and may even mediate performance. For instance, recent data suggests that sleep-wake disturbance may be relevant to both encoding and memory storage deficits in older people with depression, even after controlling for depressive symptom severity (Naismith et al. 2009a, b, 2011a, b). Additionally, inpatients tend to perform worse than outpatients (Naismith et al. 2003), and performance decrements may be particularly pronounced in those with melancholia and/or concomitant anxiety (Kizilbash et al. 2002). When evaluating memory functioning in both younger people with depression and those with late-life depression (LLD), the various subcomponents of memory require testing and consideration. That is, it is necessary to ascertain whether memory difficulties emerge at the level of 'encoding', 'storage' or 'retrieval'. Commonly, perceived memory problems are actually revealed to be 'encoding' problems when formally tested. In other words, the ability to absorb new information is affected, rather than the long-term consolidation of memory. This pattern is frequently seen in association with depression. Examining memory at this level of detail is crucial when using techniques targeting the remediation of memory.

21.1 Heterogeneity of Cognitive Deficits

Despite the prevalence of cognitive dysfunction in older people with depression, it still remains unclear in clinical practice, which patients may exhibit cognitive impairments and to what extent. In this regard, the heterogeneity of cognitive deficits in MD has received considerable attention, and cognition is likely to vary according to a range of phenotypic, genetic, neurobiological and aetiological features (Beblo et al. 2011; Naismith et al. 2003). One strategy to ascertain how cognitive impairment may vary is to characterise neurobiological changes at various stages of the lifespan and stages of illness. Baune and colleagues (2012) reviewed seven studies of young people aged 12–25 years. They showed that executive deficits were evident in only three out of seven studies, but working memory and processing speed deficits were consistently notable, being evident in three out of four studies. In a recent meta-analysis of 15 studies that examined cognitive deficits in adults (mean age = 39.4 years) with first-episode MD, Lee et al. (2012) demonstrated that cognitive deficits were mild to moderate in nature. The most robust effect-size decrements were found in the areas of psychomotor speed and memory and aspects of executive functioning including verbal fluency and mental flexibility. There were notably many contributors to heterogeneity: in addition to age and education, inpatient status, antidepressant use and symptom remission were linked to poorer cognition. Importantly, depression severity alone does not appear to mediate the extent of cognitive deficits in MD. Whilst there is certainly a correlation between severity and cognition in the domains of executive functioning, memory and processing speed (McDermott and Ebmeier 2009), effect sizes are small, and much variability remains unexplained. As noted above, other phenotypic features that have been linked to poorer cognition include bipolar disorder, anxiety, melancholia, inpatient status, sleep disturbance, later ages of onset, duration and recurrence of major depressive episodes and presence of psychosis (Naismith et al. 2003, 2009a, b, 2011a, b, 2012; Zaninotto et al. 2015). Additionally, the role of motivation and effort has been documented as a key factor to consider (Elliott 1998).

21.2 The Role of Cerebrovascular Disease

It is increasingly apparent that when attempting to understand cognition, one must also consider other medical and neurobiological features. In particular, co-morbid medical burden and concomitant brain changes are likely to underpin at least some cognitive deficits. In this regard, the presence of CVD appears to be pertinent, particularly for older people. Indeed, a wealth of clinical and epidemiological data suggests a bidirectional link between CVD and depression in later life (Schrader et al. 2005; Thomas et al. 2004). In particular, shared medical and lifestyle risk factors for both conditions include hypertension, diabetes, hypercholesterolaemia, heart disease, obesity and smoking. This is particularly relevant as research has identified the preponderance of white matter lesions (WMLs), seen as 'hyperintense' on T2-weighted magnetic resonance images in those with LLD generally, particularly for those with later ages of depression onset (Alexopoulos et al. 1997; Hickie et al. 1995; Krishnan et al. 1997; O'Brien et al. 1996).

Whilst the precise aetiology of WMLs is unclear, it is likely that they predominantly reflect underlying cerebrovascular disease including small vessel ischaemic change (Greenstein et al. 2010; Thomas et al. 2002). The strong link between WMLs, vascular risk factors (VRFs) and depression has led to the 'vascular depression' hypothesis (Alexopoulos et al. 1997; Hickie et al. 1995; Krishnan et al. 1992; Steffens et al. 1998). Approaches to characterising 'vascular depression' have on the one hand emphasised the importance of neuroimaging changes, or 'MRI-defined vascular depression' (Krishnan et al. 2004), and on the other, the role of neuropsychological deficits, including the 'depression-dysexecutive syndrome' (Alexopoulos et al. 2002). In addition to having later ages of onset, those with 'vascular depression' also tend to be older and have treatment resistance, psychomotor change, less family history of affective disorder, cognitive impairment and greater progression to dementia (Hickie and Scott 1998; Sheline et al. 2010; Steffens and Krishnan 1998; Taylor et al. 2013). In general, associations between WMLs and executive functioning have been demonstrated on measures of cognitive flexibility and verbal fluency (Breteler et al. 1994a, b; Kohler et al. 2010) as well as in the domains of processing speed (O'Brien et al. 2002) and memory (Boone et al. 1992; Gunning-Dixon and Raz 2000; Lesser et al. 1996), though one study has suggested that WMLs may impact more heavily on those cognitive tasks involving speed of processing than those involving memory (de Groot et al. 2000). In terms of linking the various cognitive deficits with specific regions of white matter damage, there is a lack of consistent evidence with this degree of regional specificity; however a recent systematic review of 14 studies suggested a greater association between periventricular WMLs and the cognitive domains of executive functioning and processing speed, compared to subcortical WMLs (Bolandzadeh et al. 2012). Some studies have shown a relationship between general cognitive impairment and subcortical hyperintensity burden (Salloway et al. 1996), whilst others have demonstrated this relationship with periventricular burden (de Groot et al. 2000).

21.3 Persistent Cognitive Change in Depression

Several studies have demonstrated that cognitive deficits in depression (particularly in older people) are not merely reflective of depressive 'state' and tend to persist despite adequate symptom resolution (Butters et al. 2000; Devanand et al. 2003; Diniz et al. 2015; Jayaweera et al. 2015a). Persistent cognitive change tends to be linked with later ages of onset and greater vascular burden (Barch et al. 2012). Furthermore, up to 75 % of older persons with a lifetime history of depression meet criteria for Mild Cognitive Impairment, a potential prodrome to dementia. Mild Cognitive Impairment in such persons is in turn linked to a higher percentage of VRFs as well as underlying neuroanatomical changes (Jayaweera et al. 2015a). Indeed, in older persons, changes in processing speed have been linked to volumes of the caudate nucleus (Naismith et al. 2002), underlying regional cerebral blood flow changes and to WMLs (Hickie et al. 2005a, b, 2007; Jayaweera et al. 2015b). Persistent memory deficits are linked to decreased size of the hippocampus as well as to spectroscopic markers of neuronal integrity (Jayaweera et al. 2015b). Additionally, as mentioned above, data suggests that persistent executive deficits may reflect permanent changes to white matter integrity linked to underlying cerebrovascular disease (Boone et al. 1992; Breteler et al. 1994a, b; Lesser et al. 1994, 1996). In older and elderly adults, early neurodegenerative changes in hippocampal and surrounding temporal regions may also contribute to the emergence and persistence of cognitive decline (Naismith et al. 2012).

21.4 Relationship Between Depression and Dementia

In recent years, depression has been recognised internationally as a prodromal feature and independent risk factor for cognitive decline (Alexopoulos 2005; Emery and Hess 2011; Panza et al. 2010; Steffens et al. 2007). Indeed, two large community-based studies recently demonstrated that increased depressive symptoms are associated with increasing risk for dementia (Saczynski et al. 2010), particularly for those with recurrent depression (Dotson et al. 2010). Of considerable interest, it appears that the risk to dementia in older persons with depression is not merely due to the presence of WMLs. This was demonstrated in a recent longitudinal study that followed participants for three years, where depression instead appeared to exert an additive or synergistic effect (Verdelho et al. 2013). The significance of the depression and dementia association has also been demonstrated in a recent meta-analysis examining modifiable risk factors for Alzheimer's disease, where it was estimated that one in ten cases of dementia worldwide is attributable to depression (Norton et al. 2014). Moreover, a recent systematic review (Barnes and Yaffe 2011) estimated that a 10% reduction in depression prevalence could potentially result in a worldwide reduction of dementia incidence by approximately 326,000 cases. Importantly, the combined effect of depression with other modifiable risk factors (predominantly including conditions associated with CVD such as diabetes, hypertension, obesity, physical inactivity and smoking) has been estimated to account for one third of all dementia cases (i.e. around 9.6 million) worldwide (Norton et al. 2014). This staggering calculation emphasises the important interplay between depression and CVD as a risk factor for cognitive decline. Crucially, these figures also emphasise the need for early intervention for holistic depression, cognition and lifestyle modification strategies.

21.5 Summary and Rationale for Targeting Cognition as a Specific Feature

Overall, it is clear from the extant literature that cognitive dysfunction in depression is a prominent feature and is likely to be linked to underlying changes in fronto-striatal circuitry, as well as in key memory circuits and in particular the hippocampus. Clinical and phenotypic features and the presence of underlying CVD are key predictors of cognitive change, and in older people, the presence of VRFs and WMLs is likely to be linked to persistence of deficits and progression to dementia syndromes. Of significance for daily functioning, cognitive changes are linked to disability and psychosocial functioning as well as activities of daily living. Efforts to improve cognition and remediate cognitive deficits are therefore vital, not only to improve daily functioning but to foster neuroplasticity and overall brain integrity. Unfortunately, whilst some antidepressant treatments (e.g. sertraline, duloxetine) appear to be linked with a degree of memory improvement (Doraiswamy et al. 2003; Raskin et al. 2007), recent epidemiological longitudinal data (with a 6-year follow-up period) suggests that global cognitive decline does not differ according to the use of antidepressants (Saczynski et al. 2015). Further, whilst the alleviation of 'state' effects may improve cognition to some degree, residual deficits often remain (Dahabra et al. 1998; Devanand et al. 2003; Portella et al. 2003) and suggest that alternative or adjunctive treatments specifically targeting cognition must be developed and empirically evaluated with respect to cognition, daily functioning and underlying neurobiology. In this regard, there is interest in a range of non-pharmacological treatments.

21.6 Improving Cognitive Functioning with Available Treatments for Depression

Several non-pharmacological treatments for depression have been widely used clinically, but have not been extensively evaluated with respect to cognitive outcomes. Psychological therapies such as cognitive behavioural therapy, problem-solving therapy and interpersonal therapy certainly improve mood symptoms (Koenig and Butters 2014), but benefits for cognitive dysfunction are not the focus, and thus, cognitive outcomes are largely unknown. It has been suggested that a modified approach to problem-solving therapy may be suitable for older adults with LLD and executive dysfunction, where the modification involves increased structure and directed assistance from the therapist in teaching the problem-solving strategies, as well as specifically addressing difficulties with affect regulation, initiation and perseveration (Alexopoulos et al. 2008); however to our knowledge this modified approach has not yet been evaluated with respect to cognitive outcomes.

Similarly, there is a burgeoning body of literature on the potential neuroplastic effects of electroconvulsive therapy (ECT), but research to date has focused on the short-term memory deficits that occur as a side effect immediately following ECT rather than cognitive enhancement. Some early research suggested that in older depressed adults, those presenting with higher levels of cognitive impairment prior to commencing ECT may be most vulnerable to developing persistent memory impairment post-treatment (Sobin et al. 1995). This increased vulnerability depending on pre-treatment cognitive status was confirmed by a more recent study investigating global cognitive change in association with ECT (Hausner et al. 2011); however, this study also showed that such cognitive decline had remitted at 6 month post-ECT cessation, across groups of depressed older adults with no cognitive impairment, Mild Cognitive Impairment or dementia at baseline. There is less specific research on ECT effects in those with CVD; however recently a retrospective chart review of 24 older patients with post-stroke depression indicated that 20/24 experienced a positive response to ECT treatment (Romanowicz et al. 2012). Additionally, none of the patients experienced exacerbation of depressive symptoms or post-stroke neurological impairment following ECT, suggesting that it may be a safe and well-tolerated treatment option in those with psychiatric symptoms related to CVD. Currently, attention is turning to the potential for ECT to enhance or even induce mechanisms of neuroplasticity. For example, both animal and some human studies have shown increased expression of BDNF following ECT (see review by Bouckaert et al. 2014). Certainly, further research is required to delineate these potential neuroplastic effects, and this research will need to overcome several methodological hurdles (e.g. sample heterogeneity; timing of BDNF or imaging samples post-ECT, etc.). However, this avenue of enquiry is particularly interesting from a rehabilitation perspective in relation to the potential for longer-term cognitive benefits.

In contrast to ECT, repetitive transcranial magnetic stimulation (rTMS) appears to be well tolerated with fewer cognitive side effects in older adults with treatment-resistant MD (Koenig and Butters 2014), and a recent meta-analysis demonstrated promising support for its utility in improving cognitive functioning in adults with treatment-resistant MD over the lifespan (Serafini et al. 2015). Specifically, 16/22 studies reporting cognitive outcomes following rTMS (typically conducted over the dorsolateral-prefrontal cortex area) reported cognitive improvements across the domains of verbal memory, verbal learning, processing speed, working memory and executive functions. Further research is now warranted to clarify whether these effects are seen specifically in older patients. Similarly, interest has grown in the potential cognitive effects of transcranial direct current stimulation (TdCS) in recent years. Whilst one review of single-session TdCS in healthy adults did not support any reliable effects on any cognitive outcomes (Horvath et al. 2015), repeated-session TdCS has been shown in some studies to improve cognition in those with depression, for example, working memory (irrespective of concurrent improvements in mood) (Fregni et al. 2006). Currently, research is being undertaken to investigate the potential for TdCS to improve cognition specifically in those with LLD (Clinical Trial #NCT02212366).

Finally, the beneficial effects of physical exercise for improving cognition as well as depressive symptoms are widely recognised in older adults, even in those already experiencing mild cognitive decline (Amoyal and Fallon 2012; Lautenschlager et al. 2008). Importantly, cognitive benefits in the domains of memory and executive functioning have also been shown specifically in older adults with MD, both acutely (i.e. immediately following 30 min of aerobic exercise (Vasques et al. 2011)) and in longer term (such as following a structured, 4-month aerobic exercise program (Khatri et al. 2001)). Importantly, physical exercise has also been associated with neuroplastic changes in areas such as the hippocampus, further emphasising its capacity to induce perhaps longer-lasting cognitive benefits (Amoyal and Fallon 2012). In light of these findings, currently research is focusing on whether physical exercise may be particularly useful in conjunction with cognitive training, to enhance cognition in older adults (e.g. the randomised controlled 'Study of Mental Activity and Regular Training (SMART)' trial (see Gates et al. 2011a, b)).

21.7 Cognitive Remediation as a Non-pharmacological Therapeutic Technique for Improving Neuropsychological Functioning in Depression

Given that neuropsychological dysfunction is a concomitant feature of depression, which can persist despite symptom resolution, and since this feature is a risk factor for dementia (Diniz et al. 2013), therapeutic interventions specifically targeting cognition and underlying neuroplasticity are paramount. In this regard, cognitive remediation approaches, although in their infancy, offer promise. In general, cognitive interventions aim to improve cognitive performance and day-to-day functional capacity. Techniques and approaches tend to vary based on the intensity of the

Table 21.1 Cognitive remediation interventions that may be used in depressed samples

Cognitive remediation			
Type	Cognitive stimulation	Cognitive training	Cognitive rehabilitation
Aim	To enhance cognitive and social functioning	To improve cognitive functioning in specific domains	To improve effectiveness in cognitive and functional capacity in everyday life
Approach	Non-specific stimulating activities	Theoretically driven; involves guided practice on tasks reflecting specific cognitive domains (e.g. memory, attention, etc.)	Identifying and targeting individual strengths and weaknesses
Techniques	Various techniques including group discussions, reminiscence, orientation, arts, music and crafts	(i) *Strategy-based training*: the use of internal (i.e. mental) and external (i.e. practical) strategies to facilitate cognitive processes or compensate for impaired cognition, e.g. mnemonic aids such as chunking, repetition and the use of a diary or whiteboard (ii) *Computer-based training*: computerised games or exercises targeting specific cognitive functions, often involving graded difficulty	Various techniques including compensatory strategies, problem-solving, psycho-education, etc.

intervention (see Table 21.1), ranging from the more diffusely focused cognitively stimulating activities, through targeted cognitive training tasks, to more functionally oriented cognitive rehabilitation. Whilst research is still in its infancy, cognitive interventions for depression are becoming increasingly popular. Most of the research in this area has employed cognitive training (CT) paradigms, incorporating computer-based approaches (Koenig and Butters 2014) rather than cognitive stimulation or rehabilitation approaches, possibly due to the more specific or targeted nature of CT.

21.7.1 Cognitive Training as a Therapeutic Technique

Cognitive training (CT) refers to targeted programs which remediate cognition by providing theoretically driven strategies and skills, usually involving 'guided practice' in compensatory or restorative techniques designed to strengthen intact cognitive functions and adapt to or improve areas of weakness (Sitzer et al. 2006).

Compensatory methods aim to bypass deficient cognitive processes and teach alternative approaches to achieving goals, including both internal (e.g. visual imagery, categorising information) and external strategies (e.g. using calendars or environmental cues). Such strategy-based CT tasks are interactive, engaging and contextually relevant to practical activities (e.g. how to remember shopping lists, appointments, conversational details or names/faces). Restorative CT methods (e.g. spaced retrieval and errorless learning) aim to improve functioning in specific domains, thus recovering impaired skills, and typically involve repetitive computer-based exercises (Gates et al. 2011b).

In recent years an increasing body of evidence has suggested that CT may be particularly promising as a therapeutic technique for improving cognitive and psychosocial functions in psychiatric groups such as those with schizophrenia (McGurk et al. 2007), in healthy older adults (Ball et al. 2002) and in groups 'at-risk' of developing dementia, including those with Mild Cognitive Impairment (Gates et al. 2011a, b; Mowszowski et al. 2010). Across the literature, improvements in memory appear to be most pronounced following CT (Mowszowski et al. 2010; Valenzuela and Sachdev 2009), although objective improvements in other domains such as attention, processing speed and reasoning have also been demonstrated in healthy older adults and individuals with Mild Cognitive Impairment (Ball et al. 2002; Kurz et al. 2009; Mowszowski et al. 2014). Additionally, several groups have reported generalised gains in psychosocial and daily functioning in these samples, such as improved performance in simulated real-life tasks (Levine et al. 2007), improved mood and sleep (Diamond et al. 2015; Kurz et al. 2009), informant-rated activities of daily living (Kurz et al. 2009) and increased knowledge and use of memory strategies in everyday life, as well as self-efficacy (Kinsella et al. 2009; Norrie et al. 2011). There is also growing evidence of sustained improvements over several months or even years following CT (Rebok et al. 2014). Importantly, one consistent finding across studies is the excellent adherence, tolerability and lack of negative effects of CT (Bahar-Fuchs et al. 2013).

In terms of potential mechanisms of action, recent evidence indicates that CT in older people with cognitive impairment is associated with neurobiological changes including increased cortical thickness, white matter connectivity and hippocampal volumes (see review by Belleville and Bherer 2012), suggesting that such programs have the potential to alter disease trajectories. However, studies examining neurobiological changes in association with CT are clearly in their infancy and tend to include small sample sizes, diverse methodologies and varied imaging sequences and training techniques. Thus, the neural mechanisms underpinning these changes have yet to be established and may vary according to the cognitive domain which improves. Presumably, given the capacity for neurogenesis in the hippocampus and observed consistent effects of CT on memory (Lampit et al. 2014), changes in the hippocampus might be expected, and indeed some preliminary studies in ageing support this hypothesis (Engvig et al. 2014). Additionally, CT may offer neuroprotection by promoting processes such as neuroplasticity and/or 'cognitive reserve'. Importantly, evidence suggests that neuroplasticity and enhancing cognitive reserve through life experiences and/or behavioural interventions can still occur later in life and that substantial restoration is possible even in the ageing brain, to delay or reverse the effects of normal ageing or neurodegenerative pathology (Mahncke et al. 2006).

Importantly, it has been suggested that CT may be particularly beneficial when implemented within a multifaceted approach such as that including relevant psycho-education or adjunctive psychological/behavioural techniques (Naismith et al. 2009a, b; Rebok et al. 2007). This is especially pertinent for older adults given the well-established links between dementia and medical/lifestyle risk factors such as depression, obesity, diabetes, hypertension and lack of exercise or sedentary behaviour (Norton et al. 2014; Walton et al. 2014). Thus, a holistic or adjunctive approach may yield more meaningful benefits to mitigate risk of cognitive decline. Moreover, CT programs are engaging, non-invasive and cost-effective and offer the opportunity for social interaction when conducted within a group format.

21.7.2 Cognitive Training in Depression

Over the last 10 years in particular, CT has attracted widespread interest as a potential therapeutic tool for neuropsychiatric groups. Much of the literature in this area has focused on schizophrenia or schizo-affective disorders, with generally promising findings indicating small to medium effects particularly in the domain of memory (Anaya et al. 2012; Vinogradov et al. 2012). However, increasingly attention is turning to whether CT may be a viable intervention strategy for affective disorders such as MD. As is the case with much of the CT literature (Vinogradov et al. 2012; Walton et al. 2014), the body of research on CT for depression is quite heterogeneous with respect to clinical factors (e.g. older versus younger adults, current versus lifetime depressive symptoms, etc.), study design (e.g. computer-based versus strategy-based CT) and outcomes (e.g. focusing on cognitive versus psychological improvements). Whilst it is therefore somewhat difficult to synthesise the literature, by far, most studies have utilised computer-based approaches to CT, and findings of these studies are summarised in Fig. 21.1. Alternatively, studies may be grouped according to predominant cognitive outcomes and/or methodological factors (such as longitudinal design or inclusion of neurobiological outcomes), also described in detail below.

21.7.3 Effects on Memory

Improvements on neuropsychological tasks of learning and memory appear to be a consistent finding across the studies that have been conducted to date (i.e. with six out of seven CT studies examining this outcome having shown positive effects), though notably the quality of the studies has been low and most have been preliminary uncontrolled studies rather than being definitive randomised controlled trials (RCTs). Nonetheless, improvements have been demonstrated utilising both computer-based and strategy-based approaches. In a series of studies conducted in this area, we developed a 10-week

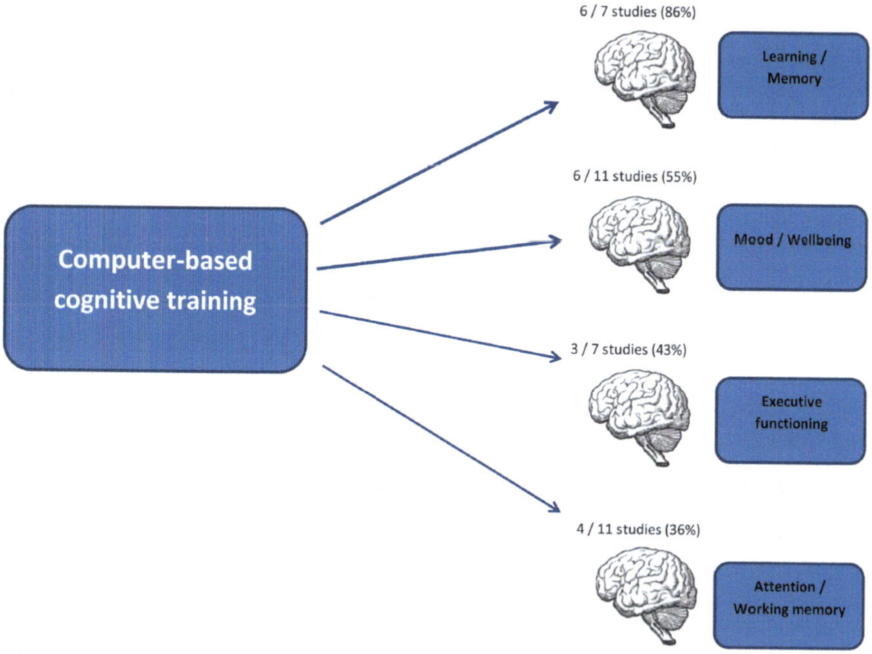

Fig. 21.1 Summary of cognitive and mood improvements following computer-based cognitive training. Studies investigating cognitive training in patients with depression across the lifespan have predominantly used computer-based training paradigms and have examined effects on learning and memory (7 studies), executive functions (7 studies), attention and working memory (11 studies) and mood or psychosocial wellbeing (11 studies). The most robust effects have been found for improvements in memory and mood/wellbeing

CT program using the Neuropsychological Educational Approach to Remediation pioneered by Medalia and colleagues (Medalia and Freilich 2008). We firstly demonstrated improved learning and memory in 16 adults with MD (mean age = 33.5) in association with this individualised computer-based CT program (Naismith et al. 2010), which maximises intrinsic motivation, graded exposure, adaptation and generalisation to real-world scenarios. We also showed this program to be effective in a mixed group of 36 young adults (mean age = 22.9 years) with either MD or first-episode psychosis (Lee et al. 2013). We then evaluated the effect of a combined computerised CT and psycho-education group program in 41 older people (mean age = 64.8 years) with a lifetime history of MD and with cognitive decline (but not meeting criteria for dementia). The psycho-education component incorporated memory and other cognitive strategies as well as information regarding management of VRFs and other modifiable risk factors for dementia (e.g. depression, sleep, exercise, anxiety, nutrition). This 10-week program was associated with significant improvements in learning and memory (but not executive functioning) (Naismith et al. 2011a, b) corresponding to medium to large effect-size changes (i.e. −0.74 to −0.82), a clinically meaningful effect. Based on participant feedback, we extended this program to be more frequent and include more sessions, resulting in a 7-week, twice-weekly program. In a RCT, 64 older adults with LLD and/or Mild Cognitive Impairment (i.e. those 'at-risk' of dementia; $n = 64$, mean age = 66.5 years; 45 % with a lifetime history or current MD) completed the program. Results again showed improved memory retention corresponding to a medium effect-size improvement (Diamond et al. 2015). Importantly, 62 % of this sample also reported CVD or a vascular risk factor associated with CVD (e.g. diabetes, hypertension, etc.). This study not only demonstrated cognitive improvements following CT but also showed improvements in self-rated depressive symptom severity and sleep quality, affirming the utility of such programs for improving psychosocial functioning in this cohort. Importantly, we have demonstrated excellent mean adherence rates of 80 % for this program across trials, indicating high acceptability for this patient group. Finally, it is worth noting that the cognitive improvements in these studies were not simply mediated by improved mood, to the extent that changes in depressive symptoms in association with CT can be partialled out statistically.

Studies employing strategy-based memory training have also proven successful in younger adults ($n = 42$; mean age = 45.67 years) with recurrent MD, as shown by Dalgleish and colleagues (2013), who compared the time-honoured 'method of loci' visual imagery technique with other mnemonic techniques such as chunking (i.e. grouping similar 'bits' of information together to facilitate encoding and retrieval) and active rehearsal of information to be remembered. After five training sessions conducted within the span of one week, participants in both conditions demonstrated improved recall of autobiographical memories, although this improvement was sustained over one week only in those who had received method of loci training, suggesting that this method may be more advantageous for longer-lasting training effects. Unfortunately, the study did not include a longer-term follow-up such as 4-weeks or 3-months, which might have strengthened this point even further. Importantly, both groups also demonstrated an improvement in self-rated depressive symptoms after receiving memory training (Dalgleish et al. 2013).

Despite these promising results, some studies have reported null findings following memory strategy training for depression. For example, a recent investigation of the efficacy of adjunctive mnemonic training (including chunking, name-face recall, method of loci, etc.) over a 4-week period in comparison to cognitive behavioural therapy alone or a waitlist control condition was reported to show no differences in subjective or objective memory performance and equivocal improvements in mood, in 53 older adults with depressive symptoms (Scogin et al. 2014). However, this study differed from those described above in its lack of face-to-face contact during delivery of the intervention, as all treatments were completed independently in a workbook format. Additionally, the authors reported an extremely high rate of attrition (52 %) at 8-week follow-up, particularly among those participants with higher rates of cognitive impairment and mood disturbance at baseline, perhaps suggesting that this approach is less useful for this group who may require a more clinically intensive, supported or extrinsically motivated intervention.

21.7.4 Effects on Working Memory

In addition to episodic memory training, several studies have focused on remediating working memory (i.e. the ability to hold and manipulate information in mind – such as calculating change at a cashier or the number of points required to win a tennis match). These studies have typically utilised computer-based training paradigms incorporating an n-back task, requiring participants to hold in mind stimuli presented *n* trials previously. One study (Iacoviello et al. 2014) utilised a 4-week training program with either neutral stimuli (shapes) or emotional faces, in 21 young adults (mean ages = 36.33 and 39.5 years per group) with current MD. Comparisons of the two training conditions indicated similar, small improvements on unrelated objective measures of working memory. Whilst both working memory training tasks resulted in reduced depressive symptoms, the task involving emotional faces resulted in a significantly greater improvement in mood, which the authors proposed may have related to additional activation of the amygdala during training in comparison to the neutral shapes which would only have activated the dorsolateral-prefrontal cortex. Another study, also involving 31 young adults (mean age of 27.72 for the experimental group and 22.63 years for the active control group) with moderate self-rated depressive symptoms showed improved working memory performance following 8-days of computerised n-back training which also transferred to improvements in information filtering efficiency on an electroencephalography (EEG) change-detection task (Owens et al. 2013) in comparison to controls. These improvements occurred alongside, but were not related to, improvements in self-rated depressive symptoms. However, other studies utilising computer-based n-back CT tasks have not demonstrated transfer to untrained cognitive tasks. For example, a study targeting rumination as a symptom of depression in 72 university undergraduates aged in their early 20's (Onraedt and Koster 2014) showed unsurprising improvements on the trained n-back task, yet these gains did not transfer to objective tests of working memory and there was no difference on measures of depression or rumination following training, nor in comparison to active or passive control conditions. However, limitations of this study include the relatively short duration of training and relatively low levels of psychopathology in comparison to other CT trials for depression. Nonetheless, another trial of computer-based n-back training (albeit in an older, midlife sample with mean age = 46.63 years) which did include a more intensive training program (six sessions per week for 4-weeks) in those with higher levels of mood disturbance (lifetime anxiety or depressive disorder) also found no improvement on objective measures of working memory or measures of depression, anxiety and rumination (Wanmaker et al. 2015). From a psychological perspective, both studies suggest that working memory training is ineffective for improving rumination, which is perhaps unsurprising given that rumination is linked to a variety of executive functions (e.g. inhibition, attentional control) and not just working memory. However, from a cognitive perspective, negative transfer of training-related gains to untrained tasks is certainly an issue of ongoing methodological and conceptual difficulty in the wider CT literature (Walton et al. 2014; Wolinsky et al. 2009).

21.7.5 Effects on Executive Functions

In terms of executive functioning, Preiss et al. (2013) recently demonstrated large effect-size improvements in set-shifting, divided attention and global executive functioning, as well as improved caregiver ratings of executive dysfunction, following an 8-week CT program involving three sessions per week of individualised CT with the commercially available *CogniFit* software, which targets a variety of cognitive domains. These improvements were evident in 15 adults (mean age = 42.87 years) compared to a group of 16 'standard care' control participants (mean age = 45.38 years), all of whom had either unipolar MD or were in the depressive phase of bipolar depression. Those who completed the computer-based CT program also reported significantly improved subjective memory performance, higher levels of satisfaction and wellbeing and reduced depressive symptoms in comparison to control participants. Despite the small sample size and lack of active control, these results suggest that a broad, multidomain, computerised CT task may offer promise for executive dysfunction in depression.

21.7.6 Multidomain Effects

Other positive cognitive effects have been reported by Elgamal et al. (2007), whereby 12 euthymic patients with unipolar MD (mean age = 50.26 years) completed twice-weekly CT sessions for 10-weeks, using a purpose-designed cognitive remediation software package targeting attention, verbal memory, psychomotor speed and executive functions. In comparison to 12 age- and gender-matched control participants with MD as well as 22 healthy control participants, the treatment group improved on a range of tests measuring attention, verbal learning and memory, psychomotor speed and executive function. Moreover, as neither the experimental nor control groups with depression improved on measures of mood at follow-up, these cognitive effects cannot be solely attributed to improved mood.

21.7.7 CT Compared to Antidepressant Treatment

Some studies have directly compared the effects of CT with those of traditional pharmacological (i.e. antidepressant) treatments. For example, Morimoto and colleagues (2014) investigated a sample of age-, cognition- and gender-matched older adults who had previously failed at least one trial of antidepressant medication, allocated to either CT ($n = 11$; mean age = 74.1 years) or escitalopram treatment for depression ($n = 33$; mean age = 73.1 years). In this study, the computer-based CT program was designed to target aspects of executive functioning known to be affected in LLD, including inhibition, initiation, cognitive flexibility and set-shifting. Results showed that the CT program was equally as effective at improving depressive symptoms in older adults; however the effect following CT was evident after 4-weeks compared to 12-weeks with escitalopram. Moreover, the CT group improved on objective (untrained) measures of executive functioning at both immediate and 3-month follow-up, although this effect did not transfer to unrelated cognitive domains such as verbal memory. Similar findings were shown in a younger group of 31 university students with MD, who were randomly allocated to either twice-weekly CT, CT with adjunctive antidepressant treatment or antidepressant treatment alone for 3-months (Alvarez et al. 2008). This CT program revolved around computerised inductive reasoning and working memory tasks. Whilst participants in all three groups demonstrated significantly reduced depressive symptomatology post-treatment, only those who received CT (alone or in conjunction with antidepressant therapy) also demonstrated improvements on neuropsychological measures of attention, verbal reasoning, visuospatial skills and global intellectual functioning.

21.7.8 Neurobiological Changes Underlying CT

It has been suggested that CT-associated improvements in cognition and psychosocial functioning may relate to non-specific effects such as clinical contact or social engagement. However, more recent research in the field of CT has investigated concurrent neurobiological effects to clarify the specificity of cognitive gains with respect to underlying neural mechanisms. For example, studies that have addressed such outcomes in healthy older adults and those with Mild Cognitive Impairment have demonstrated CT-related changes such as increased brain volume and white matter tract density as well as changes in task-related brain metabolism (see review by Belleville and Bherer 2012), usually involving the frontal lobes (Suo and Valenzuela 2012). However, further structural and functional imaging studies are required to ascertain whether the therapeutic effects of CT are restorative or compensatory in nature (Mowszowski et al. 2010). Moreover, neurobiological outcomes have yet to be sufficiently explored in groups with MD. One study (Meusel et al. 2013) has addressed this aspect of CT utilising functional magnetic resonance imaging (fMRI). This study involved 35 patients with a primary mood disorder but not with a current major depressive episode (mean age = 48.4 years), who completed a 10-week computer-based CT program targeting processing speed, attention, verbal memory and executive functions, compared to 15 healthy control participants (mean age = 39.7 years) who did not complete the CT intervention. Follow-up assessments revealed a significant improvement on a working memory task (backwards digit span) in the treatment group, in conjunction with increased activation in lateral and medial prefrontal, superior temporal and lateral parietal regions during an n-back task, and increased bilateral hippocampal activation during a memory recollection task. To our knowledge, only one study has investigated structural brain changes in association with combined strategy- and computer-based CT, in a subset of 34 'at-risk' individuals who were part of a larger RCT (mean age 66.8 years) (Diamond et al. 2015). In this sub-study (Elcombe et al. 2014a, b), 44 % had a lifetime history of MD, and four participants were currently depressed. Whilst post-CT analyses did not show significant changes in hippocampal volume, this may have related to the small sample size and broad variability in the data. Importantly, sub-analyses of the group that received CT ($n=21$) indicated that changes in hippocampal volume over the 2-month period of the intervention were associated with depressive symptoms, markers of cognitive reserve, psychosocial functioning and disability. These findings suggest that these factors must be considered in evaluating neurobiological outcomes in CT trials.

Other measures of neurobiological functions include event-related potentials (ERPs) drawn from EEG (Rossini et al. 2007). Such measures are time-locked to specific stimuli and are used to assess the speed and efficiency of information processing by examining the magnitude and latency of the waveform. Two known studies have utilised this technique to investigate CT-related changes. Using the Mismatch Negativity ERP paradigm in 40 older adults (mean age = 66.47 years) 'at-risk' of dementia (including 45 % with a lifetime history of MD and four participants with current depression), our group (Mowszowski et al. 2014) showed significantly increased fronto-central neurophysiological responses as well as improved phonemic verbal fluency and decreased self-rated memory difficulties in a treatment group ($n=25$) following a 7-week multifaceted CT program, in comparison to 15 waitlist control participants. However, there were no significant correlations between enhanced ERPs and cognitive/psychosocial outcomes, perhaps indicating that over this short time period, the training-related gains were only evident in pre-attentive information processes but had not yet translated to higher-order functions. However, such translation has been reported in other trials, such as the working memory training program described above by Owens and colleagues (Owens et al. 2013), whereby improvements in working memory were shown to transfer to improvements in information filtering efficiency on an EEG change-detection task. Such findings may have relevance in relation to expectations of higher-level structural changes (e.g. in hippocampal volume) following short-term CT programs and also underscore the importance of targeting lower-level cognitive processes during cognitive interventions (Vinogradov et al. 2012).

21.7.9 Longitudinal Relationship Between Depressive Symptoms and CT

One of the largest and seminal CT RCTs to date, the ACTIVE study, investigated the efficacy of memory, reasoning or speed-of-processing training on cognitive and psychosocial functioning in 2,832 healthy older adults aged over 65 years. Whilst primary cognitive findings were published in 2002 (Ball et al. 2002), more recent findings have been reported with respect to the relationship between each training program and depressive symptomatology. Wolinsky et al. (2009) evaluated the effects of CT on depression onset in 1,606 participants who completed 12-month follow-up assessments, as well as the effects of CT on recovery from depression in a subset of 424 participants who were considered to have clinically significant depressive symptoms at baseline. Results indicated that only the speed-of-processing CT program resulted in a significant reduction (38 %) in the likelihood of developing depression 12-months post-training compared to a no-contact control group. However, there were no significant differences among the three CT programs in terms of recovery from depression at 12-months in those older adults with depressive symptoms at baseline. A separate sub-analysis conducted by Lohman et al. (2012) investigated the impact of depressive symptom severity at baseline on memory performance in a subset of 1,401 participants who returned for follow-up after 5-years. Two hundred and ten of these participants were determined to have exhibited elevated depressive symptoms at baseline. In this 'elevated' group, baseline verbal memory performance was significantly poorer compared to those without depressive symptoms, and this difference increased significantly over 5-years of annual follow-up. Nonetheless, results of this sub-analysis also demonstrated that all participants were able to benefit from memory training to the same extent, regardless of whether they had elevated depressive symptoms at baseline or not. This indicates that CT effects on memory may be robust to the effects of depression. Finally, a recent study reported the longitudinal associations between baseline depressive symptomatology and inductive reasoning performance over a 10-year follow-up period (Parisi et al. 2014). Of the 1,375 participants who completed this longer follow-up assessment, 322 participants were shown to have had elevated depressive symptoms at baseline. Similar to those findings reported for the memory training group above, results indicated that baseline depressive symptoms were not associated with differences in immediate or annual post-training gains, again suggesting that the effects of the reasoning CT program were not affected by depressive symptomatology at the time.

21.7.10 Limitations to the Literature: Questions Remaining

The body of research on cognitive intervention for depression is marred by broad heterogeneity in study methodology, CT program design and scientific quality. Further randomised controlled CT trials for depression are now required, and such trials must also adhere to guidelines for the conceptualisation, operationalisation and implementation of complex interventions such as those set out in the CONSORT extension relating specifically to non-pharmacological intervention trials (Boutron et al. 2008). Notwithstanding these limitations, interest in the application of CT to cognition in depressive disorders is certainly growing, and there is at least an emerging, though preliminary, evidence base for this form of intervention over the short-term. In accordance with the broader CT literature across other groups (including those with schizophrenia, healthy older adults and those with Mild Cognitive Impairment), improvements in the domain of memory appear to be most consistent and have been most widely researched. However, in addition to more rigorous studies, several lines of investigation remain unclear, as outlined in Table 21.2.

Table 21.2 Key questions to be addressed in future research on cognitive training in depression

Questions remaining	Issues to be resolved
Method of CT	Is computerised CT more efficacious than strategy-based training?
	What programs should be utilised?
	What is the optimal mode of delivery?
	Multimodal vs. unimodal?
	Therapist vs. self-administered?
Dosage and time course of effects	How many sessions of CT are required in order to produce improvements?
	How often should sessions be delivered?
Generalisability and functional improvements	Do the improvements seen on objective testing and self-report translate to concurrent improvements on everyday tasks, such as household chores, conversations with friends, keeping appointments, etc.?
Sustainability of effects	Are the improvements seen following a CT program sustainable over time?
	Are booster sessions helpful to maintain benefits?
Neurobiological changes	What are the neurobiological mechanisms of action?
	Is CT associated with evidence of neuroplasticity, and if so, how is this distributed within the brain (i.e. are the benefits indicative of compensatory or restorative mechanisms)?
Individual predictors of benefit	Are there certain subgroups or individuals who may benefit more (or less) from engaging in cognitive interventions? Characteristics may relate to:
	Cognition (e.g. those with predominant memory vs. executive dysfunction)
	Personality (e.g. those with an external vs. internal locus of control)
	Psychosocial factors (e.g. extent of support network)
	Cognitive reserve (do those with greater reserve benefit preferentially from CT)
	Underlying neurobiological changes such as hippocampal atrophy, evidence of white matter lesions on neuroimaging or presence of CVD
Critical period of CT delivery	At what point in the clinical course should CT be delivered?
Role of depressive symptoms	Do patients with varying depression subtypes differ in terms of benefit from CT? Features of interest include:
	Age of onset (early vs. late onset)
	Symptom severity such as subthreshold vs. current MD episode
	Melancholic vs. psychotic depression, etc.
Accounting for CVD and underlying brain changes	Is CT useful for those with CVD but without depression? That is, can CT be utilised as a secondary intervention technique in this group who may be 'at-risk' for 'vascular depression'?

21.8 CT for Depression and Co-morbid CVD

Despite the well-established 'vascular depression' hypothesis, as evident in the above account of the literature, no CT studies have specifically targeted adults with depression and CVD. To our knowledge, only the studies conducted by our group (Diamond et al. 2015; Naismith et al. 2011a, b) have addressed vascular and other modifiable risk factors (e.g. nutrition, exercise) as part of a multifaceted intervention, combining computer based CT with psycho-education. This approach was based on the preponderance of work demonstrating cognitive decline in older people with depression and particularly those with concomitant CVD (as reviewed above). Whilst the effects of the psycho-education program may not be observed immediately, it is possible that the provision of information regarding CVD would provide longer-term preventative and CVD risk-reduction benefits.

21.8.1 Future Directions

A brief inspection of international clinical trial registries in June 2015 indicates some ongoing research into the efficacy of cognitive interventions for depression, and these studies will help to clarify the remaining questions outlined above. For example, a Canadian research team (Clinical Trial # NCT01748032) is currently conducting a pilot trial on short-term effectiveness of strategy-based CT for improving cognition and mood in older adults with current MD, whereas much of the previous literature has focused on those with a lifetime history of depression or subthreshold symptoms. Another trial currently underway in Australia is investigating the potential for computer-based CT to improve cognitive functioning and caregiver burden in older adults with Mild Cognitive Impairment, with or without concurrent mood disturbance (depression or anxiety symptoms) (ACTRN12614000335695). This trial will aid in clarifying the potential impact of concurrent mood disturbance on CT efficacy in this group 'at-risk' of dementia; however unfortunately the publicly available study protocol does not appear to include outcomes relating to the severity of the mood disturbance symptoms.

Whilst these trials are encouraging, much further research will be required in order to fully elucidate the remaining issues relating to CT efficacy in depression, particularly for those with LLD and CVD, where the risk of cognitive decline and progression to dementia is most pronounced. Moving forward, trials that offer combined cognitive remediation and exercise may have the greatest capacity to target both CVD and cognitive impairment in older persons with depression. However, it is noted that such interventions really should be delivered as early as possible, as white matter change due to underlying CVD may not be reversible (Naismith et al. 2009a, b), and therefore *prevention* of WMLs due to CVD is paramount. It is also important to consider that if WMLs are prominent and if, in turn, executive dysfunction is due to underlying structural brain change in white matter macro- and micro-architecture (Duffy et al. 2014), then remediation of executive dysfunction may be difficult to achieve. Indeed, this may even account for the lack of improvements in executive functions in trials that have been multifaceted. As described above, future trials of CT in older persons with depression should consider the presence and influence of underlying white matter/vascular change in influencing treatment outcomes. Future trials should also consider the issues outlined in Table 21.2 relating to methodology and program design in order to elicit maximum cognitive benefits, such as the intensity and duration of training, targeting lower-level (perceptual) in addition to higher-level functions and individualising or contextualising training as much as possible to facilitate generalisation (see Vinogradov et al. 2012). Finally, it is crucial that future trials also consider scientific quality. It is now time for definitive RCTs with rigorous methodology and reporting, so that optimal cognitive outcomes and personalised treatment recommendations can be advised.

Conclusions

Cognitive deficits are a major feature of depression, particularly for those with LLD where cognitive decline may reflect illness-specific factors, multiple medical co-morbidities, underlying CVD and/or emerging neurodegenerative pathology. Cognitive interventions are therefore warranted to ameliorate deficits typically seen in memory, processing speed and executive functioning, as well as to improve overall psychosocial functioning and reduce disability. In this regard, CT has been shown to be an effective intervention technique in groups such as schizophrenia, healthy older adults and those with Mild Cognitive Impairment. Only recently has CT been applied to those with depression, and whilst further rigorous research is certainly required (particularly to delineate optimal program design and longitudinal effects, as well as clarify underlying neurobiological changes), preliminary evidence does support the use of CT as a therapeutic intervention for cognitive impairment in depression, and this has important implications for early intervention strategies targeting older adults with depression.

References

Alexopoulos GS (2005) Depression in the elderly. Lancet 365(9475):1961–1970

Alexopoulos GS, Meyers BS, Young RC, Kakuma T, Silbersweig D, Charlson M (1997) Clinically defined vascular depression. Am J Psychiatry 154(4):562–565

Alexopoulos GS, Kiosses DN, Klimstra S, Kalayam B, Bruce ML (2002) Clinical presentation of the "depression-executive dysfunction syndrome" of late life. Am J Geriatr Psychiatry 10(1):98–106

Alexopoulos GS, Raue PJ, Kanellopoulos D, Mackin S, Arean PA (2008) Problem solving therapy for the depression-executive dysfunction syndrome of late life. Int J Geriatr Psychiatry 23(8):782–788

Alvarez LM, Cortés Sotres JF, León SO, Estrella J, Sánchez Sosa JJ (2008) Computer program in the treatment for major depression and cognitive impairment in university students. Comput Hum Behav 24(3):816–826

American Psychiatric Association (2013) American psychiatric association: diagnostic and statistical manual of mental disorders, 5th edn. American Psychiatric Association, Washington, DC

Amoyal N, Fallon E (2012) Physical exercise and cognitive training clinical interventions used in slow degeneration associated with mild cognitive impairment: a review of the recent literature. Top Geriatr Rehabil 28(3):208–216

Anaya C, Aran AM, Ayuso-Mateos JL, Wykes T, Vieta E, Scott J (2012) A systematic review of cognitive remediation for schizo-affective and affective disorders. J Affect Disord 142:13–21
Bahar-Fuchs A, Clare L, Woods B (2013) Cognitive training and cognitive rehabilitation for mild to moderate Alzheimer's disease and vascular dementia. Cochrane Database Syst Rev (6):CD003260
Baldwin R, Jeffries S, Jackson A, Sutcliffe C, Thacker N, Scott M, Burns A (2004) Treatment response in late-onset depression: relationship to neuropsychological, neuroradiological and vascular risk factors. Psychol Med 34(1):125–136
Ball K, Berch DB, Helmers KF, Jobe JB, Leveck MD, Marsiske M, Morris JN, Rebok GW, Smith DM, Tennstedt SL, Unverzagt FW, Willis SL, Advanced Cognitive Training for Independent and Vital Elderly Study Group (2002) Effects of cognitive training interventions with older adults: a randomized controlled trial. J Am Med Assoc 288(18):2271–2281
Barch DM, D'Angelo G, Pieper C, Wilkins CH, Welsh-Bohmer K, Taylor W, Garcia KS, Gersing K, Doraiswamy PM, Sheline YI (2012) Cognitive improvement following treatment in late-life depression: relationship to vascular risk and age of onset. Am J Geriatr Psychiatry 20(8): 682–690
Barnes DE, Yaffe K (2011) The projected impact of risk factor reduction on Alzheimer's disease prevalence. Lancet Neurol 10(9):819–828
Baune BT, Miller R, McAfoose J, Johnson M, Quirk F, Mitchell D (2010) The role of cognitive impairment in general functioning in major depression. Psychiatry Res 176(2–3):183–189
Baune BT, Smith E, Reppermund S, Air T, Samaras K, Lux O, Brodaty H, Sachdev P, Trollor JN (2012) Inflammatory biomarkers predict depressive, but not anxiety symptoms during aging: the prospective Sydney Memory and Aging Study. Psychoneuroendocrinology 37(9): 1521–1530
Beblo T, Sinnamon G, Baune BT (2011) Specifying the neuropsychology of affective disorders: clinical, demographic and neurobiological factors. Neuropsychol Rev 21(4):337–359
Belleville S, Bherer L (2012) Biomarkers of cognitive training effects in aging. Curr Transl Geriatr Exp Gerontol Rep 1:104–110
Bolandzadeh N, Davis JC, Tam R, Handy TC, Liu-Ambrose T (2012) The association between cognitive function and white matter lesion location in older adults: a systematic review. BMC Neurol 12:126
Boone KB, Miller BL, Lesser IM, Mehringer CM, Hill-Gutierrez E, Goldberg MA, Berman NG (1992) Neuropsychological correlates of white-matter lesions in healthy elderly subjects. A threshold effect. Arch Neurol 49:549–554
Bosworth HB, Hays JC, George LK, Steffens DC (2002) Psychosocial and clinical predictors of unipolar depression outcome in older adults. Int J Geriatr Psychiatry 17(3):238–246
Bouckaert F, Sienaert P, Obbels J, Dols A, Vandenbulcke M, Stek M, Bolwig T (2014) ECT: its brain enabling effects: a review of electroconvulsive therapy–induced structural brain plasticity. J ECT 30(2):143–151
Boutron I, Moher D, Altman DG, Schulz K, Ravaud P (2008) Extending the CONSORT Statement to randomized trials of nonpharmacologic treatment: explanation and elaboration. Ann Intern Med 148(4):295–309
Breteler MM, van Swieten JC, Bots ML, Grobbee DE, Claus JJ, van den Hout JH, van Harskamp F, Tanghe HL, de Jong PT, van Gijn J, Hofman A et al (1994a) Cerebral white matter lesions, vascular risk factors, and cognitive function in a population-based study: the Rotterdam Study. Neurology 44(7):1246–1252
Breteler MMB, van Amerongen NM, van Swieten JC, Claus JJ, Grobbee DE, van Gjin J, Hofman A, van Harskamp F (1994b) Cognitive correlates of ventricular enlargement and cerebral white matter lesions on MRI. The Rotterdam Study. Stroke 25:1109–1115
Butters MA, Becker JT, Nebes RD, Zmuda MD, Mulsant BH, Pollock BG, Reynolds CF (2000) Changes in cognitive functioning following treatment of late-life depression. Am J Psychiatry 157(12):1949–1954
Castrén E, Rantamäki T (2010) The role of BDNF and its receptors in depression and antidepressant drug action: reactivation of developmental plasticity. Dev Neurobiol 70(5):289–297

Dahabra S, Ashton CH, Bahrainian M, Britton PG, Ferrier IN, McAllister VA, Marsh VR, Moore PB (1998) Structural and functional abnormalities in elderly patients clinically recovered from early- and late-onset depression. Biol Psychiatry 44(1):34–46
Dalgleish T, Navrady L, Bird E, Hill E, Dunn BD, Golden AM (2013) Method-of-Loci as a mnemonic device to facilitate access to self-affirming personal memories for individuals with depression. Clin Psychol Sci 1(2):156–162
de Groot JC, de Leeuw FE, Oudkerk M, van Gijn J, Hofman A, Jolles J, Breteler MM (2000) Cerebral white matter lesions and cognitive function: the Rotterdam Scan Study. Ann Neurol 47(2):145–151
Devanand DP, Pelton GH, Marston K, Camacho Y, Roose SP, Stern Y, Sackeim HA (2003) Sertraline treatment of elderly patients with depression and cognitive impairment. Int J Geriatr Psychiatry 18(2):123–130
Diamond K, Mowszowski L, Cockayne N, Norrie L, Paradise M, Hermens DF, Lewis SJ, Hickie IB, Naismith SL (2015) Randomised controlled trial of a Healthy Brain Ageing cognitive training program: effects on memory, mood and sleep. J Alzheimer's Dis 44(4):1181–1191
Diniz BS, Butters MA, Albert SM, Dew MA, Reynolds CF III (2013) Late-life depression and risk of vascular dementia and Alzheimer's disease: systematic review and meta-analysis of community-based cohort studies. Br J Psychiatry 202(5):329–335
Diniz BS, Sibille E, Ding Y, Tseng G, Aizenstein HJ, Lotrich F, Becker JT, Lopez OL, Lotze MT, Klunk WE, Reynolds CF, Butters MA (2015) Plasma biosignature and brain pathology related to persistent cognitive impairment in late-life depression. Mol Psychiatry 20:594–601
Doraiswamy PM, Krishnan KR, Oxman T, Jenkyn LR, Coffey DJ, Burt T, Clary CM (2003) Does antidepressant therapy improve cognition in elderly depressed patients? J Gerontol A Biol Sci Med Sci 58A(12):1137–1144
Dotson VM, Beydoun MA, Zonderman AB (2010) Recurrent depressive symptoms and the incidence of dementia and mild cognitive impairment. Neurology 75(1):27–34
Duffy S, Paradise M, Hickie I, Lewis S, Naismith S, Lagopoulos J (2014) Cognitive impairment with and without depression history: an analysis of white matter microstructure. J Psychiatry Neurosci 39(2):135–143
Duman RS, Monteggia LM, Duman RS, Monteggia LM (2006) A neurotrophic model for stress-related mood disorders. Biol Psychiatry 59(12):1116–1127
Dwivedi Y (2013) Involvement of brain-derived neurotrophic factor in late-life depression. Am J Geriatr Psychiatry 21(5):433–449
Elcombe EL, Lagopoulos J, Duffy S, Lewis SJ, Norrie L, Hickie IB, Naismith SL (2014a) Hippocampal volume in older adults at risk of cognitive decline: the role of sleep, vascular risk, and depression. J Alzheimers Dis 44(4):1279–1290
Elcombe EL, Lagopoulos J, Mowszowski L, Diamond K, Paradise M, Hickie IB, Lewis SJ, Naismith SL (2014b) Clinical and cognitive correlates of structural hippocampal change in "At-Risk" older adults. J Geriatr Psychiatry Neurol 27(2):67–76
Elgamal S, McKinnon MC, Ramakrishnan K, Joffe RT, MacQueen G (2007) Successful computer-assisted cognitive remediation therapy in patients with unipolar depression: a proof of principle study. Psychol Med 37(9):1229–1238
Elliott R (1998) The neuropsychological profile in unipolar depression. Trends Cogn Sci 2(11):447–454
Emery L, Hess TM (2011) Cognitive consequences of expressive regulation in older adults. Psychol Aging 26(2):388
Engvig A, Fjell AM, Westlye LT, Skaane NV, Dale AM, Holland D, Due-Tønnessen P, Sundseth O, Walhovd KB (2014) Effects of cognitive training on gray matter volumes in memory clinic patients with subjective memory impairment. J Alzheimer's Dis 41(3):779–791
Fregni F, Boggio PS, Nitsche MA, Rigonatti SP, Pascual-Leone A (2006) Cognitive effects of repeated sessions of transcranial direct current stimulation in patients with depression. Depress Anxiety 23:482–484
Gates N, Valenzuela M, Sachdev PS, Singh NA, Baune BT, Brodaty H, Suo C, Jain N, Wilson GC, Wang Y, Baker MK, Williamson D, Foroughi N, Fiatarone Singh MA, Fiatarone

Singh MA (2011a) Study of Mental Activity and Regular Training (SMART) in at risk individuals: a randomised double blind, sham controlled, longitudinal trial. BMC Geriatr 11(1):19

Gates NJ, Sachdev PS, Fiatarone Singh MA, Valenzuela M (2011b) Cognitive and memory training in adults at risk of dementia: a systematic review. BMC Geriatr 11(1):55

Greenstein AS, Paranthaman R, Burns A, Jackson A, Malik RA, Baldwin RC, Heagerty AM (2010) Cerebrovascular damage in late-life depression is associated with structural and functional abnormalities of subcutaneous small arteries. Hypertension 56(4):734–740

Gunning-Dixon FM, Raz N (2000) The cognitive correlates of white matter abnormalities in normal aging: a quantitative review. Neuropsychology 14(2):224–232

Hausner L, Damian M, Sartorius A, Frolich L (2011) Efficacy and cognitive side effects of Electroconvulsive Therapy (ECT) in depressed elderly inpatients with coexisting mild cognitive impairment or dementia. J Clin Psychiatry 72(1):91–97

Herrmann LL, Goodwin GM, Ebmeier KP (2007) The cognitive neuropsychology of depression in the elderly. Psychol Med 37(12):1693–1702

Hickie I, Scott E (1998) Late-onset depressive disorders: a preventable variant of cerebrovascular disease? Psychol Med 28(5):1007–1013

Hickie I, Scott E, Mitchell P, Wilhelm K, Austin MP, Bennett B (1995) Subcortical hyperintensities on magnetic resonance imaging: clinical correlates and prognostic significance in patients with severe depression. Biol Psychiatry 37(3):151–160

Hickie I, Scott E, Naismith S, Ward PB, Turner K, Parker G, Mitchell P, Wilhelm K (2001) Late-onset depression: genetic, vascular and clinical contributions. Psychol Med 13(8):1403–1412

Hickie I, Naismith S, Ward P, Scott E, Mitchell P, Wilhelm K, Parker G (2005a) Vascular risk and low serum B12 predict white matter lesions in patients with major depression. J Affect Disord 85(3):327–332

Hickie I, Naismith S, Ward P, Turner K, Scott E, Mitchell P, Wilhelm K, Parker G (2005b) Reduced hippocampal volumes and memory loss occurs in patients with early- and late-onset depression. Br J Psychiatry 186(3):197–202

Hickie I, Naismith S, Ward P, Little C, Pearson M, Scott E, Mitchell P, Wilhelm K, Parker G (2007) Psychomotor slowing in older persons with major depression: relationships with blood flow in the caudate nucleus and white matter lesions. Psychiatry Res 155(3):211–220

Horvath JC, Forte JD, Carter O (2015) Quantitative review finds no evidence of cognitive effects in healthy populations from single-session Transcranial Direct Current Stimulation (tDCS). Brain Stimul 8(3):535–550

Iacoviello BM, Wu G, Alvarez E, Huryk K, Collins KA, Murrough JW, Iosifescu DV, Charney DS (2014) Cognitive emotional training as an intervention for major depressive disorder. Depress Anxiety 31(8):699–706

Jayaweera HK, Hickie IB, Duffy SL, Hermens DF, Mowszowski L, Diamond K, Terpening Z, Paradise M, Lewis SJ, Lagopoulos J, Naismith SL (2015a) Mild cognitive impairment subtypes in older people with depressive symptoms: relationship with clinical variables and hippocampal change. J Geriatr Psychiatry Neurol 28:174–83, Epub ahead of Print

Jayaweera HK, Lagopoulos J, Duffy SL, Lewis SJ G, Hermens DF, Norrie L, Hickie IB, Naismith SL (2015b) Spectroscopic markers of memory impairment, symptom severity and age of onset in older people with lifetime depression: discrete roles of N-acetyl aspartate and glutamate. J Affect Disord 183:31–38

Jeste DV, Heaton SC, Paulsen JS, Ercoli L, Harris J, Heaton RK (1996) Clinical and neuropsychological comparison of psychotic depression with nonpsychotic depression and schizophrenia. Am J Psychiatry 153(4):490–496

Khatri K, Blumenthal JA, Babyak MA, Craighead WE, Herman S, Baldewicz T, Madden DJ, Doraiswamy M, Waugh R, Krishnan KR (2001) Effects of exercise training on cognitive functioning among depressed older men and women. J Aging Phys Act 9:43–57

Kinsella GJ, Mullaly E, Rand E, Ong B, Burton C, Price S, Phillips M, Storey E (2009) Early intervention for mild cognitive impairment: a randomised controlled trial. J Neurol Neurosurg Psychiatry 80(7):730–736

Kiosses DN, Alexopoulos GS, Murphy C (2000) Symptoms of striatofrontal dysfunction contribute to disability in geriatric depression. Int J Geriatr Psychiatry 15(11):992–999

Kiosses DN, Klimstra S, Murphy C, Alexopoulos GS (2001) Executive dysfunction and disability in elderly patients with major depression. Am J Geriatr Psychiatry 9(3):269–274

Kizilbash AH, Vanderploeg RD, Curtiss G (2002) The effects of depression and anxiety on memory performance. Arch Clin Neuropsychol 17:57–67

Koenig AM, Butters MA (2014) Cognition in late life depression: treatment considerations. Curr Treat Options Psychiatry 1(1):1–14

Kohler S, Thomas AJ, Lloyd A, Barber R, Almeida OP, O'Brien JT (2010) White matter hyperintensities, cortisol levels, brain atrophy and continuing cognitive deficits in late-life depression. Br J Psychiatry 196(2):143–149

Krishnan KR, McDonald WM, Escalona PR, Doraiswamy PM, Na C, Husain MM, Figiel GS, Boyko OB, Ellinwood EH, Nemeroff CB (1992) Magnetic resonance imaging of the caudate nuclei in depression. Preliminary observations. Arch Gen Psychiatry 49(7):553–557

Krishnan KR, Hays JC, Blazer DG (1997) MRI-defined vascular depression. Am J Psychiatry 154(4):497–501

Krishnan KR, Taylor WD, McQuoid DR, MacFall JR, Payne ME, Provenzale JM, Steffens DC (2004) Clinical characteristics of magnetic resonance imaging-defined subcortical ischemic depression. Biol Psychiatry 55(4):390–397

Kurz A, Pohl C, Ramsenthaler M, Sorg C (2009) Cognitive rehabilitation in patients with mild cognitive impairment. Int J Geriatr Psychiatry 24(2):163–168

Lampit A, Hallock H, Valenzuela M (2014) Computerized cognitive training in cognitively healthy older adults: a systematic review and meta-analysis of effect modifiers. PLoS Med 11(11):e1001756

Lautenschlager NT, Cox KL, Flicker L, Foster JK, van Bockxmeer FM, Xiao J, Greenop KR, Almeida OP (2008) Effect of physical activity on cognitive function in older adults at risk for alzheimer disease: a randomized trial. J Am Med Assoc 300(9):1027–1037

Lee RSC, Hermens DF, Porter MA, Redoblado-Hodge MA (2012) A meta-analysis of cognitive deficits in first-episode major depressive disorder. J Affect Disord 140:113–124

Lee RSC, Redoblado-Hodge MA, Naismith SL, Hermens DF, Porter MA, Hickie IB (2013) Cognitive remediation improves memory and psychosocial functioning in first-episode psychiatric out-patients. Psychol Med 43(6):1161–1173

Lesser IM, Mean I, Boone KB, Miller BL, Mehringer CM, Wohl M (1994) Reduction of cerebral blood flow in older depressed patients. Arch Gen Psychiatry 51(9):677–686

Lesser IM, Boone KB, Mehringer CM, Wohl MA, Miller BL, Berman NG (1996) Cognition and white matter hyperintensities in older depressed patients. Am J Psychiatry 153(10):1280–1287

Levine B, Stuss DT, Winocur G, Binns MA, Fahy L, Mandic M, Bridges K, Robertson IH (2007) Cognitive rehabilitation in the elderly: effects on strategic behavior in relation to goal management. J Int Neuropsychol Soc 13(1):143–152

Lockwood KA, Alexopoulos GS, Kakuma T, Van Gorp WG (2000) Subtypes of cognitive impairment in depressed older adults. Am J Geriatr Psychiatry 8(3):201–208

Lohman MC, Rebok GW, Spira AP, Parisi JM, Gross AL, Kueider AM (2012) Depressive symptoms and memory performance among older adults: results from the ACTIVE memory training intervention. J Aging Health 25(8S):211–229

Mackin RS, Arean PA (2009) Impaired financial capacity in late life depression is associated with cognitive performance on measures of executive functioning and attention. J Int Neuropsychol Soc 15(5):793–798

Mahncke HW, Connor BB, Appelman J, Ahsanuddin ON, Hardy JL, Wood RA, Joyce NM, Boniske T, Atkins SM, Merzenich MM (2006) Memory enhancement in healthy older adults using a brain plasticity-based training program: a randomized, controlled study. Proc Natl Acad Sci USA 103(33):12523–12528

McDermott LM, Ebmeier KP (2009) A meta-analysis of depression severity and cognitive function. J Affect Disord 119(1):1–8

McGurk SR, Twamley EW, Sitzer DI, McHugo GJ, Mueser KT (2007) A meta-analysis of cognitive remediation in schizophrenia. Am J Psychiatry 164(12):1791–1802

Medalia A, Freilich B (2008) The Neuropsychological Educational Approach to Cognitive Remediation (NEAR) model: practice principles and outcome studies. Am J Psychiatr Rehabil 11(2):123–143
Meusel LAC, Hall GBC, Fougere P, McKinnon MC, MacQueen GM (2013) Neural correlates of cognitive remediation in patients with mood disorders. Psychiatry Res: Neuroimaging 214(2):142–152
Molendijk M, Spinhoven P, Polak M, Bus B, Penninx B, Elzinga B (2014) Serum BDNF concentrations as peripheral manifestations of depression: evidence from a systematic review and meta-analyses on 179 associations (N=9484). Mol Psychiatry 19(7):791–800
Morimoto SS, Wexler BE, Liu J, Hu W, Seirup J, Alexopoulos GS (2014) Neuroplasticity-based computerized cognitive remediation for treatment-resistant geriatric depression. Nat Commun 5:1–7
Mowszowski L, Batchelor J, Naismith SL (2010) Early intervention for cognitive decline: can cognitive training be used as a selective prevention technique? Int Psychogeriatr 22(4):537–548
Mowszowski L, Hermens DF, Diamond K, Norrie L, Cockayne N, Ward PB, Hickie IB, Lewis SJ, Batchelor J, Naismith SL (2014) Cognitive training enhances pre-attentive neurophysiological responses in older adults 'at risk' of dementia. J Alzheimer's Dis 41(4):1095–1108
Naismith S, Hickie I, Ward PB, Turner K, Scott E, Little C, Mitchell P, Wilhelm K, Parker G (2002) Caudate nucleus volumes and genetic determinants of homocysteine metabolism in the prediction of psychomotor speed in older persons with depression. Am J Psychiatry 159(12):2096–2098
Naismith SL, Hickie IB, Turner K, Little CL, Winter V, Ward PB, Wilhelm K, Mitchell P, Parker G (2003) Neuropsychological performance in patients with depression is associated with clinical, etiological and genetic risk factors. J Clin Exp Neuropsychol 25(6):866–877
Naismith SL, Hickie IB, Ward PB, Scott E, Little C (2006) Impaired implicit sequence learning in depression: a probe for frontostriatal dysfunction? Psychol Med 36(3):313–323
Naismith SL, Longley WA, Scott EM, Hickie IB (2007) Disability in major depression related to self-rated and objectively-measured cognitive deficits: a preliminary study. BMC Psychiatry 7(1):32
Naismith SL, Glozier N, Burke D, Carter PE, Scott E, Hickie IB (2009a) Early intervention for cognitive decline: is there a role for multiple medical or behavioural interventions? Early Interv Psychiatry 3(1):19–27
Naismith SL, Norrie L, Lewis SJ, Rogers NL, Scott EM, Hickie IB (2009b) Does sleep disturbance mediate neuropsychological functioning in older people with depression? J Affect Disord 116(1–2):139–143
Naismith SL, Redoblado-Hodge MA, Lewis SJ, Scott EM, Hickie IB (2010) Cognitive training in affective disorders improves memory: a preliminary study using the NEAR approach. J Affect Disord 121(3):258–262
Naismith SL, Diamond K, Carter PE, Norrie LM, Redoblado-Hodge MA, Lewis SJG, Hickie IB (2011a) Enhancing memory in late-life depression: the effects of a combined psychoeducation and cognitive training program. Am J Geriatr Psychiatry 19(3):240–248
Naismith SL, Rogers NL, Lewis SJ, Terpening Z, Ip T, Diamond K, Norrie L, Hickie IB (2011b) Sleep disturbance relates to neuropsychological functioning in late-life depression. J Affect Disord 132(1–2):139–145
Naismith S, Norrie L, Mowszowski L, Hickie I (2012) The neurobiology of depression in later-life: clinical, neuropsychological, neuroimaging and pathophysiological features. Prog Neurobiol 98(1):99–143
Norrie LM, Diamond K, Hickie IB, Rogers NL, Fearns S, Naismith SL (2011) Can older "at risk" adults benefit from psychoeducation targeting healthy brain aging? Int Psychogeriatr 23(3):413–424
Norton S, Matthews FE, Barnes DE, Yaffe K, Brayne C (2014) Potential for primary prevention of Alzheimer's disease: an analysis of population-based data. Lancet Neurol 13(8):788–794
O'Brien J, Desmond P, Ames D, Schweitzer I, Harrigan S, Tress B (1996) A magnetic resonance imaging study of white matter lesions in depression and Alzheimer's disease. Br J Psychiatry 168(4):477–485

O'Brien JT, Wiseman R, Burton EJ, Barber B, Wesnes K, Saxby B, Ford GA (2002) Cognitive associations of subcortical white matter lesions in older people. Ann N Y Acad Sci 977(1):436–444
O'Brien JT, Lloyd A, McKeith I, Gholkar A, Ferrier N (2004) A longitudinal study of hippocampal volume, cortisol levels, and cognition in older depressed subjects. Am J Psychiatry 161(11): 2081–2090
Onraedt T, Koster EHW (2014) Training working memory to reduce rumination. PLoS One 9(3):1–12
Owens M, Koster EHW, Derakshan N (2013) Improving attention control in dysphoria through cognitive training: transfer effects on working memory capacity and filtering efficiency. Psychophysiology 50(3):297–307
Panza F, Frisardi V, Capurso C, D'Introno A, Colacicco AM, Imbimbo BP, Santamato A, Vendemiale G, Seripa D, Pilotto A, Capurso A, Solfrizzi V (2010) Late-life depression, mild cognitive impairment, and dementia: possible continuum? Am J Geriatr Psychiatry 18(2):98–116
Parisi JM, Franchetti MK, Rebok GW, Spira AP, Carlson MC, Willis SL, Gross AL (2014) Depressive symptoms and inductive reasoning performance: findings from the ACTIVE reasoning training intervention. Psychol Aging 29(4):843
Pilar-Cuéllar F, Vidal R, Díaz A, Castro E, dos Anjos S, Pascual-Brazo J, Linge R, Vargas V, Blanco H, Martínez-Villayandre B, Pazos Á (2013) Neural plasticity and proliferation in the generation of antidepressant effects: hippocampal implication. Neural Plast 2013:Article ID 537265
Pisljar M, Pirtosek Z, Repovs G, Grgic M (2008) Executive dysfunction in late-onset depression. Psychiatr Danub 20(2):231–235
Portella MJ, Marcos T, Rami L, Navarro V, Gasto C, Salamero M (2003) Residual cognitive impairment in late-life depression after a 12-month period follow-up. Int J Geriatr Psychiatry 18(7):571–576
Preiss M, Shatil E, Cermakova R, Cimermanova D, Ram I (2013) Personalized cognitive training in unipolar and bipolar disorder: a study of cognitive functioning. Front Hum Neurosci 7:1–10
Raskin J, Wiltse CG, Siegal A, Sheikh J, Xu J, Dinkel JJ, Rotz BT, Mohs RC (2007) Efficacy of duloxetine on cognition, depression, and pain in elderly patients with major depressive disorder: an 8-week, double-blind, placebo-controlled trial. Am J Psychiatry 164(6):900–909
Rebok GW, Carlson MC, Langbaum JBS (2007) Training and maintaining memory abilities in healthy older adults: traditional and novel approaches. J Gerontol B Psychol Sci Soc Sci 62(Spec No 1):53–61
Rebok GW, Ball KK, Guey LT, Jones RN, Kim HY, King JW, Marsiske M, Morris JN, Tennstedt SL, Unverzagt FW, Willis SL, ACTIVE Study Group (2014) Ten-year effects of the advanced cognitive training for independent and vital elderly cognitive training trial on cognition and everyday functioning in older adults. J Am Geriatr Soc 62(1):16–24
Romanowicz M, Sutor B, Sola C (2012) Safety and efficacy of electroconvulsive therapy for depression following cerebrovascular accident. Acta Neuropsychiatrica 24(4):226–229
Rossini PM, Rossi S, Babiloni C, Polich J (2007) Clinical neurophysiology of aging brain: from normal aging to neurodegeneration. Prog Neurobiol 83(6):875–400
Saczynski JS, Beiser A, Seshadri S, Auerbach S, Wolf PA, Au R (2010) Depressive symptoms and risk of dementia: the Framingham Heart Study. Neurology 75(1):35–41
Saczynski JS, Rosen AB, McCammon RJ, Zivin K, Andrade SE, Langa KM, Vijan S, Pirraglia PA, Briesacher BA, Briesacher BA (2015) Antidepressant use and cognitive decline: the health and retirement study. Am J Med 128(7):739–746
Salloway S, Malloy P, Kohn R, Gillard E, Duffy J, Rogg J, Tung G, Richardson E, Thomas C, Westlake R (1996) MRI and neuropsychological differences in early-and late-life-onset geriatric depression. Neurology 46(6):1567–1574
Schmaal L, Veltman DJ, van Erp TG, Sämann P, Frodl T, Jahanshad N, Loehrer E, Tiemeier H, Hofman A, Niessen WJ, Vernooij MW, Ikram MA, Wittfeld K, Grabe HJ, Block A, Hegenscheid K, Völzke H, Hoehn D, Czisch M, Lagopoulos J, Hatton SN, Hickie IB, Goya-Maldonado R, Krämer B, Gruber O, Couvy-Duchesne B, Rentería ME, Strike LT, Mills NT, de Zubicaray GI,

McMahon KL, Medland SE, Martin NG, Gillespie NA, Wright MJ, Hall GB, MacQueen GM, Frey EM, Carballedo A, van Velzen LS, van Tol MJ, van der Wee NJ, Veer IM, Walter H, Schnell K, Schramm E, Normann C, Schoepf D, Konrad C, Zurowski B, Nickson T, McIntosh AM, Papmeyer M, Whalley HC, Sussmann JE, Godlewska BR, Cowen PJ, Fischer FH, Rose M, Penninx BW, Thompson PM, Hibar DP (2015) Subcortical brain alterations in major depressive disorder: findings from the ENIGMA major depressive disorder working group. Mol Psychiatry. doi:10.1038/mp.2015.69, Epub ahead of Print

Schrader G, Cheok F, Hordacre AL, Marker J, Wade V (2005) Effect of psychiatry liaison with general practitioners on depression severity in recently hospitalised cardiac patients: a randomised controlled trial. Med J Aust 182(6):272–276

Scogin F, Fairchild JK, Yon A, Welsh DA, Presnell A (2014) Cognitive bibliotherapy and memory training for older adults with depressive symptoms. Aging Ment Health 18(5):554–560

Serafini G, Pompili M, Belvederi MM, Respino M, Ghio L, Girardi P, Fitzgerald PB, Amore M (2015) The effects of repetitive transcranial magnetic stimulation on cognitive performance in treatment-resistant depression. A systematic review. Neuropsychobiology 71(3): 125–139

Sheline YI, Pieper CF, Barch DM, Welsh-Bohmer K, McKinstry RC, MacFall JR, D'Angelo G, Garcia KS, Gersing K, Wilkins C, Taylor W, Steffens DC, Krishnan RR, Doraiswamy PM (2010) Support for the vascular depression hypothesis in late-life depression: results of a 2-site, prospective, antidepressant treatment trial. Arch Gen Psychiatry 67(3): 277–285

Sheline YI, Disabato BM, Hranilovich J, Morris C, D'Angelo G, Pieper C, Toffanin T, Taylor WD, MacFall JR, Wilkins C, Barch DM, Welsh-Bohmer KA, Steffens DC, Krishnan RR, Doraiswamy PM (2012) Treatment course with antidepressant therapy in late-life depression. Am J Psychiatry 169(11):1185–1193

Simpson SW, Jackson A, Baldwin RC, Burns A (1997) Subcortical hyperintensities in late-life depression: acute response to treatment and neuropsychological impairment. Int Psychogeriatr 9(3):257–275

Sitzer DI, Twamley EW, Jeste DV (2006) Cognitive training in Alzheimer's disease: a meta-analysis of the literature. Acta Psychiatr Scand 114(2):75–90

Sneed JR, Roose SP, Keilp JG, Krishnan KR, Alexopoulos GS, Sackeim HA (2007) Response inhibition predicts poor antidepressant treatment response in very old depressed patients. Am J Geriatr Psychiatry 15(7):553–563

Sobin C, Sackeim HA, Prudic J, Devanand DP, Moody BJ, McElhiney MC (1995) Predictors of retrograde amnesia following ECT. Am J Psychiatry 152(7):995–1001

Steffens DC, Krishnan KR (1998) Structural neuroimaging and mood disorders: recent findings, implications for classification, and future directions. Biol Psychiatry 43(10):705–712

Steffens DC, Tupler LA, Ranga K, Krishnan R (1998) Magnetic resonance imaging signal hypointensity and iron content of putamen nuclei in elderly depressed patients. Psychiatry Res: Neuroimaging 83(2):95–103

Steffens DC, Potter GG, McQuoid DR, MacFall JR, Payne ME, Burke JR, Plassman BL, Welsh-Bohmer KA (2007) Longitudinal magnetic resonance imaging vascular changes, apolipoprotein E genotype, and development of dementia in the neurocognitive outcomes of depression in the elderly study. Am J Geriatr Psychiatry 15(10):839–849

Steffens DC, McQuoid DR, Payne ME, Potter GG (2011) Change in hippocampal volume on magnetic resonance imaging and cognitive decline among older depressed and nondepressed subjects in the neurocognitive outcomes of depression in the elderly study. Am J Geriatr Psychiatry 19(1):4–12

Story TJ, Potter GG, Attix DK, Welsh-Bohmer KA, Steffens DC (2008) Neurocognitive correlates of response to treatment in late-life depression. Am J Geriatr Psychiatry 16(9):752–759

Suo C, Valenzuela MV (2012) Neuroimaging outcomes of brain training trials. In: Bright P (ed) Neuroimaging – cognitive and clinical neuroscience. InTech, Croatia

Tanti A, Belzung C (2013) Neurogenesis along the septo-temporal axis of the hippocampus: are depression and the action of antidepressants region-specific? Neuroscience 252:234–252

Taylor WD, Aizenstein HJ, Alexopoulos GS (2013) The vascular depression hypothesis: mechanisms linking vascular disease with depression. Mol Psychiatry 18(9):963–974

Thomas AJ, O'Brien JT, Davis S, Ballard C, Barber R, Kalaria RN, Perry RH (2002) Ischemic basis for deep white matter hyperintensities in major depression: a neuropathological study. Arch Gen Psychiatry 59(9):785–792

Thomas AJ, Kalaria RN, O'Brien JT (2004) Depression and vascular disease: what is the relationship? J Affect Disord 79(1–3):81–95

Valenzuela M, Sachdev P (2009) Can cognitive exercise prevent the onset of dementia? Systematic review of randomized clinical trials with longitudinal follow-up. Am J Geriatr Psychiatry 17(3):179–187

Vasques PE, Moraes H, Silveira H, Deslandes AC, Laks J (2011) Acute exercise improves cognition in the depressed elderly: the effect of dual-tasks. Clinics 66(9):1553–1557

Veiel HOF (1997) A preliminary profile of neuropsychological deficits associated with major depression. J Clin Exp Neuropsychol 19(4):587–603

Verdelho A, Madureira S, Moleiro C, Ferro JM, O'Brien JT, Poggesi A, Pantoni L, Fazekas F, Scheltens P, Waldemar G, Wallin A, Erkinjuntti T, Inzitari D, LADIS Study (2013) Depressive symptoms predict cognitive decline and dementia in older people independently of cerebral white matter changes: the LADIS study. J Neurol Neurosurg Psychiatry 84(11):1250–1254

Vinogradov S, Fisher M, de Villers-Sidani E (2012) Cognitive training for impaired neural systems in neuropsychiatric illness. Neuropsychopharmacology 37(1):43–76

Walton CC, Mowszowski L, Lewis SJG, Naismith SL (2014) Stuck in the mud: time for change in the implementation of cognitive training research in ageing? Front Aging Neurosci 6:43

Wanmaker S, Geraerts E, Frangen IHA (2015) A working memory training to decrease rumination in depressed and anxious individuals: a double-blind randomized controlled trial. J Affect Disord 175:310–319

Wolinsky FD, Mahncke HW, van der Weg MW, Martin R, Unverzagt FW, Ball KK, Jones RN, Tennstedt SL (2009) The ACTIVE cognitive training interventions and the onset of and recovery from suspected clinical depression. J Gerontol 64B(5):577–585

Zaninotto L, Guglielmo R, Calati R, Ioime L, Camardese G, Janiri L, Bria P, Serretti A (2015) Cognitive markers of psychotic unipolar depression: a meta-analytic study. J Affect Disord 174:580–588

The Internet and Mobile Technology: A Platform for Behavior Change and Intervention in Depression and CVDs

22

Harald Baumeister, Yannik Terhorst, and Jiaxi Lin

Contents

Abstract

Depression often co-occurs with cardiovascular disease (CVD), affecting not only the individuals' well-being but also causing a high socioeconomic burden. Access to effective, acceptable, and cost-effective treatment of depression

H. Baumeister (✉)
Department of Clinical Psychology and Psychotherapy, Institute of Psychology and Education, University of Ulm, Albert-Einstein-Allee-47, 89081 Ulm, Germany
e-mail: harald.baumeister@uni-ulm.de

Y. Terhorst • J. Lin
Department of Rehabilitation Psychology and Psychotherapy, Institut of Psychology, University of Freiburg, Engelbergerstrasse 41, Freiburg 79085, Germany

B.T. Baune, P.J. Tully (eds.), *Cardiovascular Diseases and Depression*,
DOI 10.1007/978-3-319-32480-7_22

however is limited. Internet- and mobile-based interventions (IMIs) can provide access to effective treatments at any time at any place for many individuals simultaneously and thus have the potential to substantially improve the accessibility of mental health care for individuals with CVD.

This chapter gives an overview on IMIs in the treatment of depression in individuals with CVD. First, a description of the main characteristics of IMIs, i.e., technical implementation, human support, theory, areas of application, ethics, and data security, is provided. The evidence base is described in terms of the effectiveness and cost-effectiveness of IMIs for individuals with CVD and depression as well as an overview on potentially effect-moderating factors such as using technological and human support as adherence facilitating components of IMIs. Finally, implementation possibilities and barriers are discussed including considerations on how IMIs should be used to fully exploit their potential for individuals with CVD and depression.

22.1 Introduction

Prevalence rates of depression are increased in individuals with cardiovascular disease (CVD) (Härter et al. 2007; Baumeister et al. 2010). Therefore, the comorbidity of depression and CVD not only affects individuals' well-being (Baumeister et al. 2011a) but also poses substantial economic and societal costs (Baumeister et al. 2015; Haschke et al. 2012). Thus, effective interventions for the treatment of depression in individuals with CVD are necessary. Effectiveness has been shown for psychological and pharmacological interventions as well as for more complex collaborative and stepped-care approaches (Baumeister and Hutter 2012; Baumeister et al. 2011b; Tully and Baumeister 2014). Moreover, these interventions not only need to be effective but also available and acceptable at a public health level to substantially lower the disease burden associated with CVD-depression comorbidity, a necessity only insufficiently present in most health-care systems. Restricted access to psychotherapy, regional shortage of mental health-care offers, intolerance of drug therapy, and several other reasons can keep individuals away from depression treatment.

One promising new development of the last decade which might help to diminish the lack of available evidence-based depression interventions are Internet- and mobile-based interventions (IMIs) that can be provided 24 hours, 7 days a week to many individuals at any place. The present chapter will summarize the state of research on IMIs for individuals with CVD as one important technology-based development to facilitate depression health care in CVD. Since online intervention research is still a new discipline, the chapter focuses on the evidence on IMIs for depression in general in case of a lack of CVD-specific evidence. After reading, you will have comprehensive knowledge of how IMIs for depression work, how effective they are, and which different kinds of implementing IMIs into our health-care systems are possible.

22.2 Characterizing Internet- and Mobile-Based Interventions (IMIs)

With the help of IMIs, mental health interventions can be transferred to the virtual space. Using reliable and established psychotherapeutic techniques, IMIs target emotional, cognitive, and behavioral processes (Mohr et al. 2013; Andersson and Titov 2014). Therefore, four main aspects that characterize IMIs can be distinguished: (1) technical implementation, (2) human support, (3) theory, and (4) areas of application. Considering the development and implementation of IMIs, ethical aspects as well as aspects of data security play a central role that will be presented subsequently (Fig. 22.1).

22.2.1 Technical Implementation

IMIs consist of various technical means, such as e-mail, text message, chat or video-based communication, software programs (e.g., Internet games, virtual environment; computer games, mobile apps), or different Internet activities (e.g., blogs, podcasts, online support groups) (Mohr et al. 2013; Andersson et al. 2011; Proudfoot et al. 2011; Barak et al. 2009). As a result of the fast technological development, there are increasingly more technical opportunities to realize and shape IMIs. Especially interactive exercises (on a website or by apps), peer and expert chat rooms, and prompts (e.g., automatic e-mails and text messages) which fulfill a

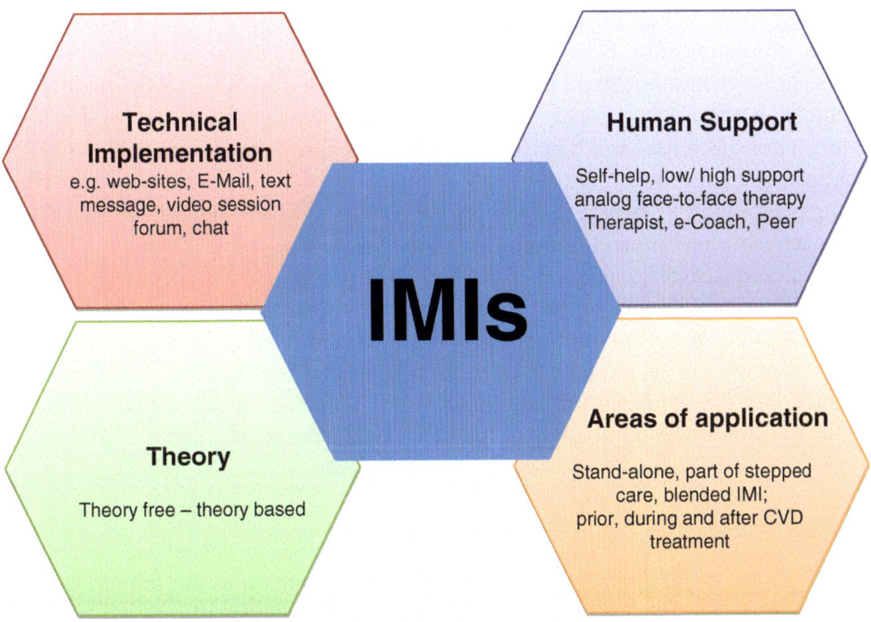

Fig. 22.1 Central parts of IMIs

reminding and reinforcing function play an important role for IMIs to be effective (Fry and Neff 2009; Ritterband et al. 2009; Webb et al. 2010; Wangberg et al. 2008). IMIs can also be supported by video and audio files, and program parts can be similar for all patients or be tailored individually for specific needs and characteristics of the participant (Carlbring et al. 2011; Johansson et al. 2012a; Andersson et al. 2009). The learn process can be supported by activation monitoring and training diaries (Mohr et al. 2013). New aspects in this area are ecological momentary interventions (EMIs), which include intervention parts in the patients' daily life by text messages via mobile or smartphone (Heron and Smyth 2010). Voice and video messages can also be used (Grassi et al. 2009). One advantage of this new technology is the possibility of an accurate data collection in relevant situations without retrospective biases (Heron and Smyth 2010). Another advantage is transferring exercises into patients' daily living and, thus, moving therapy closer to where patients' life problems occur.

22.2.2 Human Support

IMIs are mainly seen as self-help interventions without human support ("unguided self-help") or with different intensity of human support ("guided self-help") (Andersson et al. 2011; Barak et al. 2009; Baumeister et al. 2014a). In general, support includes peer support (e.g., support in forums by patients for patients) and professional support (support by e-coach). Thereby, the label "guided" refers to professional support, which mostly includes assisting users in their process and enforcing them in their improvements.

The communication between expert and participant can be synchronous (e.g., chats) or asynchronous (e.g., e-mail). In the common case of asynchronous communication, the e-coach usually needs a few minutes up to a few hours per user and intervention (as a rule 1–2 h per user and intervention) (Proudfoot et al. 2011). In contrast, patients' intervention efforts comprising of reading self-help material, doing exercises, homework, and reading and writing e-mails and text messages can be as intensive and time-consuming as in traditional face-to-face therapies (Berger and Andersson 2009; Andersson et al. 2013). The combination of technical application and minimal human support leads to increased extent of self-regulated coping and decreased intervention costs. In addition, patients' and e-coaches' flexibility and autonomy are increased by location-independent intervention, asynchronous contact, and time-independent communication. Nonetheless, the specific arrangement of communication depends on the theoretical base of the intervention.

22.2.3 Theory

IMIs are characterized by being highly structured, standardized, and methodically focused, and most of them are based on cognitive behavioral techniques and health behavior change models (Andersson and Titov 2014; Webb et al. 2010;

Andersson 2009; Barak et al. 2008; Murray 2012). However, IMIs based on other theoretical concepts such as psychodynamic therapy and acceptance and commitment therapy (ACT) can also be found (Johansson et al. 2012b; Lin et al. 2015).

Regularly, IMIs are divided up into several modules, following the session structure of evidence-based psychotherapies. These modules can be obligatory or facultative, in a predefined order or freely combinable, tailored to the specific user needs (Carlbring et al. 2011; Wanner et al. 2009). Cognitive behavioral concepts often contain psychoeducation, behavior activation, exposures, and techniques of problem solving and cognitive restructuring (Barak et al. 2009; Andersson et al. 2013; Ritterband et al. 2003). One module typically contains different tasks, which have to be completed within a specific time period, for example, within a week. Therefore, participants get automatic processed feedback by the program itself or an individual feedback given by an e-coach.

22.2.4 Areas of Application

IMIs for mental disorders have been developed for the whole range of mental disorders including mainly IMIs for depression and anxiety disorders but also IMIs for substance use disorders, bipolar disorders, obsessive-compulsive disorders, and many other mental disorders (Baumeister et al. in Press). A list of (some) existing IMIs can be found on the website www.beacon.anu.edu.au, which offers an overview on IMIs around the world (Christensen et al. 2010).

Regarding the context and setting in which IMIs are provided, they can be applied as part of a stepped-care model, as a stand-alone intervention or as blended IMIs in combination with a traditional face-to-face psychotherapy (Andersson and Titov 2014; Emmelkamp et al. 2014). Moreover, they can be used prior, during, and after specific CVD treatments to prepare, support, and taper treatments.

Stand-alone IMIs and IMIs as part of a stepped-care approach might be the main area of application for IMIs in CVD health care. Stand-alone IMIs as self-contained interventions might become a standard extension of depression care offers from general practitioners and CVD specialists, where depression drug treatment is currently often the only always available but not always indicated care offer (Baumeister 2012; Gaebel et al. 2013). In more complex treatment concepts such as collaborative care and stepped-care models, IMIs for depression offer a first low-threshold opportunity (Baumeister and Hutter 2012; Tully and Baumeister 2014; Richards 2012) prior to initiating the more resource and time-consuming treatment options of face-to-face psychotherapy and/or antidepressant drug therapy.

Blended IMIs can be used to support traditional psychotherapies by outsourcing some of the time-consuming rather standardized and less complex therapy modules such as psychoeducation, thereby saving therapist time for the more complex psychotherapeutical processes. Furthermore, blended IMIs can accompany traditional psychotherapies to shift psychotherapy more into patients' everyday life by using, e.g., mobile applications for ambulatory assessments and behavioral activation tasks (e.g., text messages reminding patients of their exercise plan).

Regarding the time of the treatment process, IMIs can be used prior to, e.g., CVD treatment to facilitate CVD outcomes. IMIs might help to overcome motivational and volitional constraints associated with depression that hamper patients' treatment adherence. During CVD treatment, comorbid depression can be treated as described before, as part of an integrated care program, or by means of a stand-alone intervention aiming to improve comorbidities that were detected but not treated in the context of CVD treatment. Finally, IMIs as step-down approach after an intensive face-to-face depression treatment might be helpful to facilitate patients' self-management competencies, thereby maintaining treatment effects over time (Lin et al. 2013; Moessner et al. 2014; Zwerenz et al. 2013).

22.2.5 Ethics and Data Security

IMIs have several ethical risks and chances that need to be taken into account when providing e-mental health care (Rochlen et al. 2004; Wells et al. 2007; Fenichel et al. 2002; Prabhakar 2013; Manhal-Baugus 2001). Central problems occur in the diagnostic and the treatment process including possible misdiagnoses, medical malpractice, and especially in the case of suicidality (Manhal-Baugus 2001). At the same time, some researchers point out that the use of Internet support for suicidal individuals and those in crisis can also be very effective as they provide relevant contact information and course of actions (Fenichel et al. 2002; Manhal-Baugus 2001). Notwithstanding, the withholding of IMIs would also be ethically problematic, as several studies reported IMIs to be as effective as treatment as usual (cf. Sect. 22.3.1). As IMIs are an opportunity for individuals, who would not use therapy otherwise, withholding IMIs would keep individuals in need of treatment away from evidence-based treatment offers.

Data security considerations are often overlooked and underfunded when IMIs are developed, delivered, and evaluated (Bennett et al. 2010). Nevertheless, a high standard of data security is crucial to the overall success of any IMI. Hence, IMIs need to be accurately developed and adapted in concordance to the legal conditions and obliged control activities of the respective legislative context. As special IT expertise is needed for the realization of data security, it is highly recommended to integrate IT staff in all stages of the development process (Bennett et al. 2010).

Thus, while there are important questions regarding data security, diagnostic accuracy, good clinical practice, and quality assurance, the question is rather how, and not if, to provide IMIs for depression in CVD health care. As long as there is no consistent quality assurance, the door will be left open for questionable offers. Important steps forward would be to develop uniform quality standards as well as to systematically examine negative effects of IMIs (Rozental et al. 2014), one aspect that is mostly missing in psychotherapy research in general.

Table 22.1 Effectiveness of Internet- and Mobile-based interventions based on selected meta-analyses

Target population	Authors	SMD	[95 % CI]	*N*
Adults				
Depression	Richards and Richardson (2012)	0.56	[−0.71, 0.41]	19
Panic disorder	Andrews et al. (2010)	0.83	[0.45, 1.21]	6
Social phobia	Andrews et al. (2010)	0.92	[0.74, 1.09]	8
Generalized anxiety disorder	Andrews et al. (2010)	1.11	[0.76, 1.47]	2
Post-traumatic stress disorder	Hedman et al. (2012)	1.23	[0.83, 1.63]	6
Sleep disorder	Cheng and Dizon (2012)	0.86[a]	[0.53, 1.18]	2
Eating disorder	Hedman et al. (2012)	0.97	[0.63, 1.30]	5
Alcohol abuse	Riper et al. (2014)	0.2	[0.13, 0.27]	16
Obsessive compulsive disorder	Paganini et al. (2016)	1.02	[0.66, 1.38]	2
Children and adolescents				
Depression	Ebert et al. (2015a)	0.76	[0.41,1.12]	4
Anxiety	Ebert et al. (2015a)	0.68	[0.45,0.92]	7

Adapted from Paganini et al. (2016)
CI confidence interval, *N* number of included primary studies, *SMD* standardized mean difference (Cohens' d/Hedges' g)
[a]Average effect of "Insomnia Severity Index"

22.3 Evidence

22.3.1 Effectiveness

There is a large evidence for mental health IMIs being effective with medium to large effect sizes when compared with treatment as usual and waiting list control groups (Table 22.1).

Regarding depression, Richards and Richardson (2012) included 19 RCTs in their meta-analysis with a total of $n=2996$ participants. Across the studies, a moderate posttreatment pooled effect size of $d=.56$ [95 %–CI: .41; .71] in favor of computer-based psychological treatments for depression compared to usual care and waitlist has been shown (Richards and Richardson 2012). Correspondingly, clinically significant improvements and remission rates were significantly superior in the computer-based intervention groups than in control groups (odds ratios: 3.68 [2.12, 6.40], 4.14 [2.01, 8.53]) (Richards and Richardson 2012). Moreover, studies that compared the effectiveness of depression interventions provided as guided IMIs against face-to-face psychotherapies indicated no significant differences between these two intervention settings (Andersson et al. 2014), suggesting that IMIs might be as effective as established, evidence-based psychotherapies for adults as well as for children and adolescents.

The positive findings for IMIs in general can also be shown for the subpopulation of chronically ill individuals. In a recent review on IMIs for comorbid depression in individuals with chronic medical diseases, Charova and colleagues (2015) reported significant improvements in depression severity (*d*=.36 [.20; .52]), based on 11 randomized and non-randomized clinical trials. As shown in a recent large-scale trial on depression treatment in individuals with diabetes, the effects of IMIs can even be expected to be higher in case of using a state-of-the-art guided IMI for depression (Nobis et al. 2013, 2015). Nobis and colleagues (2015) reported significantly lower depressive symptoms at posttreatment in the IMI group compared to an online unguided psychoeducation program for depression with a large effect of *d*=.89 [.64; 1.15].

A first study on IMIs for depression in individuals with CVD indicates that IMIs are feasible and effective in this subgroup too; however, the magnitude of the effect might be lower than in other chronic disease patient groups. Glozier and colleagues (2013) examined the effectiveness of Internet-delivered cognitive behavioral therapy (iCBT) for adults with mild to moderate depression and high cardiovascular disease risks. They compared the open access iCBT program E-couch to a group receiving an Internet-delivered attention control health information package (HealthWatch) in a large-scale RCT (*N*=562). Depression severity at posttreatment was significantly lower in the iCBT than the control group, however, with an only small to moderate effect size of *d*=.3 [.1–.5] (Charova et al. 2015; Glozier et al. 2013). An ongoing trial by Norlund and colleagues examining the effectiveness of an iCBT for depression and anxiety in patients with a recent myocardial infarction will increase the evidence base in near future (Norlund et al. 2015). The finding that effect sizes of depression treatments are lower for individuals with CVD compared to other chronic diseases are also known from psychotherapy and antidepressant drug studies on depression in individuals with coronary artery disease (CAD) or diabetes (Baumeister et al. 2011b, 2012). An explanation for these systematic differences might be that depression is rather a broad category, comprising distinct subtypes of depression with their own depression course and treatment response than a unidimensional construct (Baumeister and Parker 2012; Carney and Freedland 2012). Data from epidemiological studies indicate that we might need to look more into CVD (or at least CAD)-specific depression IMIs with a stronger focus on improving the somatic symptoms of depression (Ormel and de Jonge 2011; Roest et al. 2013).

22.3.2 Cost-Effectiveness

Cost-effectiveness of IMIs is often regarded as one of the major advantages of IMIs over established interventions, as the effectiveness seems to be comparable, and costs are presumably lower given the lower therapists' time resources needed. More surprising is the lack of studies examining the cost-effectiveness of IMIs for depression. Warmerdam and colleagues (2010) as one of the only studies that examined cost-effectiveness so far, compared the cost-effectiveness of an Internet-based cognitive behavioral therapy (iCBT) against a waiting list control group for adults with depressive symptoms. Results of the incremental cost-effectiveness ratio (ICER) analysis indicated that by offering iCBT instead of waiting list one additionally depression improved participant was associated with extra costs of 1817EUR, which can be regarded as good value for money.

With regard to IMIs and CVD, there is only one study by Keyserling et al. (2014) reporting the cost-effectiveness of a counselor-based intervention compared to an IMI for reducing the risk of CAD in a nondepression-focused IMI study. While both intervention settings were able to reduce CAD risk through 12-month follow-up, the IMI was less expensive with 207$ and 110$ per person for the counselor and the IMI intervention, respectively.

Thus, while the few studies on cost-effectiveness point in the hypothesized direction of IMIs being cost-effective, the primary conclusion is that further health economic research is highly needed. Moreover, studies should answer the question of whether IMIs are cost-effective when compared with treatment as usual, waiting list, or other established treatments such as psychotherapy, pharmacotherapy, or collaborative care. Future empirical work should also focus on the differential cost-effectiveness of IMIs varying in their level of technical and design sophistication as well as the guidance provided.

22.3.3 Effect Factors

The question on why IMIs are effective and what the effect-generating ingredients are came into the focus of research, once the effectiveness of IMIs for mental disorders had been established. In their review, Andersson and colleagues (2009) suggested that (a) a proper diagnosis prior to treatment; (b) a comprehensive treatment with a clear deadline; (c) a user friendly, not too technically advanced treatment; and (d) support are effect-facilitating features of IMIs. While most of these suggestions very likely represent significant effect factors, only the impact of support on the effectiveness of IMIs has been examined empirically to a larger extent. Therefore, support was examined as technical support by means of automatic prompts (i.e., reminders, feedback, and reinforcement automatisms) and human support.

Advantages of IMIs over face-to-face interventions are the possibility to include automatic prompts as part of the intervention. In a systematic review including 85 studies about IMIs, Webb and colleagues (2010) reported that automatic features have a small but significant effect on behavior. Titov and colleagues conducted two comparable unguided Internet-based interventions, one with prompts (Titov et al. 2009a) and one without (Titov et al. 2008). The effect in the program with prompts was almost three times as high as in the program without ($d=0.73$ vs. $d=0.28$). Most probably, the higher effect was caused by an increased treatment adherence, with a significant lower dropout rate in the intervention including prompts. Finally, Fry and colleagues (Fry and Neff 2009) and Leon et al. (2014) showed in their reviews that prompts are associated with positive outcomes. This, however, was particularly true for those interventions that combined prompts with personal contact, indicating that human support might still be an important part of IMIs being effective.

A recent systematic review by Baumeister and colleagues (2014a) summarized the current state of research on the effect of guided and unguided professional support. Their study focused on the comparison of guided and unguided interventions, dose-response relationship, qualification of e-coaches, and communication mode (Baumeister et al. 2014a). The comparison of guided and unguided interventions showed a pooled standardized mean differences (SMD) for symptom severity of −.27 (95 %–CI: −.45; −.10; $n=8$) favoring guided interventions. Moreover, the pooled mean number of completed modules (SMD: .52 (95 %–CI: .37; .67; $n=7$)) and completer rates (OR: 2.76 (95 %–CI: 1.68; 4.53; $n=6$)) was higher for guided interventions than in unguided interventions.

According to Baumeister and colleagues (2014a), only one study focused on the dose-response relationship regarding guidance with no difference regarding the effectiveness, the mean number of completed modules, and the completer rate between the groups receiving either one or three e-mail contacts per week (Klein et al. 2009). Indirect evidence on the dose-response relationship comes from several nonexperimental studies. Palmqvist and colleagues (2007) reported a direct relation between therapeutic time and treatment effectiveness and adherence. Andersson and colleagues (2009) considered a time of 100 min for each patient during a 10-week IMI as adequate. However, this should rather be seen as a preliminary estimation in the absence of empirical data on the best dose-response relationship (Baumeister et al. 2014a; Titov 2011), which in addition might depend on the specific disorder under study (Newman et al. 2011).

Next to the question whether to provide guidance, the question of who should provide guidance is of major interest. Baumeister et al. (2014a) summarized four studies that experimentally compared guided IMIs provided by e-coaches with different qualification levels. None of the studies showed a significant difference in any of the examined outcomes, indicating that the qualification of the e-coaches is rather of minor importance. Methodological limitations of the primary studies, however, limit the validity of this conclusion.

Finally, Baumeister and colleagues (2014a) investigated if the effectiveness of IMIs might vary with the communication mode used between e-coach and user. One study that experimentally examined this question did not indicate any difference between a synchronous (Internet forum) and asynchronous communication mode (telephone) (Titov et al. 2009b).

In summary, both technical and personal supports are measures likely to increase the effectiveness of IMIs. However, as yet we know little about the specifics of these effect-modifying features. Moreover, the effectiveness might also vary with regard to different patient characteristics and medical variables such as patients' subtype of depression (Roest et al. 2013; Ebert et al. 2013). Thus, it remains a question to be answered, whether the aforementioned general evidence on effect-modifying aspects of IMIs can also be found in individuals with CVD and depression and whether individuals with different types of CVD and depression would differ in the way they respond to IMIs.

22.4 Implementation

Health-care systems have to face the challenge of optimizing treatments and of assuring sustainability of treatment effects over time against the background of restricted health-care resources. Hence, IMIs are regarded as a promising option for the treatment of depression in individuals with CVD.

To successfully implement IMIs in routine CVD care, it needs to be clarified whether the target population fulfills the necessary personal and technical preconditions to use an IMI. Internet-based intervention studies aiming at children, adolescence, and adults up to an age of 60–70 years and even above indicate that a high percentage of the population fulfill at least the technical preconditions (Bond et al. 2010; Spek et al. 2007; Ye et al. 2014; Arnberg et al. 2014; Ebert et al. 2015a). In a review on technology use of cardiopulmonary outpatients, Disler and colleagues (2015) found that technological devices were a pervasive part of everyday life with respondents engaged in regular computer (82.9 %), mobile telephone (98.3 %), and Internet (86.0 %) use. Consequently, Andersson and Hedman (2013) reported in a meta-analysis of four RCTs and eight open studies that Internet-based interventions are transferable to the clinical praxis. However, to exploit the full potential of IMIs and to maximize their reach, users not only need to have Internet access but also need to be willing to use an IMI. Therefore, the common reservation of clinicians and patients toward Internet interventions might still be the major obstacle of a large-scale dissemination of IMIs (Andersson and Titov 2014), highlighting the need for active dissemination strategies (Schoenwald et al. 2012; Baumeister 2014). First studies on the impact of acceptance facilitating measures on patients' attitude toward IMIs already show that short video and face-to-face presentations on the effectiveness, characteristics, and safety issues of IMIs are able to meaningfully increase patients' acceptance of IMIs (Baumeister et al. 2014b, c; Ebert et al. 2015b). In a similar vein, clinicians' attitudes toward IMIs might be improvable by providing information material, trainings, and trial access to IMIs.

Given that IMIs are transferable to clinical practice, we further need to establish the best way to implement IMIs into routine CVD care. Integrating IMIs as a first step of collaborative and stepped-care approaches for individuals with CVD and depression seems one promising way (Baumeister and Hutter 2012; Baumeister 2012). Wildevuur and Simonse (2015) found a clear preference in favor of telemonitoring/telemedicine system interventions (71 %) versus interventions applied for connected physical care (17 %) and education (9 %) as a way to connect the patient and the health-care professionals providing advice and service. These interventions provided inter alia self-measurement of the body, self-rehabilitation exercises, telemonitoring systems, or for shared treatment decision-making (Wildevuur and Simonse 2015). Depression IMIs might easily be integrated in some of these already existing technologies for cardiovascular patients.

Another possibility would be to refer CVD patients to stand-alone IMIs if available. However, IMIs also offer the unique potential of reaching individuals who would not access depression care via the established channels of mental health-care delivery, either because they do not utilize the available offers or because they do not feel to discuss their mental health issues with their general practitioners and CVD specialists. Thus, we should also think about implementing IMIs in a way that allows individuals to self-refer to Internet interventions (Andersson and Titov 2014). This might, for example, be achievable by providing IMIs via websites of established associations for CVD and/or depression, which would probably make it necessary for several countries to think about alternative financing health-care models to integrate IMIs in the best possible way.

References

Andersson G (2009) Using the internet to provide cognitive behaviour therapy. Behav Res Ther 47:175–180
Andersson G, Hedman E (2013) Effectiveness of guided Internet-based cognitive behavior therapy in regular clinical settings. Verhaltenstherapie 23:140–148
Andersson G, Titov N (2014) Advantages and limitations of internet-based interventions for common mental disorders. World Psychiatry 13:4–11
Andersson G, Carlbring P, Berger T, Almlov J, Cuijpers P (2009) What makes internet therapy work? Cogn Behav Ther 38:55–60
Andersson G, Ljotsson B, Weise C (2011) Internet-delivered treatment to promote health. Curr Opin Psychiatry 24:168–172
Andersson G, Carlbring P, Ljótsson B, Hedman E (2013) Guided internet-based CBT for common mental disorders. J Contemp Psychother 43:223–233
Andersson G, Cuijpers P, Carlbring P, Riper H, Hedman E (2014) Guided Internet-based vs. face-to-face cognitive behavior therapy for psychiatric and somatic disorders: a systematic review and meta-analysis. World Psychiatry 13:288–295
Andrews G, Cuijpers P, Craske MG, McEvoy P, Titov N (2010) Computer therapy for the anxiety and depressive disorders is effective, acceptable and practical health care: a meta-analysis. PLoS One 5:e13196
Arnberg FK, Linton SJ, Hultcrantz M, Heintz E, Jonsson U (2014) Internet-delivered psychological treatments for mood and anxiety disorders: a systematic review of their efficacy, safety, and cost-effectiveness. PLoS One 9:e98118
Barak A, Hen L, Boniel-Nissim M, Shapira N (2008) A comprehensive review and a meta-analysis of the effectiveness of internet-based psychotherapeutic interventions. J Technol Hum Serv 26:109–160
Barak A, Klein B, Proudfoot JG (2009) Defining internet-supported therapeutic interventions. Ann Behav Med 38:4–17
Baumeister H (2012) Inappropriate prescriptions of antidepressant drugs in patients with subthreshold to mild depression: time for the evidence to become practice. J Affect Disord 139:240–243
Baumeister H (2014) Implementation research in clinical psychology, rehabilitation psychology, and psychotherapy [German]. Psychol Rundsch 65:150–158
Baumeister H, Hutter N (2012) Collaborative care for depression in medically ill patients. Curr Opin Psychiatry 25:405–414
Baumeister H, Parker G (2012) Meta-review of depressive subtyping models. J Affect Disord 139:126–140
Baumeister H, Kriston L, Bengel J, Härter M (2010) High agreement of self-report and physician-diagnosed somatic conditions yields limited bias in examining mental-physical comorbidity. J Clin Epidemiol 63:558–565

Baumeister H, Hutter N, Bengel J, Härter M (2011a) Quality of life in medically ill persons with comorbid mental disorders: a systematic review and meta-analysis. Psychother Psychosom 80:275–286

Baumeister H, Hutter N, Bengel J (2011) Psychological and pharmacological interventions for depression in patients with coronary artery disease. Cochrane Database Syst Rev 9:CD008012

Baumeister H, Hutter N, Bengel J (2012) Psychological and pharmacological interventions for depression in patients with diabetes mellitus and depression. Cochrane Database Syst Rev 12:CD008381

Baumeister H, Reichler L, Munzinger M, Lin J (2014a) The impact of guidance on internet-based mental health interventions – a systematic review. Internet Interv 1:205–215

Baumeister H, Nowoczin L, Lin J, Seifferth H, Seufert J, Laubner K et al (2014b) Impact of an acceptance facilitating intervention on diabetes patients' acceptance of internet-based interventions for depression: a randomized controlled trial. Diabetes Res Clin Pract 105: 30–39

Baumeister H, Seifferth H, Lin J, Nowoczin L, Luking M, Ebert DD (2014c) Impact of an acceptance facilitating intervention on patients' acceptance of internet-based pain interventions – a randomised controlled trial. Clin J Pain 31:528–535

Baumeister H, Haschke A, Munzinger M, Hutter N, Tully PJ (2015) Inpatient and outpatient costs in patients with coronary artery disease and mental disorders: a systematic review. BioPsychoSocial Med 9:11

Baumeister H, Lin J, Ebert DD. Internet-based health interventions. In: Koch U, Bengel J, editors. Encyclopedia of psychology: medical psychology [German]. Hogrefe, Göttingen; in Press

Bennett K, Bennett AJ, Griffiths KM (2010) Security considerations for e-mental health interventions. J Med Internet Res 12:e61

Berger T, Andersson G (2009) Internet-based psychotherapies: characteristics and empirical evidence [German]. Psychother Psychosom Med Psychol 59:159–170

Bond GE, Burr RL, Wolf FM, Feldt K (2010) The effects of a web-based intervention on psychosocial well-being among adults aged 60 and older with diabetes: a randomized trial. Diabetes Educ 36:446–456

Carlbring P, Maurin L, Torngren C, Linna E, Eriksson T, Sparthan E et al (2011) Individually-tailored, internet-based treatment for anxiety disorders: a randomized controlled trial. Behav Res Ther 49:18–24

Carney R, Freedland K (2012) Is there a high-risk subtype of depression in patients with coronary heart disease? Curr Psychiatry Rep 14:1–7

Charova E, Dorstyn D, Tully P, Mittag O (2015) Web-based interventions for comorbid depression and chronic illness: a systematic review. J Telemed Telecare 21:189–201

Cheng SK, Dizon J (2012) Computerised cognitive behavioural therapy for insomnia: a systematic review and meta-analysis. Psychother Psychosom 81:206–216

Christensen H, Murray K, Calear AL, Bennett K, Bennett A, Griffiths KM (2010) Beacon: a web portal to high-quality mental health websites for use by health professionals and the public. Med J Aust 192:S40–4

de Leon E, Fuentes LW, Cohen JE (2014) Characterizing periodic messaging interventions across health behaviors and media: systematic review. J Med Internet Res 16:e93

Disler RT, Inglis SC, Newton PJ, Currow DC, Macdonald PS, Glanville AR et al (2015) Patterns of technology use in patients attending a cardiopulmonary outpatient clinic: a self-report survey. Interact J Med Res 4:e5

Ebert DD, Gollwitzer M, Riper H, Cuijpers P, Baumeister H, Berking M (2013) For whom does it work? Moderators of outcome on the effect of a transdiagnostic internet-based maintenance treatment after inpatient psychotherapy: randomized controlled trial. J Med Internet Res 15:e191

Ebert DD, Zarski A, Christensen H, Stikkelbroek Y, Cuijpers P, Berking M et al (2015a) Internet and computer-based cognitive behavioral therapy for anxiety and depression in youth: a meta-analysis of randomized controlled outcome trials. PLoS One 10:e0119895

Ebert DD, Berking M, Cuijpers P, Lehr D, Portner M, Baumeister H (2015b) Increasing the acceptance of internet-based mental health interventions in primary care patients with depressive symptoms. A randomized controlled trial. J Affect Disord 176C:9–17

Emmelkamp PMG, David D, Beckers T, Muris P, Cuijpers P, Lutz W et al (2014) Advancing psychotherapy and evidence-based psychological interventions. Int J Methods Psychiatr Res 23(Suppl 1):58–91

Fenichel M, Suler J, Barak A, Zelvin E, Jones G, Munro K et al (2002) Myths and realities of online clinical work. Cyberpsychol Behav 5:481–497

Fry JP, Neff RA (2009) Periodic prompts and reminders in health promotion and health behavior interventions: systematic review. J Med Internet Res 11:e16

Gaebel W, Kowitz S, Fritze J, Zielasek J (2013) Use of health care services by people with mental illness: secondary data from three statutory health insurers and the German statutory pension insurance scheme. Deutsches Ärzteblatt Int 110:799–808

Glozier N, Christensen H, Naismith S, Cockayne N, Donkin L, Neal B et al (2013) Internet-delivered cognitive behavioural therapy for adults with mild to moderate depression and high cardiovascular disease risks: a randomised attention-controlled trial. PLoS One 8:e59139

Grassi A, Gaggioli A, Riva G (2009) The green valley: the use of mobile narratives for reducing stress in commuters. Cyberpsychol Behav 12:155–161

Härter M, Baumeister H, Reuter K, Jacobi F, Hofler M, Bengel J et al (2007) Increased 12-month prevalence rates of mental disorders in patients with chronic somatic diseases. Psychother Psychosom 76:354–360

Haschke A, Hutter N, Baumeister H (2012) Indirect costs in patients with coronary artery disease and mental disorders: a systematic review and meta-analysis. IJOMEH 25:319–329

Hedman E, Ljotsson B, Lindefors N (2012) Cognitive behavior therapy via the Internet: a systematic review of applications, clinical efficacy and cost-effectiveness. Expert Rev Pharmacoecon Outcomes Res 12:745–764

Heron KE, Smyth JM (2010) Ecological momentary interventions: incorporating mobile technology into psychosocial and health behaviour treatments. Br J Health Psychol 15:1–39

Johansson R, Sjöberg E, Sjögren M, Johnsson E, Carlbring P, Andersson T et al (2012a) Tailored vs. standardized internet-based cognitive behavior therapy for depression and comorbid symptoms: a randomized controlled trial. PLoS One 7:e36905

Johansson R, Ekbladh S, Hebert A, Lindström M, Möller S, Petitt E et al (2012b) Psychodynamic guided self-help for adult depression through the internet: a randomised controlled trial. PLoS One 7:e38021

Keyserling TC, Sheridan SL, Draeger LB, Finkelstein EA, Gizlice Z, Kruger E et al (2014) A comparison of live counseling with a web-based lifestyle and medication intervention to reduce coronary heart disease risk: a randomized clinical trial. JAMA Intern Med 174:1144–1157

Klein B, Austin D, Pier C, Kiropoulos L, Shandley K, Mitchell J et al (2009) Internet-based treatment for panic disorder: does frequency of therapist contact make a difference? Cogn Behav Ther 38:100–113

Lin J, Ebert D, Lehr D, Berking M, Baumeister H (2013) Internet based cognitive behavioral interventions: state of the art and implementation possibilities in rehabilitation [German]. Rehabilitation 52:155–163

Lin J, Lüking M, Ebert DD, Buhrman M, Andersson G, Baumeister H (2015) Effectiveness and cost-effectiveness of a guided and unguided internet-based acceptance and commitment therapy for chronic pain: study protocol for a three-armed randomised controlled trial. Internet Interv 2:7–16

Manhal-Baugus M (2001) E-therapy: practical, ethical, and legal issues. Cyberpsychol Behav 4:551–563

Moessner M, Bauer S, Ozer F, Wolf M, Zimmer B, Kordy H (2014) Cost-effectiveness of an internet-based aftercare intervention after inpatient treatment in a psychosomatic hospital. Psychother Res 24:496–503

Mohr DC, Burns MN, Schueller SM, Clarke G, Klinkman M (2013) Behavioral intervention technologies: evidence review and recommendations for future research in mental health. Gen Hosp Psychiatry 35:332–338

Murray E (2012) Web-based interventions for behavior change and self-management: potential, pitfalls, and progress. Med 20 1:e3

Newman MG, Szkodny LE, Llera SJ, Przeworski A (2011) A review of technology-assisted self-help and minimal contact therapies for anxiety and depression: Is human contact necessary for therapeutic efficacy? Clin Psychol Rev 31:89–103

Nobis S, Lehr D, Ebert DD, Berking M, Heber E, Baumeister H et al (2013) Efficacy and cost-effectiveness of a web-based intervention with mobile phone support to treat depressive symptoms in adults with diabetes mellitus type 1 and type 2: design of a randomised controlled trial. BMC Psychiatry 13:306

Nobis S, Lehr D, Ebert DD, Baumeister H, Snoek F, Riper H et al (2015) Efficacy of a web-based intervention with mobile phone support in treating depressive symptoms in adults with type 1 and type 2 diabetes: a randomized controlled trial. Diabetes Care 38:776–783

Norlund F, Olsson EM, Burell G, Wallin E, Held C (2015) Treatment of depression and anxiety with internet-based cognitive behavior therapy in patients with a recent myocardial infarction (U-CARE Heart): study protocol for a randomized controlled trial. Trials 16:154

Ormel J, de Jonge P (2011) Unipolar depression and the progression of coronary artery disease: toward an integrative model. Psychother Psychosom 80:264–274

Paganini S, Lin J, Ebert DD, Baumeister H (2016) Internet- and mobile-based interventions for mental disorders [German]. Neurotransmitter 27:48–55

Palmqvist B, Carlbring P, Andersson G (2007) Internet-delivered treatments with or without therapist input: does the therapist factor have implications for efficacy and cost? Expert Rev Pharmacoecon Outcomes Res 7:291–297

Prabhakar E (2013) E-therapy: ethical considerations of a changing healthcare communication environment. Pastor Psychol 62:211–218

Proudfoot J, Klein B, Barak A, Carlbring P, Cuijpers P, Lange A et al (2011) Establishing guidelines for executing and reporting internet intervention research. Cogn Behav Ther 40:82–97

Richards DA (2012) Stepped care: a method to deliver increased access to psychological therapies. Can J Psychiatry 57:210–215

Richards D, Richardson T (2012) Computer-based psychological treatments for depression: a systematic review and meta-analysis. Clin Psychol Rev 32:329–342

Riper H, Blankers M, Hadiwijaya H, Cunningham J, Clarke S, Wiers R et al (2014) Effectiveness of guided and unguided low-intensity internet interventions for adult alcohol misuse: a meta-analysis. PLoS One 9:e99912

Ritterband LM, Gonder-Frederick LA, Cox DJ, Clifton AD, West RW, Borowitz SM (2003) Internet interventions: in review, in use, and into the future. Prof Psychol Res Pract 34:527

Ritterband LM, Thorndike FP, Cox DJ, Kovatchev BP, Gonder-Frederick LA (2009) A behavior change model for internet interventions. Ann Behav Med 38:18–27

Rochlen AB, Zack JS, Speyer C (2004) Online therapy: review of relevant definitions, debates, and current empirical support. J Clin Psychol 60:269–283

Roest AM, Carney RM, Freedland KE, Martens EJ, Denollet J, de Jonge P (2013) Changes in cognitive versus somatic symptoms of depression and event-free survival following acute myocardial infarction in the Enhancing Recovery In Coronary Heart Disease (ENRICHD) study. J Affect Disord 149:335–341

Rozental A, Andersson G, Boettcher J, Ebert DD, Cuijpers P, Knaevelsrud C et al (2014) Consensus statement on defining and measuring negative effects of Internet interventions. Internet Interv 1:12–19

Schoenwald S, McHugh K, Barlow D (2012) The science of dissemination and implementation. In: McHugh R, Barlow D (eds) Dissemination and implementation of evidence-based psychological interventions. Oxford University Press, New York, pp 16–42

Spek V, Nyklicek I, Smits N, Cuijpers P, Riper H, Keyzer J et al (2007) Internet-based cognitive behavioural therapy for subthreshold depression in people over 50 years old: a randomized controlled clinical trial. Psychol Med J Res Psychiatry Allied Sci 37:1797–1806

Titov N (2011) Internet-delivered psychotherapy for depression in adults. Curr Opin Psychiatry 24:18–23

Titov N, Andrews G, Choi I, Schwencke G, Mahoney A (2008) Shyness 3: randomized controlled trial of guided versus unguided Internet-based CBT for social phobia. Aust N Z J Psychiatry 42:1030–1040

Titov N, Andrews G, Choi I, Schwencke G, Johnston L (2009a) Randomized controlled trial of web-based treatment of social phobia without clinician guidance. Aust N Z J Psychiatry 43:913–919

Titov N, Andrews G, Schwencke G, Solley K, Johnston L, Robinson E (2009b) An RCT comparing effect of two types of support on severity of symptoms for people completing Internet-based cognitive behaviour therapy for social phobia. Aust N Z J Psychiatry 43:920–926

Tully PJ, Baumeister H (2014) Collaborative care for the treatment of comorbid depression and coronary heart disease: a systematic review and meta-analysis protocol. Syst Rev 3:127

Wangberg SC, Bergmo TS, Johnsen JK (2008) Adherence in internet-based interventions. Patient Prefer Adherence 2:57

Wanner M, Martin-Diener E, Braun-Fahrländer C, Bauer G, Martin BW (2009) Effectiveness of active-online, an individually tailored physical activity intervention, in a real-life setting: randomized controlled trial. J Med Internet Res 11:e23

Warmerdam L, Smit F, van Straten A, Riper H, Cuijpers P (2010) Cost-utility and cost-effectiveness of internet-based treatment for adults with depressive symptoms: randomized trial. J Med Internet Res 12:e53

Webb TL, Joseph J, Yardley L, Michie S (2010) Using the internet to promote health behavior change: a systematic review and meta-analysis of the impact of theoretical basis, use of behavior change techniques, and mode of delivery on efficacy. J Med Internet Res 12:e4

Wells M, Mitchell KJ, Finkelhor D, Becker-Blease KA (2007) Online mental health treatment: concerns and considerations. Cyberpsychol Behav 10:453–459

Wildevuur ES, Simonse WL (2015) Information and communication technology-enabled person-centered care for the "Big Five" chronic conditions: scoping review. J Med Internet Res 17:e77

Ye X, Bapuji SB, Winters SE, Struthers A, Raynard M, Metge C et al (2014) Effectiveness of internet-based interventions for children, youth, and young adults with anxiety and/or depression: a systematic review and meta-analysis. BMC Health Serv Res 14:313

Zwerenz R, Gerzymisch K, Edinger J, Holme M, Knickenberg RJ, Spörl-Dönch S et al (2013) Evaluation of an internet-based aftercare program to improve vocational reintegration after inpatient medical rehabilitation: study protocol for a cluster-randomized controlled trial. Trials 14:26

Pharmacological Treatment and Prevention of Cardiovascular Diseases and Depression Comorbidity: Understanding Epidemiological, Clinical Trial Evidence, and the Biological Underpinnings

23

Harris A. Eyre, Malcolm Forbes, Helen Lavretsky, and Bernhard T. Baune

Contents

H.A. Eyre (✉)
Discipline of Psychiatry, School of Medicine, University of Adelaide, Adelaide, SA, Australia

Semel Institute for Neuroscience and Human Behavior, UCLA, Los Angeles, CA, USA

School of Medicine and Dentistry, James Cook University, Townsville, QLD, Australia
e-mail: harris.eyre@gmail.com

M. Forbes
School of Medicine and Dentistry, James Cook University, Townsville, QLD, Australia

H. Lavretsky
Semel Institute for Neuroscience and Human Behavior, UCLA, Los Angeles, CA, USA

B.T. Baune
Discipline of Psychiatry, School of Medicine, University of Adelaide, Adelaide, SA, Australia

B.T. Baune, P.J. Tully (eds.), *Cardiovascular Diseases and Depression*, DOI 10.1007/978-3-319-32480-7_23

Abstract

Depression and cardiovascular disease (CVD) are currently of major concern to public health and will be increasingly so in the future. These two disorders are closely interconnected both clinically and biologically. Understanding this interconnection is important to appreciating current and potential treatment and prevention platforms. There are a number of plausible biological models which may link depression and CVD together. Key models include a dysfunctional hypothalamic-pituitary-adrenal (HPA) axis, chronic elevations in pro-inflammatory cytokines, increased sympathetic tone, platelet dysfunction leading to a pro-thrombotic state, as well as reductions in arterial vessel elasticity and endothelial dysfunction. The aim of this chapter is to review the epidemiological, clinical trial, and biological literature exploring the role of pharmacological treatment and prevention of depression and CVD. Antidepressants, particularly selective serotonin reuptake inhibitors (SSRIs), do appear useful in the treatment of comorbid depression and CVD, and they appear to play a role in the prevention of adverse cardiac events. The role of serotonin-noradrenaline reuptake inhibitors (SNRIs) is poorly understood and should be treated with caution. Anti-inflammatory therapies show promise in the treatment of depression; however, there is a paucity of clinical trial data on the role of anti-inflammatory therapies for the prevention of adverse cardiac events. An emerging body of research has now begun to explore the effect of pharmacological agents on inflammation, HPA axis dysfunction, increased sympathetic tone, and vascular and platelet dysfunction. This research should be continued to better understand the underlying mechanism of effect of pharmacological agents in comorbid depression and CVD.

23.1 Introduction

Depression and cardiovascular disease (CVD) are currently of major concern to public health and will be increasingly so in the future. An assessment of the World Health Organization's (WHO) Global Burden of Disease Study between 1990 and 2010 found the burden of ischemic heart disease (IHD) and depression increased substantially over this time (Murray et al. 2012). For IHD, the burden increased by 29 % to the number 1 ranked disorder; for depression, there was a 37 % increase in burden to number 11 (Murray et al. 2012). An earlier assessment of the Global Burden of Disease Study of 2004 predicted that by 2030, these disorders will be the two most common causes of disability-adjusted life years in the world (WHO 2008). Out of a sample of community-dwelling adults in the United States of America (aged >50 years) who had major depressive disorder (MDD), two-thirds had a diagnosis of heart disease, stroke, hypertension, and/or diabetes (Gonzalez and Tarraf 2013). In the future, depression and CVD will result in increased medical costs (Sullivan et al. 2002; Rutledge et al. 2009), increased health service utilization (Egede 2007), and lost productivity (Stewart et al. 2003). These two disorders are closely interconnected both clinically and biologically (Baune et al. 2012a, b). Understanding this interconnection is important to understanding current and potential treatment and prevention platforms.

The development of depression as a consequence of CVD has been explored extensively (Baune et al. 2012a, b). This may include depression as a consequence of an acute cardiac event (e.g., acute myocardial infarction (AMI)) or a chronic disease (e.g., congestive heart failure (CHF)) (Hare et al. 2014). After AMI, mild forms of depression have been found in up to two-thirds of hospitalized patients (Cay et al. 1972). The prevalence of depression in patients with CHF has been found to be dependent upon the severity of the functional class (Rutledge et al. 2006). In asymptomatic CHF, depression is found in around 10 % of patients and found in up to 40 % of patients with severe functional impairments (Rutledge et al. 2006).

The development of CVD as a consequence of depression has also been extensively explored (Baune et al. 2012a, b). Clinical and epidemiological studies suggest depression increases the risk of subsequent CVD by an average of 1.5-fold (Nicholson et al. 2006; Lippi et al. 2009; Grippo and Johnson 2002). Depression has been found to be an independent predictor of a worse outcome after an ischemic event (Barth et al. 2004; Meijer et al. 2011; Nicholson et al. 2006). Patients with comorbid coronary artery disease (CAD) and depression have a two- to threefold increased risk of future cardiac events compared to those only cardiac disease (Frasure-Smith and Lesperance 2010; Goldston and Baillie 2008; Van der Kooy et al. 2007; Rudisch and Nemeroff 2003). Depression in CHF patients is also an independent predictor of mortality and rehospitalization (Macchia et al. 2008).

There are a number of plausible biological models which may link depression and CVD together (Baune et al. 2012a, b). Key models include a dysfunctional hypothalamic-pituitary-adrenal (HPA) axis, chronic elevations in pro-inflammatory cytokines, increased sympathetic tone, platelet dysfunction leading to a pro-thrombotic state, as well as reductions in arterial vessel elasticity and endothelial dysfunction (Baune et al. 2012a, b). Studies investigating immune system functioning in individuals with depression have found that many of these individuals manifest chronically elevated inflammatory markers, particularly C-reactive protein (CRP), interleukin-6 (IL-6), IL-1β and tumor necrosis factor (TNF)-α (Dowlati et al. 2010; Eyre et al. 2014). This pro-inflammatory state is thought to be a key link in the comorbidity of depression and CVD (Paz-Filho et al. 2010; Lippi et al. 2009). Inflammation is implicated in the pathogenesis of CVD, particularly the development of atherosclerosis. Atherosclerosis may be accelerated through these inflammatory mediators via several mechanisms including chemoattraction of pro-inflammatory leukocytes to atherosclerotic lesions, the induction of endothelial activation and expression of adhesion molecules further increasing chemotactic signaling, and the stimulation of vascular endothelial growth factor (VEGF) production (Paz-Filho et al. 2010; Lippi et al. 2009). Inflammatory signaling cascades may also accelerate thrombus formation (Paz-Filho et al. 2010; Lippi et al. 2009). Disruptions of the HPA axis may be regulated by altered expression of pro-inflammatory cytokines, suggesting a complex bidirectional biological cross talk (Sasayama et al. 2011). The contribution of the HPA axis may be mediated, partly by the loss of glucocorticoid receptors (GRs) and their negative feedback function on inflammatory signaling, again leading to a further escalation in inflammation. Dysregulation of the HPA axis may also lead to sympathoadrenal hyperactivity, or increased sympathetic tone, via central pathways. Increased sympathetic tone is associated with processes implicated in the development of CVD, such as an increase in vasoconstrictive tone, heart rate, and platelet activation (Malpas 2010; Joynt et al. 2003). Finally, increased sympathetic tone may result in reduced heart rate variability (HRV), which is associated with risk of arrhythmias (Kemp et al. 2010). Endothelial dysfunction is a recognized risk factor for CVD; it is often observed in depressed patients without CVD (Shimokawa 1999; Rybakowski et al. 2006; Bonetti et al. 2003; Cooper et al. 2011). Depression is associated with reduced arterial elasticity, in addition to an increased expression of endothelial adhesion molecules and chemokines (Rajagopalan et al. 2001; Sherwood et al. 2005). Taken together, these factors may predispose patients to atherosclerosis, thrombosis, and vasospasm.

The exploration of treatment and prevention strategies for comorbid depression and CVD is highly important given the burden of these diseases and given complexity due to biological underpinnings, as well as significant patient safety factors in the post-CVD setting. Treatments may include psychotherapy, social therapy, somatic interventions (e.g., medications or electroconvulsive therapy), lifestyle therapies (e.g., physical activity, omega-3 polyunsaturated fatty acids), or a combination. Reviews of these modes of treatment can be found here (Ramamurthy et al. 2013; Honig et al. 2007). This review will focus on monoamine- and immune-modulatory psychopharmacological agents.

Monoamine-based antidepressants have a mixed evidence base supporting their use in CVD and depression. It appears that selective serotonin reuptake inhibitor

(SSRI) medications are safe as first-line therapies (Lichtman et al. 2009; Post-Myocardial Infarction Depression Clinical Practice Guideline 2009); however, studies in this area have limitations which will be discussed in this review. Tricyclic antidepressants (TCAs) are not recommended in CVD populations given their association with adverse cardiac events (Ramamurthy et al. 2013). Serotonin-noradrenaline reuptake inhibitors (SNRIs) appear to have a paucity of research supporting their use; hence caution is recommended (Ramamurthy et al. 2013).

Anti-inflammatory medications may be a useful tool in the treatment of depression and CVD given the role of pro-inflammatory cytokines linking these diseases (Eyre et al. 2015). Early data from meta-analyses suggests anti-inflammatories may indeed by useful in the treatment of depression without CVD (Kohler et al. 2014). However, this literature is heterogeneous and requires careful description and consideration (Eyre et al. 2015). There is some evidence supporting the use of anti-inflammatories in comorbid CVD and depression; this will be reviewed here.

To understand the role of the abovementioned pharmacological agents in depression and CVD, it is important to review epidemiological, clinical, and biological data. Particularly with respect to biological data, this is an emerging literature understanding the effects of antidepressants on inflammation, the HPA axis, sympathetic tone, and vascular biology. To date, we are not aware of a review which explores this topic systematically; hence this review provides novel perspectives on this. The aim of this chapter is to review the epidemiological, clinical trial, and biological literature exploring the role of pharmacological treatment and prevention of depression and CVD.

23.2 Antidepressant Pharmacotherapy to Treat Cardiovascular Disease and Depression

Treatment of depressive symptoms comorbid with CVD is crucial given depressive symptoms are associated with worse cardiovascular prognosis and lower quality of life. To this effect, treatments for depression need to be carefully studied given variously promising and concerning findings. Some antidepressants are useful to reduce depressive symptoms and show promise for improving cardiovascular outcomes, while others are not safe for use in CVD populations. Data from epidemiological and clinical trials is useful to understand efficacy and safety of antidepressants.

23.2.1 Epidemiological Evidence

There are a number of observational studies exploring the effects of antidepressants on comorbid depression and CVD. The hypothesized biological underpinnings for these findings are outlined further below in this paper. A study by Nabi et al. (2010) used a prospective cohort design to compare the significance of depression in CVD and cerebrovascular disease, as compared to subjects with no vascular disease. These subjects were taken from the Health and Social Support Prospective Cohort

Study and included a sample of 23,282 adults aged 20–54 years; they were followed for 7 years. Fatal and first nonfatal CVD and cerebrovascular disease events were documented by linkage to national hospital discharge and mortality registers. Results show the hazard ratio (HR) for CVD was 1.66 (95 % confidence interval (CI) 1.24–2.24) for participants with mild-to-severe depressive symptoms, i.e., those scoring ≥10 on the 21-item Beck Depression Inventory (BDI), and 2.04 (95 % CI 1.27–3.27) for those who filled antidepressant prescriptions (a suggested marker for clinically significant depression) compared with those without depression markers at study baseline. No subgroup analysis was conducted on type of antidepressant used. This suggests participants who filled antidepressant prescriptions have an increased risk of CVD; however, the results should be interpreted cautiously because medication use was utilized as a marker of depression severity.

A case-control study of subjects with IHD was used to determine whether antidepressants are a risk factor for IHD (Hippisley-Cox et al. 2001). In this study, 933 IHD subjects of any age (range from <50 to >90 years) were studied along with 5,516 controls. Odds ratios (ORs) for IHD were significantly raised for patients who had ever received a prescription for TCA after full adjustment 1.56 (95 % CI 1.18–2.05). Patients who had ever taken dothiepin had a significantly raised OR for IHD after full adjustment 1.67 (95 % CI 1.17–2.36). There was no significant increase in the OR for amitriptyline, lofepramine, and SSRIs in multivariate analysis. This suggests that patients who had ever taken dothiepin had significantly increased risk of IHD, with no other antidepressants significantly associated.

A study by Whang et al. (2009) explored the association between depression and sudden cardiac death (SCD) and cardiac events among individuals with baseline CVD in the Nurses' Health Study. Patient were ages 30–55 in 1976 when the study began, and they were followed over 8 years (1992–2000). Depression was measured by the Mental Health Index (MHI-5) and also antidepressant use. Primary end points included SCD, fatal CVD, and nonfatal MI. 63,469 women were involved in this analysis. In models from 1996 onward, clinical depression was most associated with SCD in multivariable models, HR 2.33 (95 % CI 1.47–3.70), and this was primarily due to the relationship between antidepressant use and SCD. From 2000 to 2004, similar HRs were found for the two categories of medications – SSRIs HR 5.07 (95 % CI 1.73–14.8) and other antidepressants HR 3.19 (95 % CI 0.92–11.00). This therefore suggests antidepressant use in both categories was associated with SCDs.

An observational study by Rieckmann et al. (2013) explored the association between SSRI and non-SSRI second-generation antidepressant use in a patient cohort with acute coronary syndrome (ACS) (within 1 week of hospitalization). They then explored the occurrence of cardiac events and mortality over a period of 42 months in participants aged around 60 years ± 15. This study was novel given current RCTs on this topic only monitor for adverse cardiac events for up to 6 months follow-up, which is considered a short time frame for such events. Four hundred thirty-two patients were grouped according to patients not on any antidepressant ($n=354$), patients on SSRI only ($n=78$), and patients on non-SSRI second-generation antidepressants only ($n=20$). SSRI use carried an increased risk for major adverse cardiovascular events (MACE) (i.e., hospitalization for nonfatal AMI, unstable angina, or urgent/emergency percutaneous or surgical coronary revascularization/mortality) compared to no antidepressant use hazard ratio [HR] (1.83; 95 % CI 1.09–3.06; $p=0.02$); non-SSRI second-generation antidepressant use did not HR, 0.86 (95 % CI 0.31–2.42; $p=0.78$). This study therefore suggests that SSRI use may be associated with longer-term risk for adverse prognosis in ACS patients; however, low numbers in this study should be taken into account.

Another prospective cohort study by Xiong et al. (2010) examined the associa tion of perioperative coronary artery bypass grafting (CABG) bleeding risks and SSRI use prior to CABG. They explored 4,794 patients who underwent CABG surgery aged 54–72 years. Reoperation due to bleeding-related complications were not different between SSRI users OR 1.14 (95 % CI 0.52–2.47, $p=0.75$). The 30-day mortality (2.0 % in SSRI vs 2.1 % in control group; $p=0.92$) was similar. These data suggest there is no substantial increased risk of adverse events from SSRI use post-CABG surgery.

23.2.2 Clinical Trial Evidence

There are a number of clinical trials which explore the clinical and safety effects of antidepressants on patients with comorbid depression and CVD. These studies are outlined in Tables 23.1 and 23.2. Further, a number of meta-analyses have also been performed in this field. A meta-analysis by Mazza et al. (2010) explored SSRI vs control treatment in patients with recent ACS. Five RCTs (801 patients) were included, with an average age of 56.7 years. Subjects treated with SSRIs did not show a significant improvement in depression symptoms, after a median of 6 months, although there was a trend for a reduction. Subjects treated with SSRIs showed a significantly lower rate of rehospitalizations from all causes risk difference (RD) 14 % (95 % CI 5–23 %, $p=0.001$). Therapy with antidepressants was notably safe, with statistically similar rates of adverse events (i.e., MACE, death, AMI, and repeat revascularization). This suggests no effect of SSRIs on depressive symptoms, but improved or similar cardiac outcomes in patients with a recent ACS and depressive symptoms.

A Cochrane Collaboration meta-analysis (Baumeister et al. 2011) was performed to determine the effects of pharmacological and psychological interventions in CAD patients with comorbid depression. Primary outcomes were depression, mortality, and cardiac events. Secondary outcomes were healthcare costs and health-related quality of life (QoL). Eight RCTs were included with a total of 1,098 patients (see McFarlane et al. 2001; Lesperance et al. 2007; Freeman et al. 1986; Li et al. 2005; Liu and Zheng 1999; Glassman et al. 2002; Strik et al. 2000; Honig et al. 2007). The mean age of participants in these studies ranged from 54.1 to 63.6 years. It should be mentioned that the study by Freeman et al. (1986) utilized alprazolam; Li et al. utilized (2005) St. John's wort; Honig et al. (2007) utilized mirtazapine. The review provides evidence of a small beneficial effect of pharmacological interventions with SSRIs compared to placebo on depression outcomes (standardized mean difference

Table 23.1 Randomized controlled trials to evaluate the effects of antidepressant pharmacotherapy on depression in cardiovascular disease settings: depressive symptom outcomes

Ref	Aim	Population	Treatment period and groups	Outcome for depressive symptoms
Berkman et al. (2003)	To determine whether mortality and morbidity are reduced by treatment of depression and LPSS with CBT, supplemented with an SSRI	RCT; 2,481 MI patients (1,084 women, 1,397 men); minor or major depression (DSM-4); ESSI	CBT, initiated at a median of 17 days after the index MI for a median of 11 individual sessions throughout 6 months. Group therapy when feasible, with SSRIs for patients scoring higher than 24 on the HDRS or having a less than 50 % reduction in BDI scores after 5 weeks Usual care: 1,243, mean age 61 year (SD 12.5) Intervention: 1,238, mean age 61 year (SD 12.6)	Measures: HDRS; ESSI Results: improvement in psychosocial outcomes at 6 months favored treatment; mean (SD) change in HDRS score, −10.1 (7.8) in the depression and psychosocial intervention group vs −8.4 (7.7) in the depression and usual care group ($p<0.001$); mean (SD) change in ESSI score, 5.1 (5.9) in the LPSS and psychosocial intervention group vs 3.4 (6.0) in the LPSS and usual care group ($p<0.001$)
Glassman et al. (2002)	To evaluate the safety and efficacy of sertraline treatment of MDD	RCT; 369 patients with MDD DSM-4 (64 % male; mean age, 57.1 years; MI, 74 %; unstable angina, 26 %)	After a 2-week single-blind placebo run-in, patients were randomly assigned to receive sertraline ($n=186$) or placebo ($n=183$) for 24 weeks Placebo: mean age 57.6 years (SD 10.4) Sertraline: mean age 56.8 years (SD 11.1)	Measures: HAM-D scale and CGI-I Results: the CGI-I ($p=0.049$), but not the HAM-D ($p=0.14$), favored sertraline. The CGI-I responder rates for sertraline were significantly higher than for placebo in the total sample (67 % vs 53 %; $p=0.01$), in the group with at least 1 prior episode of depression (72 % vs 51 %; $p=0.003$), and in the more severe MDD group (78 % vs 45 %; $p=0.001$). In the latter 2 groups, both CGI-I and HAM-D measures were significantly better in those assigned to sertraline

Lesperance et al. (2007)	To explore efficacy of a SSRI (citalopram) and IPT in reducing depressive symptoms	RCT, 284 patients with CAD, all patients DSM-4 MDD of 4 weeks duration or longer, HAM-$D \geq 20$	12-week, parallel group; participants underwent 2 separate randomizations: (1) to receive 12 weekly sessions of IPT plus clinical management ($n=142$) or clinical management only ($n=142$) and (2) to receive 12 weeks of citalopram, 20–40 mg/day ($n=142$) or matching placebo ($n=142$)	Measures: 24-item HAM-D, BDI-II Results: citalopram was superior to placebo in reducing 12-week HAM-D scores (mean difference, 3.3 points; 96.7 % CI, 0.80–5.85; $p=0.005$), with a small to medium effect size of 0.33. Mean HAM-D response (52.8 % vs 40.1 %; $p=0.03$) and remission rates (35.9 % vs 22.5%; $p=0.01$) and the reduction in BDI-II scores (difference, 3.6 points; 98.3 % CI, 0.58–6.64; $p=0.005$; effect size=0.33) also favored citalopram. There was no evidence of a benefit of IPT over clinical management, with the mean HAM-D difference favoring clinical management (−2.26 points; 96.7 % CI, −4.78 to 0.27; $p=0.06$; effect size, 0.23). The difference on the BDI-II did not favor clinical management (1.13 points; 98.3 % CI, −1.90 to 4.16; $p=0.37$; effect size=0.11)
Blumenthal et al. (2012)	To assess the efficacy of exercise and antidepressant medication in reducing depressive symptoms and improving cardiovascular biomarkers	101 outpatients with CHD and elevated depressive symptoms; DSM-4 for MDD	Randomized to 4 months of aerobic exercise (3 times/week), sertraline, or placebo Placebo: mean age 63.5 years (SD 11.4) Sertraline: mean age 63.4 years (SD 10.2) Exercise: mean age 64.7 years (SD 11.0)	Measures: HAM-D Results: after 16 weeks, all groups showed improvement on HAM-D scores. Participants in both aerobic exercise ($M=-7.5$ [95 % CI=−9.8, −5.0]) and sertraline ($M=-6.1$ [95 % CI=−8.4, −3.9]) achieved larger reductions in depressive symptoms compared to placebo ($M=-4.5$ [95 % CI=−7.6, −1.5]; $p=0.034$); exercise and sertraline were equally effective in reducing depressive symptoms ($p=0.607$)

(continued)

Table 23.1 (continued)

Ref	Aim	Population	Treatment period and groups	Outcome for depressive symptoms
O'Connor et al. (2010)	To test the hypothesis that HF patients treated with sertraline will have lower depression scores and fewer cardiovascular events compared to placebo	RCT, sertraline vs placebo for 12 weeks, HF (LVEF ≤45 %, NYHA class IIIV), depression DSM-IV MDD	469 patients were randomized (N=234 sertraline, N=235 placebo) Placebo: mean age 61.4 years (SD 11.1) Sertraline: mean age 62.9 years (SD 10.5)	Measures: HDRS Results: the mean ± SE change from baseline to 12 weeks in the HDRS total score was −7.1 ± 0.5 (sertraline) and −6.8 ± 0.5 (placebo) ($p<0.001$ from baseline; $p=0.89$ between groups; mean change between groups −0.4, 95 % CI −1.7, 0.92)
Davidson et al. (2010)	To determine the acceptability and efficacy of enhanced depression treatment	A 3-month observation period to identify patients with ACS and persistent depressive symptoms was followed by a 6-month RCT	237 patients with ACS from 5 hospitals were enrolled, including 157 persistently depressed patients randomized to intervention (initial patient preference for problem-solving therapy and/or pharmacotherapy, then a stepped-care approach; 80 patients) or usual care (77 patients) and 80 nondepressed patients who underwent observational evaluation	Measures: patient satisfaction with depression care; BDI Results: the proportion of patients who were satisfied with their depression care was higher in the intervention group (54 % of 80) than in the usual care group (19 % of 77) (odds ratio, 5.4; 95 % CI, 2.2–12.9 [$p<0.001$]). The BDI score decreased significantly more (t (155) = 2.85 [$p=0.005$]) for intervention patients (change, −5.7; 95 % CI, −7.6 to −3.8; df = 155) than for usual care patients (change, −1.9; 95 % CI, −3.8 to −0.1; df = 155); the depression effect size was 0.59 of the standard deviation

Ye et al. (2014)	Examine cardiac events and mortality in the COPES trial through an additional 12 months of observational follow-up after the end of the 6-month treatment period	157 patients with a score of ≥10 on the BDI within 1 week of ACS hospitalization and again at 3-month follow-up. 80 enhanced treatment; 77 usual care Usual care: mean 61.1 (SD 10.6) Intervention group: mean 59.3 (SD 10.6)	Randomized to usual care or enhanced depression treatment involving stepped, patient preference-driven care with problem-solving therapy, pharmacotherapy, or both	Measures: BDI Results: at the beginning of the 12-month observational follow-up period, 58 of 77 patients (75 %) in the control group had a BDI score of ≥10, compared with 46 of 80 patients (58 %) in the intervention group ($p=0.018$), suggesting that a substantial number of participants continued to have depressive symptoms

LPSS low perceived social support, *MI* myocardial infarction, *CBT* cognitive behavioral therapy, *SSRI* selective serotonin reuptake inhibitor, *BDI* Beck Depression Inventory, *CGI-I* Clinical Global Impression Improvement, *LVEF* left ventricular ejection fraction, *IPT* interpersonal psychotherapy, *HR* hazard ratio, *COPES* Coronary Psychosocial Evaluation Studies, *ACS*, acute coronary syndrome, *RCT* randomized controlled trial, *HF* heart failure, *NYHA* New York Heart Association, *DSM-IV* Diagnostic and Statistical Manual, *HRV* heart rate variability, *IPT* interpersonal therapy, *ECG* electrocardiogram, *VPC* ventricular premature complexes, *SD* standard deviation, *ESSI* Enhancing Recovery in Coronary Heart Disease Patients (ENRICHD) Social Support Instrument (ESSI)

Table 23.2 Randomized controlled trials to evaluate the effects of antidepressant pharmacotherapy on depression in cardiovascular disease settings: cardiovascular morbidity and mortality outcomes

Ref	Aim	Population	Treatment period and groups	Outcome for cardiovascular morbidity	Outcome for mortality
Berkman et al. (2003)	To determine whether mortality and morbidity are reduced by treatment of depression and LPSS with CBT, supplemented with an SSRI	RCT; 2,481 MI patients (1,084 women, 1,397 men); minor or major depression (DSM-4); ESSI	CBT, initiated at a median of 17 days after the index MI for a median of 11 individual sessions throughout 6 months. Group therapy when feasible, with SSRIs for patients scoring higher than 24 on the HDRS or having a less than 50 % reduction in BDI scores after 5 weeks Usual care: 1,243; mean age 61 year (SD 12.5) Intervention: 1,238; mean age 61 year (SD 12.6)	Measures: recurrent MI Results: 4-year survival curves showed no significant difference between treatments in recurrence of MI Analyses of the time-dependent effect of pharmacologic therapy showed that antidepressant use was associated with a lower risk of reinfarction and/or mortality	After an average follow-up of 29 months, there was no significant difference in event-free survival between usual care (75.9 %) and psychosocial intervention (75.8 %). There were also no differences in survival between the psychosocial intervention and usual care arms in any of the 3 psychosocial risk groups (depression, LPSS, and depression and LPSS patients)

Glassman et al. (2002)	To evaluate the safety and efficacy of sertraline treatment of MDD	RCT; 369 patients with MDD DSM-4 (64 % male; mean age, 57.1 years; MI, 74 %; unstable angina, 26 %)	After a 2-week single-blind placebo run-in, patients were randomly assigned to receive sertraline ($n=186$) or placebo ($n=183$) for 24 weeks Placebo: mean age 57.6 years (SD 10.4) Sertraline: mean age 56.8 years (SD 11.1)	Measures: change from baseline in LVEF, surrogate cardiac measures, and cardiovascular adverse events Results: sertraline had no significant effect on mean (SD) LVEF (sertraline = baseline, 54 % [10 %]; week 16, 54 % [11 %]; placebo = baseline, 52 % [13 %]; week 16, 53% [13 %]), treatment-emergent increase in VPC runs (sertraline, 13.1 %; placebo, 12.9 %), QTc interval greater than 450 ms at end point (sertraline, 12 %; placebo, 13 %), or other cardiac measures. The incidence of severe cardiovascular adverse events was 14.5 % with sertraline and 22.4 % with placebo	Not detailed in paper

(continued)

Table 23.2 (continued)

Ref	Aim	Population	Treatment period and groups	Outcome for cardiovascular morbidity	Outcome for mortality
Lesperance et al. (2007)	To explore efficacy of a SSRI (citalopram) and IPT in reducing depressive symptoms	RCT, 284 patients with CAD, all patients DSM-4 MDD of 4 weeks duration or longer, HAM-$D \geq 20$	12-week, parallel group; participants underwent two separate randomizations: (1) to receive 12 weekly sessions of IPT plus clinical management ($n=142$) or clinical management only ($n=142$) and (2) to receive 12 weeks of citalopram, 20–40 mg/day ($n=142$) or matching placebo ($n=142$)	Measures: ECG, blood pressure Results: there were no differences between citalopram and placebo in any blood pressure or electrocardiographic measures, including QTc intervals. However, patients receiving IPT experienced a slight increase in systolic blood pressure at 12 weeks in comparison with a slight decrease among patients receiving clinical management alone	Not detailed in paper
Blumenthal et al. (2012)	To assess the efficacy of exercise and antidepressant medication in reducing depressive symptoms and improving cardiovascular biomarkers	101 outpatients with CHD and elevated depressive symptoms; DSM-4 for MDD	Randomized to 4 months of aerobic exercise (3 times/week), sertraline, or placebo Placebo: mean age 63.5 years (SD 11.4) Sertraline: mean age 63.4 years (SD 10.2) Exercise: mean age 64.7 years (SD 11.0)	Measures: HRV, endothelial function, baroreflex sensitivity, inflammation, platelet function Results: exercise and medication tended to result in greater improvements in HRV compared to placebo ($p=0.052$); exercise tended to result in greater improvements in HRV compared to sertraline ($p=0.093$)	Not detailed in paper

O'Connor et al. (2010)	To test the hypothesis that HF patients treated with sertraline will have lower depression scores and fewer cardiovascular events compared to placebo	RCT; sertraline vs placebo for 12 weeks; HF (LVEF ≤45 %, NYHA class II–IV); depression DSM-IV MDD	469 patients were randomized ($N=234$ sertraline, $N=235$ placebo) Placebo: mean age 61.4 years (SD 11.1) Sertraline: mean age 62.9 years (SD 10.5)	Measures: composite cardiovascular status; cardiovascular events and survival during the short-term treatment phase and long-term follow-up were also assessed Results: the proportion whose composite cardiovascular score worsened, improved, or was unchanged was 29.9 %, 40.6 %, and 29.5 % in the sertraline group and 31.1 %, 43.8 %, and 25.1 % in the placebo group ($p=0.78$)	Measures: serious adverse events Results: serious adverse events were not statistically different between the groups
Davidson et al. (2010)	To determine the acceptability and efficacy of enhanced depression treatment	A 3-month observation period to identify patients with ACS and persistent depressive symptoms was followed by a 6-month RCT	237 patients with ACS from 5 hospitals were enrolled, including 157 persistently depressed patients randomized to intervention (initial patient preference for problem-solving therapy and/or pharmacotherapy then a stepped-care approach; 80 patients) or usual care (77 patients) and 80 nondepressed patients who underwent observational evaluation	Measures: see mortality column	Measures: death and major adverse cardiac events Results: 3 intervention patients and 10 usual care patients had experienced major adverse cardiac events (4 % and 13 %, respectively; $p=0.047$), as well as 5 nondepressed patients (6 %) (for the intervention vs nondepressed cohort, $p=0.49$)

(continued)

Table 23.2 (continued)

Ref	Aim	Population	Treatment period and groups	Outcome for cardiovascular morbidity	Outcome for mortality
Ye et al. (2014)	Examine cardiac events and mortality in the COPES trial through an additional 12 months of observational follow-up after the end of the 6-month treatment period	157 patients with a score of ≥10 on the BDI within 1 week of ACS hospitalization and again at 3-month follow-up. Eighty enhanced treatment; 77 usual care Usual care: mean 61.1 (SD 10.6) Intervention group: mean 59.3 (SD 10.6)	Randomized to usual care or enhanced depression treatment involving stepped, patient preference-driven care with problem-solving therapy, pharmacotherapy, or both	Measures: major adverse cardiac events, defined as nonfatal MI or hospitalization for unstable angina Results: a significant time-by-treatment group interaction during extended follow-up ($p=0.008$). Specifically, during the 6-month treatment period, death or hospitalization for MI/unstable angina occurred in 3 participants (4 %) in the treatment group compared with 11 participants (14 %) in the usual care group (HR, 0.25; 95 % confidence interval, 0.07–0.90; $p=0.03$). In contrast, during 12 months of additional observational follow-up, 11 participants (14 %) in the treatment group experienced the composite outcome of death or hospitalization for MI/unstable angina compared with 3 participants (4 %) in the usual care group (HR, 2.91; 95 % confidence interval, 0.80–10.56; $p=0.10$)	Not detailed in paper

(SMD) of short-term depression change scores, −0.24 (−0.38–0.09), OR of short-term depression remission: 1.80 (95 % CI 1.18, 2.74)). No beneficial effects regarding mortality, cardiac events, and QoL were found. Hospitalization rates (OR of three trials, 0.58 [95 % CI 0.39, 0.85]) and emergency room visits (OR of one trial, 0.58 [95 % CI 0.34, 1.00]) were reduced in trials of pharmacological interventions compared to placebo. The authors suggest the research agenda in this field may need to explore patients based on their specific depression subtype and severity, and only few studies were available to explore outcomes for QoL, mortality, and cardiac events.

A latest quantitative analysis of this field, from Pizzi et al. (2011), was conducted to evaluate the effects of SSRIs versus placebo or no antidepressants in patients with CVD and depression. Primary outcomes were readmission for CVD (including AMI, unstable angina, and stroke) and all-cause mortality; the secondary outcome was severity of depression symptoms. Seven studies on six RCTs involving 2,461 participants were included, with a mean age similar in all trials and approximately 58 years. The four properly randomized trials constituted 734 patients (see Glassman et al. 2002; Lesperance et al. 2007; Strik et al. 2000; McFarlane et al. 2001; and Tables 23.1 and 23.2), while two other studies were categorized as "observational," i.e., RCTs with high risk of bias in randomization process – 1,727 subjects (see Taylor et al. 2005; Mohapatra et al. 2005; and Tables 23.1 and 23.2). When only the correctly randomized trials were taken into account, patients on SSRIs showed no significant differences in mortality RR 0.39 (95 % CI 0.08–2.01) or CVD readmission rates RR 0.74 (95 % CI 0.44–1.23) compared to controls. A significantly greater improvement in depression symptoms was always apparent in patients on SSRIs with all selected indicators. This study suggests SSRIs do decrease depressive symptoms and may improve CVD prognosis. This analysis suggests that a number of these trials were not adequately powered (see Glassman et al. 2002; Strik et al. 2000; Lesperance et al. 2007; Mohapatra et al. 2005; Hippisley-Cox et al. 2001). It was not possible to stratify these analyses to explore associations between various clinical outcomes and different types and doses of SSRIs.

23.2.3 Summary and Recommendation

When considering data from this field, consensus statements suggest SSRIs are recommended as first-line antidepressant treatments for depressed patients with CVD (Lichtman et al. 2009; Post-Myocardial Infarction Depression Clinical Practice Guideline 2009). It is clear given the data from epidemiological and clinical trials is conflicting when considering efficacy and safety. However, when high quality meta-analyses of RCTs are taken into account, SSRIs appear effective as a first-line antidepressant therapy for comorbid CAD and depression. The evidence of effects on mortality and morbidity is conflicting and suggests no difference to placebo. It is clear from a clinical perspective that careful follow-up is needed in the "real world" setting. Studies with longer follow-up are also required as the majority of current RCTs only follow subjects for 6 months. It is clear that TCAs do not appear safe for use in this population. There is a paucity of data on the use of SNRIs; hence caution is suggested with these medications (Ramamurthy et al. 2013). Larger studies are required to understand cardiac outcomes. A systematic review by Ramamurthy et al. (2013) highlights that an estimated 4,000 subjects are needed in RCTs to detect a 20% risk reduction in medical events from CAD. Based on this, no studies to date have been adequately powered to fully explore these changes. Finally, it is unclear in the literature how aging is associated with the efficacy and safety of antidepressants in comorbid CVD and depression.

23.3 Antidepressant Pharmacotherapy to Treat Depression and Congestive Heart Failure

23.3.1 Epidemiological Evidence

We are aware of only one epidemiological study exploring the associations between antidepressant use and outcomes in patients with CHF. In this study (Sherwood et al. 2007), 204 subjects with a diagnosis of CHF (left ventricular ejection fraction (LVEF) ≤40%) underwent baseline assessments with BDI. Depression and CHF were followed for 3 years using the BDI and B-type natriuretic peptide (BNP). Primary end points included death and CVD-related hospitalizations. The mean age at baseline was 56.8 years with a range of 27–88 years. After full adjustment, antidepressant medication use (various types) was associated with increased likelihood of death or cardiovascular hospitalization HR 1.75 (95% CI 1.14–2.68, $p=0.01$). The authors suggest patients with CHF requiring antidepressant medication should be monitored closely for adverse events. Replication of this study is clearly required.

23.3.2 Clinical Trial Evidence

We are again only aware of one clinical trial exploring the effects of antidepressants on patients with comorbid depression and CHF (see Tables 23.1 and 23.2). In an RCT by O'Connor et al. (2010), the effects of sertraline vs placebo were assessed on depression scores and cardiovascular events in patients with comorbid depression and CHF. Eligible patients were age ≥45 years with HF (LVEF ≤45%, New York Heart Association class II–IV) and clinical depression (DSM-IV criteria for current major depressive disorder). Primary end points were change in depression severity (Hamilton Depression Rating Scale, HDRS) and composite cardiovascular status at 12 weeks. Four hundred sixty-nine patients were randomized – $N=234$ for sertraline and $N=235$ for placebo. The change from baseline to 12 weeks in the HDRS total score was mean -7.1 ± 0.5 (sertraline) and -6.8 ± 0.5 (placebo) ($p<0.001$ from baseline, $p=0.89$ between groups, mean change between groups 0.92). The proportion whose composite cardiovascular score worsened, improved, or was unchanged was 29.9%, 40.6%, and 29.5% in the sertraline group and 31.1%, 43.8%, and 25.1% in the placebo group ($p=0.78$). This suggests sertraline was safe in CHF patients; however, there was no difference between sertraline and placebo in antidepressant effects.

23.3.3 Summary and Recommendation

There is a paucity of evidence in the treatment of depression and CHF; hence this is an important area for further investigation. SSRIs appear to be safe and had a minimal effect on depressive symptoms.

23.4 Antidepressant Pharmacotherapy to Prevent Cardiovascular Disease in Depressed Patients

23.4.1 Epidemiological Evidence

We are aware of one meta-analysis (Oh et al. 2014) exploring the association between antidepressant use and the risk of CVD in subjects free of CVD. In this study, 16 observational studies were included, 6 population-based case-control studies, 1 nested case-control study, 1 retrospective cohort study, and 8 prospective cohort studies. Participants were from a wide age range. Antidepressants were divided into SSRIs and TCAs. CVD outcomes were defined as fatal and nonfatal AMI and other IHD. There was no association found between SSRIs use and the risk of CVD overall OR 0.93 (95 % CI 0.65–1.33). The use of TCAs was associated with an increased risk of CVD overall OR 1.51 (95 % CI 1.07–2.12), but it was observed only in case-control studies OR 1.56 (95 % CI 1.24–1.96) and low-quality studies OR 1.49 (95 % CI 1.20–1.85) in the subgroup meta-analysis. This suggests no association between SSRI use and CVD risk; however, TCAs showed an increased risk. The rationale for this will be outlined below.

23.4.2 Clinical Trial Evidence

There are currently no published RCTs addressing antidepressant use and its effect on the development of CVD in patients without preexisting CVD.

23.5 Anti-inflammatory Pharmacotherapy to Treat Comorbid CVD and Depression

23.5.1 Background Information

As mentioned previously, inflammatory processes are suggested to play an important part in the development of depression, and it is believed that inflammation may be a promising target in the treatment and prevention of depression. Given this clinical and biological relationship between inflammation and depression, both selective cyclooxygenase (COX)-2 and nonselective COX inhibitor nonsteroidal anti-inflammatory drugs (NSAIDs) have been investigated as possible adjuncts in the treatment of depression. Our group critically and systematically reviewed the literature to determine whether selective COX-2 and nonselective COX inhibitor NSAIDs as adjunctives and monotherapies affect depressive symptoms (Eyre et al. 2015). In our analysis on adjunctive and monotherapy studies, we included six RCTs exploring the efficacy of selective COX-2 inhibitor NSAIDs on depressive symptoms with a total of 2,706 subjects. Four of the RCTs showed a significant effect of NSAIDs; two demonstrated no effect. There were a total of five studies exploring the efficacy of nonselective COX inhibitor NSAIDs on depressive symptoms with a total of 7,978 subjects. There was one RCT, three cohort studies, and one open-label pilot study. The RCT failed to show a significant result. One of the retrospective cohort studies showed a positive result, with the other two showing no effect. We concluded the efficacy of NSAIDs on depressive symptoms appears negligible; however, firm conclusions are difficult given the inconsistent findings and substantial methodological heterogeneity. Heterogeneity was derived from a variety of factors, i.e., age range, sex, presence of antidepressant use, method of depression measure, severity of depressive symptoms, duration, and study design (RCT vs cohort). A meta-analysis (Na et al. 2014) of RCTs suggests that celecoxib, a selective COX-2 inhibitor NSAID, has a therapeutic effect when used adjunctively with other antidepressants. This study utilized four RCT studies with a total of 150 patients. The patients receiving adjunctive celecoxib had significantly higher mean changes in the HDRS scores between baseline and end point measurements compared with those receiving placebo (weighted mean difference = 3.26). The adjunctive celecoxib group also showed better remission OR=6.58 and response rates OR=6.49 than the placebo group. Yet another meta-analysis by Kohler et al. (2014) explored the antidepressant effects of all anti-inflammatory interventions. Ten publications reporting on 14 trials (6,262 participants) were included; ten trials evaluated the use of NSAIDs (n=4,258; four as adjunct treatment and six as monotherapy all including celecoxib) and four investigated cytokine inhibitors (n=2,004; all studies as monotherapy). These were a mix of adjunctive (to antidepressants) and monotherapy studies. The pooled effect estimate suggested that anti-inflammatory treatment reduced depressive symptoms SMD −0.34 compared with placebo. This effect was observed in studies including patients with depression SMD −0.54 and depressive symptoms SMD −0.27. A subanalysis of celecoxib only showed a trend toward superiority to placebo (SMD −0.29). When celecoxib monotherapy studies where only examined, results were borderline significant (SMD −0.13); celecoxib adjunct studies showed significant improvement (SMD −0.82). Among the six studies reporting on adverse effects, there was no evidence of CVD events after 6 weeks of anti-inflammatory treatment compared with placebo.

Taken together, these findings suggest anti-inflammatory pharmacological agents should be studied more in the treatment of depression and CVD both as adjunctive treatment as well as monotherapy. At this stage, adjunctive celecoxib treatments appear to be most effective for the treatment of depression.

23.5.2 Epidemiological Evidence

We are only aware of one published study exploring the effects of anti-inflammatories on comorbid depression and CVD. In this observational study (Rieckmann et al. 2011), data from 168 ACS hospitalized patients were assessed along with adherence to aspirin medication. Adherence to aspirin was measured over 90 days, and rates of antidepressant use were not recorded, although present. The outcome was the 1-year first occurrence of a MACE or all-cause mortality. Controlling for age, sex, and site, baseline depressive symptoms were significantly correlated with poorer 7-day, 1-month, and 3-month aspirin adherence (all $p<0.02$). After 1 year, there had been 14 MACE/all-cause mortality events (8 %). Adjusting for age, sex, and site, poorer 7-day (HR 1.76) and 1 month aspirin adherence (HR 1.75) as well as baseline depressive symptoms (HR 1.53) were each individually associated with 1-year MACE/all-cause mortality. These findings suggest poorer aspirin adherence may account for a proportion of the excess prognostic risk associated with depressive symptoms after ACS. There is thus rational for a clinical trial in this area.

23.6 Understanding the Neurobiological Mechanisms Subserving the Effects of Antidepressants in Depression and Cardiovascular Disease

There are a number of neurobiological mechanisms potentially subserving the efficacy and safety of antidepressants in depression and CVD. These mechanisms include inflammation, HPA axis dysfunction, increased sympathetic tone, vascular dysfunction, and cardiac conduction. In the below sections, we review each of these mechanisms and explore the effect of antidepressants on them. We have aimed to distinguish the neurobiological effects of various classes of antidepressants where possible. A diagrammatic overview of this section is also provided in Fig. 23.1.

23.6.1 Inflammation

The most recent evidence from reviews and meta-analyses suggests that antidepressants may exert effects on the immune system. A meta-analysis of 22 studies by Hannestad et al. (2011) explored the effect of antidepressants on serum pro-inflammatory cytokines, TNFα, IL-1β, and IL-6, in 603 depressed subjects. This is the latest study to quantitatively explore the immune-modulatory effects of antidepressants. A stratified subgroup analysis in this meta-analysis by class of antidepressants indicated that serotonin reuptake inhibitors (SSRI) may reduce levels of IL-6 and TNFα, whereas other types of antidepressants – while efficacious for depressive symptoms – did not appear to reduce cytokine levels and showed only limited evidence in a few studies only. These data suggest that SSRIs with their prominent serotonergic functions may be more anti-inflammatory than other agents. Beyond this meta-analysis, it has been suggested that while noradrenaline reuptake inhibitor antidepressants suppress Th1-type cytokines (e.g., IFN-γ, IL-2, and TNF-α) and shift the balance toward humoral immunity, serotonin reuptake inhibitors reduce the production of Th2-type cytokines (e.g., IL-4, IL-5, IL-6, IL-9, IL-10, and IL-13) and shift the balance toward cellular immune response (Uher et al. 2014; Martino et al.

2012). These findings suggest that antidepressants do appear to be anti-inflammatory, and hence this may be one mechanism through which they reduce depressive symptoms and CVD-related health issues. However, the abovementioned data raise the possibility of differential mechanistic effects of various antidepressant classes on immune function. We caution conclusions regarding which antidepressant possesses the greater anti-inflammatory effect given methodological heterogeneity among studies and a small number of comparative studies.

23.6.2 HPA Axis

One of the most consistent biological findings in depression is a hyperactivity of the HPA axis, and there is a literature exploring the effects of antidepressants on this (Pariante and Lightman 2008). Data from both preclinical and clinical studies assists in understanding the effects of antidepressants on the HPA axis. A study by Cattaneo et al. (2013) tested leukocyte mRNA expression levels of genes in healthy controls ($n=34$) and depressed patients ($n=74$), both before and after 8 weeks of treatment with escitalopram or nortriptyline. This was conducted as part of the Genome-Based Therapeutic Drugs for Depression (GENDEP) study. Genes were explored common to both drugs. Nonresponders had higher baseline mRNA levels of IL-1β (+33 %), macrophage inhibitor factor (MIF) (+48 %), and TNF-α (+39 %). This suggests a pro-inflammatory state is associated with nonresponse. Antidepressants reduced the levels of IL-1β (−6 %) and MIF (−24 %) and increased the levels of GR (+5 %) and p11 (+8 %); however, these changes were not associated with response. Responders had a reduction in the levels of the GR-associated gene, *FKBP-5*. This suggests depression is characterized by the coexistence of higher *FKBP-5* and lower *GR*, possibly leading to GR resistance. Furthermore, successful antidepressant treatment requires normalization of GR function. In another human study, Carvalho et al. (2010) explored the effects of antidepressants (clomipramine, amitriptyline, sertraline, paroxetine, and venlafaxine) on GR function. GR function was assessed in peripheral blood cells from 33 health volunteers. GR function was measured by glucocorticoid-mediated inhibition of lipopolysaccharide (LPS)-stimulated interleukin-6 (IL-6) levels. LPS is a potent immune system activator. Compared to vehicle-treated cells, all antidepressants inhibited dexamethasone (DEX, 10–100 nM) inhibition of LPS-stimulated IL-6 levels (p values ranging from 0.007 to 0.1). The GR antagonist, RU-486, inhibited the effect of antidepressants on GR function. Research in neuronal stem cells has illustrated that antidepressants directly increase the function of the GR (Anacker et al. 2011). This was found to occur via a GR-dependent mechanism, i.e., the expression of *p11* (Anacker et al. 2011). The effect on p11 is an action that is required for the effects of antidepressants on neurogenesis (Anacker et al. 2011). These studies highlight the effects of antidepressants on the HPA axis and their role in correcting HPA axis dysfunction, which is likely associated with reducing inflammatory processes.

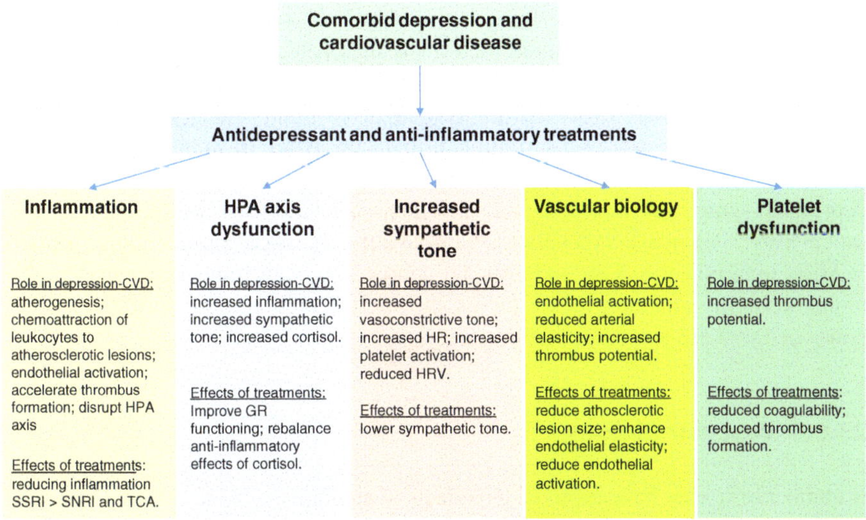

Fig. 23.1 Neurobiological mechanisms subserving the effects of antidepressants and anti-inflammatories on the treatment of depression and cardiovascular disease

23.6.3 Sympathetic Tone

HRV is a measure of sympathetic tone and is an important marker given very low-frequency (VLF) HRV may predict mortality in patients with comorbid depression and CVD (Carney et al. 2005). A prospective cohort study, the Heart and Soul Study (Zimmermann-Viehoff et al. 2014), was utilized to explore associations between antidepressant use (SSRI or TCA) and mortality in patients with CVD and HRV. Nine hundred fifty-six patients with CVD were followed for a mean duration of 7.2 years. Of 956 patients, 44 (4.6 %) used TCAs, 89 (9.3 %) used SSRIs, and 823 (86.1 %) did not use antidepressants. At baseline, TCA users exhibited lower HRV compared with SSRI users and antidepressant nonusers. At the end of the observational period, 52.3 % of the TCA users had died compared with 38.2 % in the SSRI group and 37.3 % in the control group. The adjusted HR for TCA use compared with nonuse was 1.74 ($p = 0.01$). Adjustment for measures of autonomic function rendered nonsignificant the association between TCA use and mortality. SSRI use was not associated with mortality. This suggests the associations between TCA use and mortality may be partly mediated by effects on autonomic function. A recent pilot study (Jain et al. 2014) examined the associations between resting baseline HRV and depression treatment outcomes. In this study, investigators retrospectively tested several parameters of HRV in an MDD treatment study with escitalopram ($n = 26$) as well as Iyengar yoga ($n = 16$). Lower relative power of very low-frequency (VLF) HRV at baseline predicted improvement in depressive symptoms when adjusted for age and gender ($p < 0.05$ for both treatments). This suggests VLF HRV may be a useful predictor of treatment outcome with antidepressants in depression; however, the underlying biology for this is unclear. A recent RCT by Blumenthal et al. (2012) explored the effects of aerobic exercise and sertraline in reducing depressive symptoms and certain CV biomarkers in depressed patients with CVD. One hundred participants were involved in this study and were offered 4 months of aerobic exercise, sertraline, or placebo. After 16 weeks, both the aerobic exercise group and sertraline group showed a larger reduction than placebo for depressive symptoms. Exercise and sertraline were equivalent in their antidepressant effects. Exercise and medication showed a trend toward a greater improvement in HRV than placebo. This suggests antidepressants may improve cardiovascular biomarkers. In summary, these studies show antidepressants may improve HRV; however, there are few studies in this area.

23.6.4 Vascular Biology

A number of studies have explored the effects of antidepressants of markers of vascular biology in depression. A recent case-control study (Paranthaman et al. 2012) explored the relationship between endothelial function, atherosclerosis, and treatment response to antidepressant monotherapy (various types). The study compared 25 patients with late-life depression to 21 nondepressed subjects. Vascular measures included a marker of atherosclerosis (carotid intima thickness (IMT)) and endothelial function (biopsied small artery dilatation/reactivity to acetylcholine). There was a significant group difference (responders versus nonresponders versus controls) on both IMT and endothelial function ($p<0.05$ for both). There was a gradient across groups, with control subjects having best vascular structure or function, nonresponders having the worst, and responders at an intermediate level. These findings suggest that vascular dysfunction and pathology are linked to lesser antidepressant response.

A subgroup analysis of the Sertraline Antidepressant Heart Attack Randomized Trial (SADHART) study (Serebruany et al. 2003) was used to understand the effects of sertraline on the release of platelet and endothelial biomarkers in depressed subjects with ACS. In this analysis 55 subjects were randomly assigned to sertraline ($n=23$) or placebo ($n=32$). Anticoagulants, aspirin, and clopidogrel were permitted. Twenty-six serial plasma samples collected at week 6 ($N=12$) and week 16 ($N=14$) were analyzed. Platelet factor 4 (PF4), β-thromboglobulin (β-TG), platelet/endothelial cell adhesion molecule 1 (PECAM-1), P-selectin, thromboxane B_2 (TxB_2), prostacyclin (6-keto-PGF1α), vascular cell adhesion molecule 1 (VCAM-1), and E-selectin were measured by enzyme-linked immunosorbent assay. Negative correlations were found for the plasma levels of sertraline and *N*-desmethylsertraline with PF4, β-TG, PECAM-1, P-selectin, and TxB_2. These findings allude to sertraline reducing platelet and endothelium activation.

A study by van Zyl et al. (2009) utilized an RCT framework (Canadian Cardiac Randomized Evaluation of Antidepressant and Psychotherapy Efficacy Trial (CREATE)) to explore whether treatment of depressed CAD patients with citalopram altered platelet and endothelial biomarkers. The effect of citalopram was explored on P-selectin, β-TG, soluble intercellular CAM-1 (sICAM-1), and total nitric oxide (tNO). Plasma samples were obtained at baseline and week 12 from subjects randomized to citalopram ($n=36$) or placebo ($n=21$). Anticoagulants, aspirin, and clopidogrel were permitted. Treatment with citalopram was associated with greater increase in tNO over 12 weeks compared to placebo ($p=0.005$). There were no differences for the other biomarkers. Improved endothelial function may be implied by the increased NO production in this study; however, this is not clear. Some studies show SSRIs inhibit NO (Finkel et al. 1996), and others suggest SSRIs increased NO and its metabolites (Lara et al. 2003; Chrapko et al. 2006). The differing results in this study as compared to the abovementioned SADHART subgroup analysis may be due to differing stages of CVD or the different effects of sertraline vs citalopram.

23.6.5 Platelet Dysfunction

As mentioned previously, platelet dysfunction is a potential biological mechanism connecting depression and CVD. Platelets possess receptors for serotonin (5-HT), such as 5-HT2A and 5-HT3, and also a 5-HT transporter (SERT) in their membranes (Stratz et al. 2008). 5-HT is stored in the dense granules within platelets and released during stimulation. Preclinical studies have demonstrated that 5-HT potentiates procoagulant responses of platelets and enhances the thrombogenesis on damaged vascular surfaces (Galan et al. 2009; Lopez-Vilchez et al. 2009).

An interesting exploration of the role of antidepressants in platelet function comes from an analysis of cerebral microbleeds (Aarts et al. 2014). Within the population-based Rotterdam Study, information on antidepressant use was obtained from continuously monitored pharmacy records, and brain MRIs were available in 4,945 participants between 2005 and 2011. Antidepressants were categorized based on affinity for the serotonin transporter: high, intermediate, or low. Antidepressant use with strong serotonin reuptake inhibition was not associated with microbleed presence (OR 1.03), compared with nonuse, irrespective of microbleed location in the brain. Exclusion of antithrombotic users or persons with cortical infarcts did not change these results. Furthermore, serotonergic antidepressant use was not related to ischemic vascular brain damage. This data suggests serotonin-active antidepressants do not relate to the presence of cerebral microbleeds.

A recent clinical study (Lopez-Vilchez et al. 2014) investigated the modulation of thrombogenesis by treatment with an SSRI. Modifications in a series of biomarkers of platelet and coagulation activation were evaluated in the blood from 19 patients with an MDD at the time of diagnosis, and at 8 and 24 weeks of treatment with escitalopram, 20 healthy subjects were used as controls. Response of blood aliquots recirculated through a thrombogenic surface was assessed as a thrombosis model. In comparison with controls, platelets from depression patients showed elevated clot volumes, augmented expression of GPIb, fibrinogen, factor V, and phospholipids. Clot firmness and procoagulant activity of platelet-associated tissue factor were also significantly elevated. Studies with circulating blood revealed increased fibrin formation in early diagnosed patients. After 24 weeks of treatment with escitalopram, the majority of the alterations observed were normalized, except for biomarkers of viscoelasticity and clot formation which were unaffected. This data demonstrates the pro-thrombotic state seen in depression and the effect of SSRIs in altering certain biomarkers, although not others.

23.6.6 Cardiac Conduction

Cardiac conduction is clearly crucial in understanding the effects of antidepressants on patients with depression and CVD. The effect of antidepressants on cardiac conduction systems is likely strongly related to cardiac-related adverse events.

23.6.6.1 Selective Serotonin Reuptake Inhibitors

SSRIs have been associated with very infrequent cardiac side effects, such as bradycardia and heart block (86 reported cases of the first 2.5 million taking fluoxetine (Goldberg 1998)). The Food and Drug Administration in the United States has advised that citalopram not exceed 40 mg daily to prevent prolonged QTc and associated arrhythmias. Some authors suggest benefit from serial electrocardiograms and cardiac/internal medicine consultation when adding SSRIs to patients with pre-existing arrhythmias, particularly bradycardia/atrioventricular block (Ramamurthy et al. 2013).

23.6.6.2 Serotonin Noradrenaline Reuptake Inhibitors

As mentioned previously, caution is advised with the use of SNRIs in depression and CVD. The hypothetical concern is with SNRIs increase sympathetic tone through noradrenergic action. High sympathetic tone is associated with atherogenesis (Julius 1993), cardiac remodeling post-AMI (Sabbah 2004), and arrhythmias (Hjalmarson 1997).

23.6.6.3 Tricyclic Antidepressants

Data from the Cardiac Arrhythmia Suppression Trial (CAST) (Glassman et al. 1993) published in 1993 in which post-MI patients were treated with various classes of pharmacological agents was revealing in regard to the safety of TCAs. This study showed Class 1 antiarrhythmics, where TCAs are categorized, had increased mortality.

Conclusions

The tremendous burden of depression, CVD, and their comorbid status makes the need for understanding current and developing new treatments and preventive strategies highly important. When we consider antidepressant and anti-inflammatory therapies from epidemiological and clinical trial perspectives, there are a number of interesting findings, as well as areas for further research. When considering clinical efficacy, SSRIs appear to be effective as first-line antidepressants. There is a paucity of data for SNRIs, and TCAs are not recommended. Celecoxib treatment may be useful as an adjunctive treatment, with other anti-inflammatories requiring further investigation. The effect of SSRIs on mortality and morbidity appears minimal, with a mixture of results suggesting no different to placebo and improved results to placebo. There are a number of biological systems which are implicated in the bidirectional relationship between depression and CVD, including inflammation, HPA axis dysfunction, increased sympathetic tone, and vascular and platelet dysfunction. An emerging body of research has now begun to explore the effect of pharmacological agents on these systems. More research is required to understand the effects of various drug classes on these mechanisms. In the future, we have a number of recommendations to advance this field. Larger and longer duration RCTs are required to determine the effect of various types of antidepressants on long-term CVD outcomes. Further, understanding the effects of antidepressant treatments on various types of depression (e.g., melancholic, non-melancholic, and atypical) would be helpful to understand effects on CVD outcomes. Exploration of the treatment of depression and comorbid CHF is also an area in need of further examination.

References

Aarts N, Akoudad S, Noordam R, Hofman A, Ikram MA, Stricker BH, Visser LE, Vernooij MW (2014) Inhibition of serotonin reuptake by antidepressants and cerebral microbleeds in the general population. Stroke J Cereb Circ 45(7):1951–1957. doi:10.1161/STROKEAHA.114.004990

Anacker C, Zunszain PA, Cattaneo A, Carvalho LA, Garabedian MJ, Thuret S, Price J, Pariante CM (2011) Antidepressants increase human hippocampal neurogenesis by activating the glucocorticoid receptor. Mol Psychiatry 16(7):738–750. doi:10.1038/mp.2011.26

Barth J, Schumacher M, Herrmann-Lingen C (2004) Depression as a risk factor for mortality in patients with coronary heart disease: a meta-analysis. Psychosom Med 66(6):802–813. doi:10.1097/01.psy.0000146332.53619.b2

Baumeister H, Hutter N, Bengel J (2011) Psychological and pharmacological interventions for depression in patients with coronary artery disease. Cochrane Database Syst Rev 9:CD008012. doi:10.1002/14651858.CD008012.pub3

Baune BT, Stuart M, Gilmour A, Wersching H, Arolt V, Berger K (2012a) Moderators of the relationship between depression and cardiovascular disorders: a systematic review. Gen Hosp Psychiatry 34(5):478–492. doi:10.1016/j.genhosppsych.2012.05.013

Baune BT, Stuart M, Gilmour A, Wersching H, Heindel W, Arolt V, Berger K (2012b) The relationship between subtypes of depression and cardiovascular disease: a systematic review of biological models. Transl Psychiatry 2:e92. doi:10.1038/tp.2012.18

Berkman LF, Blumenthal J, Burg M, Carney RM, Catellier D, Cowan MJ, Czajkowski SM, DeBusk R, Hosking J, Jaffe A, Kaufmann PG, Mitchell P, Norman J, Powell LH, Raczynski JM, Schneiderman N, Enhancing Recovery in Coronary Heart Disease Patients I (2003) Effects of treating depression and low perceived social support on clinical events after myocardial infarction: the Enhancing Recovery in Coronary Heart Disease Patients (ENRICHD) Randomized Trial. JAMA 289(23):3106–3116. doi:10.1001/jama.289.23.3106

Blumenthal JA, Sherwood A, Babyak MA, Watkins LL, Smith PJ, Hoffman BM, O'Hayer CV, Mabe S, Johnson J, Doraiswamy PM, Jiang W, Schocken DD, Hinderliter AL (2012) Exercise and pharmacological treatment of depressive symptoms in patients with coronary heart disease: results from the UPBEAT (Understanding the Prognostic Benefits of Exercise and Antidepressant Therapy) Study. J Am Coll Cardiol 60(12):1053–1063. doi:10.1016/j.jacc.2012.04.040

Bonetti PO, Lerman LO, Lerman A (2003) Endothelial dysfunction: a marker of atherosclerotic risk. Arterioscler Thromb Vasc Biol 23(2):168–175

Carney RM, Blumenthal JA, Freedland KE, Stein PK, Howells WB, Berkman LF, Watkins LL, Czajkowski SM, Hayano J, Domitrovich PP, Jaffe AS (2005) Low heart rate variability and the effect of depression on post-myocardial infarction mortality. Arch Intern Med 165(13):1486–1491. doi:10.1001/archinte.165.13.1486

Carvalho LA, Garner BA, Dew T, Fazakerley H, Pariante CM (2010) Antidepressants, but not antipsychotics, modulate GR function in human whole blood: an insight into molecular mechanisms. Eur Neuropsychopharmacol J Eur Coll Neuropsychopharmacol 20(6):379–387. doi:10.1016/j.euroneuro.2010.02.006

Cattaneo A, Gennarelli M, Uher R, Breen G, Farmer A, Aitchison KJ, Craig IW, Anacker C, Zunsztain PA, McGuffin P, Pariante CM (2013) Candidate genes expression profile associated with antidepressants response in the GENDEP study: differentiating between baseline 'predictors' and longitudinal 'targets'. Neuropsychopharmacology 38(3):377–385. doi:10.1038/npp.2012.191

Cay EL, Vetter N, Philip AE, Dugard P (1972) Psychological status during recovery from an acute heart attack. J Psychosom Res 16(6):425–435

Chrapko W, Jurasz P, Radomski MW, Archer SL, Newman SC, Baker G, Lara N, Le Melledo JM (2006) Alteration of decreased plasma NO metabolites and platelet NO synthase activity by paroxetine in depressed patients. Neuropsychopharmacology 31(6):1286–1293. doi:10.1038/sj.npp.1300961

Cooper DC, Tomfohr LM, Milic MS, Natarajan L, Bardwell WA, Ziegler MG, Dimsdale JE (2011) Depressed mood and flow-mediated dilation: a systematic review and meta-analysis. Psychosom Med 73(5):360–369. doi:10.1097/PSY.0b013e31821db79a

Davidson KW, Rieckmann N, Clemow L, Schwartz JE, Shimbo D, Medina V, Albanese G, Kronish I, Hegel M, Burg MM (2010) Enhanced depression care for patients with acute coronary syndrome and persistent depressive symptoms: coronary psychosocial evaluation studies randomized controlled trial. Arch Intern Med 170(7):600–608. doi:10.1001/archinternmed.2010.29

Dowlati Y, Herrmann N, Swardfager W, Liu H, Sham L, Reim EK, Lanctot KL (2010) A meta-analysis of cytokines in major depression. Biol Psychiatry 67(5):446–457. doi:10.1016/j.biopsych.2009.09.033

Egede LE (2007) Major depression in individuals with chronic medical disorders: prevalence, correlates and association with health resource utilization, lost productivity and functional disability. Gen Hosp Psychiatry 29(5):409–416. doi:10.1016/j.genhosppsych.2007.06.002

Eyre HA, Stuart MJ, Baune BT (2014) A phase-specific neuroimmune model of clinical depression. Prog Neuropsychopharmacol Biol Psychiatry 54:265–274. doi:10.1016/j.pnpbp.2014.06.011

Eyre HA, Air T, Proctor S, Rositano S, Baune BT (2015) A critical review of the efficacy of non-steroidal anti-inflammatory drugs in depression. Prog Neuropsychopharmacol Biol Psychiatry 57:11–16. doi:10.1016/j.pnpbp.2014.10.003

Finkel MS, Laghrissi-Thode F, Pollock BG, Rong J (1996) Paroxetine is a novel nitric oxide synthase inhibitor. Psychopharmacol Bull 32(4):653–658

Frasure-Smith N, Lesperance F (2010) Depression and cardiac risk: present status and future directions. Postgrad Med J 86(1014):193–196. doi:10.1136/hrt.2009.186957

Freeman AM 3rd, Fleece L, Folks DG, Sokol RS, Hall KR, Pacifico AD, McGiffin DC, Kirklin JK, Zorn GL, Karp RB (1986) Alprazolam treatment of postcoronary bypass anxiety and depression. J Clin Psychopharmacol 6(1):39–41

Galan AM, Lopez-Vilchez I, Diaz-Ricart M, Navalon F, Gomez E, Gasto C, Escolar G (2009) Serotonergic mechanisms enhance platelet-mediated thrombogenicity. Thromb Haemost 102(3):511–519. doi:10.1160/TH08-12-0810

Glassman AH, Roose SP, Bigger JT Jr (1993) The safety of tricyclic antidepressants in cardiac patients. Risk-benefit reconsidered. JAMA 269(20):2673–2675

Glassman AH, O'Connor CM, Califf RM, Swedberg K, Schwartz P, Bigger JT Jr, Krishnan KR, van Zyl LT, Swenson JR, Finkel MS, Landau C, Shapiro PA, Pepine CJ, Mardekian J, Harrison WM, Barton D, McLvor M, Sertraline Antidepressant Heart Attack Randomized Trial G (2002) Sertraline treatment of major depression in patients with acute MI or unstable angina. JAMA 288(6):701–709

Goldberg RJ (1998) Selective serotonin reuptake inhibitors: infrequent medical adverse effects. Arch Fam Med 7(1):78–84

Goldston K, Baillie AJ (2008) Depression and coronary heart disease: a review of the epidemiological evidence, explanatory mechanisms and management approaches. Clin Psychol Rev 28(2):288–306. doi:10.1016/j.cpr.2007.05.005

Gonzalez HM, Tarraf W (2013) Comorbid cardiovascular disease and major depression among ethnic and racial groups in the United States. Int Psychogeriatr/IPA 25(5):833–841. doi:10.1017/S1041610212002062

Grippo AJ, Johnson AK (2002) Biological mechanisms in the relationship between depression and heart disease. Neurosci Biobehav Rev 26(8):941–962

Hannestad J, Dellagioia N, Bloch M (2011) The effect of antidepressant medication treatment on serum levels of inflammatory cytokines: a meta-analysis. Neuropsychopharmacology 36(12):2452–2459. doi:10.1038/npp.2011.132, npp2011132 [pii]

Hare DL, Toukhsati SR, Johansson P, Jaarsma T (2014) Depression and cardiovascular disease: a clinical review. Eur Heart J 35(21):1365–1372. doi:10.1093/eurheartj/eht462

Hippisley-Cox J, Pringle M, Hammersley V, Crown N, Wynn A, Meal A, Coupland C (2001) Antidepressants as risk factor for ischaemic heart disease: case-control study in primary care. BMJ 323(7314):666–669

Hjalmarson A (1997) Effects of beta blockade on sudden cardiac death during acute myocardial infarction and the postinfarction period. Am J Cardiol 80(9B):35J–39J

Honig A, Kuyper AM, Schene AH, van Melle JP, de Jonge P, Tulner DM, Schins A, Crijns HJ, Kuijpers PM, Vossen H, Lousberg R, Ormel J, Investigators M-I (2007) Treatment of post-myocardial infarction depressive disorder: a randomized, placebo-controlled trial with mirtazapine. Psychosom Med 69(7):606–613. doi:10.1097/PSY.0b013e31814b260d

Jain FA, Cook IA, Leuchter AF, Hunter AM, Davydov DM, Ottaviani C, Tartter M, Crump C, Shapiro D (2014) Heart rate variability and treatment outcome in major depression: a pilot study. Int J Psychophysiol Off J Int Organ Psychophysiol 93(2):204–210. doi:10.1016/j.ijpsycho.2014.04.006

Joynt KE, Whellan DJ, O'Connor CM (2003) Depression and cardiovascular disease: mechanisms of interaction. Biol Psychiatry 54(3):248–261

Julius S (1993) Corcoran Lecture. Sympathetic hyperactivity and coronary risk in hypertension. Hypertension 21(6 Pt 2):886–893

Kemp AH, Quintana DS, Gray MA, Felmingham KL, Brown K, Gatt JM (2010) Impact of depression and antidepressant treatment on heart rate variability: a review and meta-analysis. Biol Psychiatry 67(11):1067–1074. doi:10.1016/j.biopsych.2009.12.012

Kohler O, Benros ME, Nordentoft M, Farkouh ME, Iyengar RL, Mors O, Krogh J (2014) Effect of anti-inflammatory treatment on depression, depressive symptoms, and adverse effects: a systematic review and meta-analysis of randomized clinical trials. JAMA Psychiatry 71(12):1381–1391. doi:10.1001/jamapsychiatry.2014.1611

Lara N, Archer SL, Baker GB, Le Melledo JM (2003) Paroxetine-induced increase in metabolic end products of nitric oxide. J Clin Psychopharmacol 23(4):408–412. doi:10.1097/01.jcp.0000085416.08426.1d

Lesperance F, Frasure-Smith N, Koszycki D, Laliberte MA, van Zyl LT, Baker B, Swenson JR, Ghatavi K, Abramson BL, Dorian P, Guertin MC, Investigators C (2007) Effects of citalopram and interpersonal psychotherapy on depression in patients with coronary artery disease: the Canadian Cardiac Randomized Evaluation of Antidepressant and Psychotherapy Efficacy (CREATE) trial. JAMA 297(4):367–379. doi:10.1001/jama.297.4.367

Li YM, Li GY, Wang XL, Yu LF (2005) Rehabilitation effect of San John's Wort extract on depression and myocardial function after coronary artery bypass grafting: a randomized grouping, placebo-control and blind evaluation [Chinese]. Zhongguo Linchuang Kangfu 9:28–29

Lichtman JH, Bigger JT Jr, Blumenthal JA, Frasure-Smith N, Kaufmann PG, Lesperance F, Mark DB, Sheps DS, Taylor CB, Froelicher ES (2009) AHA science advisory. Depression and coronary heart disease. Recommendations for screening, referral, and treatment. A science advisory from the American Heart Association Prevention Committee to the Council on Cardiovascular Nursing,

Council on Clinical Cardiology, Council on Epidemiology and Prevention, and Interdisciplinary Council on Quality of Care Outcomes Research. Endorsed by the American Psychiatric Association. Prog Cardiovasc Nurs 24(1):19–26. doi:10.1111/j.1751-7117.2009.00028.x

Lippi G, Montagnana M, Favaloro EJ, Franchini M (2009) Mental depression and cardiovascular disease: a multifaceted, bidirectional association. Semin Thromb Hemost 35(3):325–336. doi: 10.1055/s-0029-1222611

Liu JD, Zheng H (1999) Efficacy of fluoxetine in the treatment of depression in patients with acute myocardial infarction [Chinese]. J Clin Psychol Med 9:210–211

Lopez-Vilchez I, Diaz-Ricart M, White JG, Escolar G, Galan AM (2009) Serotonin enhances platelet procoagulant properties and their activation induced during platelet tissue factor uptake. Cardiovasc Res 84(2):309–316. doi:10.1093/cvr/cvp205

Lopez-Vilchez I, Serra-Millas M, Navarro V, Rosa Hernandez M, Villalta J, Diaz-Ricart M, Gasto C, Escolar G, Galan AM (2014) Prothrombotic platelet phenotype in major depression: downregulation by antidepressant treatment. J Affect Disord 159:39–45. doi:10.1016/j.jad.2014.02.022

Macchia A, Monte S, Pellegrini F, Romero M, D'Ettorre A, Tavazzi L, Tognoni G, Maggioni AP (2008) Depression worsens outcomes in elderly patients with heart failure: an analysis of 48,117 patients in a community setting. Eur J Heart Fail 10(7):714–721. doi:10.1016/j.ejheart.2008.05.011

Malpas SC (2010) Sympathetic nervous system overactivity and its role in the development of cardiovascular disease. Physiol Rev 90(2):513–557. doi:10.1152/physrev.00007.2009

Martino M, Rocchi G, Escelsior A, Fornaro M (2012) Immunomodulation mechanism of antidepressants: interactions between serotonin/norepinephrine balance and Th1/Th2 balance. Curr Neuropharmacol 10(2):97–123. doi:10.2174/157015912800604542

Mazza M, Lotrionte M, Biondi-Zoccai G, Abbate A, Sheiban I, Romagnoli E (2010) Selective serotonin reuptake inhibitors provide significant lower re-hospitalization rates in patients recovering from acute coronary syndromes: evidence from a meta-analysis. J Psychopharmacol 24(12):1785–1792. doi:10.1177/0269881109348176

McFarlane A, Kamath MV, Fallen EL, Malcolm V, Cherian F, Norman G (2001) Effect of sertraline on the recovery rate of cardiac autonomic function in depressed patients after acute myocardial infarction. Am Heart J 142(4):617–623. doi:10.1067/mhj.2001.116766

Meijer A, Conradi HJ, Bos EH, Thombs BD, van Melle JP, de Jonge P (2011) Prognostic association of depression following myocardial infarction with mortality and cardiovascular events: a meta-analysis of 25 years of research. Gen Hosp Psychiatry 33(3):203–216. doi:10.1016/j.genhosppsych.2011.02.007

Mohapatra PK, Kar N, Kar GC, Behera M (2005) Effectiveness of sertraline in treatment of depression in a consecutive sample of patients with acute myocardial infarction: six month prospective study on outcome. Clin Pract Epidemiol Ment Health CP & EMH 1:26. doi:10.1186/1745-0179-1-26

Murray CJ, Vos T, Lozano R, Naghavi M, Flaxman AD, Michaud C, Ezzati M, Shibuya K, Salomon JA, Abdalla S, Aboyans V, Abraham J, Ackerman I, Aggarwal R, Ahn SY, Ali MK, Alvarado M, Anderson HR, Anderson LM, Andrews KG, Atkinson C, Baddour LM, Bahalim AN, Barker-Collo S, Barrero LH, Bartels DH, Basanez MG, Baxter A, Bell ML, Benjamin EJ, Bennett D, Bernabe E, Bhalla K, Bhandari B, Bikbov B, Bin Abdulhak A, Birbeck G, Black JA, Blencowe H, Blore JD, Blyth F, Bolliger I, Bonaventure A, Boufous S, Bourne R, Boussinesq M, Braithwaite T, Brayne C, Bridgett L, Brooker S, Brooks P, Brugha TS, Bryan-Hancock C, Bucello C, Buchbinder R, Buckle G, Budke CM, Burch M, Burney P, Burstein R, Calabria B, Campbell B, Canter CE, Carabin H, Carapetis J, Carmona L, Cella C, Charlson F, Chen H, Cheng AT, Chou D, Chugh SS, Coffeng LE, Colan SD, Colquhoun S, Colson KE, Condon J, Connor MD, Cooper LT, Corriere M, Cortinovis M, de Vaccaro KC, Couser W, Cowie BC, Criqui MH, Cross M, Dabhadkar KC, Dahiya M, Dahodwala N, Damsere-Derry J, Danaei G, Davis A, De Leo D, Degenhardt L, Dellavalle R, Delossantos A, Denenberg J, Derrett S, Des Jarlais DC, Dharmaratne SD, Dherani M, Diaz-Torne C, Dolk H, Dorsey ER, Driscoll T, Duber H, Ebel B, Edmond K, Elbaz A, Ali SE, Erskine H, Erwin PJ, Espindola P, Ewoigbokhan SE, Farzadfar F, Feigin V, Felson DT, Ferrari A, Ferri CP, Fevre EM, Finucane MM, Flaxman S, Flood L, Foreman K,

Forouzanfar MH, Fowkes FG, Fransen M, Freeman MK, Gabbe BJ, Gabriel SE, Gakidou E, Ganatra HA, Garcia B, Gaspari F, Gillum RF, Gmel G, Gonzalez-Medina D, Gosselin R, Grainger R, Grant B, Groeger J, Guillemin F, Gunnell D, Gupta R, Haagsma J, Hagan H, Halasa YA, Hall W, Haring D, Haro JM, Harrison JE, Havmoeller R, Hay RJ, Higashi H, Hill C, Hoen B, Hoffman H, Hotez PJ, Hoy D, Huang JJ, Ibeanusi SE, Jacobsen KH, James SL, Jarvis D, Jasrasaria R, Jayaraman S, Johns N, Jonas JB, Karthikeyan G, Kassebaum N, Kawakami N, Keren A, Khoo JP, King CH, Knowlton LM, Kobusingye O, Koranteng A, Krishnamurthi R, Laden F, Lalloo R, Laslett LL, Lathlean T, Leasher JL, Lee YY, Leigh J, Levinson D, Lim SS, Limb E, Lin JK, Lipnick M, Lipshultz SE, Liu W, Loane M, Ohno SL, Lyons R, Mabweijano J, MacIntyre MF, Malekzadeh R, Mallinger L, Manivannan S, Marcenes W, March L, Margolis DJ, Marks GB, Marks R, Matsumori A, Matzopoulos R, Mayosi BM, McAnulty JH, McDermott MM, McGill N, McGrath J, Medina-Mora ME, Meltzer M, Mensah GA, Merriman TR, Meyer AC, Miglioli V, Miller M, Miller TR, Mitchell PB, Mock C, Mocumbi AO, Moffitt TE, Mokdad AA, Monasta L, Montico M, Moradi-Lakeh M, Moran A, Morawska L, Mori R, Murdoch ME, Mwaniki MK, Naidoo K, Nair MN, Naldi L, Narayan KM, Nelson PK, Nelson RG, Nevitt MC, Newton CR, Nolte S, Norman P, Norman R, O'Donnell M, O'Hanlon S, Olives C, Omer SB, Ortblad K, Osborne R, Ozgediz D, Page A, Pahari B, Pandian JD, Rivero AP, Patten SB, Pearce N, Padilla RP, Perez-Ruiz F, Perico N, Pesudovs K, Phillips D, Phillips MR, Pierce K, Pion S, Polanczyk GV, Polinder S, Pope CA 3rd, Popova S, Porrini E, Pourmalek F, Prince M, Pullan RL, Ramaiah KD, Ranganathan D, Razavi H, Regan M, Rehm JT, Rein DB, Remuzzi G, Richardson K, Rivara FP, Roberts T, Robinson C, De Leon FR, Ronfani L, Room R, Rosenfeld LC, Rushton L, Sacco RL, Saha S, Sampson U, Sanchez-Riera L, Sanman E, Schwebel DC, Scott JG, Segui-Gomez M, Shahraz S, Shepard DS, Shin H, Shivakoti R, Singh D, Singh GM, Singh JA, Singleton J, Sleet DA, Sliwa K, Smith E, Smith JL, Stapelberg NJ, Steer A, Steiner T, Stolk WA, Stovner LJ, Sudfeld C, Syed S, Tamburlini G, Tavakkoli M, Taylor HR, Taylor JA, Taylor WJ, Thomas B, Thomson WM, Thurston GD, Tleyjeh IM, Tonelli M, Towbin JA, Truelsen T, Tsilimbaris MK, Ubeda C, Undurraga EA, van der Werf MJ, van Os J, Vavilala MS, Venketasubramanian N, Wang M, Wang W, Watt K, Weatherall DJ, Weinstock MA, Weintraub R, Weisskopf MG, Weissman MM, White RA, Whiteford H, Wiebe N, Wiersma ST, Wilkinson JD, Williams HC, Williams SR, Witt E, Wolfe F, Woolf AD, Wulf S, Yeh PH, Zaidi AK, Zheng ZJ, Zonies D, Lopez AD, AlMazroa MA, Memish ZA (2012) Disability-adjusted life years (DALYs) for 291 diseases and injuries in 21 regions, 1990–2010: a systematic analysis for the Global Burden of Disease Study 2010. Lancet 380(9859):2197–2223. doi:10.1016/S0140-6736(12)61689-4

Na KS, Lee KJ, Lee JS, Cho YS, Jung HY (2014) Efficacy of adjunctive celecoxib treatment for patients with major depressive disorder: a meta-analysis. Prog Neuropsychopharmacol Biol Psychiatry 48:79–85. doi:10.1016/j.pnpbp.2013.09.006

Nabi H, Kivimaki M, Suominen S, Koskenvuo M, Singh-Manoux A, Vahtera J (2010) Does depression predict coronary heart disease and cerebrovascular disease equally well? The Health and Social Support Prospective Cohort Study. Int J Epidemiol 39(4):1016–1024. doi:10.1093/ije/dyq050

Nicholson A, Kuper H, Hemingway H (2006) Depression as an aetiologic and prognostic factor in coronary heart disease: a meta-analysis of 6362 events among 146 538 participants in 54 observational studies. Eur Heart J 27(23):2763–2774. doi:10.1093/eurheartj/ehl338

O'Connor CM, Jiang W, Kuchibhatla M, Silva SG, Cuffe MS, Callwood DD, Zakhary B, Stough WG, Arias RM, Rivelli SK, Krishnan R, Investigators S-C (2010) Safety and efficacy of sertraline for depression in patients with heart failure: results of the SADHART-CHF (Sertraline Against Depression and Heart Disease in Chronic Heart Failure) trial. J Am Coll Cardiol 56(9):692–699. doi:10.1016/j.jacc.2010.03.068

Oh SW, Kim J, Myung SK, Hwang SS, Yoon DH (2014) Antidepressant use and risk of coronary heart disease: meta-analysis of observational studies. Br J Clin Pharmacol 78(4):727–737. doi:10.1111/bcp.12383

Paranthaman R, Greenstein A, Burns AS, Heagerty AM, Malik RA, Baldwin RC (2012) Relationship of endothelial function and atherosclerosis to treatment response in late-life depression. Int J Geriatr Psychiatry 27(9):967–973. doi:10.1002/gps.2811

Pariante CM, Lightman SL (2008) The HPA axis in major depression: classical theories and new developments. Trends Neurosci 31(9):464–468. doi:10.1016/j.tins.2008.06.006

Paz-Filho G, Licinio J, Wong ML (2010) Pathophysiological basis of cardiovascular disease and depression: a chicken-and-egg dilemma. Rev Bras Psiquiatr 32(2):181–191

Pizzi C, Rutjes AW, Costa GM, Fontana F, Mezzetti A, Manzoli L (2011) Meta-analysis of selective serotonin reuptake inhibitors in patients with depression and coronary heart disease. Am J Cardiol 107(7):972–979. doi:10.1016/j.amjcard.2010.11.017

Post-Myocardial Infarction Depression Clinical Practice Guideline P (2009) AAFP guideline for the detection and management of post-myocardial infarction depression. Ann Fam Med 7(1):71–79. doi:10.1370/afm.918

Rajagopalan S, Brook R, Rubenfire M, Pitt E, Young E, Pitt B (2001) Abnormal brachial artery flow-mediated vasodilation in young adults with major depression. Am J Cardiol 88(2):196–198, A197

Ramamurthy G, Trejo E, Faraone SV (2013) Depression treatment in patients with coronary artery disease: a systematic review. Prim Care Companion CNS Disord 15(5). doi:10.4088/PCC.13r01509

Rieckmann N, Burg MM, Kronish IM, Chaplin WF, Schwartz JE, Davidson KW (2011) Aspirin adherence, depression and one-year prognosis after acute coronary syndrome. Psychother Psychosom 80(5):316–318. doi:10.1159/000323168

Rieckmann N, Kronish IM, Shapiro PA, Whang W, Davidson KW (2013) Serotonin reuptake inhibitor use, depression, and long-term outcomes after an acute coronary syndrome: a prospective cohort study. JAMA Intern Med 173(12):1150–1151. doi:10.1001/jamainternmed.2013.910

Rudisch B, Nemeroff CB (2003) Epidemiology of comorbid coronary artery disease and depression. Biol Psychiatry 54(3):227–240

Rutledge T, Reis VA, Linke SE, Greenberg BH, Mills PJ (2006) Depression in heart failure a meta-analytic review of prevalence, intervention effects, and associations with clinical outcomes. J Am Coll Cardiol 48(8):1527–1537. doi:10.1016/j.jacc.2006.06.055

Rutledge T, Vaccarino V, Johnson BD, Bittner V, Olson MB, Linke SE, Cornell CE, Eteiba W, Sheps DS, Francis J, Krantz DS, Bairey Merz CN, Parashar S, Handberg E, Vido DA, Shaw LJ (2009) Depression and cardiovascular health care costs among women with suspected myocardial ischemia: prospective results from the WISE (Women's Ischemia Syndrome Evaluation) study. J Am Coll Cardiol 53(2):176–183. doi:10.1016/j.jacc.2008.09.032

Rybakowski JK, Wykretowicz A, Heymann-Szlachcinska A, Wysocki H (2006) Impairment of endothelial function in unipolar and bipolar depression. Biol Psychiatry 60(8):889–891. doi:10.1016/j.biopsych.2006.03.025

Sabbah HN (2004) Biologic rationale for the use of beta-blockers in the treatment of heart failure. Heart Fail Rev 9(2):91–97. doi:10.1023/B:HREV.0000046363.59374.23

Sasayama D, Hori H, Iijima Y, Teraishi T, Hattori K, Ota M, Fujii T, Higuchi T, Amano N, Kunugi H (2011) Modulation of cortisol responses to the DEX/CRH test by polymorphisms of the interleukin-1beta gene in healthy adults. Behav Brain Funct BBF 7:23. doi:10.1186/1744-9081-7-23

Serebruany VL, Glassman AH, Malinin AI, Nemeroff CB, Musselman DL, van Zyl LT, Finkel MS, Krishnan KR, Gaffney M, Harrison W, Califf RM, O'Connor CM, Sertraline AntiDepressant Heart Attack Randomized Trial Study G (2003) Platelet/endothelial biomarkers in depressed patients treated with the selective serotonin reuptake inhibitor sertraline after acute coronary events: the Sertraline AntiDepressant Heart Attack Randomized Trial (SADHART) Platelet Substudy. Circulation 108(8):939–944. doi:10.1161/01.CIR.0000085163.21752.0A

Sherwood A, Hinderliter AL, Watkins LL, Waugh RA, Blumenthal JA (2005) Impaired endothelial function in coronary heart disease patients with depressive symptomatology. J Am Coll Cardiol 46(4):656–659. doi:10.1016/j.jacc.2005.05.041

Sherwood A, Blumenthal JA, Trivedi R, Johnson KS, O'Connor CM, Adams KF Jr, Dupree CS, Waugh RA, Bensimhon DR, Gaulden L, Christenson RH, Koch GG, Hinderliter AL (2007) Relationship of depression to death or hospitalization in patients with heart failure. Arch Intern Med 167(4):367–373. doi:10.1001/archinte.167.4.367

Shimokawa H (1999) Primary endothelial dysfunction: atherosclerosis. J Mol Cell Cardiol 31(1):23–37. doi:10.1006/jmcc.1998.0841

Stewart WF, Ricci JA, Chee E, Hahn SR, Morganstein D (2003) Cost of lost productive work time among US workers with depression. Jama 289(23):3135–3144. doi:10.1001/jama.289.23.3135

Stratz C, Trenk D, Bhatia HS, Valina C, Neumann FJ, Fiebich BL (2008) Identification of 5-HT3 receptors on human platelets: increased surface immunoreactivity after activation with adenosine diphosphate (ADP) and thrombin receptor-activating peptide (TRAP). Thromb Haemost 99(4):784–786. doi:10.1160/TH07-10-0630

Strik JJ, Honig A, Lousberg R, Lousberg AH, Cheriex EC, Tuynman-Qua HG, Kuijpers PM, Wellens HJ, Van Praag HM (2000) Efficacy and safety of fluoxetine in the treatment of patients with major depression after first myocardial infarction: findings from a double-blind, placebo-controlled trial. Psychosom Med 62(6):783–789

Sullivan M, Simon G, Spertus J, Russo J (2002) Depression-related costs in heart failure care. Arch Intern Med 162(16):1860–1866

Taylor CB, Youngblood ME, Catellier D, Veith RC, Carney RM, Burg MM, Kaufmann PG, Shuster J, Mellman T, Blumenthal JA, Krishnan R, Jaffe AS, Investigators E (2005) Effects of antidepressant medication on morbidity and mortality in depressed patients after myocardial infarction. Arch Gen Psychiatry 62(7):792–798. doi:10.1001/archpsyc.62.7.792

Uher R, Tansey KE, Dew T, Maier W, Mors O, Hauser J, Dernovsek MZ, Henigsberg N, Souery D, Farmer A, McGuffin P (2014) An inflammatory biomarker as a differential predictor of outcome of depression treatment with escitalopram and nortriptyline. Am J Psychiatry. doi:10.1176/appi.ajp.2014.14010094

Van der Kooy K, van Hout H, Marwijk H, Marten H, Stehouwer C, Beekman A (2007) Depression and the risk for cardiovascular diseases: systematic review and meta analysis. Int J Geriatr Psychiatry 22(7):613–626. doi:10.1002/gps.1723

van Zyl LT, Lesperance F, Frasure-Smith N, Malinin AI, Atar D, Laliberte MA, Serebruany VL (2009) Platelet and endothelial activity in comorbid major depression and coronary artery disease patients treated with citalopram: the Canadian Cardiac Randomized Evaluation of Antidepressant and Psychotherapy Efficacy Trial (CREATE) biomarker sub-study. J Thromb Thrombolysis 27(1):48–56. doi:10.1007/s11239-007-0189-3

Whang W, Kubzansky LD, Kawachi I, Rexrode KM, Kroenke CH, Glynn RJ, Garan H, Albert CM (2009) Depression and risk of sudden cardiac death and coronary heart disease in women: results from the Nurses' Health Study. J Am Coll Cardiol 53(11):950–958. doi:10.1016/j.jacc.2008.10.060

WHO (2008) Global burden of disease: 2004 update

Xiong GL, Jiang W, Clare RM, Shaw LK, Smith PK, O'Connor CM, Ranga K, Krishnan R, Kristin Newby L (2010) Safety of selective serotonin reuptake inhibitor use prior to coronary artery bypass grafting. Clin Cardiol 33(6):E94–E98. doi:10.1002/clc.20621

Ye S, Shaffer JA, Rieckmann N, Schwartz JE, Kronish IM, Ladapo JA, Whang W, Burg MM, Davidson KW (2014) Long-term outcomes of enhanced depression treatment in patients with acute coronary syndromes. Am J Med 127(10):1012–1016. doi:10.1016/j.amjmed.2014.05.004

Zimmermann-Viehoff F, Kuehl LK, Danker-Hopfe H, Whooley MA, Otte C (2014) Antidepressants, autonomic function and mortality in patients with coronary heart disease: data from the Heart and Soul Study. Psychol Med 44(14):2975–2984. doi:10.1017/S003329171400066X

Anti-inflammatory Agents for the Treatment of Depression in the Light of Comorbid Cardiovascular Disease

24

Ole Köhler and Christiane Gasse

Contents

Abstract

A growing body of evidence supports the role of inflammation as a common etiological factor of the pathophysiology of depression and cardiovascular diseases. Recent clinical studies have indicated that different anti-inflammatory agents may yield antidepressant treatment effects, both as add-on and monotherapy.

O. Köhler
Psychosis Research Unit, Aarhus University Hospital, Skovagervej 2, Risskov 8240, Denmark

C. Gasse (✉)
National Center for Register-based Research (NCRR), Department of Economics and Business Economics, Aarhus BSS, Aarhus University, Aarhus, Denmark
e-mail: cg@econ.au.dk

B.T. Baune, P.J. Tully (eds.), *Cardiovascular Diseases and Depression*, DOI 10.1007/978-3-319-32480-7_24

However, cardiac side effects emphasize cautious use of several agents, whereas other agents might have beneficial effects on both depression and cardiovascular disease. The current chapter aims to review the most promising anti-inflammatory agents that have been studied in depressed individuals and other patient groups including their potential underlying mechanisms. The most frequently investigated agents are nonsteroidal anti-inflammatory drugs (NSAIDs), monoclonal antibodies, and polyunsaturated fatty acids, but antidepressant properties were also observed for statins, minocycline, pioglitazone, cortisol, modafinil, and angiotensin-2 receptor antagonists. In addition, this chapter will discuss important clinical aspects for identifying patient groups which will be most likely to benefit of anti-inflammatory treatment, such as biological markers potentially predicting antidepressant treatment effects of anti-inflammatory intervention, timing and duration of anti-inflammatory intervention, and targeting specific depressive symptoms. Finally, we will discuss which anti-inflammatory agents, e.g., statins and low-dose acetylsalicylic acid, may represent relevant add-on treatment strategies in patients suffering of comorbid depression and cardiovascular diseases.

24.1 Introduction

In spite of a number of treatment options in depression, response and remissions rates are far from optimal, which has resulted in recent initiatives emphasizing the need for further research translating suggested patho-etiological findings with regard to major depression into effective alternative treatments (Collins et al. 2011; O'Leary et al. 2015). One of these potential therapeutic alternatives is anti-inflammatory therapy of the suggested inflammatory component of depression (Maes 1995). Inflammation is a suggested common etiological factor of the pathophysiology of depression and cardiovascular disease (CVD), mediated predominantly via pro-inflammatory cytokines, and the hypothalamic-pituitary-adrenal (HPA) axis (Dantzer et al. 2008; Bechter et al. 2010; Krishnadas and Cavanagh 2012; Rosenblat et al. 2014; Baune 2015). Therefore, anti-inflammatory agents may be candidates to target inflammation in both disorders and may affect the association between depression and CVD potentially preventing their co-occurrence or mitigating their severity (Muller et al. 2006).

The aim of the current chapter is to provide an overview of the antidepressant potential of anti-inflammatory agents. More specifically, we will review clinical trials that have investigated the use of anti-inflammatory agents in the prevention and treatment of depression (see Table 24.1) with a focus on those anti-inflammatory agents with the most promising antidepressant potential. Furthermore, we will discuss whether anti-inflammatory agents may also be beneficial in terms of preventing CVD-depression comorbidity.

Table 24.1 Baseline characteristics and treatment effects of identified clinical trials investigating anti-inflammatory treatment in depression

Study	Patient population (placebo group/intervention group-1/intervention group-2)					Diagnosis	Treatment (N)	Treatment effect
	N (female)	Mean age, years (SD)	Mean depressive episodes (SD)	Duration current episode	Comorbidity			
NSAIDs								
Add-on treatment								
Muller et al. (2006)	20 (12)/20 (8)	44.3 (13.5)/44.5 (11.6)	2.4 (1.2)/2.5 (2.3)	18.7 weeks (20.8)/17.0 weeks (21.7)	None	$HAMD_{17}$ 15–38	6 weeks NARI + placebo (20) vs. NARI + celecoxib 400 mg (20)	Celecoxib superior
Akhondzadeh et al. (2009)	20 (12)/20 (13)	34.2 (4.96)/34.65 (6.76)	3.52 (0.84)/3.40 (0.70)	n.a.	None	$HAMD_{17}$ ≥18	6 weeks SSRI + placebo (20) vs. SSRI + celecoxib 400 mg (20)	Celecoxib superior
Hashemian et al. (2011)	20 (20)/20 (20)	36.20 (12.79)/34.78 (7.39)	First-episode patients	Antidepressant naive	None	$HAMD_{17}$ 18–36	8 weeks SSRI + placebo (20) vs. SSRI + celecoxib 200 mg (20)	Celecoxib superior
Abbasi et al. (2012)	20 (6)/20 (7)	34.2 (6.9)/35.1 (8.0)	3.6 (0.9)/3.7 (0.8)	2.7 months (1.0)/2.4 months (0.9)	None	$HAMD_{17}$ ≥18	6 weeks SSRI + placebo (20) vs. SSRI + celecoxib 400 mg (20)	Celecoxib superior. IL-6 predicted response

(continued)

Table 24.1 (continued)

Study	Patient population (placebo group/intervention group-1/intervention group-2)					Diagnosis	Treatment (N)	Treatment effect
	N (female)	Mean age, years (SD)	Mean depressive episodes (SD)	Duration current episode	Comorbidity			
Monotherapy								
Fields et al. (2012)	1,083 (488)/726 (342)/719 (330)	74.4/74.5/74.5	Only depressive symptoms	Not relevant	Family history of dementia	GDS	12 months placebo (1,038) vs. celecoxib 400 mg (726) vs. naproxen 440 mg (719) daily	No difference
Iyengar et al. (2013)	297 (199)/593 (409)/607 (413)	61/61/61	Only depressive symptoms	Not relevant	Active osteoarthritis	PHQ-9	6 weeks placebo (297) vs. ibuprofen 2,400 mg or naproxen 1,000 mg (593) vs. celecoxib 200 mg (607)	Celecoxib, naproxen, and ibuprofen superior to placebo
Cytokine inhibitors – monotherapy								
Tyring et al. (2006)	307 (93)/311 (108)	45.6 (12.1)/45.8 (12.8)	Only depressive symptoms	Not relevant	Stable psoriasis	$HAMD_{17}$ BDI	12 weeks placebo (309) vs. etanercept 50 mg (311) injections twice weekly	Etanercept superior
Menter et al. (2010)	52 (18)/44 (13)	43.3 (13.1)/45.6 (11.7)	Only depressive symptoms	Not relevant	Psoriasis	ZDS	12 weeks placebo (52) vs. adalimumab 40 mg (44) injections every other week	Adalimumab superior

Langley et al. (2010)	410 (127)/820 (263)	47.0 (12.5)/46.0 (12.1)	Only depressive symptoms	Not relevant	Psoriasis	HADS-D	24 weeks placebo (410) vs. ustekinumab 45 mg (409) vs. ustekinumab 90 mg (411)	Ustekinumab superior
Raison et al. (2013)	30 (20)/30 (20)	44.3 (9.4)/42.5 (8.2)	8.7 (24.8)/7.8 (24.8)		None	$HAMD_{17}$	12 weeks three infusions placebo (30) vs. infliximab 5 mg/kg (30)	Infliximab superior if CRP>5 mg/L
Statins – add-on treatment								
Ghanizadeh and Hedayati (2013)	34 (21)/34 (22)	32.5 (10.2)/31.7 (9.3)	n.a.	n.a.	None	$HAMD_{17}$ ≥18	6 weeks SSRI + placebo (34) vs. SSRI + lovastatin 30 mg (34)	Lovastatin superior
Gougol et al. (2015)	22 (16)/22 (13)	34.2 (10.8)/36.4 (8.1)	n.a.	n.a.	None	$HAMD_{17}$ ≥22	6 weeks SSRI + placebo (22) vs. SSRI + simvastatin 20 mg (22)	Simvastatin superior
Minocycline – add-on treatment								
Miyaoka et al. (2012)	25 (12)	46.9 (10.2)	n.a.	58.6 (46.8)	None	$HAMD_{21}$ ≥25	Open-label, not placebo-controlled: 6 weeks SSRI + 150 mg minocycline	Minocycline showed safe antidepressant effects

(continued)

Table 24.1 (continued)

Pioglitazone								
Add-on treatment								
Sepanjnia et al. (2012)	20 (15)/20 (14)	32.7 (5.4)/31.4 (5.4)	3.5 (0.8)/3.6 (0.8)	n.a.	None	HAMD$_{17}$ ≥22	6 weeks SSRI + placebo (20) vs. SSRI + pioglitazone 30 mg (20)	Pioglitazone superior
Monotherapy								
Kashani et al. (2013)	20 (20)/20 (20)	20.3 (4.6)/21.2 (3.3)	Only depressive symptoms	Not relevant	PCOS, obesity (BMI≥27)	HAMD$_{17}$ ≤19	6 weeks metformin 1,500 mg (25) vs. pioglitazone 30 mg (25)	Pioglitazone superior to metformin
Polyunsaturated fatty acids – monotherapy								
Mischoulon (2015)	59 (35)/60 (38)/58 (32)	45.0 (12.1)/46.2 (11.8)/46.3 (13.7)	n.a.	n.a.	None	HAMD$_{17}$ ≥15	8 weeks placebo (59) vs. EPA-enriched omega-3 1,000 mg/day (60) vs. DHA-enriched omega-3 1,000 mg/day (58)	No difference
Gharekhani et al. (2014)	20 (8)/25 (12)	57.2 (15.19)/56.8 (13.09)	Only depressive symptoms	Not relevant	Maintenance dialysis patients	BDI	4 months placebo (20) vs. omega-3 1,800 mg/day (25)	Omega-3 superior
Bloch and Hannestad (2012); Martins et al. (2012)	Meta-analyses suggesting a small antidepressant effect of omega-3 polyunsaturated fatty acids, which may depend on EPA levels							

Corticosteroids – monotherapy								
Arana et al. (1995)	18/19	Age range 20 to 67 years	n.a.	n.a.	None	$HAMD_{21}$ ≥21	4 days placebo (18) vs. dexamethasone 4 mg (19)	Dexamethasone superior at day 14
DeBattista et al. (2000)	10 (7)/6 (3)/6 (3)	39.8 (10.1)/46.7 (18.0)/35.0 (10.5)	n.a.	n.a.	None	$HAMD_{21}$ ≥21	One infusion placebo (10) vs. CRH 1 μg/kg (6) vs. hydrocortisone 15 mg (6)	Hydrocortisone superior
Modafinil								
Abolfazli et al. (2011)	23 (11)/23 (12)	33.27 (6.08)/33.13 (7.53	3.91 (0.92)/3.85 (0.83)	n.a.	None	$HAMD_{17}$ ≥18	6 weeks SSRI + placebo (23) vs. SSRI + modafinil 40 mg (23)	Modafinil superior
Goss et al. (2013)	Meta-analysis suggesting that modafinil is an effective augmentation strategy for acute depressive episodes, including for symptoms of fatigue, in both unipolar and bipolar disorders							

^*n.a.* data not available, *BDI* Beck Depression Inventory, *CRH* corticotropin-releasing hormone, *GDS* 30-item Geriatric Depression Score, *HADS-D* Hospital Anxiety and Depression Scale for Depression, *HAMD* Hamilton Depression Scale, *NARI* noradrenaline reuptake inhibitor, *PHQ* Patient Health Questionnaire-9, *SSRI* selective serotonin reuptake inhibitor, *ZDS* Zung Self-Rating Depression Scale

24.2 Anti-inflammatory Drugs with Potential Antidepressant Properties

24.2.1 Nonsteroidal Anti-inflammatory Drugs (NSAIDs)

The class of anti-inflammatory drugs, which has been studied most extensively in relation to depression, are the nonsteroidal anti-inflammatory drugs (NSAIDs), particularly the selective cyclooxygenase-2 (COX-2) inhibitors and acetylsalicylic acid (ASA). The first randomized controlled clinical trial (RCT) showing adjunctive antidepressant properties of the selective cyclooxygenase-2 (COX-2) inhibitor celecoxib was published in 2006 (Muller et al. 2006). Findings from subsequent RCTs supported the antidepressant properties for add-on treatment with celecoxib (Akhondzadeh et al. 2009; Abbasi et al. 2012; Hashemian et al. 2011). Furthermore, RCTs among patients with osteoarthritis have found that monotherapy with either celecoxib, naproxen, or ibuprofen decreased depressive symptoms compared to placebo independently of their pain-relieving effects (Iyengar et al. 2013). Similarly, ASA has been associated with adjunctive antidepressant effects, even at low doses (Mendlewicz et al. 2006). Moreover, ASA has been discussed to possibly yield a more favorable benefit-risk ratio (Fond et al. 2013) and potentially better antidepressant treatment effects (Berk et al. 2013) than the selective COX-2 inhibitors.

However, the findings of further clinical and observational studies on NSAIDS as a therapeutic class or analyzing individual compounds are not homogenous: For example, in two cohort studies, NSAID use during treatment with antidepressants was associated with deteriorated effects on depression (Warner-Schmidt et al. 2011; Gallagher et al. 2012) while a clinical study found neutral effects of adjunctive NSAID use in depressed individuals (Uher et al. 2012). No antidepressant effects were detected in a study investigating antidepressant properties of monotherapy with celecoxib or naproxen regarding onset of depressive symptoms among nondepressed individuals aged 70 years or older (Fields et al. 2012). Hence, it seems important to differentiate between specific NSAID compounds rather than to attribute their potential antidepressant effects to NSAIDs as a class (Knights et al. 2010). This heterogeneity was further illustrated by a recent pharmaco-epidemiological study on SSRI users, where effectiveness and safety outcomes varied across individual NSAIDs (Köhler et al. 2015). In this study, low-dose ASA and ibuprofen were associated with decreased risks for psychiatric hospitalizations, while the selective COX-2 inhibitors were associated with increased risks for psychiatric hospitalizations and suicide attempts (Köhler et al. 2015). In summary, several studies have found promising results regarding use of individual NSAIDs in the treatment of depression, but as discussed in recent reviews including clinical and observational studies published by September 2013 (Baune 2015; Eyre et al. 2015), the studies showed high methodological heterogeneity, making firm conclusions difficult, and emphasized the need of methodological improvements in future trials.

Moreover, NSAID use should always be balanced against their well-known risk for adverse events. For example, NSAIDs increase the risk for gastrointestinal (de Abajo and Garcia-Rodriguez 2008) and cardiovascular (Schjerning Olsen et al. 2011, 2014) adverse events. In particular, the use of the selective COX-2 inhibitors has been associated with an increased risk for myocardial infarction and thromboembolic events (Solomon et al. 2008), resulting in partial withdrawal of this drug class from the market. However, other studies have suggested that adverse effects of the selective COX-2 inhibitors may not represent a class effect, since only rofecoxib, but not celecoxib, has been associated with increased risk for acute cardiovascular events (Solomon et al. 2006). A recent review and meta-analysis evaluated the effect of NSAID intervention on both depression outcomes and side effects based on ten randomized clinical trials including 4,258 patients (Köhler et al. 2014). NSAIDs significantly reduced depressive symptoms by a standard mean difference (SMD) of −0.27 (95 %–CI=−0.45; −0.08) indicating overall a small effect. By convention, SMDs of −0.2, −0.4, and −0.8 are considered to represent small, medium, and large effects, respectively. Notably, add-on treatment with celecoxib was associated with large antidepressant effects (SMD=−0.82 (95 %–CI=−1.17; −0.46)). Only four of the included studies reported on adverse events, and no evidence for an increased number of cardiovascular or gastrointestinal adverse events during 6 weeks of NSAID treatment was detected compared to placebo. Thus, the meta-analysis appears to serve as a proof of concept concerning the beneficial potential of NSAIDs in the treatment of depression. However, the studies currently available for meta-analysis are quite heterogeneous, and the findings should therefore be interpreted with caution (Baune 2015; Fond et al. 2013; Berk et al. 2013; Eyre et al. 2015; Köhler et al. 2014).

The suggested mechanisms of antidepressant actions of NSAIDs include direct inhibition of peripheral pro-inflammatory cytokines which may serve as the basis for the antidepressant effects of NSAIDs (Abbasi et al. 2012). On the contrary, it has been suggested that NSAIDs may inhibit antidepressant treatment by antagonizing induction of p11 in several areas of the brain (Warner-Schmidt et al. 2011), a protein which interacts with specific serotonin receptors and may be necessary for sufficient antidepressant response. Furthermore, oxidative and nitrosative stress pathways may be associated with the etiology of depression (Anderson et al. 2013), and reduction of these pathways has been proposed to explain acetylsalicylic acids antidepressant properties (Berk et al. 2013).

Peripheral inflammation can affect the kynurenine pathway, contributing to decreased serotonin levels (Muller et al. 2011) and production of neurotoxic compounds, such as COX-2 expression (Wichers et al. 2005), which may partly explain the antidepressant effects of selective COX-2 inhibitors (Muller et al. 2011). Selective COX-2 inhibitors may furthermore exert antidepressant effects via increment of central serotonin levels (Sandrini et al. 2002) and prevention of increase of pro-inflammatory cytokines and cortisol (Casolini et al. 2002). COX-2 inhibitors may thereby also affect the pro-inflammatory cytokine macrophage migration inhibition factor (MIF), which upregulates COX-2 mRNA (Sampey et al. 2001). MIF was found elevated in depressed individuals as compared to healthy controls (Musil et al. 2011). In CVD, MIF has been associated with inflammatory pathogenesis of atherosclerosis and its consequences, namely, unstable plaque formation, remodeling after arterial injury, aneurysm formation, myocardial infarction, or ischemia-reperfusion injury (Zernecke et al. 2008).

24.2.2 Cytokine Inhibitors

Monoclonal antibodies, such as infliximab, etanercept, ustekinumab, and adalimumab, are potent cytokine inhibitors, which have shown antidepressant effects in comparison with placebo in depressed individuals without somatic comorbidity (Raison et al. 2013) and in patients with psoriasis suffering of single depressive symptoms (Tyring et al. 2006; Menter et al. 2010; Langley et al. 2010). However, one trial found no overall antidepressant effect of treatment with infliximab, but in subgroup analyses, individuals with CRP levels >5 mg/L showed better response compared to individuals with CRP <5 mg/L (Raison et al. 2013). In a recent meta-analysis, cytokine inhibitors did not reduce depressive symptoms significantly, although indicating a tendency toward an antidepressant effect (standard mean difference (SMD) = −0.38 (95%–CI=−0.88; 0.12)) (Köhler et al. 2014). Regarding side effects, cytokine inhibitors have been shown to increase the risk for infections (Toussi et al. 2013), but no evidence for an increased number of infections during 12 weeks of cytokine inhibitor treatment could be found compared to placebo (Köhler et al. 2014).

Direct inhibition of peripheral pro-inflammatory cytokines may serve as the basis for the antidepressant effects of cytokine inhibitors (Raison et al. 2013; Tyring et al. 2006).

24.2.3 Statins

Statins (HMG-CoA reductase inhibitors) are used extensively for their lipid-lowering properties in the prevention of CVD (Reiner 2013). However, statins also have anti-inflammatory effects that are mediated both via and independently of the HMG-CoA reductase inhibition (Weitz-Schmidt 2002). The anti-inflammatory properties of statins may be explained by blocking lymphocyte function-associated antigen-1 (LFA-1), which has an important role in the pathophysiology of inflammatory and autoimmune diseases (Weitz-Schmidt et al. 2001).

Based on the assumption that inflammation may be part of the etiology of depression, the knowledge of the statins' anti-inflammatory potential has led researchers to investigate whether this class of drugs could have antidepressant effects. Epidemiological studies of this aspect have shown highly mixed results; some studies have indicated that statins worsen depression (You et al. 2013) or have neutral effects (Mansi et al. 2013; Glaus et al. 2015), while others have supported the notion that statins may have direct antidepressant effects (Parsaik et al. 2014; Otte et al. 2012; Young-Xu et al. 2003; Redlich et al. 2014). The latter inspired Ghanizadeh and Hedayati to test the antidepressant effect of lovastatin (30 mg/day) in combination with the selective serotonin reuptake inhibitor (SSRI) fluoxetine (up to 40 mg/day) against fluoxetine+placebo in a RCT of patients with major depressive disorder (Ghanizadeh and Hedayati 2013). Despite a small sample size ($n = 68$, divided on the two treatment arms), the results of the study by Ghanizadeh and Hedayati indicated that the combination of fluoxetine with lovastatin had superior antidepressant effect compared to fluoxetine and placebo (Ghanizadeh and Hedayati 2013). Another recent placebo-controlled RCT in patients with moderate to severe depression concomitantly treated with fluoxetine and simvastatin over 6 weeks found a decrease in depressive symptoms, while remission rates were not different between the verum and the placebo group (Gougol et al. 2015). However, these are the only placebo-controlled trials of statins in the treatment of depression and are by no means conclusive, so more and larger studies should be conducted in the future. This would not only be necessary to establish the antidepressant effect of the statins but also to ensure safety. Indeed, it has been suggested that lowering cholesterol levels, for instance, via statin treatment, may increase the risk for suicidal ideation (De Berardis et al. 2012; Vevera et al. 2005). Therefore, using statins to treat patients with depression, who are already at relatively increased risk of suicidal behavior, could be hazardous. Consequently, suicidal ideation/behavior should ideally be included as secondary outcome measures in future trials of statins in depression. Also, other potential side effects of statins (Foody 2010; Goldstein and Mascitelli 2009; Hippisley-Cox and Coupland 2010) should be taken into consideration when evaluating the antidepressant properties of this class of drugs.

24.2.4 Minocycline

The second-generation tetracyclic antibiotic minocycline is an agent with pleiotropic properties that targets multiple proteins and cellular processes implicated in the patho-etiology of mood disorders and heart disease (Soczynska et al. 2012; Garrido-Mesa et al. 2013). It has gained interest during the last decade because it is able to cross the blood-brain barrier more easily than the other tetracycline antibiotics (Tomas-Camardiel et al. 2004) and may exert potential antidepressant effects through its robust neuroprotective activities, which include neurogenesis, antioxidation, anti-glutamate excitotoxicity, and regulation of pro-inflammatory agents (Miyaoka et al. 2012). Smaller clinical trials in depression have been conducted and more clinical trials are currently under way (Soczynska et al. 2012; Miyaoka et al. 2012; Dean et al. 2014). For example, a small non-randomized open-label trial including 25 adult inpatients with major depression with psychotic features taking minocycline (150 mg/day) in combination with antidepressants (fluvoxamine, paroxetine, and sertraline) found significant improvement in depression (Miyaoka et al. 2012). In vitro and animal studies indicate further potential target mechanisms of minocycline, such as inhibition of brain retinoic acid metabolism, a molecule which exhibits a great variety of anti-inflammatory and neuroprotective properties in the adult CNS (Regen et al. 2015), as well as modulation of microglial activation and the central expression of inflammatory mediators (Burke et al. 2014).

24.2.5 Other Anti-inflammatory Agents with Potential Antidepressant Effect

Furthermore, RCTs have found antidepressant effects for other agents, where the anti-inflammatory properties are of more speculative nature. For instance, both the antidiabetic drug pioglitazone (Sepanjnia et al. 2012; Kashani et al. 2013) and polyunsaturated fatty acids (Gharekhani et al. 2014) improved antidepressant effects when compared to placebo. Regarding polyunsaturated fatty acids, recent meta-analyses have suggested that they have a minor antidepressant effect (Bloch and Hannestad 2012; Martins et al. 2012), which may depend on the content of eicosapentaenoic acid (EPA). An analysis of studies using ≥60 % EPA resulted in a highly significant pooled SMD estimate, whereas studies using ≤60 % EPA found no significant antidepressant effects (Martins et al. 2012). Moreover, synthetic cortisol compounds may have acute antidepressant effects (Arana et al. 1995; DeBattista et al. 2000), but due to cortisol's broad effects, these results should be interpreted cautiously. In addition, preliminary data indicate that angiotensin receptor blockers (AT2 inhibitors), such as valsartan, affecting the renin-angiotensin system (RAS) as a central pro-inflammatory pathway, exert an antidepressant/antianxiety-like effect (Kalra et al. 2015; de Gois Queiroz et al. 2013; Ping et al. 2014). This may potentially be due to promoting the hippocampus neurogenesis and the brain-derived neurotrophic factor (BDNF) expression as suggested from animal models (Kalra et al. 2015; de Gois Queiroz et al. 2013; Ping et al. 2014). Finally, another emerging drug is the antiepileptic drug modafinil, which has been associated with anti-inflammatory properties (Jung et al. 2012) and furthermore shown effective antidepressant effects in augmentation strategies for acute depressive episodes, including symptoms of fatigue, in both unipolar and bipolar disorders (Abolfazli et al. 2011; Goss et al. 2013).

24.3 Targeted Anti-inflammatory Treatment of Depression: The Right Agent for the Right Patient at the Right Time for the Right Duration

As described above, several anti-inflammatory agents may have antidepressant properties, which may be independent of their primary intended pharmacological effects. However, the risk for side effects associated with some of these agents emphasizes cautious use. Therefore, identifying the patients, which will benefit from anti-inflammatory treatment for depression, is of utmost importance, in particular with regard to timing and duration of such treatment.

24.3.1 Acute Treatment Phase of Depressive Episodes

Clinical trials have shown adjunctive antidepressant effects of celecoxib (Muller et al. 2006; Akhondzadeh et al. 2009; Abbasi et al. 2012; Hashemian et al. 2011) and statin (Ghanizadeh and Hedayati 2013; Gougol et al. 2015) treatment among acute depressed patients already after 4–6 weeks without increased risk for cardiovascular or gastrointestinal adverse events (Köhler et al. 2014). In particular, acutely developed depressive episodes may be associated with a more pronounced inflammatory response (Howren et al. 2009; Setiawan et al. 2015). Concerning side effects, studies have indicated that treatment with rofecoxib, but not celecoxib, increases the risk for acute cardiovascular outcomes within the first 60 days (Solomon et al. 2006). Also monotherapy with monoclonal antibodies has shown better antidepressant treatment effects compared to placebo after 12 (Raison et al. 2013; Tyring et al. 2006; Menter et al. 2010) and 24 weeks (Langley et al. 2010) without increased risks for infections (Köhler et al. 2014). This may indicate that intervention only lasting a few weeks may be beneficial in the acute treatment of depressive episodes while also minimizing the risk for adverse events (Eyre et al. 2014; Krogh et al. 2014).

24.3.2 Predictive Value of Pro-inflammatory Markers

Few studies have tested whether peripheral levels of pro-inflammatory markers among depressed individuals can be used to predict the antidepressive effects of anti-inflammatory drugs. It has been shown that increased IL-6 levels (Abbasi et al. 2012) are associated with higher remission rates and better response among depressed individuals treated with celecoxib add-on. Similarly, depressed patients with CRP >5 mg/L responded better to infliximab treatment compared to patients with CRP <5 mg/L (Raison et al. 2013).

The significance of the level of inflammatory markers may also help in the choice of standard antidepressant drugs. A recent study of data from 241 adults with depression indicated that among patients with CRP >1 mg/L, the tricyclic antidepressant nortriptyline was associated with better antidepressant effects compared to the SSRI escitalopram, whereas escitalopram was associated with better antidepressant effects among patients with CRP <1 mg/L (Uher et al. 2014). These results may be explained by differential effects of norepinephrine and serotonin antidepressants on the immune system (Martino et al. 2012).

In addition, specific somatic comorbidities, possibly indicating that an active inflammatory process is part of the depressive etiology, may predict better treatment response (Table 24.1). Monotherapy with celecoxib, naproxen, and ibuprofen showed better antidepressant effects compared to placebo among patients with active osteoarthritis (Iyengar et al. 2013) but not among healthy individuals aged 70 years or above (Fields et al. 2012). Similarly, monotherapy with the monoclonal antibodies etanercept (Tyring et al. 2006), ustekinumab (Langley et al. 2010), and adalimumab (Menter et al. 2010) showed better antidepressant treatment effects on depressive symptoms among psoriasis patients as compared to placebo. Also, antidepressive effects have been found for pioglitazone among obese women (BMI ≥27) with polycystic ovarian syndrome (Kashani et al. 2013) and for omega-3 fatty acids among patients undergoing maintenance dialysis (Gharekhani et al. 2014).

24.3.3 Specific Depressive Symptoms

Evidence whether anti-inflammatory agents may decrease specific depressive symptoms is still missing. In schizophrenia though, celecoxib has been found to have beneficial effects on cognition – a core feature of depression (Muller et al. 2005). In a rat model of depression, infliximab prevented cognitive decline, i.e., spatial and emotional memory impairments, which was accompanied by prevention of reduction of hippocampal brain-derived neurotrophic factor (BDNF) (Sahin et al. 2015). Another cardinal symptom in depression is fatigue. In multiple sclerosis (MS) patients, NSAID treatment lowered fatigue (Wingerchuk et al. 2005), potentially through their antipyretic effects as elevated body temperature has been associated with worse fatigue (Sumowski and Leavitt 2014). In summary, antidepressants effects of inflammatory agents on specific symptoms, such as fatigue or cognition, and body temperature as a potential marker, still need to be explored in depressed individuals.

In conclusion, the abovementioned results suggest potential for targeting increased inflammatory response during acute depressive episodes (Howren et al. 2009; Setiawan et al. 2015), an effect on specific depressive symptoms (Muller et al. 2005; Wingerchuk et al. 2005), and assessment of markers of systemic inflammation to predict better response seems highly relevant (Abbasi et al. 2012; Raison et al. 2013; Sumowski and Leavitt 2014). Anti-inflammatory treatment lasting only a few weeks may improve antidepressant treatment effects among acutely depressed individuals (Muller et al. 2006; Akhondzadeh et al. 2009; Abbasi et al. 2012; Hashemian et al. 2011; Raison et al. 2013; Ghanizadeh and Hedayati 2013; Gougol et al. 2015) and among individuals with somatic diseases suffering of single depressive symptoms (Iyengar et al. 2013; Tyring et al. 2006; Menter et al. 2010; Langley et al. 2010). These findings should encourage future clinical trials to further investigate potential subgroups and markers possibly predicting timing of intervention and better treatment response.

24.4 Can Anti-inflammatory Agents "Treat" the Bidirectional CVD-Depression Relationship?

The following paragraph will address the questions whether anti-inflammatory treatment can decrease the risk of CVD in patients with depression while attenuating depression and whether anti-inflammatory agents may prevent depression in patients with coronary heart disease. Currently, patients with comorbid depression and CVD are treated mainly with standard antidepressant therapy, i.e., under particular considerations of the cardiac risk profile of some of the contraindicated antidepressants, such as MAO inhibitors and tricyclic antidepressants (please see also Chap. 22 (Pharmacological treatment of depression in cardiac conditions)) (Yekehtaz et al. 2013). SSRIs by contrast may themselves influence cardiac functioning through serotonin-mediated and collagen-mediated platelet aggregation, thereby reducing inflammatory mediator levels and improving endothelial function (Andrade et al. 2013).

Among patients with depression and established CVD, SSRI use may act cardioprotective in patients with ischemic heart disease but less clearly in patients with heart failure (Andrade et al. 2013). Among patients with established CVD without depression, SSRIs have been shown to decrease mortality but not depression onset (Zuidersma et al. 2013).

Antidepressants have also been previously associated with cardiac risks. A recent meta-analysis though, based on observational studies conducted in patients with depression but without manifested CVD, found that neither use of TCAs nor SSRIs was associated with increased risk of cardiovascular disease (Oh et al. 2014). Though protective effects regarding risk of cardiovascular disease were not in the focus of the meta-analyses, the results also do not indicate a decreased risk of CVD in SSRI users. Thus, currently there is some evidence that antidepressants may improve cardiac outcomes among patients with established CVD, but beneficial influence of antidepressants on new onset of heart disease has not been observed yet.

Turning to the suggested anti-inflammatory drugs with potential antidepressant effects, as discussed above, serious side effects on the cardiovascular system caution the clinical value of NSAIDs and their widespread application, in particular among patients with preexisting cardiovascular disease (Schjerning Olsen et al. 2014). Therefore, in light of the well-described comorbidity between depression and CVD, the use of cardioprotective agents would be preferable, such as statins (Ghanizadeh and Hedayati 2013; Köhler et al. 2016), low-dose ASA (Mendlewicz et al. 2006; Köhler et al. 2015), drugs affecting the renin-angiotensin system (RAS) as a central pro-inflammatory pathway (Kalra et al. 2015; de Gois Queiroz et al. 2013), or polyunsaturated fatty acids (Gharekhani et al. 2014).

There have been few studies in this area investigating the effects of anti-inflammatory treatment on the bidirectional relationship between depression and CVD. RCTs have mainly focused on the prevention or treatment of depression by anti-inflammatory drugs while cardiac effects have not been assessed (Muller et al. 2006; Akhondzadeh et al. 2009; Abbasi et al. 2012; Hashemian et al. 2011; Ghanizadeh and Hedayati 2013) (Table 24.1); particularly cardiac effects are rather long-term effects and are basically not detectable in small or short-term clinical trials. Observational studies by contrast may serve as a source for testing the suggested protective or improving properties of anti-inflammatory drugs in different study populations with different disease status. However, in observational studies, mostly register-based studies, it should be noted that cardioprotective drugs, such as low-dose aspirin and statins are mainly used by individuals with risk factors for CVD or established CVD, whereas antidepressants such as SSRIs are used by people with depression or a variety of other psychiatric conditions. In an epidemiological study in patients using SSRIs, low-dose ASA was associated with a lowered risk of psychiatric contacts in those using SSRIs concomitantly compared to SSRI monotherapy but showed an increased risk for CVD hospitalizations and mortality indicating confounding by indication (Köhler et al. 2015). In another observational study among individuals without established depression, the use of aspirin or statins during a 6-month period prior to inclusion into the study (thus at baseline) was not associated with a decreased risk of depression during a mean follow-up of approximately 5 years (Glaus et al. 2015). By contrast, another epidemiological study measuring exposure to statins during the complete follow-up period of up to 3 years found decreased risk of depression among users of statins aged 40 years or older (Redlich et al. 2014).

Angiotensin II receptor blockers of the central RAS system and polyunsaturated fatty acids are further potential cardioprotective drugs which potential use though is still under investigation.

Conclusion

Increasing evidence suggests inflammatory processes as a common etiological factor in depression and cardiovascular diseases (CVD). Based on these findings, clinical trials have indicated antidepressant treatment effects among depressed individuals for a range of anti-inflammatory drugs, whereas less evidence exists on treatment of comorbid depression and CVD. The most frequently investigated agents are nonsteroidal anti-inflammatory drugs (NSAIDs) and cytokine inhibitors. Moreover, studies have identified clinically relevant predictors for timing and duration concerning anti-inflammatory intervention. However, despite promising findings for several anti-inflammatory drugs, the risk for adverse events emphasizes caution regarding widespread use, in particular, for NSAIDs. Relevant anti-inflammatory agents for patients with comorbid depression and CVD still need to be identified, but cardioprotective agents such as statins, low-dose acetylsalicylic acid, and polyunsaturated fatty acids may represent promising agents. Thus, the field of personalized treatment with anti-inflammatory agents in depression and possibly comorbid CVD has attracted increasing interest, but the presented findings are still preliminary and under investigation and should therefore be regarded with caution. Future high-quality clinical trials on larger patient samples, including predictors for anti-inflammatory intervention, assessment of adverse events, and the importance of comorbid somatic diseases, are warranted.

References

Abbasi SH, Hosseini F, Modabbernia A, Ashrafi M, Akhondzadeh S (2012) Effect of celecoxib add-on treatment on symptoms and serum IL-6 concentrations in patients with major depressive disorder: randomized double-blind placebo-controlled study. J Affect Disord 141:308–314

Abolfazli R, Hosseini M, Ghanizadeh A, Ghaleiha A, Tabrizi M, Raznahan M, Golalizadeh M, Akhondzadeh S (2011) Double-blind randomized parallel-group clinical trial of efficacy of the combination fluoxetine plus modafinil versus fluoxetine plus placebo in the treatment of major depression. Depress Anxiety 28:297–302

Akhondzadeh S, Jafari S, Raisi F, Nasehi AA, Ghoreishi A, Salehi B, Mohebbi-Rasa S, Raznahan M, Kamalipour A (2009) Clinical trial of adjunctive celecoxib treatment in patients with major depression: a double blind and placebo controlled trial. Depress Anxiety 26:607–611

Anderson G, Berk M, Dean O, Moylan S, Maes M (2013) Role of immune-inflammatory and oxidative and nitrosative stress pathways in the etiology of depression: therapeutic implications. CNS Drugs 28:1–10

Andrade C, Kumar CB, Surya S (2013) Cardiovascular mechanisms of SSRI drugs and their benefits and risks in ischemic heart disease and heart failure. Int Clin Psychopharmacol 28:145–155

Arana GW, Santos AB, Laraia MT, McLeod-Bryant S, Beale MD, Rames LJ, Roberts JM, Dias JK, Molloy M (1995) Dexamethasone for the treatment of depression: a randomized, placebo- controlled, double-blind trial. Am J Psychiatry 152:265–267

Baune BT (2015) Inflammation and neurodegenerative disorders: is there still hope for therapeutic intervention? Curr Opin Psychiatry 28:148–154

Bechter K, Reiber H, Herzog S, Fuchs D, Tumani H, Maxeiner HG (2010) Cerebrospinal fluid analysis in affective and schizophrenic spectrum disorders: identification of subgroups with immune responses and blood-CSF barrier dysfunction. J Psychiatr Res 44:321–330

Berk M, Dean O, Drexhage H, McNeil JJ, Moylan S, O'Neil A, Davey CG, Sanna L, Maes M (2013) Aspirin: a review of its neurobiological properties and therapeutic potential for mental illness. BMC Med 11:74, 7015-11-74

Bloch MH, Hannestad J (2012) Omega-3 fatty acids for the treatment of depression: systematic review and meta-analysis. Mol Psychiatry 17:1272–1282

Burke NN, Kerr DM, Moriarty O, Finn DP, Roche M (2014) Minocycline modulates neuropathic pain behaviour and cortical M1-M2 microglial gene expression in a rat model of depression. Brain Behav Immun 42:147–156

Casolini P, Catalani A, Zuena AR, Angelucci L (2002) Inhibition of COX-2 reduces the age-dependent increase of hippocampal inflammatory markers, corticosterone secretion, and behavioral impairments in the rat. J Neurosci Res 68:337–343

Collins PY, Patel V, Joestl SS, March D, Insel TR, Daar AS, Scientific Advisory B, the Executive Committee of the Grand Challenges on Global Mental Health, Anderson W, Dhansay MA, Phillips A, Shurin S, Walport M, Ewart W, Savill SJ, Bordin IA, Costello EJ, Durkin M, Fairburn C, Glass RI, Hall W, Huang Y, Hyman SE, Jamison K, Kaaya S, Kapur S, Kleinman A, Ogunniyi A, Otero-Ojeda A, Poo MM, Ravindranath V, Sahakian BJ, Saxena S, Singer PA, Stein DJ (2011) Grand challenges in global mental health. Nature 475:27–30

Dantzer R, O'Connor JC, Freund GG, Johnson RW, Kelley KW (2008) From inflammation to sickness and depression: when the immune system subjugates the brain. Nat Rev Neurosci 9:46–56

de Abajo FJ, Garcia-Rodriguez LA (2008) Risk of upper gastrointestinal tract bleeding associated with selective serotonin reuptake inhibitors and venlafaxine therapy: interaction with nonsteroidal anti-inflammatory drugs and effect of acid-suppressing agents. Arch Gen Psychiatry 65:795–803

De Berardis D, Marini S, Piersanti M, Cavuto M, Perna G, Valchera A, Mazza M, Fornaro M, Iasevoli F, Martinotti G, Di Giannantonio M (2012) The relationships between cholesterol and suicide: an update. ISRN Psychiatry 2012:387901

de Gois Queiroz AI, Medeiros CD, Ribeiro BM, de Lucena DF, Macedo DS (2013) Angiotensin receptor blockers for bipolar disorder. Med Hypotheses 80:259–263

Dean OM, Maes M, Ashton M, Berk L, Kanchanatawan B, Sughondhabirom A, Tangwongchai S, Ng C, Dowling N, Malhi GS, Berk M (2014) Protocol and rationale-the efficacy of minocycline as an adjunctive treatment for major depressive disorder: a double blind, randomised, placebo controlled trial. Clin Psychopharmacol Neurosci 12:180–188

DeBattista C, Posener JA, Kalehzan BM, Schatzberg AF (2000) Acute antidepressant effects of intravenous hydrocortisone and CRH in depressed patients: a double-blind, placebo-controlled study. Am J Psychiatry 157:1334–1337

Eyre HA, Stuart MJ, Baune BT (2014) A phase-specific neuroimmune model of clinical depression. Prog Neuropsychopharmacol Biol Psychiatry 54:265–274

Eyre HA, Air T, Proctor S, Rositano S, Baune BT (2015) A critical review of the efficacy of non-steroidal anti-inflammatory drugs in depression. Prog Neuropsychopharmacol Biol Psychiatry 57:11–16

Fields C, Drye L, Vaidya V, Lyketsos C (2012) Celecoxib or naproxen treatment does not benefit depressive symptoms in persons age 70 and older: findings from a randomized controlled trial. Am J Geriatr Psychiatry 20:505–513

Fond G, Hamdani N, Kapczinski F, Boukouaci W, Drancourt N, Dargel A, Oliveira J, Le Guen E, Marlinge E, Tamouza R, Leboyer M (2013) Effectiveness and tolerance of anti-inflammatory drugs' add-on therapy in major mental disorders: a systematic qualitative review. Acta Psychiatr Scand 129:163–179

Foody J (2010) Statin use associated with increased risk of cataract, myopathy, liver dysfunction and acute renal failure with varying numbers needed to harm. Evid-Based Med 15:187–188

Gallagher PJ, Castro V, Fava M, Weilburg JB, Murphy SN, Gainer VS, Churchill SE, Kohane IS, Iosifescu DV, Smoller JW, Perlis RH (2012) Antidepressant response in patients with major depression exposed to NSAIDs: a pharmacovigilance study. Am J Psychiatry 169:1065–1072

Garrido-Mesa N, Zarzuelo A, Galvez J (2013) What is behind the non-antibiotic properties of minocycline? Pharmacol Res 67:18–30

Ghanizadeh A, Hedayati A (2013) Augmentation of fluoxetine with lovastatin for treating major depressive disorder, a randomized double-blind placebo controlled-clinical trial. Depress Anxiety 30:1084–1088

Gharekhani A, Khatami MR, Dashti-Khavidaki S, Razeghi E, Noorbala AA, Hashemi-Nazari SS, Mansournia MA (2014) The effect of omega-3 fatty acids on depressive symptoms and inflammatory markers in maintenance hemodialysis patients: a randomized, placebo-controlled clinical trial. Eur J Clin Pharmacol 70:655–665

Glaus J, Vandeleur CL, Lasserre AM, Strippoli MP, Castelao E, Gholam-Rezaee M, Waeber G, Aubry JM, Vollenweider P, Preisig M (2015) Aspirin and statin use and the subsequent development of depression in men and women: results from a longitudinal population-based study. J Affect Disord 182:126–131

Goldstein MR, Mascitelli L (2009) Do statins decrease cardiovascular disease at the expense of increasing cancer? Int J Cardiol 133:254–255

Goss AJ, Kaser M, Costafreda SG, Sahakian BJ, Fu CH (2013) Modafinil augmentation therapy in unipolar and bipolar depression: a systematic review and meta-analysis of randomized controlled trials. J Clin Psychiatry 74:1101–1107

Gougol A, Zareh-Mohammadi N, Raheb S, Farokhnia M, Salimi S, Iranpour N, Yekehtaz H, Akhondzadeh S (2015) Simvastatin as an adjuvant therapy to fluoxetine in patients with moderate to severe major depression: a double-blind placebo-controlled trial. J Psychopharmacol 29:575–581

Hashemian F, Majd M, Hosseini SM, Sharifi A, Panahi MVS, Bigdeli O (2011) A randomized, double-blind, placebo-controlled trial of celecoxib augmentation of sertraline in the treatment of a drug-naive women with major depression. Klin Psikofarmakol Bull 21:S183–S184

Hippisley-Cox J, Coupland C (2010) Unintended effects of statins in men and women in England and Wales: population based cohort study using the QResearch database. BMJ 340:c2197

Howren MB, Lamkin DM, Suls J (2009) Associations of depression with C-reactive protein, IL-1, and IL-6: A meta-analysis. Psychosom Med 71:171–186

Iyengar RL, Gandhi S, Aneja A, Thorpe K, Razzouk L, Greenberg J, Mosovich S, Farkouh ME (2013) NSAIDs are associated with lower depression scores in patients with osteoarthritis. Am J Med 126:1017.e11–8

Jung JC, Lee Y, Son JY, Lim E, Jung M, Oh S (2012) Simple synthesis of modafinil derivatives and their anti-inflammatory activity. Molecules 17:10446–10458

Kalra J, Prakash A, Kumar P, Majeed AB (2015) Cerebroprotective effects of RAS inhibitors: beyond their cardio-renal actions. J Renin Angiotensin Aldosterone Syst 16:459–468

Kashani L, Omidvar T, Farazmand B, Modabbernia A, Ramzanzadeh F, Tehraninejad ES, Ashrafi M, Tabrizi M, Akhondzadeh S (2013) Does pioglitazone improve depression through insulin-sensitization? results of a randomized double-blind metformin-controlled trial in patients with polycystic ovarian syndrome and comorbid depression. Psychoneuroendocrinology 38:767–776

Knights KM, Mangoni AA, Miners JO (2010) Defining the COX inhibitor selectivity of NSAIDs: implications for understanding toxicity. Expert Rev Clin Pharmacol 3:769–776

Köhler O, Benros ME, Nordentoft M, Farkouh ME, Iyengar RL, Mors O, Krogh J (2014) Effect of anti-inflammatory treatment on depression, depressive symptoms, and adverse effects: a systematic review and meta-analysis of randomized clinical trials. JAMA Psychiatry 71:1381–1391

Köhler O, Petersen L, Mors O, Gasse C (2015) Inflammation and depression: combined use of selective serotonin-reuptake inhibitors and NSAIDs or paracetamol and psychiatric outcomes. Brain Behav 5:e00338

Köhler O, Gasse C, Petersen L, Nierenberg A, Mors O, Østergaard S (2016) The effect of concomitant treatment with selective serotonin reuptake inhibitors and statins: a population-based study. Am J Psychiatry May 3:appiajp201615040463

Krishnadas R, Cavanagh J (2012) Depression: an inflammatory illness? J Neurol Neurosurg Psychiatry 83:495–502

Krogh J, Benros ME, Jorgensen MB, Vesterager L, Elfving B, Nordentoft M (2014) The association between depressive symptoms, cognitive function, and inflammation in major depression. Brain Behav Immun 35:70–76

Langley RG, Feldman SR, Han C, Schenkel B, Szapary P, Hsu M, Ortonne J, Gordon KB, Kimball AB (2010) Ustekinumab significantly improves symptoms of anxiety, depression, and skin-related quality of life in patients with moderate-to-severe psoriasis: results from a randomized, double-blind, placebo-controlled phase III trial. J Am Acad Dermatol 63:457–465

Maes M (1995) Evidence for an immune response in major depression: a review and hypothesis. Prog Neuropsychopharmacol Biol Psychiatry 19:11–38

Mansi I, Frei CR, Pugh MJ, Mortensen EM (2013) Psychologic disorders and statin use: a propensity score-matched analysis. Pharmacotherapy 33:615–626

Martino M, Rocchi G, Escelsior A, Fornaro M (2012) Immunomodulation mechanism of antidepressants: interactions between Serotonin/Norepinephrine balance and Th1/Th2 balance. Curr Neuropharmacol 10:97–123

Martins JG, Bentsen H, Puri BK (2012) Eicosapentaenoic acid appears to be the key omega-3 fatty acid component associated with efficacy in major depressive disorder: a critique of Bloch and hannestad and updated meta-analysis. Mol Psychiatry 17:1144–1149; discussion 1163–7

Mendlewicz J, Kriwin P, Oswald P, Souery D, Alboni S, Brunello N (2006) Shortened onset of action of antidepressants in major depression using acetylsalicylic acid augmentation: a pilot open-label study. Int Clin Psychopharmacol 21:227–231

Menter A, Augustin M, Signorovitch J, Yu AP, Wu EQ, Gupta SR, Bao Y, Mulani P (2010) The effect of adalimumab on reducing depression symptoms in patients with moderate to severe psoriasis: a randomized clinical trial. J Am Acad Dermatol 62:812–818

Mischoulon D, Nierenberg AA, Schettler PJ, Kinkead BL, Fehling K, Martinson MA, Hyman Rapaport M (2015) A double-blind, randomized controlled clinical trial comparing eicosapentaenoic acid versus docosahexaenoic acid for depression. J Clin Psychiatry 76:54–61

Miyaoka T, Wake R, Furuya M, Liaury K, Ieda M, Kawakami K, Tsuchie K, Taki M, Ishihara K, Araki T, Horiguchi J (2012) Minocycline as adjunctive therapy for patients with unipolar psychotic depression: an open-label study. Prog Neuro-Psychopharmacol Biol Psychiatry 37:222–226

Muller N, Riedel M, Schwarz MJ, Engel RR (2005) Clinical effects of COX-2 inhibitors on cognition in schizophrenia. Eur Arch Psychiatry Clin Neurosci 255:149–151

Muller N, Schwarz MJ, Dehning S, Douhe A, Cerovecki A, Goldstein-Muller B, Spellmann I, Hetzel G, Maino K, Kleindienst N, Moller HJ, Arolt V, Riedel M (2006) The cyclooxygenase-2 inhibitor celecoxib has therapeutic effects in major depression: Results of a double-blind, randomized, placebo controlled, add-on pilot study to reboxetine. Mol Psychiatry 11:680–684

Muller N, Myint AM, Schwarz MJ (2011) Inflammatory biomarkers and depression. Neurotox Res 19:308–318

Musil R, Schwarz MJ, Riedel M, Dehning S, Cerovecki A, Spellmann I, Arolt V, Muller N (2011) Elevated macrophage migration inhibitory factor and decreased transforming growth factor-beta levels in major depression--no influence of celecoxib treatment. J Affect Disord 134:217–225

O'Leary OF, Dinan TG, Cryan JF (2015) Faster, better, stronger: towards new antidepressant therapeutic strategies. Eur J Pharmacol 753:32–50

Oh SW, Kim J, Myung SK, Hwang SS, Yoon DH (2014) Antidepressant use and risk of coronary heart disease: meta-analysis of observational studies. Br J Clin Pharmacol 78:727–737

Otte C, Zhao S, Whooley MA (2012) Statin use and risk of depression in patients with coronary heart disease: longitudinal data from the heart and soul study. J Clin Psychiatry 73:610–615
Parsaik AK, Singh B, Hassan Murad M, Singh K, Mascarenhas SS, Williams MD, Lapid MI, Richardson JW, West CP, Rummans TA (2014) Statins use and risk of depression: a systematic review and meta-analysis. J Affect Disord 160:62–67
Ping G, Qian W, Song G, Zhaochun S (2014) Valsartan reverses depressive/anxiety-like behavior and induces hippocampal neurogenesis and expression of BDNF protein in unpredictable chronic mild stress mice. Pharmacol Biochem Behav 124:5–12
Raison CL, Rutherford RE, Woolwine BJ, Shuo C, Schettler P, Drake DF, Haroon E, Miller AH (2013) A randomized controlled trial of the tumor necrosis factor antagonist infliximab for treatment-resistant depression: the role of baseline inflammatory biomarkers. JAMA Psychiatry 70:31–41
Redlich C, Berk M, Williams LJ, Sundquist J, Sundquist K, Li X (2014) Statin use and risk of depression: a Swedish national cohort study. JAMA Psychiatry 14:348, 014-0348-y
Regen F, Le Bret N, Hildebrand M, Herzog I, Heuser I, Hellmann-Regen J (2015) Inhibition of brain retinoic acid catabolism: a mechanism for minocycline's pleiotropic actions? World J Biol Psychiatry June 5:1–7
Reiner Z (2013) Statins in the primary prevention of cardiovascular disease. Nat Rev Cardiol 10:453–464
Rosenblat JD, Cha DS, Mansur RB, McIntyre RS (2014) Inflamed moods: a review of the interactions between inflammation and mood disorders. Prog Neuropsychopharmacol Biol Psychiatry 53C:23–34
Sahin TD, Karson A, Balci F, Yazir Y, Bayramgurler D, Utkan T (2015) TNF-alpha inhibition prevents cognitive decline and maintains hippocampal BDNF levels in the unpredictable chronic mild stress rat model of depression. Behav Brain Res 292:233–240
Sampey AV, Hall PH, Mitchell RA, Metz CN, Morand EF (2001) Regulation of synoviocyte phospholipase A2 and cyclooxygenase 2 by macrophage migration inhibitory factor. Arthritis Rheum 44:1273–1280
Sandrini M, Vitale G, Pini LA (2002) Effect of rofecoxib on nociception and the serotonin system in the rat brain. Inflamm Res 51:154–159
Schjerning Olsen AM, Fosbol EL, Lindhardsen J, Folke F, Charlot M, Selmer C, Lamberts M, Bjerring Olesen J, Kober L, Hansen PR, Torp-Pedersen C, Gislason GH (2011) Duration of treatment with nonsteroidal anti-inflammatory drugs and impact on risk of death and recurrent myocardial infarction in patients with prior myocardial infarction: a nationwide cohort study. Circulation 123:2226–2235
Schjerning Olsen AM, Fosbol EL, Gislason GH (2014) The impact of NSAID treatment on cardiovascular risk - insight from danish observational data. Basic Clin Pharmacol Toxicol 115:179–184
Sepanjnia K, Modabbernia A, Ashrafi M, Modabbernia M, Akhondzadeh S (2012) Pioglitazone adjunctive therapy for moderate-to-severe major depressive disorder: randomized double-blind placebo-controlled trial. Neuropsychopharmacology 37:2093–2100
Setiawan E, Wilson AA, Mizrahi R, Rusjan PM, Miler L, Rajkowska G, Suridjan I, Kennedy JL, Rekkas PV, Houle S, Meyer JH (2015) Role of translocator protein density, a marker of neuroinflammation, in the brain during major depressive episodes. JAMA Psychiatry 72:268–275
Soczynska JK, Mansur RB, Brietzke E, Swardfager W, Kennedy SH, Woldeyohannes HO, Powell AM, Manierka MS, McIntyre RS (2012) Novel therapeutic targets in depression: minocycline as a candidate treatment. Behav Brain Res 235:302–317
Solomon DH, Avorn J, Sturmer T, Glynn RJ, Mogun H, Schneeweiss S (2006) Cardiovascular outcomes in new users of coxibs and nonsteroidal antiinflammatory drugs: high-risk subgroups and time course of risk. Arthritis Rheum 54:1378–1389
Solomon SD, Wittes J, Finn PV, Fowler R, Viner J, Bertagnolli MM, Arber N, Levin B, Meinert CL, Martin B, Pater JL, Goss PE, Lance P, Obara S, Chew EY, Kim J, Arndt G, Hawk E (2008) Cross trial safety assessment group: cardiovascular risk of celecoxib in 6 randomized placebo-controlled trials: the cross trial safety analysis. Circulation 117:2104–2113

Sumowski JF, Leavitt VM (2014) Body temperature is elevated and linked to fatigue in relapsing-remitting multiple sclerosis, even without heat exposure. Arch Phys Med Rehabil 95:1298–1302
Tomas-Camardiel M, Rite I, Herrera AJ, de Pablos RM, Cano J, Machado A, Venero JL (2004) Minocycline reduces the lipopolysaccharide-induced inflammatory reaction, peroxynitrite-mediated nitration of proteins, disruption of the blood-brain barrier, and damage in the nigral dopaminergic system. Neurobiol Dis 16:190–201
Toussi SS, Pan N, Walters HM, Walsh TJ (2013) Infections in children and adolescents with juvenile idiopathic arthritis and inflammatory bowel disease treated with tumor necrosis factor-alpha inhibitors: systematic review of the literature. Clin Infect Dis 57:1318–1330
Tyring S, Gottlieb A, Papp K, Gordon K, Leonardi C, Wang A, Lalla D, Woolley M, Jahreis A, Zitnik R, Cella D, Krishnan R (2006) Etanercept and clinical outcomes, fatigue, and depression in psoriasis: double-blind placebo-controlled randomised phase III trial. Lancet 367:29–35
Uher R, Carver S, Power RA, Mors O, Maier W, Rietschel M, Hauser J, Dernovsek MZ, Henigsberg N, Souery D, Placentino A, Farmer A, McGuffin P (2012) Non-steroidal anti-inflammatory drugs and efficacy of antidepressants in major depressive disorder. Psychol Med 42:2027–2035
Uher R, Tansey KE, Dew T, Maier W, Mors O, Hauser J, Dernovsek MZ, Henigsberg N, Souery D, Farmer A, McGuffin P (2014) An inflammatory biomarker as a differential predictor of outcome of depression treatment with escitalopram and nortriptyline. Am J Psychiatry 171:1278–1286
Vevera J, Fisar Z, Kvasnicka T, Zdenek H, Starkova L, Ceska R, Papezova H (2005) Cholesterol-lowering therapy evokes time-limited changes in serotonergic transmission. Psychiatry Res 133:197–203
Warner-Schmidt JL, Vanover KE, Chen EY, Marshall JJ, Greengard P (2011) Antidepressant effects of selective serotonin reuptake inhibitors (SSRIs) are attenuated by antiinflammatory drugs in mice and humans. Proc Natl Acad Sci U S A 108:9262–9267
Weitz-Schmidt G (2002) Statins as anti-inflammatory agents. Trends Pharmacol Sci 23:482–486
Weitz-Schmidt G, Welzenbach K, Brinkmann V, Kamata T, Kallen J, Bruns C, Cottens S, Takada Y, Hommel U (2001) Statins selectively inhibit leukocyte function antigen-1 by binding to a novel regulatory integrin site. Nat Med 7:687–692
Wichers MC, Koek GH, Robaeys G, Verkerk R, Scharpe S, Maes M (2005) IDO and interferon-alpha-induced depressive symptoms: a shift in hypothesis from tryptophan depletion to neurotoxicity. Mol Psychiatry 10:538–544
Wingerchuk DM, Benarroch EE, O'Brien PC, Keegan BM, Lucchinetti CF, Noseworthy JH, Weinshenker BG, Rodriguez M (2005) A randomized controlled crossover trial of aspirin for fatigue in multiple sclerosis. Neurology 64:1267–1269
Yekehtaz H, Farokhnia M, Akhondzadeh S (2013) Cardiovascular considerations in antidepressant therapy: an evidence-based review. J Tehran Heart Cent 8:169–176
You H, Lu W, Zhao S, Hu Z, Zhang J (2013) The relationship between statins and depression: a review of the literature. Expert Opin Pharmacother 14:1467–1476
Young-Xu Y, Chan KA, Liao JK, Ravid S, Blatt CM (2003) Long-term statin use and psychological well-being. J Am Coll Cardiol 42:690–697
Zernecke A, Bernhagen J, Weber C (2008) Macrophage migration inhibitory factor in cardiovascular disease. Circulation 117:1594–1602
Zuidersma M, Conradi HJ, van Melle JP, Ormel J, de Jonge P (2013) Depression treatment after myocardial infarction and long-term risk of subsequent cardiovascular events and mortality: a randomized controlled trial. J Psychosom Res 74:25–30

The Use of Complementary Alternative and Integrative Medicine (CAIM) for Treatment and Prevention of Late-Life Depression and Cardiovascular Disease

25

Taya Varteresian and Helen Lavretsky

Contents

Abstract

This chapter discusses cardiovascular disease in older adults including hypertension, congestive heart failure, and myocardial infarctions and diverse preventive and treatment options including nutrition, exercise, and mind-body approaches as well as natural product. We discuss integrative approaches to treatment and prevention of depression and cardiovascular disease. The discussion is based on the analysis of the more rigorously examined approaches for both depression and cardiovascular disease.

T. Varteresian, DO, MS
Psychiatrist LA County Department of Mental Health, University of California, Irvine, CA, USA

H. Lavretsky, MD, MS (✉)
Late-Life Mood, Stress, and Wellness Research Program, Semel Institute for Neuroscience and Human Behavior, Geffen School of Medicine at University of California, Los Angeles, CA, USA
e-mail: hlavretsky@mednet.ucla.edu

B.T. Baune, P.J. Tully (eds.), *Cardiovascular Diseases and Depression*,
DOI 10.1007/978-3-319-32480-7_25

25.1 Introduction

This chapter discusses the relationship between depression and cardiovascular disease in older adults, as well as treatment and prevention of these disorders through traditional approaches including psychotherapy and antidepressants, and Complementary and Integrative Medicine (CIM) interventions with emphasis placed on strategies which are mutually beneficial.

25.2 Depression and Cardiovascular Disease

The relationship between depression and cardiovascular disease is complex and worth discussing due to its bidirectional relationship. Depression increases the risk for cardiovascular disease. A large epidemiologic study involving thousands of middle-aged and older adults in the United States demonstrated that depression increased the risk for developing cardiovascular disease compared to age-matched controls without clinical depression (Xiang and An 2015). In particular, a part of this increased risk for cardiovascular disease in individuals suffering from depression comes from modifiable lifestyle factors such as inactivity, poor nutrition, and increased incidence of smoking tobacco (Lebowitz 2011). Other psychosocial stressors can influence the adverse effect of depression on cardiovascular disease as occurs in depressed adults with a history of childhood trauma or current stress. Recently, a 2-year longitudinal cohort study conducted in the Netherlands demonstrated a correlation between increased arterial stiffness and history of childhood trauma and/or recent life stress, thereby demonstrating the interconnection between environment and cardiovascular disease (Bomhof-Roordink et al. 2015). This correlation between social history and disease state is commonly seen in psychiatry. Depression and cardiovascular disease share multiple risk factors.

However, there does still appear to be an independent risk factor of depression on cardiovascular disease. The relative risk of developing CAD in an individual suffering from depression is 1.5 (Rudisch and Nemeroff 2003). Some proposed mechanisms for linking depression and cardiovascular disease have been heart rate variability, inflammation, and hypercoagulability (Joynt and O'Connor 2005). There is a definite impact of depression impacting cardiovascular disease.

Co-occurrence of late-life depression and vascular disease has been coined "vascular depression." Initially, Alexopoulos et al. (1997) coined the term vascular depression to describe the influence of cerebrovascular disease on the development and course of depression. Krishnan et al. (1997) identified the radiologic findings in a subtype of depression demonstrating a significant amount of deep white-matter hyperintensities (WMH) or subcortical gray-matter hyperintensities on MRI. Vascular depression has been associated with late age at onset of depression, older age, anhedonia, functional disability, and limited family history compared to depression occurring in individuals without cerebrovascular impairments (Krishnan et al. 1997). Later, Alexopoulos et al. (1999) further described cerebrovascular disease to increase the risk for a vascular depression which appears different from previously described forms of depression in that it stems from damage to the cortico-striato-pallido-thalamo-cortical pathways, thereby leading to cognitive impairment in addition to depression. More recent research demonstrates that cerebral small vessel ischemic disease as measured by subcortical infarct and atrophy was related to more depressive symptoms (Van Stolen et al. 2015). Therefore it is important to highlight a subtype of late-life depression due to its pathophysiologic and treatment response differences from other forms of depression.

The treatment of cardiovascular disease and its risk factors are influential on the management of depression. Patients suffering from hypertension, diabetes, coronary disease, and stroke have a high prevalence of depression (Alexopoulos et al. 1997). The standard mortality rates for various epidemiologic studies range from 1.6 to 2.2 for cardiovascular mortality while suffering from depression or bipolar disorder (Fiedorowicz 2014). Given the construct of vascular depression, the interrelationship between reducing vascular disease risk factors lends additional preventative nature to depression as well. For example, the treatment of hypertension and hypercholesterolemia can directly reduce chances of developing vascular depression by reducing the occurrence of cardiovascular disease (Alexopoulos et al. 1999). Additionally in individuals suffering from atrial fibrillation, anticoagulation may reduce the risk of stroke, thereby also preventing vascular depression (Alexopoulos et al. 1999).

Multiple neurotransmitter systems and circuits may be affected in vascular depression that may be helped by augmentation with stimulants and dual-action antidepressants (Alexopoulos et al. 1999). In our recently published randomized controlled trial (RCT) of 146 older adults with major depression, the combination of methylphenidate with citalopram led to improved response and remission compared to either drug alone (Lavretsky et al. 2015). In depressed older adults, vascular risk factors, including age, elevated systolic blood pressure, diabetes, smoking, history of cerebrovascular accident (CVA), atrial fibrillation, and left ventricular hypertrophy, all contributed to cognitive impairment (Schneider et al. 2012). Therefore addressing and treating cardiovascular disease and risk factors can have a beneficial effect on the mental health conditions.

Mechanisms connecting depression and cardiovascular disease have been summarized to include hormonal and sympathetic nervous system arousal. Fiedorowicz (2014) summarized the relationship between hyperactivity of the hypothalamic pituitary axis (HPA) and depression, including risks factors such as elevated cortisol levels. Additionally, the autonomic nervous system, with particular focus on reduced heart rate variability in depression, provides a link between depression and worsening cardiovascular status (Fiedorowicz 2014). Another proposed mechanism attributed to the interaction between depression and heart disease involves an impact on endothelia functioning as measured by arterial flow. Multiple studies have been reviewed demonstrating the correlation between endothelial dysfunction and depression (Fiedorowicz 2014). In older females suffering from chest pain, coronary angiogram demonstrated the presence of coronary artery disease (CAD) to be more common in individuals with elevated Beck Depression Inventory scores (Cho et al. 2015). Systemic inflammation is commonly seen as a risk factor in the development of cardiovascular disease in particular atherosclerosis and is also seen to be elevated during depressive episodes. Studies have found that apathy, which is often involved in late-life depression, in particular vascular depression is correlated with elevated marker of inflammation. In a cross-sectional study of over 2,000 older adults without known cardiovascular disease, apathy was associated with elevated C-reactive protein levels (CRP) and thought to further mediate the adverse effect of depressive symptoms on cardiovascular disease (Eurelings et al. 2015). Depression also appears to be related to CAD risk factors as well. Type 2 diabetes mellitus (DM2) is a common risk factor for CAD and has been related to increased platelet activation in individuals suffering from major depressive disorder (MDD) (Zahn et al. 2015).

25.3 Cardiovascular Disease and Diet

The Mediterranean diet includes a higher concentration of unsaturated fats, usually monounsaturated fats including olive oil as well as fruits, vegetables, whole grains, nuts, and legumes, as well as moderate alcohol consumption (Widmer et al. 2015). Evidence from meta-analysis and RCTs supports the Mediterranean diet being an effective intervention for cardiovascular disease and various risk factors (Table 25.1). Among noteworthy studies, the PREDIMED (Preventiòn con dieta Mediterrànea) study compared the impact of a low-fat diet to a Mediterranean diet. Interestingly, the study had to be prematurely terminated due to the Mediterranean diet showing such a large improvement in terms of reducing future cardiovascular events compared to the low-fat diet (Estruch et al. 2013). Further evidence to support the cardiovascular benefits of the Mediterranean diet comes from the Lyon Heart Study, which was a prospective randomized single-blinded secondary prevention trial. The Lyon Heart Study showed the Mediterranean diet reduced the development of future cardiovascular disease in those individuals who had already suffered a myocardial infarction (MI) (de Lorgeril et al. 1999). The Mediterranean diet utilized in the study was enriched with alpha-linolenic acid due to the findings that lowest rates of cardiovascular disease are found in individuals consuming high amounts of alpha-linolenic acid such as the Japanese and Cretans who consume high amounts of canola oil and soybeans as well as purslane and walnuts (de Lorgeril et al. 1999). In addition to preventing disease, the Mediterranean diet appears to improve risk factors for cardiovascular disease. A meta-analysis showed a significant improvement in reduction of cardiovascular risk factor including waist circumference, lipids, metabolic syndrome, glucose, and blood pressure (Kastorini et al. 2011). There is consistent support that the Mediterranean diet is a beneficial adjunctive treatment for the prevention of cardiovascular disease. Table 25.1 includes a summary of the various dietary interventions for cardiovascular disease.

There are multiple components of the Mediterranean diet, and some but not all components have been evaluated and isolated in research studies. Fish oil or omega-3 polyunsaturated fatty acids are a main component of the Mediterranean diet. Interestingly the American Heart Association and American College of Cardiology recommend consuming one to two servings of fish per week for those

Table 25.1 Summary of CAIM interventions for treatment of cardiovascular disease and depression

Study	Sample	Design	Cardiovascular effects	Mental health effects
Omega-3				
Rondanelli et al. *J Nutrition, Health & Aging* (2011)	$N=42$ Older females in SNF Pretreatment GDS-LF 17.1 ± 3.6 (Mildly depressed)	RCT		Antidepressant effect of omega-3 monotherapy Posttreatment GDS-LF mean 12.7, difference from placebo −3.2 CI −5.9, −0.6, ($p=0.017$)
Giltay et al. *Am J Clin Nutr* (2011)	$N=4{,}116$ $N=36$ dep on meds Older adults post-MI Pretreatment GDS-SF 1.2–1.4 (Not depressed)	RCT		No improvement in depressive symptoms in general sample In those with depression on antidepressants, omega-3 served as an augmentation strategy
Zimmer et al. *J. Clin Psych* (2013)	$N=2{,}081$ $N=33$ MDD on meds Older adults post-MI	RCT		No improvement in depressive symptoms in general sample In those with depression on antidepressants, omega-3 provided an antidepressant effect BDI-II 20.9 (7.1) vs. 24.9(8.5), $p<0.05$

(continued)

Table 25.1 (continued)

Study	Sample	Design	Cardiovascular effects	Mental health effects
L-methylfolate				
Papakostas et al. *Am J Psychiatry* (2012)	$N=148$ Partial responders of SSRI w/ MDD	RCT		15 mg l-methylfolate improved HAMD scores (5.6 points) as augmentation strategy to SSRI
SAMe				
Papakostas et al. *Am J Psychiatry* (2012)	$N=73$ SSRI nonresponders w/ MDD	RCT		HAMD scores SAMe (mean: 11.1 [SD=6.1]) versus placebo-treated patients (mean: 15.8 [SD=6.2])
St. John's Wort (SJW)				
Linde *Cochrane database of systematic reviews* (2008)	23 RCTs General adult	Meta-analysis		SJW is an effective antidepressant Combined response rates 1.28–1.87
Kasper et al. *International clinical psychopharmacology* (2010)	15 RCT placebo 6 RCT TCA 12 RCT SSRI	Review		SJW has comparable efficacy to traditional antidepressants and better tolerability
Harrer et al. *Arzneimittel-Forschung* (1999)	$N=149$ Older adults with mild-to-moderate depression	RCT		SJW is equally effective to fluoxetine, HAMD scores decreased by ½
Mannel et al. *J. Psych Res* (2010)	$N=100$ Older adults with moderate depression	RCT		SJW did not improve HAMD; however it did improve subset of symptoms indicated in atypical depression

CoQ10				
Burke et al. *Southern Medical Journal* (2001)	*N* = 73 Isolated systolic hypertension SBP >140	RCT	Significant reduction in systolic blood pressure 17.8 ± 7.3 mmHg	
Horse chestnut				
Pittler and Ernst. *Cochrane Collaboration* (2012)	17 RCTs	Meta-analysis	Improvement in CVI, leg pain, edema, and pruritus	
Hawthorn				
Pittler et al. *Cochrane Collaboration* (2008)	10 trials, *N* = 855 with CHF	Meta-analysis	Improved exercise tolerance (WMD 122.76, 95 % CI 32.74–212.78) Decreased pressure-heart rate product (WMD −19.22, 95 % CI −30.46, −7.98) Improved shortness of breath (WMD −547, 95 % CI −8.68, −2.26) Improved fatigue (WMD −5.47, 95 % CI −8.68, 2.26)	
Acupuncture				
Li et al. *International Journal of Clinical Acupuncture* (1994)	*N* = 21 Older adults with post-stroke depression	Case series		Acupuncture improved mood

(continued)

Table 25.1 (continued)

Study	Sample	Design	Cardiovascular effects	Mental health effects
Williams and Grahm. *International Journal of Geriatric Psychiatry* (2006)	$N = 13$ Older adults with depression	Pilot study		Acupuncture was feasibly provided in a geriatric population Acupuncture was relaxing and improved mood
Li et al. *Evidence-Based Complementary and Alternative Medicine* (2014)	4 RCTs	Meta-analysis	Acupuncture did not change or affect HTN unless patient was on antihypertensive med	
Macklin et al. *Hypertension* (2006)	$N = 192$ Middle-aged adults with HTN weaned off antihypertensive meds	RCT	Acupuncture was no more effective than sham acupuncture at reducing blood pressure	
Meditation				
Anderson et al. (2008)	9 RCT	Meta-analysis	Decreased SBP –4.7 mmHg and DBP –3.2 mmHg	
Yoga				
Yang. *Evidence-Based Complement Alternative Med* (2007)	32 studies	Review	Decreased weight Improved cholesterol Improved glycemic control Decreased blood pressure	

Yogendra et al. *J Assoc Physicians India* (2004)	*N*=113	Controlled open-label study	Decreased total cholesterol 23.3 % Decreased HDL by 26 % Regression of coronary lesions improved myocardial perfusion	
Bonura and Teenbaum. *J Phys Act Health* (2014)	*N*=89 Older adults in SNF	RCT		Improved depression
Patel et al. J *Alternative Complementary Medicine* (2012)	18 studies *N*=649	Meta-analysis		Yoga improved self-rated health status, aerobic fitness, and strength Mixed effect of yoga on depression
Chan et al. *Alternative Therapy Health Medicine* (2012)	*N*=14 History of stroke	RCT		No significant differences in antidepressant effect between depression in exercise group and yoga group
Shaidi et al. *International J Geriatric Psych* (2010)	*N*=70 depressed older women	RCT		Laughter yoga is as effective as group exercise in improving depression and life satisfaction
Tai Chi				
Lan et al. *Evidence-Based Complementary and Alternative Medicine* (2013)	11 RCTs	Review	Decreased BP Improved glycemic control	

(continued)

Table 25.1 (continued)

Study	Sample	Design	Cardiovascular effects	Mental health effects
Tsai et al. J *Alternative and Complementary Medicine* (2003)	$N=76$ Stage I hypertension	RCT	Improved BP Improved lipids	Improved anxiety
Mediterranean diet				
Sanchez-Villegas et al. *Public Health Nutrition* (2006)	9,670 general adults	Cross-sectional analysis of prospective cohort study		Folate intake inversely related to depression Vitamin B12 inversely related to depression in women Omega-3 fatty acids protective for women
De Lorgeril et al. *Lancet* (1994)	605 participants after MI	Prospective randomized single-blinded secondary prevention trial	Reduced mortality in Mediterranean diet (RR 0.30, 95 % CI 0.11–0.82)	
DASH diet				
Torres and Nowson. *Nutrition* (2012)	95 healthy postmenopausal women	Randomized parallel intervention modified DASH diet vs. healthy diet		Improvement in mood
Nowson et al. *Nutrition Research* (2009)	95 healthy postmenopausal women with hypertension	Randomized parallel intervention modified DASH diet vs. healthy diet	Those taking antihypertensive meds + DASH diet showed decrease SBP (6.5 ± 2.5 mmHg) and DBP (4.6 ± 1.4 mmHg)	

Exercise				
Drenowatz et al. *Journal of Science and Medicine in Sport* (2014)	*N*=7,321 women	Cross-sectional study	Resistance training was associated with reduced body fat, better glycemic control, and lower total cholesterol	
Blumenthal et al. *Arch Intern Med* (1999)	*N*=156 older adults with MDD	RCT		Exercise was equally effective as antidepressant over time
Tea				
Peters et al. *American J. Epidemiology* (2001)	Ten cohort studies and seven case-control studies	Meta-analysis	Tea decreased MI by 11 % In the United Kingdom, increased risk MI/CHD 1.73 (CI 0.97, 3.08) In Europe (not the United Kingdom), decreased risk MI/CHD 0.27 (CI 0.14, 0.50)	
Alcohol				
Di Castenuovo et al. *Archives of Internal Medicine* (2006)	34 studies *N*=1,015,835	Meta-analysis	Reducing in total mortality in women drinking 1–2 drinks per day and men drinking 2–4 drinks per day but increased consumption showed increased mortality	

(continued)

Table 25.1 (continued)

Study	Sample	Design	Cardiovascular effects	Mental health effects
Mente et al. *Archives of Internal Medicine* (2009)	70 cohorts studies light/moderate $N = 1{,}747{,}107$	Meta-analysis	Light-moderate alcohol RR 0.71 (CI 95 % 0.67–0.75)	
	64 cohort studies heavy $N = 1{,}693{,}893$		Heavy alcohol 0.69 (0.64–0.75)	

RCT randomized controlled trial, *RR* relative risk, *GDS-LF* geriatric depression scale – long form, *GDS- SF* geriatric depression scale – short form, *N* sample size, *CI* confidence interval, *p* significance value, *SSRI* selective serotonin reuptake inhibitor, *MDD* major depressive disorder, *MI* myocardial infarction, *BDI-II* Beck Depression Inventory 2, *HAMD* Hamilton depression scale, *SAMe* S-adenosyl-L-methionine, *CHF* congestive heart failure, *WMD* weighted mean difference, *HTN* hypertension, *HDL* high-density lipoprotein, *SJW* St. John's Wort, *DASH* Dietary Approaches to Stop Hypertension, *BP* blood pressure, *CVI* chronic venous insufficiency, *SBP* systolic blood pressure, *DBP* diastolic blood pressure, *CHD* coronary heart disease, *CoQ10* coenzyme Q10, *SNF* skilled nursing facility, *TCA* tricyclic antidepressant, *RR* Relative Risk with a history of cardiovascular disease in order to reduce subsequent events (Kris-Etherton et al. 2002). In a systematic review Mente et al. (2009) demonstrated a reduction in cardiovascular disease with the intake of fish (RR 0.81) and marine fatty acid (RR 0.86); interestingly the risk reduction was seen more so for those who had already suffered from a cardiovascular event, lending evidence to encourage dietary interventions at multiple stages of the disease process.

Olive oil is an unsaturated fatty acid and makes up another component of a Mediterranean diet. Interestingly studies are able to isolate the essential therapeutic component of olive oil which is its phenolic compounds that serve as antioxidants, free-radical scavengers, and enzyme modulators (Widmer et al. 2015). RCTs examining the impact of olive oil on cardiovascular risks appear to reduce markers of cardiovascular disease including inflammation such as a reduction in platelet activation (Widmer et al. 2015). It appears that olive oil can have an impact, but it is difficult to evaluate whether it is the influential component of the Mediterranean diet that is contributing to the most benefit and therefore cannot be as confidently recommended in isolation of the Mediterranean diet for the prevention or treatment of cardiovascular disease. Fruits and vegetables are generally considered part of most healthy diets and therefore are not limited to the Mediterranean diet; however they do make up a large component. Studies do show that higher consumption of fruits and vegetables was associated with lower blood pressure, lower BMI, and reduction in cardiovascular disease (Widmer et al. 2015). A systematic review of cohort studies and RCTs demonstrated that there was a reduction in coronary heart disease with the consumption of vegetables (RR 0.77) and fruits (RR 0.80) (Mente et al. 2009). Whole grains include oats and barley, and high-fiber content makes up another component of the Mediterranean diet. It is assumed that fiber reduces absorption of lipids which thereby reduces cardiovascular disease. A RCT demonstrated an improvement in blood pressure and lipids in individuals consuming a diet consisting whole grains compared to refined carbohydrates (Tighe et al. 2010). A meta-analysis of seven cohort studies showed that consumption of 2.5 servings per day of whole grains reduced the risk of cardiovascular events by 21 % (Mellen et al. 2008). In a systematic review, whole grains (RR 0.81) and fiber (RR 0.78) were associated with reduction in risk for coronary heart disease (Mente et al. 2009). Therefore, whole grains appear to demonstrate a significant impact on cardiovascular disease outside of the Mediterranean diet.

Nuts and legumes are another component of the Mediterranean diet which has been studied in isolation. There is data to support consumption of nuts on reduction of cardiovascular disease. In their review, Mente et al. (2009) demonstrated a reduction in cardiovascular risk by 0.67. Additionally, a meta-analysis demonstrated that walnut consumption reduced LDL cholesterol (Banel and Hu 2009). At the present time, there is insufficient evidence to support legumes in reducing cardiovascular disease (Widmer et al. 2015); however the consumption of nuts in particular walnuts both with and without the Mediterranean diet appears to provide reduction in risk for cardiovascular disease. After reviewing multiple studies looking at the Mediterranean diet, Widmer et al. (2015) concluded that there is sufficient evidence for both primary and secondary prevention of cardiovascular disease with the

Mediterranean diet; however when reviewed in isolation, there was no individual component in isolation that showed equal efficacy to the Mediterranean diet as a whole, but the consumption of fresh fruits, vegetables, nuts, and whole grains.

Another approach for optimizing certain cardiovascular disease risk factors has been Dietary Approaches to Stop Hypertension (DASH). The theory behind the DASH diet in reducing hypertension is based on premise that a high consumption of fruits and vegetables produces fewer bicarbonate or acid precursors (Nowson et al. 2008). Additionally the DASH diet includes low-fat dairy products and low saturated fat. In a randomized parallel dietary intervention study of the DASH, diet with low sodium (60–70 mmol/day) along with the addition of lean red meat showed a significant reduction in systolic blood pressure (Nowson et al. 2008). The landmark study which utilized the DASH diet demonstrated a significant decrease in blood pressure in individuals (SBP 5.5 mmHg and DBP 3 mmHg) and a more robust decrease in blood pressure in those suffering from hypertension (SBP 11.5 mmHg and DBP 5.5 mmHg) (Appel et al. 1997). The amount of sodium consumed by the general US population is significantly more than the recommended necessary amount, which is 500 mg per day (Sinatra and Houston 2011). It is well established that sodium can increase blood pressure, and diets with reduced sodium show decreases in blood pressure. Sacks et al. (2001) combined the successful components of the DASH diet with a reduction in sodium intake to produce a significant decrease in systolic and diastolic blood pressure in both individuals with and without hypertension. In conclusion, low-sodium diets and the DASH diet with large amounts of fruits and vegetables and low amounts of fats could both prevent and treat hypertension.

Consumption of tea is thought to have a beneficial effect on cardiovascular disease due to its constituents including polyphenolic flavonoids that have an antioxidant effect (Peters et al. 2001). A meta-analysis consisting of ten cohort studies and seven case-control studies demonstrated that consumption of three cups of tea was helpful at reducing occurrence of myocardial infarction by 11 % (Peters et al. 2001). However there was a regional difference in results showing an actual increase in cardiovascular disease in the United Kingdom and an increase in Australia in terms of stroke. There was insufficient evidence in the type of tea which showed the benefit. The regional difference in risk reduction between the United States and the combination of the United Kingdom and Australia was suggested to be related to the common occurrence of milk being added to tea in those regions which could reduce the antioxidant effect of tea. Furthermore there may be a confounding variable that tea consumption in the United States is more commonly consistent with a healthier lifestyle compared to tea consumption in Australia and the United Kingdom.

Additional dietary interventions include the consumption of alcohol. A review of alcohol consumption and general mortality in mixed-aged populations demonstrated a J shape (Di Castenuovo et al. 2006). Women drinking one to two drinks per day and men drinking two to four drinks per day showed a reduction in total mortality, but higher levels of alcohol consumption increased mortality (Di Castenuovo et al. 2006). Furthermore, light to moderate alcohol consumption is associated with a reduction in risk for CHD (Mente et al. 2009). Interestingly younger men can drink up to four drinks per day and younger women up to two drinks per day; however the strongest risk reduction appeared to occur at one-half of a drink per day (Kloner and Rezkalla 2007). It does not appear that they have found the exact mechanism of action which alcohol reduces cardiovascular mortality, but it does appear that there is an elevation in high-density lipoprotein (HDL), an anti-inflammatory effect and antioxidant effect (Kloner and Rezkalla 2007). As with any intervention, the risk versus benefit must be weighted, but it appears that regular consumption of alcohol is protective for cardiovascular health. Therefore in summary there are multiple dietary interventions that can serve as prevention and treatment of cardiovascular disease including the Mediterranean diet, DASH diet, nuts, fruits, vegetables, whole grains, tea, and moderate alcohol consumption, some of which can serve as appropriate adjunctive treatments for various cardiovascular diseases.

25.4 Cardiovascular Disease and Exercise

The American Heart Association recommends physical activity to reduce the risk for cardiovascular disease (Darden et al. 2013). Evidence supports both aerobic exercise and also resistance exercise as being effective for cardiovascular disease and also for the primary and secondary prevention of CAD (Table 25.1). A cross-sectional study of over 7,000 women demonstrated resistance training reducing body fat, fasting glucose, and total cholesterol (Drenowatz et al. 2014). In a study of over 5,000 individuals with a history of coronary heart disease, cardiac rehabilitation, which involved physical activity, improved survival (Darden et al. 2013). Studies show that in congestive heart failure (CHF) (New York Heart Association class III or IV), aerobic exercise improved survival and also reduced future hospitalizations due to heart failure (Darden et al. 2013). There appears to be a balance between aerobic activities for individuals with cardiovascular disease. Williams and Thompson (2014) demonstrated an increase in cardiovascular mortalities for running more than 7.1 miles/day or walking briskly above 10.7 km/day. Therefore, physical activity can improve cardiovascular disease but is not without its consequences.

25.5 Cardiovascular Disease and Mind-Body Approaches

It is well established that there is a link between increased sympathetic tone and hypertension in states of psychological distress. It is understandable therefore that approaches that connect the mind and body would reduce sympathetic tone and impact both mental and physical well-being. Approaches including Tai Chi, yoga, and acupuncture are considered integrative in terms of the body and mind and have effects on both depression and cardiovascular disease (Table 25.1).

Tai Chi is a Chinese martial art form that has demonstrated improvements in various disease states (Abbott and Lavretsky 2013). A review of Tai Chi showed multiple cardiovascular benefits including lowering blood pressure, better glycemic control in diabetes, and lower cholesterol (Lan et al. 2013). Another study demonstrated a significant improvement in blood pressure as well as anxiety with the use of Tai Chi (Tsai et al. 2003). Further interventions regarding Tai Chi and mental health will be discussed in the mental health discussion later in this chapter. However based on the available evidence, there is empiric evidence that Tai Chi can modulate certain aspects of cardiovascular disease especially by lowering blood pressure.

Alternatively yoga is another mind-body-based intervention which has applications to treating hypertension. Yoga demonstrates reductions in blood pressure when practiced 30–60 min per day (Sinatra and Houston 2011). Additionally less physically demanding interventions of mind-body-based approaches include transcendental meditation (TM). TM originated in India and involves repetitive vocalizations called mantras. A meta-analysis of TM demonstrated a significant reduction in blood pressure (Anderson et al. 2008). Kaback et al. (2011) identified the intricate relationship between stress response and CHF exacerbations and therefore recommend mind-body techniques such as meditation, yoga, and Tai Chi for better cardiovascular outcomes. Modifications for older adults have been successfully applied in previous studies. Lee et al. (2010) demonstrated positive mental and physical effects of Tai Chi on older adults living in a skilled nursing facility (SNF).

Acupuncture is another form of mind-body techniques that is a form of traditional Chinese medicine, which has been utilized for health and wellness for thousands of years. It utilizes meridians or acupoints throughout the body that are thought to tap into an energy called Qi (Longhurst 2011). In general acupuncture does not create a significant change in blood pressure in individuals who are normotensive; however in those individuals who suffer from hypertension, acupuncture is thought to reduce sympathetic tone, thereby reducing blood pressure (Longhurst 2011). The studies examining acupuncture for hypertension are mixed. However a recent meta-analysis examining four RCTs comparing acupuncture to sham acupuncture did not show a significant reduction in blood pressure (Li et al. 2014). Interestingly the authors did find a significant reduction in blood pressure in those individuals who were already taking a hypertensive medication. Therefore, acupuncture might serve as a useful adjunctive treatment to hypertension in those individuals who are already undergoing traditional treatment. The authors of the largest RCT called the SHARP trial (Stop Hypertension with the Acupuncture Research Program) conduced in the United States examined almost 200 individuals suffering from stage 2 hypertension (SBP/DBP 140/90–179/109 mmHg) and included a comparison placebo arm of sham acupuncture but failed to reveal a significant impact of acupuncture on blood pressure (Macklin et al. 2006). The authors do suggest that longer trials, beyond 6 weeks, might be more effective at detecting a significant benefit on blood pressure. Therefore, the data do not support using acupuncture for severe hypertension without traditional therapies, but might be helpful for less severe hypertension (i.e., prehypertension 120/80–139/89 mmHg) as also an adjunctive treatment along with traditional antihypertensive medications.

Many of our traditional Western medications have been derived from plants making it responsible to continue to look toward natural products for effective treatment interventions. For example, *Rauvolfia serpentina* is a biologically based product which is often used when other more traditional forms of antihypertensive medication are not available as it has reserpine within it which functions as a an antihypertensive medication by reducing sympathetic tone via noradrenergic inhibition (Low Dog 2011).

This section will discuss the data regarding five different forms of natural products for the treatment of cardiovascular disease. Horse chestnut seed (*Aesculus hippocastanum*) is a proposed treatment for chronic venous insufficiency. A Cochrane database review including six RCTs and over 500 participants concluded that horse chestnut seed improved symptoms of leg pain, edema, and pruritis associated with chronic venous insufficiency (Pittler and Ernst 2012). Horse chestnut works by thinning blood, and therefore monitoring for excessive bleeding should be done; however it is generally otherwise well tolerated.

Another biological-based product called Hawthorn extract has been proposed to treat CHF due to its effect on relaxing blood vessels. A Cochrane database review examined 14 RCTs and concluded that Hawthorn extract is a reasonable adjunctive treatment for CHF in combination with conventional treatments (Pittler and Ernst 2013). Hawthorn extract demonstrated significant benefit in exercise tolerance as well as cardiac oxygen consumption. Recommended dosages of Hawthorn extract for therapeutic effect on CHF range from 600 to 1,800 mg/day (Kaback et al. 2011).

Coenzyme Q10 (CoQ10) also called ubiquinone is an essential component of mitochondria and therefore plays a key role in energy production. Levels of coenzyme Q10 are known to be reduced with hypertension, CAD, high cholesterol, diabetes, and atherosclerosis (Sinatra and Houston 2011). A RCT of 60 mg of CoQ10 showed a significant reduction in systolic blood pressure (Burke et al. 2001). CoQ10 is an evidenced-based alternative approach to reducing blood pressure.

As mentioned previously the consumption of fatty fish is related to reduced cardiovascular disease; additionally there also appears to be a benefit of omega-3 fatty acid supplementation. The GISSI-HF trial demonstrated a reduction in mortality when individuals with CHF were given 1 g of omega-3 fatty acid per day (Gissi-HF investigators et al. 2008). Therefore the regular consumption of fatty fish as well as supplemental omega-3 fatty acids provides cardiovascular protection.

25.6 Treatment of Depression and Cardiovascular Disease

Cardiovascular disease increases the risk for depression. Approximately 20 % of individuals who have suffered an MI have major depressive disorder (Thombs et al. 2005). Detecting and treating depression in individuals who have suffered an MI are essential due to the fact that depression increases mortality and morbidity. Studies show that depression can double the risk of cardiac events after an MI (Lichtman et al. 2008). Fortunately, studies show that depression in individuals suffering from cardiovascular disease is treatable and improves cardiovascular outcomes. Results from the SADHART study (Sertraline Antidepressant Heart Attack Randomized Trial) demonstrated the safety of sertraline 50–200 mg in treating individuals who have recently suffered an MI or have unstable angina (Glassman et al. 2002). Surprisingly, the SADHART study demonstrated a nonsignificant trend toward reducing incidence of death, myocardial infarction, congestive heart failure, stroke, and recurrent angina (Joynt and O'Connor 2005). Medications are not the only evidence-based treatment approach to treating the complications of depression on cardiovascular disease. The ENRICHD (Enhancing Recovery in Coronary Heart Disease) study examined the impact of Cognitive Behavioral Therapy (CBT) on depression after suffering an MI. The results demonstrated CBT was effective at treating depression after 6 months, but the results did not persist at 30-month follow-up and there was no trend to impacting survival (ENRICHD 2003). Therefore, depression in the context of cardiovascular disease is treatable and should be addressed as both mental and physical benefits can develop from such treatment.

Many epidemiological studies have shown a link between inflammation and disorders such as depression or heart disease. Consuming a diet with limited amounts of fruits, vegetables, and whole grains and high amounts of refined grains, processed meat, sugar, and saturated- and trans-fatty acids promotes inflammation (Kiecolt-Glaser et al. 2010), which can lead to diseases such as depression and cardiovascular disease. Interleukin-6 (IL-6) and C-reactive protein (CRP) are two inflammatory markers in the body that are increased with the consumption of meals with high amounts of fat (Kiecolt-Glaser et al. 2010). Nutrition is an integrative treatment approach to preventing various diseases based on minimizing inflammation that contributes to the development of heart disease and also depression.

The impact on nutrition on mental health is a growing field. There is an impact of heart healthy diets, such as DASH as also having an impact on mental illness (Torres and Nowson 2012). A meta-analysis demonstrated the Mediterranean diet reduces the risk for development of depression (RR 0.68) (Psaltopoulou et al. 2013). Additionally, low dietary consumption of seafood is associated with increased risk in the development of depression and bipolar disorder (Hibbeln and Gow 2014), while regular fish consumption decreased the risk of depression and suicidal ideation (Hibbeln and Gow 2014). Low levels of omega-3 fatty acids are implicated in depression due to a reduction in the serotonin and dopamine systems as seen through animal studies (Hibbeln and Gow 2014). A meta-analysis demonstrated the antidepressant effect of providing omega-3 fatty acid supplementation (Sublette et al. 2011). Therefore the Mediterranean diet and moderate consumption of fish oil appear to prevent depression as well as previously mentioned risk reduction for cardiovascular disease.

Folate is abundant in foods and is generally considered part of a healthy diet which includes large quantities of fruits and vegetables, and because of this overlap, it is difficult to discern how much of the benefit from the healthy diet on mood is actually coming from folate versus other nutrients. Nevertheless, depression occurs more commonly in individuals with low levels of folate, and treatment with standard antidepressants is not very successful with folate deficiencies (Papakostas et al. 2012). In a trial of individuals suffering from depression, l-methylfolate supplementation provided better response when being treated with a selective serotonin reuptake inhibitor (SSRI) (Papakostas et al. 2012). Therefore, evidence supports the use of folate supplementation in the treatment of depression.

25.7 Exercise

In addition to the cardiovascular benefits of exercise, there appears to be a significant impact of exercise on mental health as well (Table 25.1). Aerobic exercise conveys an antidepressant and anxiolytic effect that can impact aging outcomes as well (Salmon 2001). Studies from both human and animals have shown a connection between exercise and brain health. In older adults exercise affects memory and learning thereby affecting neurodegeneration as well as depression. Given the connection between vascular disease and depression and neurodegeneration in the elderly, it is not surprising that exercise can benefit these disease states. Late-life depression is oftentimes related to cognitive decline for which cardiovascular disease is a risk factor (Cotman et al. 2007). Studies have demonstrated a significant impact of exercise on multiple brain areas, however, most consistently have been the hippocampus (Cotman et al. 2007). Both aerobic exercise and resistance training improve depression in geriatric individuals as well as younger adults with results comparable to traditional antidepressants (Blumenthal et al. 1999). Taken together with the previously discussed benefits of exercise on cardiovascular disease and the antidepressant effect of exercise, clinicians should encourage exercise for better mental and physical results in their patients.

25.8 Mind-Body Approaches and Depression

There are several studies showing some improvement in mood with acupuncture. A pilot study of acupuncture and late-life depression demonstrated an antidepressant effect (Williams and Graham 2006). Another study in China demonstrated an antidepressant effect of "mind-refreshing antidepressive" acupuncture was as effective as doxepin and more effective than acupuncture alone in a group of approximately 100 adults with "post-wind stroke depression," which is a traditional Chinese diagnosis (Li et al. 1994). The evidence is growing for the role of acupuncture as an antidepressant treatment for late-life depression.

Tai Chi is effective in treating late-life depression. A shortened and manual-based version of Tai Chi called Tai Chi Chih showed an antidepressant effect and improvement in both cognition and physical functioning as well as a reduction in the inflammatory marker CRP when compared to a control group consisting of a health education classes (Lavretsky et al. 2011). Therefore, Tai Chi offers an effective intervention for physical and mental well-being in older adults.

25.9 Biologically Based Products and Depression

Omega-3 fatty acid has both cardiovascular benefits and antidepressant effects (Table 25.1). Low levels of omega-3 fatty acids have been implicated in individuals suffering from suicidal ideation and depression (Hibbeln 1998; Tanskanen et al. 2001; Timonen et al. 2004). Diagnosis of a clinical depression as opposed to minor depressive symptoms appears to benefit the most from omega-3 fatty acid supplementation (Appleton et al. 2010). It appears that a higher concentration of EPA (≥60 % of EPA) versus DHA provided a better therapeutic effect on depression (Sublette et al. 2011). The data supporting an antidepressant effect of omega-3 fatty acids is less extensive in the geriatric population, however still promising. A RCT was performed in older adults living in an SNF and demonstrated a benefit to depression as well as quality of life (Rondanelli et al. 2011). Additionally an RCT of older adults who had suffered an MI showed an antidepressant effect of omega-3 fatty acid supplementation only when they had a clinical episode of depression, not simply depressive symptoms (Giltay et al. 2011). There is an effect of omega-3 fatty acid supplementation in late-life depression.

St. John's Wort (SJW) (*Hypericum perforatum*) is a well-substantiated alternative treatment for depression in the general adult and older adult populations (Table 25.1). There are several standardized extracts available that have been studied in various trials. A Cochrane database review of 23 randomized trials of adults with mild-to-moderate depression demonstrated an antidepressant effect of SJW (Linde et al. 2008). The typical dosage of SJW was 300–1,000 mg daily. An additional meta-analysis demonstrated the antidepressant effect of SJW to be comparable to standard antidepressants such as tricyclic antidepressants and SSRIs (Kasper 2010). As with all depression treatments, there are fewer trials involving older adults and SJW. However of the available trials, there does appear to be some antidepressant effect of standard extracts of SJW. A 6-week RCT showed SJW to be equally effective to treating depression as fluoxetine in moderately depressed older adults (Harrer et al. 1999). In an additional trial consisting of mixed-aged adults, SJW treated atypical depression (Mannel et al. 2010). Therefore, the few studies available which include older adults support the use of SJW for depression. In general, SJW is well tolerated when used alone; however there are several noteworthy interactions. SJW acts as a monoamine oxidase inhibitor (MAOI) making its combination with standard antidepressants concerning for precipitating a serotonin syndrome. SJW is also an inducer of cytochrome P-450 3A4 liver enzyme system which leads to reductions in multiple medications such as coumadin, methadone, alprazolam, clopidogrel, cyclosporine, and verapamil. SJW has also been seen to precipitate a manic episode (Kaustubh and Faubion 2005). SJW is an alternative natural remedy for mild-to-moderate depression, but the potential side effects should be monitored similar to a traditional treatment approach.

S-adenosyl-L-methionine (SAMe) is a biologically based product which is involved in the metabolic pathway involving folic acid and vitamin B12 (Mischoulon and Fava 2002; Papakostas 2009). SAMe is a cofactor in the development of serotonin, norepinephrine, and dopamine and therefore plays a role in depression

(Paul et al. 2004). Furthermore individuals suffering from depression appear to have lower levels of SAMe compared to nondepressed individuals, and treatment has been shown to increase these deficiencies (Bottiglieri et al. 1990). In the general adult population, meta-analyses have demonstrated parenteral SAMe to be equally effective as TCAs and superior to placebo (Bressa 1994). In terms of oral formulations of SAMe, an open trial in a mixed-aged population demonstrated SAMe to be an effective augmentation strategy in participants taking conventional antidepressants (Alpert et al. 2004). A study looking at late-life depression in the context of Parkinson's disease showed an antidepressant effect of SAMe (DiRocco et al. 2007). Most studies demonstrated a therapeutic effect of SAMe in the range of 800–1,600 mg/day (Mischoulon and Fava 2002), but dosages up to 3,600 mg/day have been successfully administered in late-life depression (DiRocco et al. 2007). SAMe is fairly well tolerated but should be cautiously used if at all in individuals with bipolar disorder due to the possibility of triggering a manic episode or suicidal ideation (Carney et al. 1987; Chitiva et al. 2012). SAMe is an alternative antidepressant for mildly depressed patients or patient with difficulty tolerating multiple side effects to medications (Mischoulon and Fava 2002).

Conclusion

Depression is an unfortunate consequence of cardiovascular disease and both often co-occur with aging. Preventative and treatment interventions for both depression and cardiovascular disease oftentimes overlap. Nutritional approaches including the Mediterranean diet, DASH diet, and consumption of fatty fish appear to reduce both depression and cardiovascular disease. Additionally several integrative approaches including acupuncture and Tai Chi have been seen to improve outcomes in both conditions. There are also various natural products and supplements which can be utilized to treat depression and cardiovascular disease, some of which overlap such as omega-3 fatty acids while others do not. Table 25.1 demonstrates a summary of treatment approaches for depression and cardiovascular disease. Having an understanding of the various treatment and preventative approaches to targeting these serious disease states can help older adults feel empowered about their treatment.

References

Abbott R, Lavretsky H (2013) Tai Chi and Qigong for the treatment and prevention of mental disorders. Psychiatr Clin North Am 36(1):109–119

Alexopoulos GS, Meyers BS, Young RC, Campbell S, Silbersweig D, Charlson M (1997) 'Vascular depression' hypothesis. Arch Gen Psychiatry 54(10):915–922

Alexopoulos GS, Bruce M, Silbersweig D, Kalayam B, Stern E (1999) Vascular depression: a new view of late-onset depression. Dialogues Clin Neurosci 11(2):68–80

Alpert JE et al (2004) S-adenosyl-L-methionine (SAMe) as an adjunct for resistant major depressive disorder. J Clin Psychopharmacol 24(6):661–664

Anderson JW, Liu C, Krysico RJ (2008) Blood pressure response to transcendental meditation. Am. J. Hypertension 21:310–316

Appel L, Moore T, Obarzanek E et al (1997) Clinical trial of the effects of dietary patterns on blood pressure. N Engl J Med 336(16):1117–1124
Appleton KM, Rogers PJ, Ness AR (2010) Updated systematic review and meta-analysis of the effects of n-3 long-chain polyunsaturated fatty acids on depressed mood. Am J Clin Nutr 91:757–770
Banel D, Hu FB (2009) Effects of walnut consumption on blood lipids and other cardiovascular risk factors: a meta-analysis and systematic review. Am J Clin Nutr 90(1):56–63
Blumenthal JA, Babyak MA, Moore KA, Craighead WE, Herman S, Khatri P et al (1999) Effects of exercise training on older patients with major depression. Arch Intern Med 159:2349–2356
Bomhof-Roordink H, Seldenrijk A, van Hout H et al (2015) Associations between life stress and subclinical cardiovascular disease are partly medicated by depressive and anxiety symptoms. J Psychosom Res 78:332–339
Bonura KB, Tenenbaum G (2014) Effects of yoga on psychological health in older adults. Phys Act Health 11(7):1334–1341
Bottiglieri T et al (1990) Cerebrospinal fluid S-adenosylmethionine in depression and dementia: effects of treatment with parenteral and oral S-adenosylmethionine. J Neurol Neurosurg Psychiatry 53:1096–1098
Bressa GM (1994) S-adenosyl-l-methionine (SAMe) as antidepressant: meta-analysis of clinical studies. Acta Neurol Scand Supplementum 154:7–14
Burke BE, Neuenschwander R, Olson R (2001) Randomized, double-blind placebo-controlled trial of Coenzyme Q10 in isolated systolic hypertension. South Med J 94(11):1112–1117
Carney MW, Chary TK, Bottiglieri T, Reynolds EH, Toone BK (1987) Switch mechanism in affective illness and oral S-adenosylmethionine (SAM). Br J Psychiatry: J Ment Sci 150: 724–725
Chitiva H, Audivert F, Alvarez C (2012) Suicide attempt by self-burning associated with ingestion of S-adenosylmethionine. J Nerv Ment Dis 200:99–101
Cho KI, Shim WJ, Park SM, Dim MA, Kim HL, Son JW (2015) Association of depression with coronary artery disease and QTc interval prolongation in women with chest pain: data from the KoRean wOmen's chest pain REgistry (KoROSE) study. Physiol Behav 143:45–50
Cotman CW, Berchtold NC, Christie LA (2007) Exercise builds brain health: key roles of growth factor cascades and inflammation. Trends Neurosci 30:464–472
Darden D, Richardson C, Jackson EA (2013) Physical activity and exercise for secondary prevention among patients with cardiovascular disease. Curr Cardiovasc Risk Rep 7(6):446–452
de Lorgeril M, Renaud S, Mamelle N et al (1994) Mediterranean alpha-linolenic acid-rich diet in secondary prevention of coronary heart disease. Lancet 343:1454–1459
de Lorgeril M, Salen P, Martin JL, Monjaud I, Delaye J, Mamelle N (1999) Mediterranean diet, traditional risk factos, and the rate of cardiovascular complications after myocardial infarction. Circulation 99:779–785
Di Castenuovo A, Costanzo S, Bagnardi V et al (2006) Alcohol dosing and total mortality in men and women. Arch Intern Med 166:2437–2445
DiRocco A et al (2007) S-adenosyl-methionine improves mdepression in patients with Parkinson's disease in an open-label clinical trial. Mov Disord 15(6):1225–1229
Drenowatz C, Sui X, Fritz S et al (2014) The association between resistance exercise and cardiovascular disease risk in women. J Sci Med Sport 23:1207–1208
ENRICHD writing committee (2003) Effects of treating depression and low perceived social support on clinical events after myocardial infarction. JAMA 289:3106–3116
Estruch R, Ros E, Salas-Salvado J et al (2013) Primary prevention of cardiovascular disease with a Mediterranean diet. N Engl J Med 368(14):1279–1290
Eurelings L, Richard E, Eikelenboom P et al (2015) Low-grade inflammation differentiates between symptoms of apathy and depression in community-dwelling older individuals. Int Psychogeriatr 27(4):639–647
Fiedorowicz JG (2014) Depression and cardiovascular disease: an update on how course of illness may influence risk. Curr Psychiatry Rep 16(10):492

Giltay E, Geleijinse JM, Dromhout D (2011) Effects of n-3 fatty acids on depressive symptoms and dispositional optimism after myocardial infarction. Am J Clin Nutr 94:1442–1450

Gissi-HF Investigators, Tavazzi L, Maggioni AP, Marchioli R et al (2008) Effect of n-3 polyunsaturated fatty acids in patients with chronic heart failure (the GISSI-HF trial): a randomized, double-blind, placebo-controlled trial. Lancet 372:1223–1230

Glassman AH, O'Connor CM, Califf RM et al (2002) Sertraline treatment of major depression in patients with acute MI or unstable angina. JAMA 288(6):1701–1720

Harrer G, Schmidt U, Kuhn U, Biller A (1999) Comparison of equivalence between the St. John's wort extract LoHyp-57 and fluoxetine. Arzneimittelforschung 49:289–296

Hibbeln JR (1998) Fish consumption and major depression. Lancet 351:1213

Hibbeln JR, Gow RV (2014) The potential for military diets to reduce depression, suicide, and impulsive aggression: a review of current evidence for omega-3 and omega-6 fatty acids. Mil Med 179(11):117–128

Joynt KE, O'Connor CM (2005) Lessons from SADHART, ENRICH and other trials. Psychosom Med 67S:563–566

Kaback E, Lipsenthal L, Guarneri M (2011) In: Devries S, Dalen JE (eds) Integrative approaches to heart failure in integrative cardiology. Oxford University, New York, pp 265–288

Kastorini CM, Milionis HJ, Esposito K, Giugliano D, Goudevenos JA, Panagiotakos DB et al (2011) The effect of Mediterranean diet on metabolic syndrome and its components: a meta-analysis of 50 studies and 534,906 individuals. J Am Coll Cardiol 15(57):1299–1313

Kasper S, Gastpar M, Moller HJ, Muller WE, Volz HP, Dienel A, Kieser M (2010) Better tolerability of St. John's wort extract WS 5570 compared to treatment with SSRIs: a reanalysis of data from controlled clinical trials in acute major depression. Int Clin Psychopharmacol 25:204–213

Kaustubh JG, Faubion MD (2005) Mania and psychosis associated with St. John's wort and ginseng. Psychiatry 2:56–61

Kiecolt-Glaser JK, Christian L, Preston H, Houts CR, Malarkey WB, Emery CF et al (2010) Stress, inflammation, and yoga practice. Psychosom Med 72:113–121

Kloner RA, Rezkalla SH (2007) To drink or not to drink? That is the question. Circulation 116:1306–1317

Kris-Etherton P, Harris WS, Appel LJ (2002) American Heart Association. Nutrition Committee. Fish consumption, fish oil, omega 3 fatty acids and cardiovascular disease. Circulation 106(21):2747–2757

Krishnan K, Hayes J, Blazer (1997) MRI-defined vascular depression. Am J Psychiatry 154:497–501

Lan C, Chen SY, Wong MK, Lai JS (2013) Tai Chi Chuan for patients with cardiovascular disease. Evid Based Complement Alternat Med 2013:1–9

Lavretsky H, Alstein LL, Olmstead RE, Ercoli LM, Riparetti-Brown M, Cyr NS et al (2011) Complementary use of tai chi chih augments escitalopram treatment of geriatric depression: a randomized controlled trial. Am J Geriatr Psychiatry 19(10):839–850

Lavretsky H, Reinlieb M, St Cyr N, Siddarth P, Ercoli L, Senturk D (2015) Citalopram, methylphenidate, or their combination in geriatric depression: a randomized, double-blind, placebo-controlled trial. Am J Psychiatry 55:1–9

Lebowitz KR (2011) Cardiac behavioral medicine: mind-body approaches to heart health. In: Devries S, Dalen JE (eds) Integrative cardiology. Oxford University, New York, pp 135–168

Lee LY, Lee DT, Woo J (2010) The psychosocial effect of Tai Chi on nursing home residents. J Clin Nurs 19:927–938

Li CD, Huang Y, Li YK, Hu KM, Jiang ZY (1994) Treating post-stroke depression with "mind-refreshing antidepressive" acupuncture therapy: a clinical study of 21 cases. Int J Clin Acupunct 5:389–393

Li DZ, Zhou Y, Yang YN et al (2014) Acupuncture for essential hypertension: a meta-analysis of randomized sham-controlled clinical trials. Evid Based Complement Alternat Med 9:1–7

Lichtman JH, Bigger JT, Blumenthal JA et al (2008) Depression and coronary heart disease recommendations for screening, referral, and treatment. Prog Cardiovasc Nurs 118:1768–1775

Linde K, Berner MM, Kriston L (2008) St John's wort for major depression. Cochrane Database Syst Rev 8:CD000448
Longhurst J (2011) Acupuncture in cardiovascular medicine. In: Devries S, Dalen JE (eds) Integrative cardiology. Oxford University, New York, pp 100–116
Low Dog T (2011) Botanical medicine and cardiovascular disease. In: Devries S, Dalen JE (eds) Integrative cardiology. Oxford University, New York, pp 55–69
Macklin EA, Wayne PM, Kalish LA et al (2006) Stop hypertension with the acupuncture research program (SHARP) results from a randomized controlled clinical trial. Hypertension 48:838–845
Mannel M, Kuhn U, Schmidt U, Ploch M, Murck H (2010) St. John's wort extract L160 for the treatment of depression with atypical features-a double-blind randomized, and placebo-controlled trial. J Psychiatr Res 44:760–767
Mente A, de Koning L, Shannon HS et al (2009) A systematic review if the evidence supporting a causal link between dietary factors and coronary heart disease. Arch Intern Med 169(7):659–669
Mellen PB, Walsh TF, Herrington DM (2008) Whole grain intake and cardiovascular disease: a meta-analysis. Nutr Metab Cardiovasc Dis 18:283–290
Mischoulon D, Fava M (2002) Role of S-adenosyl-L-methionine in the treatment of depression: a review of the evidence. Am J Clin Nutr 76:1158S–1161S
Nowson CA, Wattanapenpaiboon N, Pachett A (2008) Low-sodium dietary approaches to stop hypertension-type diet including lean red meat lowers blood pressure in postmenopausal women. Nutr Res 29:8–18
Papakostas GI (2009) Evidence for S-adenosyl-L-methionine (SAM-e) for the treatment of major depressive disorder. J Clin Psychiatry 70(Suppl 5):18–22
Papakostas GI et al (2012) L-methylfolate as adjunctive therapy for SSRI-resistant major depression : results of two randomized, double blind, parallel-sequential trials. Am J Psychiatry 169(12):1267–1274
Patel NK, Newstead AH, Ferrer RL (2012) The effects of yoga on physical functioning and health related quality of life in older adults : a systematic review and meta-analysis. J Alternat Complement Med 18(10):902–917
Paul RT, McDonnell AP, Kelly CB (2004) Folic acid: neurochemistry, metabolism and relationship to depression. Hum Psychopharmacol 19:477–488
Peters U, Poole C, Arab L (2001) Does tea affect cardiovascular disease? A meta-analysis. Am J Epidemiol 154(6):496–503
Pittler MH, Ernst E (2012) Horse chestnut seed extract for chronic venous insufficiency. Cochrane Collab 11:CD003230
Pittler MH, Ernst E (2013) Hawthorn extract for treating chronic heart failure. Cochrane Collab 8:57–109
Pittler MH, Guo R, Ernst E (2008). Hawthorn extract for treating chronic heart failure. Cochrane Database Syst Rev (1):CD005312.
Psaltopoulou T, Sergentanis TN, Panagiotakos DB et al (2013) Mediterranean diet, stroke, cognitive impairment, and depression: a meta-analysis. Ann Neurol 74(4):580–591
Rondanelli M, Giacosa A, Opizzi A et al (2011) Long chain omega 3 polyunsaturated fatty acids supplementation in the treatment of elderly depression: effects on depressive symptoms, on phospholipids fatty acids profile and on health-related quality of life. J Nutr Health Aging 15:37–44
Rudisch B, Nemeroff CB (2003) Epidemiology of cormorbid coronary artery disease and depression. Biol Psychiatry 54:227–240
Sacks FM, Svetkey LP, Vollmer WM et al (2001) Effects on blood pressure of reduced dietary sodium and the dietary approaches to stop hypertension (DASH) diet. N Engl J Med 344(1):3–10
Salmon P (2001) Effects of physical exercise on anxiety, depression, and sensitivity to stress: a unifying theory. Clin Psychol Rev 21:33–61

Schneider B, Ercoli L, Siddarth P, Lavretsky H (2012) Vascular burden and cognitive functioning in depressed older adults. Am J Geriatr Psychiatry 20(8):673–681
Sinatra ST, Houston MC (2011) The integrative approach to hypertension. In: Devries S, Dalen JE (eds) Integrative cardiology. Oxford University, New York, pp 224–246
Sublette ME, Steven PE, Gleant AL, Mann JJ (2011) Meta-analysis of the effects of eicosapentaenoic acid (EPA) in clinical trials in depression. J Clin Psychiatry 72:1577–1584
Tanskanen A, Hibbeln JR, Hintikka J, Haatainen K, Honkalampi K, Viinamaki H (2001) Fish consumption, depression, and suicidality in a general population. Arch Gen Psychiatry 58:512–513
Tighe P, Duthie G, Vaughan N et al (2010) Effect of increased consumption of whole-grain foods on blood pressure and other cardiovascular risk markers in healthy middle-aged persons: a randomized controlled trial. Am J Clin Nutr 92(4):733–740
Timonen M, Horrobin D, Jokelainen J, Laitinen J, Herva A, Rasanen P (2004) Fish consumption and depression: the northern Finland 1966 birth cohort study. J Affect Disord 82:447–452
Torres SJ, Nowson CA (2012) A moderate-sodium DASH-type diet improves mood in postmenopausal women. Nutrition 28:896–900
Thombs BD, Bass EB, Ford DE, Stewart KJ, Konstantinos KT, Patel U et al (2005) Prevalence of depression in survivors of acute myocardial infarction. J Gen Intern Med 21:30–38
Tsai JC, Wang WH, Chan P et al (2003) The beneficial effects of Tai Chi Chuan on blood pressure and lipid profile and anxiety status in a randomized controlled trial. J Altern Complement Med 9(5):747–754
Van Sloten TT, Sigurdsson S, van Buchem MA et al (2015) Cerebral small vessel disease and association with higher incidence of depressive symptoms in a general elderly population: the AGES-Reykavik Study. Am J Psychiatry 1–9
Widmer RJ, Flammer AJ, Lerman LO, Lerman A (2015) The Mediterranean diet, its components, and cardiovascular disease. Am J Med 128(3):229–238
Williams PT, Thompson PD (2014) Increased cardiovascular disease mortality associated with excessive exercise in heart attack survivors. Mayo Clin Proc 89(9):1187–1194
Williams J, Grahm C (2006) Acupuncture for older adults with depression–a pilot study to assess acceptability and feasibility. Int J Geriatr Psychiatry 21(6):599–600
Xiang X, An R (2015) Depression and onset of cardiovascular disease in the US middle-aged and older adults. Aging Ment Health 19(12):1084–1092
Yang K (2007) A review of yoga programs for four leading risk factors of chronic disease. Evid Based Complement Alternat Med 4(4):487–491
Yogendra J, Yogendra HJ, Ambardekar S et al (2004) Beneficial effects of yoga lifestyle on reversibility of ischaemic heart disease: caring heart project of International Board of Yoga. J Assoc Physicians India 52:283–289
Zahn D, Petrak F, Franke L et al (2015) Cortisol, platelet serotonin content and platelet activity in patients with major depression and type 2 diabetes: an exploratory investigation. Psychosom Med 77:145–155
Zimmer R, Riemer T, Rauch B, Schneider S, Schiele R, Gohlke H et al (2013) Effects of 1-year treatment with highly purified omega-3 fatty acids on depression after myocardial infarction: results from OMEGA trial. J Clin Psychiatry 74(11):e1037–e1045

An Integrative Psychosomatic Approach to the Treatment of Patients with Cardiovascular Diseases: Concepts and Experiences of a Dedicated Psychocardiology Ward at the University of Göttingen Medical Center

26

Marvin Olewinski, Anne-Maria Paschke, Anahit Mohebbi, Christoph Herrmann-Lingen, and Christina Kleiber

Contents

Abstract

Mental comorbidity adversely affects quality of life, health behavior, and prognosis in cardiac patients. While this comorbidity goes untreated in many patients, others typically receive outpatient treatment with psychotherapy, antidepressant medication, or collaborative care. However, severity of heart disease or the

M. Olewinski • A.-M. Paschke • A. Mohebbi • C. Herrmann-Lingen (✉) • C. Kleiber
Department of Psychosomatic Medicine and Psychotherapy, University of Göttingen Medical Center, Von-Siebold-Str. 5, 37075 Gottingen, Germany
e-mail: marvin.olewinski@posteo.de; cherrma@gwdg.de

B.T. Baune, P.J. Tully (eds.), *Cardiovascular Diseases and Depression*,
DOI 10.1007/978-3-319-32480-7_26

mental disorders sometimes interferes with continuous outpatient treatment. For severely ill patients, simultaneous inpatient treatment of heart disease and mental comorbidity may become necessary. In the German healthcare system, statutory health insurance covers inpatient psychosomatic treatment if medically indicated. This chapter describes a model of integrated inpatient psychocardiology treatment as implemented on a dedicated ward at University of Göttingen Medical Center. The different components of the therapeutic program are outlined and vignettes of typical cases are presented. Clinical impressions and first evaluation results suggest that the psychocardiology ward closes an important gap in the care of patients with severe comorbid heart disease and mental disorders or cardiac somatization.

26.1 Introduction

Psychocardiology is a young interdisciplinary area of research and patient care. Although the epidemiological relevance of the interrelation between cardiovascular diseases and mental stress or disorders is well known, treatment attempts are often either purely somatic (as in most cardiology departments), or in some cases psychiatric/psychotherapeutic. Therefore, whole-patient care in psychocardiology still poses a challenge, even in the German healthcare system offering broad health insurance coverage for psychiatry and psychotherapy as well as for specialized psychosomatic medicine. A quick look at historical and structural backgrounds might be helpful to understand the reasons for this difficulty.

26.1.1 Psychosomatic Medicine in the German Healthcare System

Since the early twentieth century, psychotherapy wards were established in Germany, mostly in psychiatric hospitals. This development was interrupted during the Nazi regime in Germany from 1933 to 1945, when many leading psychotherapists were forced to exile. After the end of World War II, in 1950 the first German inpatient department of psychosomatic medicine was founded in Heidelberg and chaired by the psychoanalyst Alexander Mitscherlich (Hoffmann et al. 1999). This event marked the beginning of a clinical separation between psychosomatic and psychiatric institutions. Psychiatry on the one side often had a rather neurobiological view of the patients' diseases, while psychosomatic medicine, on the other side, often identified itself with psychotherapy rather than somatic medicine. In the early 1970s, courses in psychosomatic medicine and psychotherapy became mandatory for medical students. In the 1990s the field of psychosomatic medicine and psychotherapy (formerly called psychotherapeutic medicine) was acknowledged as a distinct medical specialty, requiring training in internal medicine, psychiatry, and psychosomatic medicine itself (Hoffmann et al. 1999).

Junior physicians are trained on specialized psychosomatic wards, in dedicated outpatient clinics, and consultation-liaison services and acquire profound skills and knowledge in psychotherapy with either a psychodynamic or cognitive-behavioral focus.

26.1.2 Outpatient and Inpatient Psychotherapy in Germany

The public healthcare system in Germany offers payment by statutory health insurance companies for both outpatient and inpatient psychotherapy, if patients suffer from a disorder that can effectively be treated by psychotherapy according to the available evidence. The most frequent diagnoses of patients receiving psychotherapy are anxiety disorders and depression. The classical forms of outpatient psychotherapy paid by health insurance are psychodynamic psychotherapy (both short-term psychodynamic psychotherapy and classical psychoanalysis) and (cognitive) behavioral therapy. Providers are both psychologists and physicians with a special training and board approval in psychotherapy. The choice of treatment method depends on the patient's diagnosis, on the nature of underlying personality or psychosocial problems, and also on patient preferences and the availability of therapists trained in a specific method. After up to five initial ("probatory") sessions, the indication for outpatient psychotherapy has to be confirmed by a blinded assessor at the base of an anonymized case report and treatment plan written by the therapist.

Inpatient psychotherapy is only indicated if severity and complexity of the individual case make the success of outpatient therapy unlikely at a given point of time or if outpatient treatment has already failed. Inpatient psychotherapy is typically provided in a structured format on specialized wards located in general or psychiatric hospitals or in hospitals or rehabilitation centers entirely dedicated to psychosomatic medicine (Schauenburg and Hildenbrand 2011). The decision for inpatient psychotherapy is typically made after referral of a patient by his or her GP or by another specialist (including community-based psychiatrists or psychotherapists) and an initial ambulatory encounter between the patient and hospital psychotherapist. Case conferences are often used to discuss and confirm the indication for hospital admission.

Inpatient psychotherapy is typically offered by multidisciplinary teams and combines different psychotherapeutic and medical approaches in an individualized manner. Its effects and cost-effectiveness have repeatedly been documented (Schauenburg and Hildenbrand 2011). In patients with complex disorders often seen in psychocardiology, such a multimodal and interdisciplinary approach appears essential for therapeutic progress. This can be more easily initiated in an inpatient setting, where the patient can benefit from synergies of medical, psychological, and complementary therapies. Typical weekly schedules include 20 h or more of different therapies and the typical length of stay varies between 4 and 10 weeks, which is considered necessary for initiating sustainable behavior change and symptom improvement in these severely ill patients.

After discharge from the hospital, an additional series of outpatient psychotherapy sessions is often recommended to stabilize the achieved changes and help patients back into daily life and work.

Example: A physically healthy patient suffering from a mild depressive disorder and asking for psychotherapeutic support would be treated in an outpatient setting by his or her GP and possibly a psychotherapist working in private practice. In contrast, a patient with major depression after a myocardial infarction persisting after several weeks of primary care, with several relevant comorbidities, unhealthy behavior patterns, little insight into psychosomatic aspects of his heart disease, and low motivation for psychotherapy would benefit from an integrative, multimodal inpatient treatment before eventually utilizing additional outpatient psychotherapy to complement cardiological treatment.

26.1.3 Barriers to Integrating Psychosomatic Medicine and Cardiology

At the same time when psychosomatic aspects of heart diseases started being recognized more systematically, technical developments in cardiology such as cardiac catheterization and stenting or implantable devices provided exciting and often lifesaving new therapeutic options, which strengthened a technically orientated self-image in cardiology.

For a long time, this seemed to widen the gap between the disciplines of cardiology and psychosomatic medicine. This often went – and still goes – along with mutual misunderstanding and distrust. While cardiologists often look at psychotherapists as poorly skilled mystics, psychotherapists sometimes see cardiologists as inhumane technicians.

While basic training in psychosomatic medicine has long been a mandatory part of specialty training in German gynecology and family medicine, no such training is required for internists or cardiologists. On the other hand, as mentioned above, many psychotherapists have little knowledge of heart diseases and their treatment.

Additionally, clinical work in cardiology happens under ever-increasing time pressure, and physicians or hospitals receive far better payments for technical procedures than for personal attention and verbal interventions. Under these adverse circumstances, only few physicians specialized in psychosomatic medicine or psychologists trained in psychotherapy as well as somatically trained physicians have attempted to overcome the traditional gap between mind and body in cardiology. The way to establish psychocardiology in Germany was therefore long and sometimes complicated (Herrmann-Lingen 2011a), but it finally resulted in several interdisciplinary projects such as development of medical guidelines and training courses in basic psychocardiology for cardiologists and psychologists/psychiatrists (Herrmann-Lingen 2011b) and also in the formation of interdisciplinary treatment models. One of these models is the psychocardiology ward at our university hospital, which opened in 2009.

26.1.4 The Psychocardiology Ward at University of Göttingen Medical Center

The Department of Psychosomatic Medicine and Psychotherapy at University of Göttingen Medical Center understands itself as complementary to the biomedical hi-tech medicine offered in the university hospitals' heart center. With its focus on psychocardiology, it is actively involved in numerous research projects and clinical work on psychosomatic aspects of cardiovascular diseases (Herrmann-Lingen 2011a, b).

The psychocardiology ward provides integrated medical care and multimodal psychotherapy (Kleiber and Herrmann-Lingen 2011, 2015). On the one hand, and in contrast to most psychosomatic hospitals or wards in Germany, all human and technical resources of the biomedical heart center are available and actively involved in the treatment wherever needed. Patients can be transferred directly from cardiology wards during treatment of acute heart diseases, e.g., post-MI, or referred by external hospitals or physicians in the more chronic phase of heart disease, such as chronic heart failure. Besides treatment for their cardiac conditions, patients receive up to 6 weeks of intense psychotherapy as outlined below. Patients are admitted for inpatient treatment when severity and complexity of the biomedical and psychosocial situation do not allow sufficient outpatient treatment. Frequent indications for treatment on this ward are, for example, severe anxiety and depression after myocardial infarction, supportive treatment in emotionally distressed patients with severe heart failure before and after heart transplant, or panic disorder/post-traumatic stress disorder in patients with malignant cardiac arrhythmias after multiple shocks delivered by an implanted defibrillator. Other indications include repeated emergency admissions for cardiac somatization or hypertensive crises and maladaptive behavior patterns interfering with the treatment of heart diseases.

The ward is jointly led by the departments of psychosomatic medicine and cardiology and senior physicians from both departments share final responsibility for patient care. The team consists of physicians trained in psychosomatic medicine and psychotherapy, one physician in training for cardiology, and one or two psychologists. Furthermore, two part-time physiotherapists, one art therapist, and one part-time social worker belong to the team. Nine full-time posts for nurses guarantee continuous availability of support. While most patients are more or less mobile and able to perform basic self-care activities, nurses play an important part both in the medical and psychotherapeutic treatment process by arranging medical diagnostics, offering crisis intervention, and leading patient groups and relaxation training.

The psychosomatic treatment program comprises on the one hand biomedical diagnostics and treatment as needed. While some patients are too frightened to undergo medically indicated and prognostically important procedures and need much reassurance or even personal company by a familiar team member in order to consent to an invasive procedure or magnetic resonance scan, others demand medically useless repeated diagnostics for reassurance, which is often short-lived. On the other hand, the program consists of an intensive psychotherapy regime integrating psychodynamic, cognitive-behavioral, bio-psychological, and complementary elements. It is based on detailed biopsychosocial assessment including a thorough case history, from which a detailed behavior analysis or psychodynamic hypothesis is generated, serving as a prerequisite for agreeing with the patient on individual therapeutic goals. Diagnoses are made by diagnostic interview according to ICD-10. In addition, patients fill in validated psychometric questionnaires at admission and before discharge. The instruments used include the German version of the Brief Symptom Inventory (BSI; Franke 2000) covering a variety of psychological symptoms such as anxiety and depressive symptoms, the short version of the Gießen symptom checklist (GBB; Brähler et al. 2000) assessing bodily symptoms, the European Quality of Life Questionnaire (EQ-5D; Greiner et al. 2005) as a global measure of health-related quality of life, and the General Self-Efficacy Scale (GSE-6; Romppel et al. 2013). Individual and group psychotherapy is offered with either a cognitive-behavioral or a psychodynamic focus. Psychoeducation provides information about relevant topics such as stress, sleep, depression, anxiety, and cardiovascular diseases. Complementary therapies such as art therapy and body therapy help to express and modify emotions by mainly nonverbal methods. These therapies are combined with relaxation training such as progressive muscle relaxation and biofeedback. The latter are used for altering individual cardiovascular stress responses to emotional stressors. Physical activation and training and – if individually indicated – physiotherapy are used to help patients regain confidence into the regular functioning of their bodies. Based on patients' and therapists' experiences during the different treatment modules, the team and patient develop a common understanding of individual problems, resources, and realistic solutions. For this purpose, continuous and reliable communication among all team members and with the patient is essential. Regular team conferences, patient groups, and ward rounds are useful for this purpose.

A typical weekly therapy schedule for a particular patient is shown in Table 26.1 (medical treatments and procedures are often difficult to schedule and typically take place during blank time slots or sometimes instead of a scheduled therapeutic session):

The combination of different therapies and the simultaneous and equal consideration of both physical and psychosocial aspects of health and disease often help the patient to gain better cognitive and emotional insight into his or her individual situation, reinforcing sense of coherence and feelings of self-efficacy. It helps to improve emotional awareness and competence in dealing with the heart disease. Maladaptive behavior or interaction patterns can be observed and often reshaped immediately. Long-lasting behaviors such as smoking or overwork can be discussed and motivation for sustainable change can be built up. Before discharge, achievement of initial goals and next steps are discussed with the patient. In addition, symptomatic improvement can be quantified by the psychometric scales completed again before discharge.

Table 26.1 Example of a 1-week patient schedule

Example for patient schedule			Group A		Slot A5
Time	Monday	Tuesday	Wednesday	Thursday	Friday
7:45–8:45	Morning meeting Walking group	Meeting with physician Walking group	Morning meeting Walking group	Meeting with physician Walking group	Morning meeting Walking group
09:00–10:00	**Ward round 9–9:30**		**Ward round with (vice) Med. Dir. 9–9:30**		**Ward round 9:40–10:10**
10:00–11:00			**Exercise training**		
11:00–12:00	Group psychotherapy	**Individual psychotherapy**		Group psychoeducation	Group psychotherapy
12:00–13:00	*Lunch break*	*Lunch break*	*Lunch break*	*Lunch break*	*Lunch break*
13:00–14:00	**Individual art therapy**				
14:00–15:00	Group body therapy 14:00–15:15			Group art therapy 14:30–16:10	**Individual psychotherapy**
15:00–16:00					
16:00–17:00					
17:00–17:30	Evening meeting	Evening meeting	Evening meeting	Evening meeting	Evening meeting
17:30–18:00	Relaxation training	Relaxation training	Relaxation training	Relaxation training	Relaxation training
18:30–19:00	*Supper break*	*Supper break*	*Supper break*	*Supper break*	*Supper break*
19:15–19:45	Walking group	Walking group	Walking group	Walking group	Walking group

26.2 Case Vignettes

The following case vignettes are intended to illustrate individually different clinical approaches to psychocardiological problems.

26.2.1 Case 1: Cardiac Arrhythmias, Anxiety, and Depression

Mrs. B., a 45-year-old patient with complete situs inversus, suffers from sick sinus syndrome with symptomatic bradycardia and paroxysmal tachyarrhythmic atrial fibrillation. A cardiac pacemaker had been implanted 2 years ago. Her recent cardiac and general medical status has been stable. She was referred by her outpatient cardiologist due to unclear vertigo attacks, drowsiness, nausea, and subjective cardiac irregularity going along with a feeling of pressure in her throat. Recently, she had consulted several physicians, especially cardiologists. The possibility of an ablation therapy was discussed but, due to her situs inversus and an inconsistency of clinical complaints and objective arrhythmia, not realized. Mrs. B. had developed increased anxiety related to her symptoms and had become unable to continue working as a committed nurse. Social withdrawal and avoidance behavior furthermore led to significant depressive symptoms.

In a first contact, she appears graceful, friendly, and insecure. Her social situation reveals that she is divorced and has not had a close partnership for many years. Her grown-up daughter recently moved out to pursue her academic studies. There is only little contact with her family members, especially no contact to her mother. Her brothers and sisters are reported to have alcohol-related problems. The patients' father is unknown. The ex-husband refuses to support the patient and her daughter adequately. Biography reveals that the patient grew up in Eastern Europe and came to Germany at age 25. Her mother was single, appears to have had emotionally unstable personality traits, and showed little affection for the patient.

During the therapeutic process, it was possible to discuss relations between Mrs. B.'s psychosocial situation, her biography, and her current medical illness. It appeared that the patient had developed a high altruistic motivation with a lack of capabilities to recognize her own individual limits and needs. The lack of appreciation for her altruism in the context of reduced capacities due to her medical situation and the recent move-out of her daughter have led to destabilization with increased somatic symptoms, anxiety, and depression.

Mrs. B. was diagnosed with a secondary somatoform disorder of the cardiovascular system and major depression. Psychotherapy included individual and group therapy with psychodynamic and cognitive-behavioral elements. Together with complementary therapies such as art therapy and body psychotherapy, this helped the patient to improve her emotional self-perception and pay more attention to her needs. Parallel cardiac diagnostics were completed and a cardiac CT showed no signs of coronary alterations, which was very relieving for the patient.

At discharge her symptoms (vertigo, drowsiness, low mood) had significantly improved, and she could relate remaining symptoms to underlying emotions (such as suppressed anger) rather than the heart disease. The complexity of the case made an initial inpatient therapy necessary and helpful. In the course of inpatient treatment, she could be motivated to look for additional outpatient psychotherapy after discharge.

26.2.2 Case 2: Recurrent Ventricular Tachycardia with ICD Shocks

Mr. A., a 50-year-old man, had experienced repeated ventricular tachycardias after myocarditis. He had been implanted with a cardioverter defibrillator (ICD) that sometimes succeeded in terminating tachycardias by antitachycardic pacing (ATP). However, after ATP failure the patient had also received several DC shocks from the device. These shocks were perceived as traumatic events by the patient. He had frequent ventricular extrasystoles which he experienced as quite frightening, since he interpreted them as harbingers of new tachycardias and ICD shocks. Finally, he had been unable to leave his home, avoided any physical activity, and completely withdrew from his social contacts. Quality of life was perceived as maximally reduced. Before the arrhythmic events, the patient had led an active life, and even after the myocarditis, he had loved traveling. However, he had given up traveling after he had been frightened by an arrhythmic episode occurring in a foreign country and by the subsequent hospitalization far from home.

His main treatment goals were to reduce his anxiety, increase his mobility, and resume his physical activities and social contacts. For this purpose, stabilizing interventions and education were used as a first step to induce a feeling of security in the patient. The hospital environment and the availability of medical emergency care around the clock contributed to relieving the patients' anxiety and hyperarousal. He was better able to distinguish harmless bodily sensations such as extrasystoles from possibly dangerous arrhythmias and started regaining better confidence in his body.

In the next step, graded exposure therapy was started. Unlike typical exposure therapy with physically healthy patients, Mr. A. had to live with the possibility that indeed new tachycardias might be triggered by activity. Nevertheless, it was possible to develop with the patient an individual model of his anxiety, in which he could develop a personal understanding of his thoughts, feelings, and physical symptoms and their interdependencies. In a process of balancing possible (real) risks of inducing new arrhythmias against the benefits of a more active life, the patient became motivated to undertake first steps toward more activity. Given the real risk of cardiac complications, it was important to move ahead slowly during exposure therapy in order to not overburden the patient and trigger malignant arrhythmias. Exposure was prepared by psychoeducational group sessions on anxiety and anxiety management. It began on the lowest level of the patient's hierarchy of anxieties, namely, by walking alone in the hospital park.

For Mr. A. it was important to feel his anxiety rise during exposure and at the same time realize that no ICD shock was triggered by the situation. He could learn that anxiety increases but can be tolerated and abates after a while without further adverse consequences, such as defibrillator shocks. Developing tolerance to hardly tolerable anxiety is a key element of exposure. Many patients (and in case of cardiac comorbidity even therapists) avoid correct exposure by fighting down anxiety or leaving the frightening situation prematurely. Given the real risks involved, this is understandable, especially if no medical emergency care is easily available. However, this turns exposure ineffective and cannot induce habituation, because patients cannot make the experience that anxiety decreases by itself. In these cases, anxiety tends to persist and flare up as soon as external security provided by a safe environment is no longer available or internal mechanisms of anxiety control fail.

Once Mr. A. had understood this principle, he was able to practice on his own and increase the demand of situations to which he exposed himself. However, good preparation of exposure and discussion of experiences from the exposure with the therapist was important for guiding the process. With increasing physical activity, it also became important to discuss with a cardiologist his current cardiac status, which was re-assessed during the inpatient treatment and showed that usual physical activity was not dangerous from a somatic point of view – although no cardiologist could ever assure the patient that he would never again experience new ventricular tachycardias. The patient practiced several times per week and experienced a decline in anxiety with repeated exposure to similar situations, encouraging him to increase the difficulty of situations.

At the end of treatment, Mr. A. felt stabilized and able to perform moderate physical activities. He identified a personally appropriate limit of his physical capacity and felt confident to resume daily activities after returning home.

26.2.3 Case 3: Coronary Heart Disease, Myocardial Infarction, Depression, and Anxiety

Mr. S., a 60-year-old teacher with known three-vessel coronary heart disease who had suffered from myocardial infarction (MI) 4 years ago, was admitted for recurrent angina pectoris-like complaints combined with an intense fear of suffering another MI. The complaints did not respond to nitroglycerine. He had already undergone 12 coronary angiographies within 4 years. All invasive diagnostics showed an acceptable coronary status and no further progression of coronary atherosclerosis. The patient suffered from severe exhaustion, high inner tension, and feelings of "burnout" and guilt toward his colleagues. He felt unable to recover on weekends or during vacations and felt insufficient at work, where he was frequently confronted with children with conduct disorders. He additionally suffered from a fear of getting a malignancy or other severe disease and permanently experienced an icy cold feeling on his tongue and in his throat. Comprehensive diagnostics had not shown any evidence of a somatic cause for these symptoms. On admission he appeared slowed down and showed a tendency to ruminate. His affect was depressed with a sense of despair. Affective modulation and energy were reduced.

Treatment focused on the appropriate investigation of his medical status on the one hand and on exploring the psychosocial situation as well as individual developmental circumstances on the other hand. It was noticed that he experienced a decrease of his "heartache" immediately after admission. With this initial improvement, he tended to get into a helping position for his ward mates and showed little sense for his emotional and physical limits and exhaustion. He also could not easily show feelings of sadness and unfulfilled needs. When confronted with his strong striving for achievement, his low self-perception and self-care and feelings of shame and guilt became visible, and his heartache increased again without a somatic correlate. After spending a weekend at home for therapeutic reasons, he found several inner and outer factors that triggered his symptoms. The awareness of his lifelong pattern to ignore his personal needs and demands gave him a glimpse into the reason for his deep unhappiness and depression. He became aware of the buried parts of his self that obviously led to a chronic sense of insufficiency and depression, expressing themselves in an overly altruistic behavior, which finally resulted in severe exhaustion and may have contributed to his coronary disease. The confrontation with his inner conflicts and emotional states only became possible when the patient could find a safe environment allowing him to face his life-threatening fears and his biographically shaped essential need for security.

Consequently, he could let go of his suspicious attention to his inner bodily sensations. When he was discharged, he had gained a more meaningful life perspective, dedicating more time to his inner needs. His recurrent heartache had decreased considerably. He applied for our outpatient group therapy and began regular individual psychotherapy.

26.2.4 Summary

These vignettes illustrate typical psychocardiological cases. While outpatient treatment such as collaborative care, combining expertise from cardiology and psychotherapy or psychiatry, is very helpful for many patients, other patients do not benefit sufficiently from outpatient care but can improve markedly with interdisciplinary inpatient treatment, addressing physical and psychosocial dimensions in an integrative treatment concept and providing a safe environment, including facilities for arrhythmia monitoring, immediate cardiopulmonary resuscitation, or other cardiac interventions. Patients admitted to our ward typically have undertaken several attempts to overcome their problems. Many have had repeated hospitalizations or emergency admissions before but still the subjective burden had not diminished or even increased. Cost-effectiveness analyses studying psychosomatic inpatient treatments in other German patient groups have shown that the high cost of inpatient treatment is more than offset by future savings in both direct medical and indirect costs, such as absence from work or early retirement (Schauenburg and Hildenbrand 2011). In our own evaluation study of the psychocardiology inpatient treatment, physical symptoms (measured by the GBB) and psychological distress (measured by the BSI) decreased, while overall quality of life on the EQ-5D improved substantially during the 5–6 weeks of treatment. The improvement was widely maintained over 1–2 years of follow-up (Herrmann-Lingen et al. 2015). In detail, cardiac symptoms decreased by $d=0.84$ for pre-post and $d=0.59$ for baseline vs. 1.5-year follow-up. Effect sizes on the global severity index of the BSI were $d=0.65$ for pre-post and $d=0.45$ for baseline vs. follow-up. Global quality of life increased by $d=0.57$ during inpatient treatment and was still improved by $d=0.46$ 18 months later (all $p<0.001$). Improvement during inpatient treatment significantly predicted follow-up well-being.

26.3 What Makes Clinical Psychocardiology So Challenging?

Cardiovascular patients coming to our ward often tend to have a somatically orientated concept of their disease. And they often were not told anything else by their physicians for years or even decades. A crucial part of our work therefore is to help the patients to develop a comprehensive concept of their disease and give them back the experience of self-efficacy.

In many other psychosomatic hospitals, patients come with some basic – though often ambivalent – ideas of psychosomatic processes affecting their current illness. In contrast, patients in psychocardiology often show an extensive ambivalence. In the delicate early stages, the treating therapist must "contain" this high level of ambivalence and resulting tensions, especially in patients with structural personality deficits and somatic or somatoform disorders.

Most people suffering from "heart disease" initially expect a treatment in which they can stay passive and do not need to contribute much more than taking a medication and wait for its effect without making a conscious effort. Even medication adherence is often low (Chowdhury et al. 2013), and the demand to change one's lifestyle, especially when it goes beyond increasing levels of exercise or dietary change, often leads to resistance or frank refusal, as long as patients do not get a deeper understanding of the inner benefit they can derive from living a more health-conscious life.

26.4 The Importance of an Integrative, Multi-professional Approach

In this context, the multi-professional approach appears most helpful and important (Perk et al. 2012). Many cardiac patients have a profound though sometimes denied fear of dying and little access to their inner world. Reliable medical care and nurse support create a safe environment enabling patients to face their fears. Nonverbal therapies such as art therapy, relaxation training, and body awareness therapy open avenues for better self-perception and self-expression and help with adaptive ways of emotion regulation. Physical therapy, based on the individual goals of each patient, offers the opportunity for recovering physical strength, cardiovascular fitness, increased self-confidence, and better perception of the body as an "indicator" of feelings and emotional states. Exercise and relaxation can also be used to demonstrate cardiovascular effects of daily life situations. Psychophysiological assessment offers the opportunity to visualize effects of emotional arousal or relaxation on heart rate, blood pressure, and autonomic balance. Art therapy allows access to hidden emotions on a nonverbal level. It can also help to (re-)discover creative potential, to imagine and depict symbolic solutions (such as healing the wounded heart), and to find inner stability against traumatic intrusions. The social worker can help with putting necessary changes to the working or housing situation into practice (Bjarnason-Wehrens et al. 2007). All these elements can be reflected upon during verbal psychotherapy sessions to create a comprehensive understanding of heart-mind associations and healthy ways to deal with them.

Psychosomatic medicine in our understanding typically works as relationship medicine – both by illustrating the relationship between emotions, behavior, and bodily processes as indicated above and by building on the therapeutic relationship as a powerful therapeutic agent. In practice, the first contact may take place through the psychosomatic consultation-liaison service, often providing the first experience of a professional explicitly acknowledging the patient's suffering and distress, which is often missed in today's somatic departments because of structural factors, insufficient training of physicians, and lack of time.

This experience can encourage patients to overcome withdrawal or aggressive ways of coping and develop a sense of validation and new hope. At the same time, the perspective to have both partners for reliable communication and immediate access to diagnostic and interventional facilities whenever needed is often very much appreciated in patients feeling emotionally and physically unstable. Typical psychiatric or psychosomatic departments usually cannot provide the intensity of medical care needed for treating these subjectively and often also objectively critically ill patients. On the other hand, cardiologists often lack the skills and time to get a deeper understanding of the patients' individuality, their "non-somatic" symptoms, and available treatment options.

Effective delivery of treatment therefore requires a competent and appreciative multidisciplinary team willing to reflect their collaboration with each other and their countertransference toward their patients. Specific factors of high importance include an interdisciplinary biopsychosocial understanding between the somatic and psychosomatic clinicians as well as psychologists, nurses, and other therapists. The nursing team plays a key role as the first contact persons and sources of support for the patients. In this function, nurses often have to buffer frequent expressions of negative affect and medical urgencies. A good perception and first appraisal of critical somatic or affective events is therefore expected from the nursing team, and they are held responsible for maintaining a helpful working environment on the ward. Shaping the relationship between patients and the nursing team represents a significant diagnostic and therapeutic element, which needs regular super- and inter-vision with the team of physicians and therapists including daily opportunities for exchange, weekly team conferences discussing each individual patient, detailed case conferences for difficult or demanding patients, external supervision, etc.

With such a competent multidisciplinary team, which is often acknowledged by patients as a core factor for their symptomatic improvement, also severe emotional and physical instability can be absorbed and transformed into new learning opportunities for both patients and individual team members.

Conclusions

Integrated cardiac care and psychotherapy can successfully be implemented and delivered at a tertiary care center to treat severely ill patients with cardiac and mental comorbidity. However, treating this group of patients requires a highly competent multi-professional team. It needs sufficient funding to pay for treatments lasting several weeks. While cost-effectiveness of this concept still needs to be demonstrated, studies of psychosomatic inpatient treatments in general show promising clinical results and possibly even cost savings on the long run.

References

Bjarnason-Wehrens B, Held K, Hoberg E, Karoff M, Rauch B (2007) Deutsche Leitlinie zur Rehabilitation von Patienten mit Herz-Kreislauferkrankungen (DLL-KardReha). Clin Res Cardiol 96(Suppl 2):III/1–III/54

Brähler E, Schumacher J, Brähler C (2000) Erste gesamtdeutsche Normierung der Kurzform des Giessener Beschwerdebogens GBB-24. Psychother Psychosom Med Psychol 50:14–21

Chowdhury R, Khan H, Heydon E, Shroufi A, Fahimi S, Moore C, Stricker B, Mendis S, Hofman A, Mant J, Franco OH (2013) Adherence to cardiovascular therapy: a meta-analysis of prevalence and clinical consequences. Eur Heart J 34:2940–2948

Franke GH (2000) Brief symptom inventory von L. R. Derogatis (Kurzform der SCL-90-R): BSI Manual – Deutsche Version. Belz Test, Göttingen

Greiner W, Claes C, Busschbach JJ, von der Schulenburg JM (2005) Validating the EQ-5D with time trade off for the German population. Eur J Health Econ 6:124–130

Herrmann-Lingen C (2011a) Steps towards integrated psychosomatic medicine – the example of psychocardiology. J Psychosom Res 70:111–115

Herrmann-Lingen C (2011b) Interdisziplinäre Kursfortbildung Psychokardiologische Grundversorgung. Psychother Psych Med 61:489–490

Herrmann-Lingen C, Löser K, Kleiber C (2015) Predictors of persistent improvement in symptoms and quality of life after inpatient treatment for comorbid cardiovascular and mental illness. Psychosom Med 77:A35–A36, abstract

Hoffmann SO, Liedtke R, Schneider W, Senf W (1999) Psychosomatishce Medizin und Psychotherapie. Denkschrift zur Lage des Faches an den Hochschulen der Bundesrepublik Deutsschland. Schattauer, Stuttgart

Kleiber C, Herrmann-Lingen C (2011) Mit Herz und Seele: Psychokardiologische Konsiliar- und Liaisonarbeit. Verhaltensther Verhaltensmed 32:39–43

Kleiber C, Herrmann-Lingen C (2015) Psychokardiologie im Herzzentrum – somatische und psychotherapeutische Herausforderungen. Ärztl Psychother 10:151–155

Perk J, De Backer G, Gohlke H, Graham I, Reiner Z, Verschuren M, Albus C, Benlian P, Boysen G, Cifkova R, Deaton C, Ebrahim S, Fisher M, Germano G, Hobbs R, Hoes A, Karadeniz S, Mezzani A, Prescott E, Ryden L, Scherer M, Syvänne M, op Reimer WJ S, Vrints C, Wood D, Zamorano JL, Zannad F, European Association for Cardiovascular Prevention & Rehabilitation (EACPR), ESC Committee for Practice Guidelines (CPG) (2012) European Guidelines on cardiovascular disease prevention in clinical practice (version 2012). The Fifth Joint Task Force of the European Society of Cardiology and Other Societies on Cardiovascular Disease Prevention in Clinical Practice (constituted by representatives of nine societies and by invited experts). Eur Heart J 33:1635–1701

Romppel M, Herrmann-Lingen C, Wachter R, Edelmann F, Düngen H, Pieske B, Grande G (2013) A short form of the general self-efficacy scale (GSE-6): development, psychometric properties and validity in an intercultural non-clinical sample and a sample of patients at risk for heart failure. GMS Psychosoc Med 10:1–7

Schauenburg H, Hildenbrand G (2011) Stationäre Psychotherapie und Psychosomatik. In: Adler RH, Herzog W, Joraschky P, Köhle K, Langewitz W, Söllner W, Wesiack W (eds) Uexküll – Psychosomatische Medizin, 7th edn. Urban & Fischer, Munich, pp 561–571

Prevention of CVD in Depression

27

Kate Margaret Scott

Contents

Abstract

People with depression history develop cardiovascular diseases at a higher rate than people without depression, suggesting that current CVD prevention guidelines are less effective for this patient group. There are several reasons for this, including that screening for behavioural and biological CVD risk factors is less likely to occur among those with depression; that screening, when it does occur, comes years after depression onset allowing decades for CVD-potentiating lifestyles to become habitual; and that depression-CVD biological mediators (e.g. HPA axis dysregulation) are not a specific focus of attention in either primary care or specialist mental health services. Ways to improve CVD prevention approaches among those with depression are discussed. These include commencing screening earlier in the life (and depressive disorder) course, using

K.M. Scott, MA (Clin. Psych.), PhD
Department of Psychological Medicine, Dunedin School of Medicine, University of Otago, PO Box 913, Dunedin, New Zealand
e-mail: kate.scott@otago.ac.nz

B.T. Baune, P.J. Tully (eds.), *Cardiovascular Diseases and Depression*,
DOI 10.1007/978-3-319-32480-7_27

integrative and collaborative care approaches developed for SMI to simultaneously address physical and mental health needs in depressed patients and making greater use of psychological treatments that incorporate stress reduction components.

27.1 Introduction

This chapter takes as a starting point the well-established finding that people with depression history are at higher risk of developing cardiovascular diseases (CVD: coronary heart disease, other types of heart disease or heart failure and stroke) (Wulsin and Singla 2003; Nicholson et al. 2006; Van der Kooy et al. 2007; Scott et al. 2013). Given this elevated risk of CVD, policies and programmes aimed at prevention of CVD are of particular importance to people with depressive disorder. In this chapter current CVD prevention guidelines are discussed in terms of their application to people with depression. Suggestions for changes to improve the prevention of CVD in depression are then proposed that have implications for primary care and specialist mental health services.

The distinction between primary and secondary prevention of CVD is now seen as less useful because of the long, insidious trajectory of atherosclerosis (Perk et al. 2012). For clarity, however, this chapter is concerned with what would previously have been referred to as primary prevention of CVD: that is, interventions or approaches that are aimed at reducing incidence (number of new cases) of CVD. Prevention can be differentiated into three levels: universal approaches that are targeted at the general population, selective approaches that are targeted at population subgroups considered at high risk and indicated approaches aimed at people with signs or symptoms of the condition (Muñoz et al. 2010). Prevention of CVD in depression would therefore entail selective (focused on those with depression as the high-risk subgroup) and/or indicated (focused on depressed individuals with CVD risk factors) approaches. The first question to consider is why a selective approach focused on depression is even necessary given the existence of very comprehensive guidelines on CVD prevention in general practice (Perk et al. 2012; Mosca et al. 2011).

27.2 Why Are CVD Prevention in General Practice Guidelines Not Working for People with Depression?

Existing CVD prevention guidelines detail the parameters of the classical CVD risk factors (smoking, physical activity, BMI, waist circumference, blood pressure, total and LDL cholesterol and blood glucose/diabetes) that elevate risk. Some guidelines also discuss the contribution that psychosocial factors (low SES, depression, anxiety, hostility, stress) may make to risk with recommendation that such factors should be screened for (Perk et al. 2012). Recent developments in these guidelines emphasise the use of total risk estimation by considering the combined effect of differing combinations of risk factors including age and sex, with scoring algorithms that can calculate 10-year risk of a CVD event (Perk et al. 2012). Evidently though, such guidelines are not working well for those with depression given their elevated risk of CVD events relative to those without depression.

There are several reasons why CVD prevention guidelines may be proving less effective in the population with depression. One component of the guidelines is assessing and providing advice on the behavioural risk factors for CVD (obesity, smoking, lack of physical activity, poor diet and heavy alcohol consumption). These behaviours are known to be more prevalent among those with depression than those without (Scott et al. 2006; Bonnet et al. 2005; Appelhans et al. 2012; Payne et al. 2012), suggesting that there is a greater need for lifestyle advice in this group. In practice though, research suggests that depressed people are *less* likely to receive lifestyle advice than those without depression, either because of the competing demands of addressing both mental and physical health in the primary care consultation (Jaen et al. 1994), the GP's perception that depression is the higher priority (Jaen et al. 2001) or the GP's view that behaviour changes should not be attempted until a depressive episode has remitted (Coleman et al. 2000). Given that only around a third of depressive episodes do fully remit (Rush et al. 2006), a strategy of avoiding the topic of lifestyle change until remission of depression may allow unhealthy behaviours to become further entrenched.

A second key component of CVD prevention guidelines is screening by general practitioners for key biomarkers: lipids, blood pressure and blood glucose. Research suggests that screening may be less likely to occur among people with depression (Johnson et al. 2012; Osborn 2001) and that even when screening does occur, less aggressive interventions may be pursued (Kendrick 1996). That said, most research in this area has been conducted in relation to 'serious mental illness (SMI)', a category that predominantly consists of psychotic and bipolar disorders, so more studies are needed to determine the extent to which nonpsychotic depression affects general practice approaches to CVD biomarker screening and treatment. However, even if screening is undertaken, there remains a question around whether the timing of screening (within the lifespan) is appropriate to those with depression. In most guidelines the recommendation is that biomarker screening be commenced in middle age, for example, men >40 and women >50 (Perk et al. 2012). This is many years after the median age of onset of depression (Kessler et al. 2007), and even in young people, it is evident that depression is associated with concurrent and subsequent poor physical health (McCloughen et al. 2012; Aarons et al. 2008; Rottenberg et al. 2014). So commencing screening in middle age may actually be decades later than would be optimal for this patient group. Earlier identification of risk factors is also likely to improve adherence to prescribed medication or lifestyle advice. Treatment adherence tends to be lower among those with depression but particularly among older patients with multi-morbidity (Katon 2003).

Another reason why current CVD prevention guidelines are less effective in those with depression may be because they do not address specific biological factors that mediate the association between depression and CVD. Dysregulation of the physiological systems for handling stress, the sympathetic-adrenal-medullary

(SAM) axis and the hypothalamic-pituitary-adrenocortical (HPA) axis, has been associated with depression (Stetler and Miller 2011; Cowen 2010). This biological state of chronic stress that appears to accompany depression has a range of adverse metabolic, cardiovascular and immune system effects that contribute to atherosclerosis and CVD (Miller et al. 2002; Chrousos and Kino 2007). Some researchers view depression itself as the source of chronic stress (McEwen 2003); depression can also be the consequence of early life stress that confers a lower threshold and heightened response to subsequent stressors (Heim et al. 2000). In either case, current CVD guidelines offer no recommendation for interventions that could address the apparent heightened stress response among those with depression, leaving these direct biological pathways between depression and CVD unaltered.

A further factor that may reduce the effectiveness of CVD prevention guidelines among those with depression is the possible association between antidepressant medications and increased risk of heart disease and stroke (Brunoni et al. 2012; Shah et al. 2011; Licht et al. 2010; Wu et al. 2011; Hackam and Mrkobrada 2012). The research on this question is far from clear cut because observational studies cannot completely adjust for the many differences between depressed individuals who are treated versus untreated with medication. But given that antidepressants are the main treatment that most of those who seek treatment for depression will receive, the possibility that they might have deleterious effects on the cardiovascular system is a significant concern. This further underscores the need for a targeted approach to CVD prevention in depression.

27.3 What Could Be Done to Improve CVD Prevention Among People with Depression?

27.3.1 Start Screening Earlier in the Depression Course

One important principle is that prevention efforts should occur as early as possible in the course of depressive disorder. As noted above, depression typically first occurs relatively early in life and has the capacity to affect physical health from a young age. Moreover, depression is typically preceded by an even earlier history of anxiety disorder (Kessler and Walters 2002), and anxiety is also reliably associated with subsequent CVD (Scott et al. 2013; Tully et al. 2015; Janszky et al. 2010). Atherosclerosis is a slowly developing disease that also often begins in young adulthood or earlier (Magnussen et al. 2013; Joseph et al. 1993; Strong et al. 1999). This means that although the clinical manifestation of depression and CVD is often decades apart, the underlying connection between the two may be tracking from adolescence. This may be one reason why the treatment of depression in those with existing CVD has been largely unsuccessful in improving CVD prognosis (Glassman et al. 2002; The ENRICHD Investigators 2003): these interventions may be occurring too late in the course of the depression-heart disease comorbidity to be effective. Targeted CVD prevention for those with depression in primary care could therefore include recommendations that screening for CVD behavioural and biological risk factors should begin at least 10 years earlier than in the general population. In those with severe or recurrent depression history, who will often be seen in specialist mental health services, screening should be undertaken at the first opportunity. Awareness among general practitioners needs to be developed that mental disorders in their patients should cue greater, rather than less, attention to physical health and health behaviours.

27.3.2 Move to Integrative or Collaborative Care

Where treatment is undertaken in specialist mental health services, it is usually considered the responsibility of the primary practitioner to monitor physical health. This splitting of the mental and physical health aspects of depression across separate services does not appear to be working well. There is clear awareness now that mental health services must monitor and coordinate interventions concerning the physical health of those with SMI (Lawrence and Kisely 2010) and that this needs to be commenced early in the course of the disorder (Bailey et al. 2012). There is also evidence that such interventions work, improving a range of CVD risk factors (Green et al. 2015; Laursen et al. 2014). This kind of awareness and approach now needs to be extended to those with depression (as well as other nonpsychotic disorders). This could be done in a variety of ways (some of which are already being implemented with SMI): mental health clinicians could be upskilled to undertake some aspects of this work, mental health teams could be extended to include health psychologists and physicians specialising in working with the mentally ill or collaborative care approaches could be implemented that link mental and general health care more closely.

Collaborative care approaches can be utilised to improve the physical health of patients seen in mental health service settings as suggested here, but they can also be utilised to improve the mental health of primary care patients. A recent trial of collaborative care for depression in primary care (Stewart et al. 2014) demonstrated substantially reduced risk of a subsequent CVD event among those randomised to the depression treatment compared to those receiving usual care. However, this cardioprotective effect was confined to those without CVD at baseline: depression treatment had no cardioprotective benefit over and above usual care in those with CVD at baseline. This trial is consistent with other studies (Glassman et al. 2002; The ENRICHD Investigators 2003) in demonstrating that treating comorbid depression among those with existing CVD has no impact on CVD prognosis, but it does offer hope that depression treatment may prevent or delay CVD-related events if undertaken prior to the first clinical manifestation of CVD.

27.3.3 Make Greater Use of Treatment Approaches that Simultaneously Improve Mental and Physical Health

The evidence that depression is often associated with a heightened or dysregulated stress response, coupled with the possibility that the medications usually prescribed for depression may increase CVD risk, argues for a greater use of psychological treatments that incorporate a stress reduction component. Mindfulness-based CBT has proven effective with recurrent depression (Piet and Hougaard 2011; Segal et al. 2012); this approach or mindfulness-based stress reduction (Fjorback et al. 2011) could be helpful in reducing risk of subsequent CVD. If such an approach were augmented with a focus on health-related behaviour, this package could further help offset CVD risk. The great promise of this kind of treatment package is not just that it could help reduce future physical illness but that it could enhance current mental health through the antidepressant effects of increased physical activity and improved diet and sleep. Future research could assess how this kind of CBT + stress reduction + health behaviour package impacts on mental and physical health both at end of depression treatment and over the longer term.

Conclusion

People with depression history develop cardiovascular diseases at a higher rate than people without depression, providing evidence that current CVD prevention guidelines are to some extent failing this patient group. There are several reasons why this might be: screening for behavioural and biological CVD risk factors is less likely to occur among those with depression; screening, when it does occur, comes years after depression onset allowing decades for CVD-potentiating lifestyles to become habitual; and depression-CVD biological mediators (e.g. HPA axis dysregulation) are not being directly addressed in either primary care or specialist mental health services.

There are a range of options for improving this situation and making prevention of CVD in depression a real possibility. In primary care, patients with depression need effective treatment of depression combined with targeted screening for CVD risk factors; these interventions should be commenced in early adulthood, not middle age. The kind of awareness that has developed among mental health clinicians and primary care physicians that treatment of SMI must integrate attention to physical health now needs to be extended to people with severe or recurrent depression. Dual attention to physical and mental health may be best accomplished in integrative or collaborative care approaches. In terms of depression treatment, some types of treatment may have more CVD prevention potential than others. There are effective psychological treatments for depression that have stress reduction effects; these could be further enhanced by a behaviour change component. This kind of treatment approach would not only reduce risk of CVD (as well as other chronic diseases) but further improve mental health through the positive feedback effects of healthier lifestyle on mood. The need to address the physical health needs of depressed patients should not be viewed by clinicians as yet another thing to do but as an opportunity to simultaneously enhance both quality and quantity of life in this vulnerable patient group.

References

Aarons GA, Monn AR, Leslie LK, Garland AF, Lugo L, Hough RL et al (2008) Association between mental and physical health problems in high-risk adolescents: a longitudinal study. J Adolesc Health 43(3):260–267

Appelhans BM, Whited MC, Schneider KL, Ma Y, Oleski JL, Merriam PA et al (2012) Depression severity, diet quality, and physical activity in women with obesity and depression. J Acad Nutr Diet 112(5):693–698

Bailey S, Gerada C, Lester H, Shiers D (2012) The cardiovascular health of young people with severe mental illness: addressing an epidemic within an epidemic. Psychiatrist 36(10): 375–378

Bonnet F, Irving K, Terra J-L, Nony P, Berthezène F, Moulin P (2005) Anxiety and depression are associated with unhealthy lifestyle in patients at risk of cardiovascular disease. Atherosclerosis 178(2):339–344

Brunoni AR, Lotufo PA, Benseñor IM (2012) Are antidepressants good for the soul but bad for the matter? Using noninvasive brain stimulation to detangle depression/antidepressants effects on heart rate variability and cardiovascular risk. Biol Psychiatry 71:e27–e28

Chrousos GP, Kino T (2007) Glucocorticoid action networks and complex psychiatric and/or somatic disorders. Stress 10:213–219

Coleman T, Murphy E, Cheater F (2000) Factors influencing discussion of smoking between general practitioners and patients who smoke: a qualitative study. Br J Gen Pract 50(452):207–210

Cowen P (2010) Not fade away: the HPA axis and depression. Psychol Med 40(01):1–4

Fjorback L, Arendt M, Ørnbøl E, Fink P, Walach H (2011) Mindfulness-based stress reduction and mindfulness-based cognitive therapy–a systematic review of randomized controlled trials. Acta Psychiatr Scand 124(2):102–119

Glassman AH, O'Connor CM, Califf RM, Swedberg K, Schwartz P, Bigger JT Jr et al (2002) Sertraline treatment of major depression in patients with acute MI or unstable angina. JAMA 288(6):701–709

Green CA, Yarborough BJH, Leo MC, Yarborough MT, Stumbo SP, Janoff SL et al (2015) The STRIDE weight loss and lifestyle intervention for individuals taking antipsychotic medications: a randomized trial. Am J Psychiatry 172:71–81

Hackam DG, Mrkobrada M (2012) Selective serotonin reuptake inhibitors and brain hemorrhage a meta-analysis. Neurology 79(18):1862–1865

Heim C, Newport DJ, Heit S, Graham YP, Wilcox M, Bonsall R et al (2000) Pituitary-adrenal and autonomic responses to stress in women after sexual and physical abuse in childhood. JAMA 284:592–597

Jaen CR, Stange KC, Nutting PA (1994) Competing demands of primary care: a model for the delivery of clinical preventive services. J Fam Pract 38:166–171

Jaen CR, Mcilvain H, Pol L, Phillips R, Flocke S, Crabtree BF (2001) Tailoring tobacco counseling to the competing demands in the clinical encounter. J Fam Pract 50(10):859–863

Janszky I, Ahnve S, Lundberg I (2010) Early-onset depression, anxiety and risk of subsequent coronary heart disease. J Am Coll Cardiol 56:31–37

Johnson HM, Thorpe CT, Bartels CM, Pandhi N, Sheehy AM, Smith MA (2012) Predictors of undiagnosed hypertension among young adults with regular primary care use. Circulation 126(21 Supplement):A16557

Joseph A, Ackerman D, Talley JD, Johnstone J, Kupersmith J (1993) Manifestations of coronary atherosclerosis in young trauma victims—an autopsy study. J Am Coll Cardiol 22(2):459–467

Katon WJ (2003) Clinical and health services relationships between major depression, depressive symptoms, and general medical illness. Biol Psychiatry 54(3):216–226

Kendrick T (1996) Cardiovascular and respiratory risk factors and symptoms among general practice patients with long-term mental illness. Br J Psychiatry 169:733–739

Kessler RC, Walters EE (2002) The national comorbidity survey. In: Tsuang MT, Tohen M (eds) Textbook in psychiatric epidemiology, 2nd edn. Wiley-Liss, New York

Kessler RC, Angermeyer M, Anthony JC, De Graaf R, Demyttenaere K, Gasquet I et al (2007) Lifetime prevalence and age-of-onset distributions of mental disorders in the World Health Organization's World Mental Health Surveys. World Psychiatry 6:168–176

Laursen TM, Nordentoft M, Mortensen PB (2014) Excess early mortality in schizophrenia. Annu Rev Clin Psychol 10:425–448

Lawrence D, Kisely S (2010) Review: inequalities in healthcare provision for people with severe mental illness. J Psychopharmacol 24(4 suppl):61–68

Licht CMM, de Geus EJC, van Dyck R, Penninx BWJH (2010) Longitudinal evidence for unfavorable effects of antidepressants on heart rate variability. Biol Psychiatry 68(9):861–868

Magnussen CG, Smith KJ, Juonala M (2013) When to prevent cardiovascular disease? As early as possible: lessons from prospective cohorts beginning in childhood. Curr Opin Cardiol 28(5):561–568

McCloughen A, Foster K, Huws-Thomas M, Delgado C (2012) Physical health and wellbeing of emerging and young adults with mental illness: an integrative review of international literature. Int J Ment Health Nurs 21(3):274–288

McEwen BS (2003) Mood disorders and allostatic load. Biol Psychiatry 54:200–207

Miller GE, Cohen S, Ritchey AK (2002) Chronic psychological stress and the regulation of pro-inflammatory cytokines: a glucocorticoid resistance model. Health Psychol 21:536–541

Mosca L, Benjamin EJ, Berra K, Bezanson JL, Dolor RJ, Lloyd-Jones DM et al (2011) Effectiveness-based guidelines for the prevention of cardiovascular disease in women—2011 update: a guideline from the American Heart Association. J Am Coll Cardiol 57(12):1404–1423

Muñoz RF, Cuijpers P, Smit F, Barrera AZ, Leykin Y (2010) Prevention of major depression. Annu Rev Clin Psychol 6:181–212

Nicholson A, Kuper H, Hemingway H (2006) Depression as an aetiological and prognostic factor in coronary heart disease: a meta-analysis of 6362 events among 146 538 participants in 54 observational studies. Eur Heart J 27:2763–2774

Osborn DP (2001) Topics in review: the poor physical health of people with mental illness. West J Med 175(5):329

Payne ME, Steck SE, George RR, Steffens DC (2012) Fruit, vegetable, and antioxidant intakes are lower in older adults with depression. J Acad Nutr Diet 112(12):2022–2027

Perk J, De Backer G, Gohlke H, Graham I, Reiner Ž, Verschuren M et al (2012) European Guidelines on cardiovascular disease prevention in clinical practice (version 2012). Eur Heart J 33(13):1635–1701

Piet J, Hougaard E (2011) The effect of mindfulness-based cognitive therapy for prevention of relapse in recurrent major depressive disorder: a systematic review and meta-analysis. Clin Psychol Rev 31(6):1032–1040

Rottenberg J, Yaroslavsky I, Carney RM, Freedland KE, George CJ, Baji I et al (2014) The association between major depressive disorder in childhood and risk factors for cardiovascular disease in adolescence. Psychosom Med 76(2):122–127

Rush A, Trivedi MH, Wisniewski SR, Nierenberg AA, Stewart JW, Warden D et al (2006) Acute and longer-term outcomes in depressed outpatients requiring one or several treatment steps: a STAR*D report. Am J Psychiatry 163(11):1905–1917

Scott KM, Oakley Browne MA, McGee MA, Wells JE (2006) Mental-physical comorbidity in Te Rau Hinengaro: the New Zealand Mental Health Survey (NZMHS). Aust N Z J Psychiatry 40:882–888

Scott K, De Jonge P, Alonso J, Viana M, Liu Z, O'Neill S et al (2013) Associations between DSM-IV mental disorders and subsequent heart disease onset: beyond depression. Int J Cardiol 168:5293–5299

Segal ZV, Williams JMG, Teasdale JD (2012) Mindfulness-based cognitive therapy for depression. Guilford Press, New York

Shah AJ, Veledar E, Shallenberger L, Murrah NV, Jawed F, Bremner D et al (2011) Association of antidepressant medications with carotid intima media thickness in middle aged veteran twins. J Am Coll Cardiol 57(14, Supplement):E1588

Stetler C, Miller GE (2011) Depression and hypothalamic-pituitary-adrenal activation: a quantitative summary of four decades of research. Psychosom Med 73:114–126

Stewart JC, Perkins AJ, Callahan CM (2014) Effect of collaborative care for depression on risk of cardiovascular events: data from the IMPACT randomized controlled trial. Psychosom Med 76(1):29–37

Strong JP, Malcom GT, McMahan CA, Tracy RE, Newman WP III, Herderick EE et al (1999) Prevalence and extent of atherosclerosis in adolescents and young adults: implications for prevention from the Pathobiological Determinants of Atherosclerosis in Youth Study. JAMA 281(8):727–735

The ENRICHD Investigators (2003) Effects of treating depression and low perceived social support on clinical events after myocardial infarction. J Am Med Assoc 289:3106–3116

Tully PJ, Turnbull DA, Beltrame J, Horowitz J, Cosh S, Baumeister H et al (2015) Panic disorder and incident coronary heart disease: a systematic review and meta-regression in 1 131 612 persons and 58 111 cardiac events. Psychol Med. In press:1–12

Van der Kooy K, Van Hout H, Marwijk H, Marten H, Stehouwer C, Beekman A (2007) Depression and the risk for cardiovascular diseases: systematic review and meta analysis. Int J Geriatr Psychiatry 22:613–626

Wu C-S, Wang S-C, Cheng Y-C, Gau SS-F (2011) Association of cerebrovascular events with antidepressant use: a case-crossover study. Am J Psychiatry 168(5):511–521

Wulsin LR, Singla BM (2003) Do depressive symptoms increase the risk for the onset of coronary disease: a systematic quantitative review. Psychosom Med 65:201–210

Screening for Depression in Coronary Heart Disease: Detection of Early Disease States

28

Malcolm P. Forbes and Harris A. Eyre

Contents

Abstract

There is a high prevalence of depression in patients with coronary heart disease (CHD) that is often undetected. Around 15 % of patients are diagnosed with major depressive disorder (MDD) after acute myocardial infarction (AMI) or coronary artery bypass grafts (CABG), and 22 % of patients with congestive heart failure (CHF) have MDD. Rates of depression are higher in patients with CHF who are admitted to hospital. Screening aims to identify disease in the community early, enabling early intervention to reduce suffering. Screening programmes for depression in patients with cardiovascular disease (CVD) exist in a number of countries

M.P. Forbes
School of Medicine and Dentistry, James Cook University, Townsville, Australia

H.A. Eyre (✉)
School of Medicine and Dentistry, James Cook University, Townsville, Australia

Discipline of Psychiatry, School of Medicine, University of Adelaide, Adelaide, Australia

Semel Institute for Neuroscience and Human Behavior, UCLA, Los Angeles, CA, USA
e-mail: harris.eyre@gmail.com

B.T. Baune, P.J. Tully (eds.), *Cardiovascular Diseases and Depression*,
DOI 10.1007/978-3-319-32480-7_28

around the world. There is good evidence to suggest that screening programmes increase rates of diagnosis of depression. However, while rates of diagnosis are increased, there is limited evidence to show that patients diagnosed with depression through screening have improved outcomes. Given the evidence available, screening for depression in patients with cardiovascular disease should be cautiously supported when appropriate referral and treatment pathways are in place. There are a number of screening tools that can be used to screen patients for depression. Clinicians should use the Patient Health Questionnaire-9 (PHQ-9) to screen patients for depression, as this is recommended by international guidelines. If time pressure is an issue, the shorter Patient Health Questionnaire-2 (PHQ-2) can be used followed by the PHQ-9 if the PHQ-2 is positive.

28.1 Introduction

There is a high prevalence of depression in patients with CHD as well as congestive heart failure (CHF) that is often undetected. Rates of major depressive disorder (MDD) of around 15 % have been reported in patients after acute myocardial infarction (AMI) or coronary artery bypass grafts (CABG) (Thombs et al. 2006; Carney and Freedland 2003). Depression has an adjusted odds ratio of 1.4 for CHD (Patten et al. 2005). Certain individuals with CHD are at higher risk of experiencing depression. The UK UPBEAT study found that individuals living alone (odds ratio (OR) 2.08, $p=0.02$), experiencing current chest pain (OR 5.44, $p<0.001$), having greater than two comorbid illness (i.e. diabetes mellitus, osteoarthritis, chronic obstructive pulmonary disease, chronic renal disease, asthma, hypertension or active cancer) (OR 6.00, $p=0.005$) and experiencing social problems such as problems living alone (OR 8.73, $p<0.001$) or more than one disability (i.e. mobility problems, self-care problems, problems with usual activities or problems with pain or discomfort) (OR 7.48, $p<0.001$) were at an increased risk for depression (Walters et al. 2014). The prevalence of depression in patients with CHF has been reported to be around 22 %, however, ranging from 11 to 35 % in outpatients and 35–70 % among inpatients (Rutledge et al. 2006; Angermann et al. 2011; Luttik et al. 2011). Interestingly, these figures have been confirmed in diverse populations (Adewuya et al. 2006) and in implanted cardioverter-defibrillator recipients (Freedenberg et al. 2011).

It has been suggested that the presence of comorbid MDD doubles the risk of major cardiac events and death in patients with documented cardiovascular disease (CVD) and triples the risk of hospitalisation (O'Connor et al. 2008; Jiang et al. 2001). The longer-term impact of depression has been closely correlated with post-acute coronary events and 12-month physical health status (Thombs et al. 2008a). The comorbidity between depression and CHD has also been found for both systolic and diastolic cardiac dysfunction (Kato et al. 2012), and patients with higher severity of left ventricular dysfunction have been showing an increased risk for CVD-related mortality and all-cause mortality in patients with depression (van den Broek et al. 2011). On the contrary, these trends do not hold for adults with congenital heart disease since these individuals have rates of depression similar to that seen in the general population. This reflects the observation that adults with congenital heart disease, while they may face potential medical complications, are generally asymptomatic (Rayner et al. 2014).

Screening is the process of identifying individuals who may have a condition or be at risk of a condition but do not currently demonstrate signs or symptoms. A number of effective screening programmes are in place for a variety of disorders; however, the value of screening programmes is often controversial. This chapter will review and evaluate the value of screening for depression in coronary heart disease (CHD) and investigate, if screening leads to earlier treatment of depression in CHD. It will discuss the risk of overtreatment and will discuss international screening guidelines currently in existence.

28.2 Current Recommendations for Depression Screening in Coronary Heart Disease Patients

Depression identification in CHD is a component of international cardiology guidelines and recommendations (Lichtman et al. 2008; Orth-Gomer et al. 2005; Albus et al. 2004; McMurray et al. 2012; Lainscak et al. 2011; Colquhoun et al. 2013) based on a number of screening algorithms (Lichtman et al. 2008; Holzapfel et al. 2007). The American Heart Association (AHA) guidelines recommend that all patients with CHD disease should be screened with a two-item Patient Health Questionnaire (PHQ-2) at a minimum (see Fig. 28.1). In case of a screen positive result, it is recommended to administer the longer Patient Health Questionnaire (PHQ-9) (see Fig. 28.2). While patients with a score <10 on the PHQ-9 should be provided with additional clinical support, education and follow-up within 1 month, patients with a score >10 should be referred for more comprehensive clinical evaluation by a professionally qualified practitioner in the diagnosis and management of depression (Lichtman et al. 2008).

The National Heart Foundation of Australia (NHFA) guidelines largely reflect the AHA guidelines. The NHFA gives a Grade A recommendation for routine screening, which describes the body of evidence informing this recommendation as 'trusted to guide practice'. The National Health and Medical Research Council (NHMRC) gives a level of evidence of I for routine screening, which infers that a systematic review of randomised controlled trials (RCTs) has been completed. The NHFA guidelines recommend a simple tool such as the PHQ-2 to be incorporated into routine screening of patients with CHD disease. These guidelines also offer suggested time points at which screening should occur. These time points are at first presentation, at the next follow-up appointment, around the 2–3 months after the first presentation and annually thereafter. The NHFA goes further than the AHA guidelines in that they recommend consideration to be given to screening of the partner or spouse of patients with CHD for depression (Colquhoun et al. 2013). Serial screening is supported by evidence that finds high annual incidence rates of depression in heart failure patients initially free of depression (Lossnitzer et al. 2013).

Further screening guidelines exist to suggest that all primary care patients should be screened for depression. The United States Preventive Services Task Force

Patient Health Questionnaire: 2 items (PHQ-2) *

Over the past 2 weeks, how often have you been bothered by any of the following problems?

1) Little interest or pleasure in doing things.
2) Feeling down, depressed or hopeless.

* If the answer is "yes" to either question, then refer for more comprehensive clinical evaluation by a professional qualified in the diagnosis and management of depression or screen with PHQ-9.

* Alternative scoring system: Questions are scored: not at all –0; several days –1; more than half the days –2; and nearly every day –3. Add together the item scores to get a total score for depression severity

Fig. 28.1 Patient Health Questionnaire: two items (PHQ-2) (Modified from (Lichtman et al. 2008)

Patient Health Questionnaire: 9 items (PHQ-9) *

Over the past 2 weeks, how often have you been bothered by any of the following problems?

1) Little interest or pleasure doing things.
2) Feeling down, depressed, or hopeless.
3) Trouble falling asleep, staying asleep, or sleeping too much.
4) Feeling tired or having little energy.
5) Poor appetite or overeating.
6) Feeling bad about yourself, feeling that you are a failure, or feeling that you have let yourself or your family down.
7) Trouble concentrating on things such as reading the newspaper or watching television.
8) Moving or speaking so slowly that other people could have noticed. Or being so fidgety or restless that you have been moving around a lot more than usual.
9) Thinking that you would be better off dead or that you want to hurt yourself in some way.

* Questions are scored: not at all –0; several days –1; more than half the days –2; and nearly every day –3. Add together the item scores to get a total score for depression severity.

Interpretation

- 0 – 4 minimal depression
- 5 – 9 mild depression
- 10 – 14 moderate depression
- 15 – 19 moderately severe depression
- 20 – 27 severe depression

Fig. 28.2 Patient Health Questionnaire: nine items (PHQ-9) (Modified from Angermann et al. 2011)

(USPSTF) (Force UPST 2009) recommends such screening for all primary care patients in circumstances where resources are in place to assure accurate diagnosis, effective treatment and follow-up. This recommendation is based on examination of the evidence on the benefits and harm of screening primary care patients for depression, including direct evidence that depression screening programmes improve health outcomes. Specifically, the USPSTF found good evidence that treating depressed adults identified through screening in primary care settings with antidepressants, psychotherapy, or both, decreases clinical morbidity (Force UPST 2009). This recommendation was a Grade B recommendation – indicating there is high certainty that the net benefit is moderate or there is moderate certainty that the net benefit is moderate to substantial (Force UPST 2009).

28.2.1 Critique of Current Recommendations

Guidelines have been critiqued for a multitude of reasons. For example, criticism of this USPSTF recommendation has been raised due to the lack of RCTs testing whether screening would be more effective than not screening (Thombs and Ziegelstein 2014a). In contrast, the United Kingdom National Institute of Health and Clinical Excellence does not recommend routine screening in primary care (Thombs et al. 2012), citing reasons including the high rate of false-positive results, the lack of empirical evidence of benefits to patients, the likelihood that most people identified only by screening would have relatively mild symptoms of depression and often recover without formal intervention, the high cost and large number of resources involved in identifying people who might gain little in terms of improvements to their mental health, and the diversion of resources away from people with more serious cases of depression whose care is already often inadequate. In addition, the National Heart Foundation of Australia (NHFA) guidelines have also been criticised since it was thought that these guidelines do not adequately consider the potential benefits versus the potential harms of screening (Thombs and Ziegelstein 2014b). Thombs and Ziegelstein (2014b) have criticised the NHFA guidelines as not being based on current evidence. In their critique, they explain that no RCTs have found evidence that patients undergoing screening for depression have better depression outcomes than similar patients who have not been screened for depression, when comparable treatment resources are provided to depressed patients in both groups (Thombs and Ziegelstein 2013). Further criticism of these guidelines is outlined in the section below.

Comment has been made on the applicability of research findings to real-world practice. Tully et al. (2014) found that the implementation of routine depression screening protocols in cardiology settings may underestimate the severity and complexity of psychiatric needs in heart failure patients such as comorbid personality disorders, alcohol/substance use, suicide risk and anxiety disorders. RCTs often exclude patients with comorbid psychiatric conditions, despite comorbid psychiatric conditions being common in psychiatric patients.

28.3 Screening Tools for Depression in Coronary Heart Disease

A variety of tools have been made available to screen patients with CHD for depression. Of these, Hospital Anxiety and Depression Scale (HADS) (Albus et al. 2004; Bambauer et al. 2005; Turner et al. 2010), Beck Depression Inventory (BDI) and Beck Depression Inventory-II (BDI-II) (Jiang et al. 2001; Valkamo et al. 2001; Ketterer et al. 2002; Parakh et al. 2008; Lett et al. 2009), and Patient

Health Questionnaire-2 (PHQ-2) and Patient Health Questionnaire-9 (PHQ-9) (Elderon et al. 2011; McManus et al. 2005; Rollman et al. 2012) are the most commonly used in clinical practice. Evidence for these tools is outlined in the section below and in Table 28.1. Other screening tools are outlined in Box 28.1.

Table 28.1 Details of commonly used screening tools for depression in coronary heart disease

Screening tool	Details
Hospital Anxiety and Depression Scale (HADS)	Description: scored out of 21
	Utility: A score of 11 has a sensitivity of 52 % and specificity of 94 % for MDD (Bambauer et al. 2005). The cut-off for depression differs according to population. In an older population with heart failure, with a score of 6, it had a sensitivity and specificity of 77 % and 89 %, respectively (Haworth et al. 2007). This scale has been used successfully in non-English-speaking settings (Barth and Martin 2005; Wang et al. 2006; Martin et al. 2008)
Beck Depression Inventory (BDI)	Description: widely in research on screening for depression in CHD. It is a 21-question multiple choice self-report inventory. The BDI scores each question from 0 to 4, with a higher total score indicating greater severity of depression
	Utility: Delisle et al. found that somatic symptoms accounted for the majority of the BDI score in patients with post-myocardial infarction (Delisle et al. 2012a, b). It was concluded that the second iteration of the BDI, the BDI-II, is preferable to the BDI in post-myocardial infarction patients
Beck Depression Inventory-II (BDI-II)	Description: as above
	Utility: the BDI-II uses the same scoring system but has a number of reworded items and replaces items involving changes in body image and hypochondria. It also asks participants to assess their mood over 2 weeks as opposed to one
Patient Health Questionnaire-2 (PHQ-2)	Description: asks whether an individual has had (Thombs et al. 2006) little interest or pleasure in doing things and if they have been (Carney and Freedland 2003) feeling down, depressed or hopeless, over the past 2 weeks. An assessment is positive if the patient answers in the affirmative to one or both questions and is negative if they deny both
	Utility: the validity of PHQ-2 screening tool has been assessed in a range of populations of varying age groups and ethnicity. In cardiac patients, it has been shown to have a sensitivity of 80–90 % and specificity of 70–80 % for major depressive disorder (Elderon et al. 2011; McManus et al. 2005). It has also been shown to be associated with an elevated 12-month mortality risk in patients with heart failure (Rollman et al. 2012). When the PHQ-2 is positive, the 9-item Patient Health Questionnaire (PHQ-9) is necessary, and a diagnosis of depression should not be made based on the results of a PHQ-2 alone. The PHQ-2 screening time was reported to be 1.4 min on average (Sowden et al. 2010). Both the PHQ-2 and PHQ-9 can be self-administered, have been tested in inpatient cardiac units and found to be feasible, well-accepted by staff and not resource intensive
	In a community setting, the administration of the screening tool takes longer than in inpatient settings (O'Reilly et al. 2015)

Table 28.1 (continued)

Screening tool	Details
Patient Health Questionnaire-9 (PHQ-9)	Description: as above
	Utility: a score ≥ 10 on the PHQ-9 has a sensitivity of 88 % and specificity of 88 % for major depressive disorder. Scores of 5, 10, 15 and 20 represent mild, moderate, moderately severe and severe depression, respectively (Newhouse and Jiang 2014). Other studies have found a similar specificity (90 %) but a reduced sensitivity (54 %), with a positive likelihood ratio of 5.4 (McManus et al. 2005). In Australian indigenous populations with CHD disease, a modified version of the PHQ-9 has been validated (Esler et al. 2008). Razykov et al. (2012) have found high correlation between the PHQ-9 and a modified version removing the final question about passive thoughts of death and active thoughts of self-harm (PHQ-8); with a Pearson's coefficient of 0.997, the authors have suggested that the final question may not add much in patients with CHD disease. The PHQ-9 has also been used in community settings, with an Australian study showing that pharmacists are capable of screening and risk assessment services for depression and making referrals to appropriate health-care professionals when required

Box 28.1. List of Commonly Used Screening Tools for Depression in Coronary Heart Disease

Inventory to Diagnose Depression (IDD)
Beck Depression Inventory (BDI)
Beck Depression Inventory-II (BDI-II)
Patient Health Questionnaire-2 (PHQ-2)
Patient Health Questionnaire-9 (PHQ-9)
Geriatric Depression Scale
Primary Care Evaluation of Mental Disorders (PRIME-MD) questionnaire
Centre for Epidemiological Studies Depression Scale
Medical Outcomes Study-Depression questionnaire
Depression in the Medically Ill (DMI-18 and DMI-10)
Mental Health Index (MH-5)

A number of screening tools, including the HADS and PHQ, can be administered with a computer-adaptive model enabling completion in more flexible models (Fischer et al. 2014).

In a meta-analysis of depression screening tools, Thombs et al. (2008b) found that with predefined cut-off scores, the sensitivity of tools ranged from 39 to 100 % and specificity from 58 to 94 %. A more recent meta-analysis by Ren et al. (2015) (Doerfler et al. 1997) found sensitivity of tools ranged from 34 to 96 % and specificity ranged from 69 to 95 %.

28.4 Benefits of Routine Screening for Depression in Coronary Heart Disease

Evaluations of screening programmes in real-life settings suggest that integrated models of care involving depression screening using PHQ are feasible and can result in increased referral rates for appropriate mental health follow-up (Subramanian and Hopayian 2008; Ski et al. 2012; Kang et al. 2015). In a large elderly and predominantly male population, screening with PHQ-2 yielded 20.1 % positive depression screens. Among the PHQ-2 positive screens, 59.8 % scored 10 or higher on the PHQ-9 scale (Yano et al. 2012). In a large retrospective cohort study of patients with diabetes or CHD disease, Burton et al. (2013) found that the number needed to routinely screen for a new diagnosis of depression was 976. A cross-sectional study in primary care in the UK found that depression screening using HADS had relatively low uptake, despite incentivisation (Jani et al. 2013). An Australian study looking at 12-month outcomes of patients with CHD screened for depression found that while a short depression screening tool had good predictive validity, a screening and referral tool alone was not enough to achieve optimal disease management, with rates of depression remaining relatively stable at 1, 3, 6 and 12 months after diagnosis (Ski et al. 2015). Evidence from Australia has found that education programmes can improve nursing staff understanding of depression and boost screening rates for depression in a tertiary hospital (Worrall-Carter et al. 2012). The introduction of screening for depression in patients with CHD disease is not simple due to lack of time and resources and disagreement over screening protocols (Maxwell et al. 2013).

Numerous studies have shown that treatment of depression leads to improvement in adherence of pharmacological therapy, which in turn may decrease CHD events and improve survival (Rieckmann et al. 2006; Glassman et al. 2009; Bauer et al. 2012). It has been shown successfully that screening allows the opportunity to pick up previously undiagnosed cases supported by a study, where 70 % of the CHF inpatients had a diagnosis of MDD that was previously unknown (Angermann et al. 2011). In contrast, screening only those patients that the physician believes are depressed and are at high risk has been demonstrated to be unsuccessful. Ziegelstein et al. (2005) found little correlation between standardised depression test scores and clinician assessment of depression, with a false-negative rate (doctor or nurse missing a diagnosis of depression in a patient with depression) of 75 %.

Screening may be most beneficial in some populations who appear more responsive to treatment than others as they will be more likely to achieve significant treatment response. For example, in the SADHART-CHF study (Jiang et al. 2011), men with heart failure and mild depression had almost a 2.5-fold greater chance of achieving depression remission with sertraline when compared with the rest of the study population, i.e. men with moderate and severe depression, and women. In the same study, patients with greater somatic presentations of their depression were less likely to remit after treatment with sertraline. Mourad et al. (2012) found that patients with symptomatic CHD disease and depression had utilised most healthcare services vs. individuals with one condition or the other.

Screening for depression may not depend on whether treatment improves cardiac outcomes. This given depression is a chronic, disabling condition with a major impact on quality of life. Hence, authors suggest improved depression-related reductions in quality of life may be considered as important as cardiac outcomes (Thombs and Ziegelstein 2008). Furthermore, Elderon and Whooley and the authors of the NHFA guidelines support this notion and argue that whether treatment depression improves CHD outcomes is moot, as treatment for depression is necessary anyway (Elderon and Whooley 2013; Tatoulis 2014).

28.5 Criticisms of Routine Screening for Depression in Coronary Heart Disease

Screening programmes can only be successful if three factors are met: patients not already known to have depression agree to be screened; a substantial number of new cases are identified with relatively few false-positive screens; and newly identified patients engage in treatment with successful outcomes (Thombs and Ziegelstein 2014a). Thombs and Ziegelstein (2014a) advance the point that studies of routine depression screening programmes do not meet these three factors, and the evidence used to advocate for routine depression screening is not supported by RCTs that meet these three key criteria. Hitherto, there is no directly relevant evidence from RCTs to support screening of patients for depression in primary care (Thombs et al. 2014), and the two systematic reviews that have been completed have concluded that there has not been any RCT that has tested whether depression screening is effective in CHD care settings (Thombs et al. 2008b, 2013).

Other concerns include routine screening potentially diverting existing mental health resources away from patients in need of existing services (Thombs and Ziegelstein 2014a; Ziegelstein and Thombs 2011). Further, there may be insufficient mental health resources to ensure adequate further management after depression is detected by screening (Ziegelstein and Thombs 2011). Inappropriate treatments may be started by clinicians not experienced in mental health but who note 'positive' depression screening, i.e. cardiologists may give patients a diagnosis of depression and start the patient on antidepressants on the basis of a screening tool alone (Ziegelstein et al. 2009). This may result in the patient experiencing unnecessary stigma of a diagnosis of depression and unnecessary risk of adverse effects from antidepressant agents (Ziegelstein et al. 2009).

Other complicating factors for screening of depression in CHD include (a) the inherently clinical nature of psychiatric diagnosis, requiring detailed history; (b) stigma leading to patient denial or minimisation of symptoms; (c) lack of training of CHD medical staff in psychiatric diagnosis; (d) the frequent presence of pseudo-depression/distress attributable to medical illness or therapy and (e) the symptomatic overlap of psychological distress and cardiac illness (Ketterer and Knysz 2009). While no relevant adverse effects of the process of screening itself exist (Collins et al. 2011), negative consequences of screening including primarily unintended harms, such as adverse effects from medication and stigma of a diagnosis of depression, and cost have been reported. Another limitation is that depression screening may also occur in clinical settings without appropriate referral pathways or patient follow-up. For example, specialist referral is probably required to meet CHD patient needs who endorse the PHQ-9 suicidality item (Tully and Baker 2012).

28.6 Future Directions

At present, literature is lacking to give an unequivocal answer on whether screening translates into improved outcomes. Further large-scale clinical trials will do much to settle this debate. A cluster RCT is underway in general practice to assess if a treatment model involving collaborative care can improve patient outcomes for patients with diabetes and/or CHD who have been screened and diagnosed with depression (Coventry et al. 2012). A longitudinal, multicentre observational study based in general practice is also underway to determine the association between screening for depression and quality of life, hospitalisation and mortality (Eisele et al. 2013). The results of these studies will inform next update of recommendations by major health bodies.

28.7 Summary

Disagreement about the benefit of screening for depression of patients with CHD remains. However, the majority of guidelines recommend that screening should occur, and the majority of the literature supports screening in environments with resources to enable proper management once diagnosis is made. Given the evidence available, we believe screening for depression in patients with cardiovascular disease should be cautiously supported. There are a number of screening tools that can be used to screen patients for depression. Clinicians could use the PHQ-9 to screen patients for depression, as this is recommended by international guidelines. If time pressure is an issue, the shorter PHQ-2 can be used followed by the PHQ-9, if the PHQ-2 is positive. Screening already occurs around the world. In Australia, three in ten cardiologists screen for depression often or always. However, very few use a standard screening tool, largely due to unawareness of the existence of available screening tools (Stewart et al. 2010). Greater knowledge of existing guidelines may result in increased use of screening tools with the best accuracy. Once diagnosis occurs, it is essential that it is followed up with appropriate referral and management.

Disclosures and Acknowledgements All authors declare that there are no conflicts of interest or financial disclosures.

References

Adewuya AO, Ola BA, Ajayi OE, Oyedeji AO, Balogun MO, Mosaku SK (2006) Prevalence and correlates of major depressive disorder in Nigerian outpatients with heart failure. Psychosomatics 47(6):479–485. Epub 2006/11/23. eng

Albus C, Jordan J, Herrmann-Lingen C (2004) Screening for psychosocial risk factors in patients with coronary heart disease-recommendations for clinical practice. Eur J Cardiovasc Prev Rehabil Off J Eur Soc Cardiol Work Groups Epidemiol Prev Cardiac Rehabil Exerc Physiol 11(1):75–79. Epub 2004/05/29. eng

Angermann CE, Gelbrich G, Stork S, Schowalter M, Deckert J, Ertl G et al (2011) Somatic correlates of comorbid major depression in patients with systolic heart failure. Int J Cardiol 147(1):66–73. PubMed PMID: WOS:000287443300018. English

Bambauer KZ, Locke SE, Aupont O, Mullan MG, McLaughlin TJ (2005) Using the hospital anxiety and depression scale to screen for depression in cardiac patients. Gen Hosp Psychiatry 27(4):275–284. Epub 2005/07/05. eng

Barth J, Martin CR (2005) Factor structure of the Hospital Anxiety and Depression Scale (HADS) in German coronary heart disease patients. Health Qual Life Outcomes 3:15. Pubmed Central PMCID: Pmc555847, Epub 2005/03/18. eng

Bauer LK, Caro MA, Beach SR, Mastromauro CA, Lenihan E, Januzzi JL et al (2012) Effects of depression and anxiety improvement on adherence to medication and health behaviors in recently hospitalized cardiac patients. Am J Cardiol 109(9):1266–1271

Burton C, Simpson C, Anderson N (2013) Diagnosis and treatment of depression following routine screening in patients with coronary heart disease or diabetes: a database cohort study. Psychol Med 43(3):529–537. Epub 2012/07/19. eng

Carney RM, Freedland KE (2003) Depression, mortality, and medical morbidity in patients with coronary heart disease. Biol Psychiatry 54(3):241–247

Collins RE, Lopez LM, Marteau TM (2011) Emotional impact of screening: a systematic review and meta-analysis. BMC Public Health 11:603. Pubmed Central PMCID: Pmc3223929, Epub 2011/07/30. eng

Colquhoun DM, Bunker SJ, Clarke DM, Glozier N, Hare DL, Hickie IB et al (2013) Screening, referral and treatment for depression in patients with coronary heart disease. Med J Aust 198(9):483–484. Epub 2013/05/21. eng

Coventry PA, Lovell K, Dickens C, Bower P, Chew-Graham C, Cherrington A et al (2012) Collaborative Interventions for Circulation and Depression (COINCIDE): study protocol for a cluster randomized controlled trial of collaborative care for depression in people with diabetes and/or coronary heart disease. Trials 13:139. Pubmed Central PMCID: Pmc3519809, Epub 2012/08/22. eng

Delisle VC, Abbey SE, Beck AT, Dobson KS, Dozois DJ, Grace SL et al (2012a) The influence of somatic symptoms on Beck Depression Inventory scores in hospitalized postmyocardial infarction patients. Can J Psychiatry Rev Can Psychiatr 57(12):752–758

Delisle VC, Beck AT, Ziegelstein RC, Thombs BD (2012b) Symptoms of heart disease or its treatment may increase Beck Depression Inventory Scores in hospitalized post-myocardial infarction patients. J Psychosom Res 73(3):157–162

Doerfler LA, Pbert L, DeCosimo D (1997) Self-reported depression in patients with coronary heart disease. J Cardiopulm Rehabil 17(3):163–170. Epub 1997/05/01. eng

Eisele M, Blozik E, Stork S, Trader JM, Herrmann-Lingen C, Scherer M (2013) Recognition of depression and anxiety and their association with quality of life, hospitalization and mortality in primary care patients with heart failure – study protocol of a longitudinal observation study. BMC Fam Pract 14:180. Pubmed Central PMCID: Pmc4222561, Epub 2013/11/28. eng

Elderon L, Whooley MA (2013) Depression and cardiovascular disease. Prog Cardiovasc Dis 55(6):511–523. Epub 2013/04/30. eng

Elderon L, Smolderen KG, Na B, Whooley MA (2011) Accuracy and prognostic value of American Heart Association: recommended depression screening in patients with coronary heart disease: data from the Heart and Soul Study. Circ Cardiovasc Qual Outcomes 4(5):533–540. Epub 2011/08/25. eng

Esler D, Johnston F, Thomas D, Davis B (2008) The validity of a depression screening tool modified for use with Aboriginal and Torres Strait Islander people. Aust N Z J Public Health 32(4):317–321. Epub 2008/09/11. eng

Fischer HF, Klug C, Roeper K, Blozik E, Edelmann F, Eisele M et al (2014) Screening for mental disorders in heart failure patients using computer-adaptive tests. Qual Life Res Int J Qual Life Asp Treat Care Rehabil 23(5):1609–1618. Epub 2013/12/18. eng

Force UPST (2009) Screening for depression in adults: US preventive services task force recommendation statement. Ann Intern Med 151(11):784–W256. PubMed PMID: WOS:000272727900004. English

Freedenberg V, Thomas SA, Friedmann E (2011) Anxiety and depression in implanted cardioverter-defibrillator recipients and heart failure: a review. Heart Fail Clin 7(1):59–68. Epub 2010/11/27. eng

Glassman AH, Bigger JT Jr, Gaffney M (2009) Psychiatric characteristics associated with long-term mortality among 361 patients having an acute coronary syndrome and major depression: seven-year follow-up of SADHART participants. Arch Gen Psychiatry 66(9): 1022–1029

Haworth JE, Moniz-Cook E, Clark AL, Wang M, Cleland JG (2007) An evaluation of two self-report screening measures for mood in an out-patient chronic heart failure population. Int J Geriatr Psychiatry 22(11):1147–1153. Epub 2007/04/26. eng

Holzapfel N, Zugck C, Muller-Tasch T, Lowe B, Wild B, Schellberg D et al (2007) Routine screening for depression and quality of life in outpatients with congestive heart failure. Psychosomatics 48(2):112–116. Epub 2007/03/03. eng

Jani BD, Purves D, Barry S, Cavanagh J, McLean G, Mair FS (2013) Challenges and implications of routine depression screening for depression in chronic disease and multimorbidity: a cross sectional study. PLoS One 8(9):e74610. Pubmed Central PMCID: Pmc3772931. Epub 2013/09/24. eng

Jiang W, Alexander J, Christopher E, Kuchibhatla M, Gaulden LH, Cuffe MS et al (2001) Relationship of depression to increased risk of mortality and rehospitalization in patients with congestive heart failure. Arch Intern Med 161(15):1849–1856

Jiang W, Krishnan R, Kuchibhatla M, Cuffe MS, Martsberger C, Arias RM et al (2011) Characteristics of depression remission and its relation with cardiovascular outcome among patients with chronic heart failure (from the SADHART-CHF Study). Am J Cardiol 107(4):545–551. PubMed PMID: WOS:000287892100009. English

Kang HJ, Stewart R, Bae KY, Kim SW, Shin IS, Hong YJ et al (2015) Effects of depression screening on psychiatric outcomes in patients with acute coronary syndrome: findings from the K-DEPACS and EsDEPACS studies. Int J Cardiol 190:114–121. PubMed PMID: WOS:000355112400031. English

Kato N, Kinugawa K, Shiga T, Hatano M, Takeda N, Imai Y et al (2012) Depressive symptoms are common and associated with adverse clinical outcomes in heart failure with reduced and preserved ejection fraction: the differential relevance of beta-blockers for reducing depressive symptoms. J Am Coll Cardiol 59(13):E1035-E. PubMed PMID: WOS:000302326701146. English

Ketterer MW, Knysz W (2009) Screening, diagnosis & monitoring of depression/distress in CHF patients. Heart Fail Rev 14(1):1–5. Epub 2007/08/02. eng

Ketterer MW, Denollet J, Goldberg AD, McCullough PA, John S, Farha AJ et al (2002) The big mush: psychometric measures are confounded and non-independent in their association with age at initial diagnosis of Ischaemic Coronary Heart Disease. J Cardiovasc Risk 9(1):41–48. Epub 2002/05/02. eng

Lainscak M, Blue L, Clark AL, Dahlstrom U, Dickstein K, Ekman I et al (2011) Self-care management of heart failure: practical recommendations from the Patient Care Committee of the Heart Failure Association of the European Society of Cardiology. Eur J Heart Fail 13(2):115–126

Lett HS, Blumenthal JA, Babyak MA, Catellier DJ, Carney RM, Berkman LF et al (2009) Dimensions of social support and depression in patients at increased psychosocial risk recovering from myocardial infarction. Int J Behav Med 16(3):248–258. Pubmed Central PMCID: Pmc2752492, Epub 2009/03/17. eng

Lichtman JH, Bigger JT Jr, Blumenthal JA, Frasure-Smith N, Kaufmann PG, Lesperance F et al (2008) Depression and coronary heart disease: recommendations for screening, referral, and treatment: a science advisory from the American Heart Association Prevention Committee of the Council on Cardiovascular Nursing, Council on Clinical Cardiology, Council on Epidemiology and Prevention, and Interdisciplinary Council on Quality of Care and Outcomes Research: endorsed by the American Psychiatric Association. Circulation 118(17):1768–1775. Epub 2008/10/01. eng

Lossnitzer N, Herzog W, Stork S, Wild B, Muller-Tasch T, Lehmkuhl E et al (2013) Incidence rates and predictors of major and minor depression in patients with heart failure. Int J Cardiol 167(2):502–507. Epub 2012/02/22. eng

Luttik ML, Jaarsma T, Sanderman R, Fleer J (2011) The advisory brought to practice: routine screening on depression (and anxiety) in coronary heart disease; consequences and implications. Eur J Cardiovasc Nurs J Work Group Cardiovasc Nurs Eur Soc Cardiol 10(4):228–233. Epub 2010/09/30. eng

Martin CR, Thompson DR, Barth J (2008) Factor structure of the Hospital Anxiety and Depression Scale in coronary heart disease patients in three countries. J Eval Clin Pract 14(2):281–287. Epub 2008/02/21. eng

Maxwell M, Harris F, Hibberd C, Donaghy E, Pratt R, Williams C et al (2013) A qualitative study of primary care professionals' views of case finding for depression in patients with diabetes or coronary heart disease in the UK. BMC Fam Pract 14:46. Pubmed Central PMCID: Pmc3623815, Epub 2013/04/06. eng

McManus D, Pipkin SS, Whooley MA (2005) Screening for depression in patients with coronary heart disease (data from the Heart and Soul Study). Am J Cardiol 96(8):1076–1081. Pubmed Central PMCID: Pmc2776683, Epub 2005/10/11. eng

McMurray JJ, Adamopoulos S, Anker SD, Auricchio A, Bohm M, Dickstein K et al (2012) ESC guidelines for the diagnosis and treatment of acute and chronic heart failure 2012: The Task Force for the Diagnosis and Treatment of Acute and Chronic Heart Failure 2012 of the European Society of Cardiology. Developed in collaboration with the Heart Failure Association (HFA) of the ESC. Eur J Heart Fail 14(8):803–869

Mourad G, Jaarsma T, Hallert C, Stromberg A (2012) Depressive symptoms and healthcare utilization in patients with noncardiac chest pain compared to patients with ischemic heart disease. Heart Lung J Crit Care 41(5):446–455. Epub 2012/06/02. eng

Newhouse A, Jiang W (2014) Heart failure and depression. Heart Fail Clin 10(2):295–304. Epub 2014/03/25. eng

O'Connor CM, Jiang W, Kuchibhatla M, Mehta RH, Clary GL, Cuffe MS et al (2008) Antidepressant use, depression, and survival in patients with heart failure. Arch Intern Med 168(20):2232–2237. Pubmed Central PMCID: 3889122

O'Reilly CL, Wong E, Chen TF (2015) A feasibility study of community pharmacists performing depression screening services. Res Social Adm Pharm 11(3):364–381

Orth-Gomer K, Albus C, Bages N, DeBacker G, Deter HC, Herrmann-Lingen C et al (2005) Psychosocial considerations in the European guidelines for prevention of cardiovascular diseases in clinical practice: third joint task force. Int J Behav Med 12(3):132–141

Parakh K, Thombs BD, Fauerbach JA, Bush DE, Ziegelstein RC (2008) Effect of depression on late (8 years) mortality after myocardial infarction. Am J Cardiol 101(5):602–606

Patten SB, Beck CA, Kassam A, Williams JV, Barbui C, Metz LM (2005) Long-term medical conditions and major depression: strength of association for specific conditions in the general population. Can J Psychiatry Rev Can de Psychiatr 50(4):195–202. Epub 2005/05/19. eng

Rayner L, Matcham F, Hutton J, Stringer C, Dobson J, Steer S et al (2014) Embedding integrated mental health assessment and management in general hospital settings: feasibility, acceptability and the prevalence of common mental disorder. Gen Hosp Psychiatry 36(3):318–324. Epub 2014/03/19. eng

Razykov I, Ziegelstein RC, Whooley MA, Thombs BD (2012) The PHQ-9 versus the PHQ-8 – is item 9 useful for assessing suicide risk in coronary artery disease patients? Data from the Heart and Soul Study. J Psychosom Res 73(3):163–168

Ren Y, Yang H, Browning C, Thomas S, Liu M (2015) Performance of screening tools in detecting major depressive disorder among patients with coronary heart disease: A Systematic Review. Med Sci Monit 21:646–653. PMCID: PMC4354444. doi:10.12659/MSM.892537

Rieckmann N, Gerin W, Kronish IM, Burg MM, Chaplin WF, Kong G et al (2006) Course of depressive symptoms and medication adherence after acute coronary syndromes: an electronic medication monitoring study. J Am Coll Cardiol 48(11):2218–2222

Rollman BL, Herbeck Belnap B, Mazumdar S, Houck PR, He F, Alvarez RJ et al (2012) A positive 2-item Patient Health Questionnaire depression screen among hospitalized heart failure patients is associated with elevated 12-month mortality. J Card Fail 18(3):238–245. Pubmed Central PMCID: Pmc3298032, Epub 2012/03/06. eng

Rutledge T, Reis VA, Linke SE, Greenberg BH, Mills PJ (2006) Depression in heart failure a meta-analytic review of prevalence, intervention effects, and associations with clinical outcomes. J Am Coll Cardiol 48(8):1527–1537

Ski CF, Page K, Thompson DR, Cummins RA, Salzberg M, Worrall-Carter L (2012) Clinical outcomes associated with screening and referral for depression in an acute cardiac ward. J Clin Nurs 21(15–16):2228–2234. Epub 2012/01/25. eng

Ski CF, Worrall-Carter L, Cameron J, Castle DJ, Rahman MA, Thompson DR. Depression screening and referral in cardiac wards: A 12-month patient trajectory. European journal of cardiovascular nursing : journal of the Working Group on Cardiovascular Nursing of the European Society of Cardiology. 2015 Apr 20.

Sowden G, Mastromauro CA, Januzzi JL, Fricchione GL, Huffman JC (2010) Detection of depression in cardiac inpatients: feasibility and results of systematic screening. Am Heart J 159(5): 780–787. Epub 2010/05/04. eng

Stewart AGO, Driscol A, Hare DL (2010) National survey of australian cardiologists beliefs and practice regarding screening, diagnosis and management of depression in cardiac patients. Eur Heart J 31:232. PubMed PMID: WOS:000281531901392. English

Subramanian DN, Hopayian K (2008) An audit of the first year of screening for depression in patients with diabetes and ischaemic heart disease under the Quality and Outcomes Framework. Qual Prim Care 16(5):341–344. Epub 2008/11/01. eng

Tatoulis J (2014) The rationale for depression screening in patients with coronary heart disease. On behalf of the Psychosocial Risk Factors Expert Working Group of the National Heart Foundation of Australia. J Psychosom Res 76(2):172–173. Epub 2014/01/21. eng

Thombs BD, Ziegelstein RC (2008) Retrospective screening of patients for age of initial diagnosis of coronary artery disease: shouldn't we just ask? J Cardiovasc Nurs 23(1):79–81; author reply -3

Thombs BD, Ziegelstein RC (2013) Depression screening in patients with coronary heart disease: does the evidence matter? J Psychosom Res 75(6):497–499. Epub 2013/12/03. eng

Thombs BD, Ziegelstein RC (2014a) Does depression screening improve depression outcomes in primary care? BMJ 348:g1253

Thombs BD, Ziegelstein RC (2014b) Evidence does matter – and evidence does not support the National Heart Foundation of Australia's consensus statement on depression screening. J Psychosom Res 76(2):173–174

Thombs BD, Bass EB, Ford DE, Stewart KJ, Tsilidis KK, Patel U et al (2006) Prevalence of depression in survivors of acute myocardial infarction. J Gen Intern Med 21(1):30–38. Pubmed Central PMCID: 1484630

Thombs BD, Ziegelstein RC, Stewart DE, Abbey SE, Parakh K, Grace SL (2008a) Usefulness of persistent symptoms of depression to predict physical health status 12 months after an acute coronary syndrome. Am J Cardiol 101(1):15–19

Thombs BD, de Jonge P, Coyne JC, Whooley MA, Frasure-Smith N, Mitchell AJ et al (2008b) Depression screening and patient outcomes in cardiovascular care: a systematic review. JAMA 300(18):2161–2171

Thombs BD, Coyne JC, Cuijpers P, de Jonge P, Gilbody S, Ioannidis JP et al (2012) Rethinking recommendations for screening for depression in primary care. CMAJ 184(4):413–418. Pubmed Central PMCID: 3291670

Thombs BD, Roseman M, Coyne JC, de Jonge P, Delisle VC, Arthurs E et al (2013) Does evidence support the American Heart Association's recommendation to screen patients for depression in cardiovascular care? An updated systematic review. PLoS One 8(1):e52654. Pubmed Central PMCID: Pmc3538724. Epub 2013/01/12. eng

Thombs BD, Ziegelstein RC, Roseman M, Kloda LA, Ioannidis JP (2014) There are no randomized controlled trials that support the United States Preventive Services Task Force Guideline on screening for depression in primary care: a systematic review. BMC Med 12:13. Pubmed Central PMCID: 3922694

Tully PJ, Baker RA (2012) Depression, anxiety, and cardiac morbidity outcomes after coronary artery bypass surgery: a contemporary and practical review. J Geriatr Cardiol JGC 9(2):197–208. Pubmed Central PMCID: 3418911

Tully PJ, Wittert G, Selkow T, Baumeister H (2014) The real world mental health needs of heart failure patients are not reflected by the depression randomized controlled trial evidence. PLoS One 9(1):e85928. Pubmed Central PMCID: Pmc3901664. Epub 2014/01/30. eng

Turner A, Phillips L, Hambridge JA, Baker AL, Bowman J, Colyvas K (2010) Clinical outcomes associated with depression, anxiety and social support among cardiac rehabilitation attendees. Aust N Z J Psychiatry 44(7):658–666. Epub 2010/06/22. eng

Valkamo M, Hintikka J, Niskanen L, Koivumaa-Honkanen H, Honkalampi K, Viinamaki H (2001) Depression and associated factors in coronary heart disease. Scand Cardiovasc J SCJ 35(4):259–263. Epub 2002/01/05. eng

van den Broek KC, DeFilippi CR, Christenson RH, Seliger SL, Gottdiener JS, Kop WJ (2011) Predictive value of depressive symptoms and B-type natriuretic peptide for new-onset heart failure and mortality. Am J Cardiol 107(5):723–729. PubMed PMID: WOS:000287837200015. English

Walters P, Barley EA, Mann A, Phillips R, Tylee A (2014) Depression in primary care patients with coronary heart disease: baseline findings from the UPBEAT UK study. PLoS One 9(6):e98342. Pubmed Central PMCID: 4055485

Wang W, Lopez V, Martin CR (2006) Structural ambiguity of the Chinese version of the Hospital Anxiety and Depression Scale in patients with coronary heart disease. Health Qual Life Outcomes 4:6. Pubmed Central PMCID: Pmc1360658, Epub 2006/01/28. eng

Worrall-Carter L, Ski CF, Thompson DR, Davidson PM, Cameron J, Castle D et al (2012) Recognition and referral of depression in patients with heart disease. Eur J Cardiovasc Nurs J Work Group Cardiovasc Nurs Eur Soc Cardiol 11(2):231–238. Epub 2011/05/27. eng

Yano EM, Chaney EF, Campbell DG, Klap R, Simon BF, Bonner LM et al (2012) Yield of practice-based depression screening in VA primary care settings. J Gen Intern Med 27(3):331–338. Pubmed Central PMCID: Pmc3286554, Epub 2011/10/07. eng

Ziegelstein RC, Thombs BD (2011) Is routine screening a parachute for heart disease patients with depression? J Psychosom Res 71(1):3–5. Epub 2011/06/15. eng

Ziegelstein RC, Kim SY, Kao D, Fauerbach JA, Thombs BD, McCann U et al (2005) Can doctors and nurses recognize depression in patients hospitalized with an acute myocardial infarction in the absence of formal screening? Psychosom Med 67(3):393–397

Ziegelstein RC, Thombs BD, Coyne JC, de Jonge P (2009) Routine screening for depression in patients with coronary heart disease never mind. J Am Coll Cardiol 54(10):886–890. Pubmed Central PMCID: Pmc2749208, Epub 2009/08/29. eng

The manufacturer's authorised representative in the EU is Springer Nature Customer Service Centre GmbH, Europaplatz 3, 69115 Heidelberg, Germany. If you have any concerns regarding our products, please contact ProductSafety@springernature.com

Printed and bound by CPI Group (UK) Ltd, Croydon, CR0 4YY
25/09/2026
02222880-0002